Handbook of Cancer Treatment-Related Toxicities

FIRST EDITION

Handbook of Cancer Treatment-Related Toxicities

VAMSI VELCHETI, MD, FACP, FCCP
Medical Director, Thoracic Oncology Program
NYU Grossman School of Medicine
NYU Langone Health - Laura and Isaac Perlmutter Cancer Center
New York, New York

SALMAN R. PUNEKAR, MD
NYU Grossman School of Medicine
NYU Langone Health - Laura and Isaac Perlmutter Cancer Center
New York, New York

ELSEVIER

ELSEVIER

1600 John F. Kennedy Blvd.
Ste 1800, Philadelphia, PA 19103-2899

HANDBOOK OF CANCER TREATMENT-RELATED TOXICITIES   ISBN: 978-0-323672412

Notices

Library of Congress Control Number:

Content Strategist: Robin R. Carter
Content Development Specialist: Angie Breckon
Publishing Services Manager: Deepthi Unni
Project Manager: Radjan Lourde Selvanadin
Design Direction: Amy Buxton

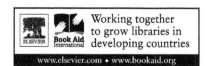

Working together to grow libraries in developing countries

www.elsevier.com • www.bookaid.org

Printed in the United States of America
Last digit is the print number: 9   8   7   6   5   4

We dedicate this effort to our patients who trusted us with the one thing most valuable to them, their health. We are deeply appreciative of everything that they have taught us over the years.

Mohammed Abazeed, MD, PhD
Associate Professor, Department of Radiation
Oncology, Director, Center for Precision
Radiotherapy, Scientific Director,
Lung Cancer Program, The Robert H.
Lurie Comprehensive Cancer Center,
Northwestern University, Evanston, Illinois
MECHANISMS OF RADIATION-RELATED
TOXICITIES

Nadine Abdallah, MD
Department of Medicine, Wayne State
University, Detroit, Michigan
MECHANISMS OF TOXICITIES ASSOCIATED WITH
TARGETED THERAPIES

Cassandra Calabrese, DO
Cleveland Clinic Foundation, Department of
Rheumatologic and Immunologic Diseases,
Cleveland, Ohio
RHEUMATOLOGICAL TOXICITIES OF
IMMUNOTHERAPY

Alison Carulli, PharmD, BCOP
Cleveland Clinic, Department of Pharmacy,
Cleveland, Ohio
ORAL MUCOSITIS, NEUROLOGICAL
COMPLICATIONS

Tahmida Chowdhury, MD
Department of Oncology, Barbara Ann
Karmanos Cancer Institute, Wayne
State University School of Medicine,
Detroit, Michigan
GASTROINTESTINAL TOXICITY OF TARGETED
THERAPY

Marc S. Ernstoff, MD
ITO, Department of Medicine, Roswell
Park Comprehensive Cancer Center,
Buffalo, New York
ENDOCRINE TOXICITY OF IMMUNOTHERAPY,
GASTROINTESTINAL TOXICITIES OF
IMMUNOTHERAPIES, NEUROLOGICAL
COMPLICATIONS OF IMMUNOTHERAPY,
IMMUNOTHERAPY-INDUCED CARDIOTOXICITIES

Bassam Estfan, MD
Cleveland Clinic, Taussig Cancer Institute,
Cleveland, Ohio
ORAL MUCOSITIS, GASTROINTESTINAL
COMPLICATIONS OF CHEMOTHERAPY,
NEUROLOGICAL COMPLICATIONS,
DERMATOLOGICAL COMPLICATIONS OF
CHEMOTHERAPY, CARDIOTOXICITIES OF
CHEMOTHERAPY

Christopher W. Fleming, MD
Taussig Cancer Center, Radiation Oncology,
Cleveland Clinic, Cleveland, Ohio
MECHANISMS OF RADIATION-RELATED
TOXICITIES

Shipra Gandhi, MD
Assistant Professor of Medicine, Department
of Medicine, Roswell Park Comprehensive
Cancer Center, Buffalo, New York
GASTROINTESTINAL TOXICITIES OF
IMMUNOTHERAPIES, IMMUNOTHERAPY-
INDUCED CARDIOTOXICITIES

Itivrita Goyal, MBBS
Fellow, Endocrinology, Diabetes, and
Metabolism, University at Buffalo,
Buffalo, New York
ENDOCRINE TOXICITY OF IMMUNOTHERAPY

Aman Gupta, MD
Department of Medicine, Division of General
Internal Medicine, University of Pittsburgh
Medical Center, Pittsburgh, Pennsylvania
GASTROINTESTINAL TOXICITIES OF
IMMUNOTHERAPIES, IMMUNOTHERAPY-
INDUCED CARDIOTOXICITIES

Arjun Khunger, MD
Department of Hematology and Oncology,
Taussig Cancer Institute, Cleveland Clinic
Foundation, Cleveland, Ohio
GASTROINTESTINAL COMPLICATIONS
OF CHEMOTHERAPY, DERMATOLOGICAL
COMPLICATIONS OF CHEMOTHERAPY,
CARDIOTOXICITIES OF CHEMOTHERAPY

Melissa King, MSN, APRN, FNP-C
Cleveland Clinic, Taussig Cancer Institute,
  Cleveland, Ohio
ORAL MUCOSITIS, NEUROLOGICAL
COMPLICATIONS

Subhakar Mutyala, MD
Department of Interdisciplinary Oncology,
  University of Arizona College of
  Medicine, Arizona Oncology Associates,
  Phoenix, Arizona
RADIATION THERAPY-RELATED DERMATOLOGIC
TOXICITIES

Misako Nagasaka, MD
Department of Oncology, Barbara Ann
  Karmanos Cancer Institute, Wayne State
  University School of Medicine, Detroit
  Michigan, Department of Advanced
  Medical Innovation, St. Marianna
  University Graduate School of Medicine,
  Kawasaki, Japan
MECHANISMS OF TOXICITIES ASSOCIATED WITH
TARGETED THERAPIES, GASTROINTESTINAL
TOXICITY OF TARGETED THERAPY,
DERMATOLOGICAL TOXICITIES OF TARGETED
THERAPY, CARDIOVASCULAR TOXICITY OF
TARGETED THERAPY

Tanmay S. Panchabhai, MD, FACP, FCCP
John and Doris Norton Thoracic Institute,
  St. Joseph's Hospital and Medical Center,
  Associate Professor, Creighton University
  School of Medicine, Phoenix, Arizona
PULMONARY TOXICITIES OF CYTOTOXIC
CHEMOTHERAPY, PULMONARY
TOXICITIES OF MOLECULAR TARGETED
THERAPIES, PULMONARY TOXICITIES OF
IMMUNOTHERAPEUTIC AGENTS, PULMONARY
TOXICITY FROM RADIATION THERAPY

Manu Pandey, MBBS
Fellow, Department of Medicine, Roswell
  Park Comprehensive Cancer Institute,
  Buffalo, New York
ENDOCRINE TOXICITY OF IMMUNOTHERAPY,
NEUROLOGICAL COMPLICATIONS OF
IMMUNOTHERAPY

Rahul Pansare, MD
Department of Internal Medicine, St. Mary
  Mercy Livonia, Livonia, Michigan
DERMATOLOGICAL TOXICITIES OF TARGETED
THERAPY

Shyamal Patel, MD
Assistant Clinical Professor, University
  of Arizona College of Medicine,
  Creighton University School of Medicine,
  Department of Radiation Medicine,
  University of Arizona Cancer Center at
  Dignity Health, St. Joseph's Hospital and
  Medical Center, Phoenix, Arizona
RADIATION-INDUCED CARDIOTOXICITIES

Pradnya D. Patil, MD, FACP
Department of Hematology and Oncology,
  Taussig Cancer Institute, Cleveland Clinic,
  Cleveland, Ohio
PULMONARY TOXICITIES OF CYTOTOXIC
CHEMOTHERAPY, PULMONARY TOXICITIES
OF MOLECULAR TARGETED THERAPIES,
MECHANISM OF IMMUNE-RELATED ADVERSE
EVENTS, PULMONARY TOXICITIES OF
IMMUNOTHERAPEUTIC AGENTS, CUTANEOUS
TOXICITIES OF IMMUNOTHERAPEUTIC AGENTS

Salman R. Punekar, MD
Perlmutter Cancer Center, NYU Langone
  Health, New York, New York
MECHANISMS OF CANCER-DIRECTED
THERAPIES, CANCER TREATMENT-RELATED
THROMBOCYTOPENIA

Igor Puzanov, MD
Professor of Medicine, Roswell Park
  Comprehensive Cancer Center,
  Buffalo, New York
IMMUNOTHERAPY-INDUCED CARDIOTOXICITIES

Dale Shepard, MD, PhD
Director, Taussig Phase I and Sarcoma
  Programs, Hematology/Medical Oncology,
  Cleveland Clinic, Cleveland, Ohio
NEUTROPENIC COMPLICATIONS OF
CHEMOTHERAPY, CHEMOTHERAPY-INDUCED
ANEMIA

Ammar Sukari, MD
Department of Oncology, Barbara Ann
  Karmanos Cancer Institute, Wayne
  State University School of Medicine,
  Detroit, Michigan
MECHANISMS OF TOXICITIES ASSOCIATED WITH
TARGETED THERAPIES, GASTROINTESTINAL
TOXICITY OF TARGETED THERAPY,
DERMATOLOGICAL TOXICITIES OF TARGETED
THERAPY, CARDIOVASCULAR TOXICITY OF
TARGETED THERAPY

Alankrita Taneja, MBBS
Resident Physician, Internal Medicine,
   Detroit Medical Center, Wayne
   State University School of Medicine,
   Detroit, Michigan
NEUTROPENIC COMPLICATIONS OF
CHEMOTHERAPY, CHEMOTHERAPY-INDUCED
ANEMIA

Nitika Thawani, MD
Associate Professor, Department of
   Radiation Medicine, University of
   Arizona Cancer Center at Dignity Health,
   St. Joseph's Hospital and Medical Center,
   Phoenix, Arizona
RADIATION-INDUCED MUCOSITIS AND
ESOPHAGITIS, RADIATION THERAPY-RELATED
DERMATOLOGIC TOXICITIES, PULMONARY
TOXICITY FROM RADIATION THERAPY,
RADIATION-INDUCED CARDIOTOXICITIES

Pankit Vachhani, MD
Roswell Park Comprehensive Cancer Center,
   Buffalo, New York
IMMUNOTHERAPY-INDUCED CARDIOTOXICITIES

Vamsidhar Velcheti, MD
Department of Hematology and Oncology,
   Perlmutter Cancer Center, New York
   University Langone, New York, New York
MECHANISM OF IMMUNE-RELATED ADVERSE
EVENTS, CUTANEOUS TOXICITIES OF
IMMUNOTHERAPEUTIC AGENTS

Sharanya Vemula, BPharm, MS, PhD
Medical Writer, Clinical Research, Alexion,
   Twerksbury, Massachusetts
MANAGEMENT OF CANCER TREATMENT
INFUSION REACTIONS

Shilpa Vyas, MD
Radiation Oncologist, Rochester Regional
   Health/Lipson Cancer Institute,
   Rochester, New York
RADIATION-INDUCED MUCOSITIS AND
ESOPHAGITIS

Sri Yadlapalli, MD
Department of Hematology and Oncology,
   Ascension Providence Hospital Medical
   Center, Southfield, Michigan
CARDIOVASCULAR TOXICITY OF TARGETED
THERAPY

Oncology is a rapidly evolving field. In the last few years, we have seen a dramatic improvement in the outcomes for patients with cancer with the advent of new modalities for treatment, particularly with immunotherapy. We have seen multiple new therapeutic approvals for several cancers. We are amid a dramatic shift in our treatment paradigms with a significant impact on survival—even for cancer types that seemed incurable, we have seen durable responses and survivals in the metastatic setting.

As we develop more effective therapeutics and extend survival in patients with cancer, we are faced with unique challenges with the management of potential toxicities with these treatments. It is imperative that oncology providers and providers who manage patients with cancer are aware of the mechanisms of these complications as well as the appropriate diagnostic and treatment approaches.

In this handbook, disease area specialists with expertise in managing cancer treatment-related adverse events have covered many aspects of oncology, from basic pathophysiology of the toxicities to the current state-of-the-art management of these treatment-related toxicities. This succinct handbook provides a quick guide to understand the pathophysiology and the management of cancer treatment-related toxicities, therefore it will serve as a practical guide for any professionals involved in the care of cancer patients.

We would like to acknowledge our teachers and mentors over the years. Those who cultivated our passion for service to mankind and our yearning towards medicine.

CONTENTS

CHAPTER 1

Mechanisms of Cancer-Directed Therapies

Salman R. Punekar, MD

Mechanisms of Cancer-Directed Therapies

Cancer has been prevalent for centuries and humans have been concerned with the treatment of cancer for a seemingly equal time. Breast cancer was first described thousands of years ago and was first reported to be treated with surgery in 500 BCE. In the 18th and 19th centuries, surgical resection for the treatment of cancer started to gain popularity, but it was only in the early 1900s that chemotherapy entered the picture.[1] It was post-World War II that chemotherapy began to become widely used with cures of leukemia and lymphoma described in the 1960s.[2] While oncologists became the purveyors of chemotherapy, they equally began managing complications of these same treatments. Thus, a mechanistic understanding is essential to the prediction and treatment of complications stemming from cancer-directed therapies.

CATEGORIES OF CANCER-DIRECTED THERAPY

- **Cytotoxic chemotherapy:** The term chemotherapy arises from the concept of treating disease with chemicals. Traditional chemotherapy was developed in the early 1900s and is still a part of the treatment program for most cancers. Some common types of chemotherapy include pyrimidine analogs, purine analogs, anthracyclines, antifolates, alkylating agents, platinum derivatives, DNA topoisomerase inhibitors, taxanes, vinca alkaloids, hypomethylating agents, and proteasome inhibitors, among others.
- **Targeted therapy:** Targeted therapies come in various forms but are generally monoclonal antibodies or small molecules that interact with a specific molecule known to be implicated in cancer growth. Some examples include imatinib targeting BCR-ABL, bevacizumab targeting VEGF, trastuzumab targeting HER2, and erlotinib targeting EGFR, among an ever-increasing number of drugs.
- **Immunotherapy:** Immunotherapy is a relatively new form of cancer-directed therapy, encompassing vaccine, cellular, cytokine, anti-CTLA-4, and anti-PD-1 therapies. Examples of the most commonly used therapies are pembrolizumab, ipilimumab, and nivolumab.
- **Radiation therapy:** Radiation therapy can be divided into two types, based on the source of radiation. External beam radiation refers to radiation in which the source comes from outside the patient. Internal beam radiation, also known as brachytherapy, refers to radiation in which the source is placed next to, or within, a tumor. Complications from radiation therapy arise from radiation exposure to non-tumor cells and are based on the type and location of cells that are affected.

References

1. Mukherjee S. *The Emperor of All Maladies: A Biography of Cancer*. 1 ed. New York: Scribner; 2010.
2. DeVita VT, Chu E. A history of cancer chemotherapy. *Cancer Res*. 2008;68(21):8643–8653.

CHAPTER 2

Neutropenic Complications of Chemotherapy

Alankrita Taneja, MBBS ▪ Dale Shepard, MD, PhD

Introduction

- Neutrophils, eosinophils, and basophils are a subset of white blood cells characterized by the presence of granules and collectively referred to as granulocytes. Granulocytopenia is a decrease in the absolute count of these three cell lines while neutropenia is a decrease in only the absolute neutrophil count (ANC). However, for practical purposes the terms granulocytopenia and neutropenia are often used interchangeably.
- It is important to understand normal physiology in order to understand neutropenia and its complications. Most neutrophils reside in the bone marrow[1] in mitotic (myeloblasts, promyelocytes, myelocytes) and postmitotic (metamyelocytes, bands, and then neutrophils) stages. Of the neutrophils in the circulation, an equal proportion make up the marginal and the nonmarginal pool.[2] From the circulation, neutrophils enter tissue as a result of proinflammatory trafficking cytokines. Neutropenia is a reduction in the nonmarginal pool of neutrophils which constitute only 4% to 5% of total neutrophil stores.

> Neutropenia is defined as an absolute neutrophil count (ANC) of less than 1500 cells/μL; ANC of less than 1000 cells/μL is considered moderate neutropenia and ANC of less than 500 cells/μL is considered severe neutropenia. The risk of infection is greatest with severe neutropenia.[3]

Etiology of Neutropenia

- Neutropenia is a common complication seen in various malignant conditions. There are many contributing factors that should be considered in patients with malignancy. Table 2.1[4] describes causes of neutropenia commonly seen in patients with malignancy. Although neutropenia is the most common dose limiting toxicity (DLT) of chemotherapy,[5] it is important to consider the differential diagnosis to determine the appropriate management for each patient.
- There are several ways in which chemotherapy predisposes to infections. While neutropenia is an important etiology, chemotherapy can also impair physical barriers created by mucosal surfaces, the first line of defense against infections. Classic signs of inflammation including dolor (pain), calor (heat), rubor (redness), tumor (swelling), and functio laesa (loss of function) may be dampened in such patients due to blunting of the function of neutrophils. Thus increasing the chance of infections to be missed. Fever is usually the only sign of infection in neutropenic infections and thus warrants special vigilance.[4]

TABLE 2.1 ■ Causes of Neutropenia in Cancer Patients[4]

Causes of Neutropenia in Malignancy	Mechanism
Chemotherapy (the chemotherapy regimen remains the strongest determinant in the likelihood of developing neutropenia)	Myelosuppressive effects due to cytotoxicity
Chronic lymphoproliferative disorders – natural killer cell lymphomas (large granular lymphocytic leukemia), hairy cell leukemia, and chronic lymphocytic leukemia (CLL)	Bone marrow infiltration
Radiation	**Cytotoxic Effects**
Autoimmune conditions: Systemic lupus erythematosus (SLE), aplastic anemia, Crohn's disease	Presence of antineutrophil antibodies
Rheumatoid arthritis (Felty's syndrome)	Hypersplenism
Granulomatous infections	Bone marrow infiltration
Viral infections (e.g., CMV, EBV, HIV)	Bone marrow suppression
Parasitic infections (e.g., malaria)	Hypersplenism, multifactorial
Bacterial infections (e.g., typhoid, tuberculosis)	Multifactorial
Hemophagocytic lymphohistiocytosis (HLH)	Infiltration of bone marrow, hypersplenism
Antibiotic-induced isolated neutropenia (e.g., quinidine, hydralazine, β-lactams)	Maturation arrest of myeloid lineage
Benign ethnic neutropenia (BEN; also known as constitutional neutropenia)	Inherited predisposition
Cyclic neutropenia (21-day cycling of neutrophils)	Inherited (autosomal dominant, ELA2 gene) and acquired causes

CMV, Cytomegalovirus; *EBV,* Epstein-Barr virus.

Risk Assessment of Adults With Chemotherapy-Induced Neutropenia

■ It is helpful to stratify patients into different risk categories for effective management. This risk assessment should be conducted prior to the first cycle of chemotherapy and revisited with subsequent cycles as needed. Although all patients with febrile neutropenia require antibiotics, the route of antibiotic therapy (oral vs. intravenous), the setting (outpatient vs. inpatient), and the duration of such therapy is decided after assessing the risk of febrile neutropenia. The decision about whether to give prophylactic granulocyte colony stimulating factor (G-CSF) is also made after assessing the risk of febrile neutropenia. Such a risk may be affected by patient, disease, or treatment-related factors (Table 2.2).[6–13]

■ The importance of neutropenia cannot be understated. One of the feared complications of chemotherapy-induced neutropenia is febrile neutropenia which predisposes to high risk infections with high mortality.[5] There are different universally followed risk assessment criteria for stratifying patients into low- and high-risk categories. The level of risk thus implies risk of serious complications, including prolonged hospitalizations and death in patients with neutropenic fever.

■ **The Multinational Association for Supportive Care in Cancer (MASCC) Score**[13]
The MASCC score is an internationally validated score to stratify patients by risk. A MASCC risk-index score ≥21 identifies low-risk patients with a positive predictive value of 91%, a specificity of 68%, and a sensitivity of 71%. This risk score is incorporated into the National Comprehensive Cancer Network (NCCN) guidelines for management of patients with neutropenic fever.[14]

TABLE 2.2 ■ **Risk Factors Associated with Development of Neutropenia**

Patient-Related Risk Factors	Disease-Related Risk Factors	Treatment-Related Risk Factors
Age (>65 years)[5]	Advanced stage of malignancy[13]	Time since last chemotherapy (<7 days)[6]
Gender (female)[7]	Lymphopenia[8,9]	High-dose chemotherapy[5,10]
High body surface area[11]	Bone marrow involvement by malignancy[12]	Higher number of planned cycles[10]
Comorbidities[11]	Raised lactate dehydrogenase level in lymphomas[12]	Colony-stimulating factor prophylaxis (inverse relationship)[10]
Nutritional status (malnourishment, including serum albumin ≤3.5 mg/dL)[6,11]	Absolute neutrophil count (inverse relationship)[6]	Low baseline and first-cycle nadir blood counts
Poor performance status	C-reactive protein concentration >15 mg/dL	Longer hospital stay >10 days
	Hematological malignancy as compared with solid organ malignancies	

MASCC uses the following criteria to calculate a score[15]:
- **Burden of illness**
  - No or mild symptoms (5 points)
  - Moderate symptoms (3 points)
  - Severe symptoms (0 points)
- **Comorbidities**
  - No hypotension (systolic blood pressure >90 mmHg) (5 points)
  - No chronic obstructive pulmonary disease (4 points)
  - Solid tumor or hematologic malignancy with no history of previous fungal infections (4 points)
  - No dehydration requiring parenteral fluids (3 points)
- **Status**
  - Outpatient status at the time of onset of the neutropenic fever syndrome (3 points)
- **Age**
  - Lesser than 60 years (2 points)
  - ≥ 60 years (0 points)
  - Depending on the total score, patients can be stratified into low (21–26 points) or high-risk (0–20 points) categories. Patients with a low MASCC score may be treated in the outpatient setting with oral antibiotics. On the other hand, patients with a score of less than 21 are at high risk of infections and complications and should be treated in the inpatient setting with broad spectrum intravenous antibiotics. Although the MASCC score is widely used, it has some potential limitations. First, it may not be applicable to more stable patients in the outpatient setting.[16] Second, the duration of neutropenia, an important criteria in the NCCN risk assessment, is not incorporated into the MASCC score.[17]

NCCN risk assessment
- A more commonly used approach is the NCCN risk assessment, which is described in Table 2.3. The NCCN assessment categorizes patients into low risk, intermediate risk, and high risk based on clinical features. In general, low-risk patients can be treated in the outpatient setting with oral antibiotics and high-risk patients should be treated in the inpatient setting with IV antibiotics. Intermediate-risk patients should receive individualized assessments regarding therapy.

TABLE 2.3 ■ The National Comprehensive Cancer Network (NCCN) Risk Assessment

Low Risk (No High-Risk Factors and Most of the Following Factors)	Intermediate Risk (Any of These Factors)	High Risk (Any of These Factors)
Outpatient status at the time of development of fever	Autologous HCT	Inpatient status at the time of development of fever
No associated acute comorbid illness, which could be an independent factor necessitating inpatient treatment	Lymphoma	Significant comorbid illness
Anticipated short duration of severe neutropenia (<100 cells/μL for <7 days)	Chronic lymphocytic leukemia	Anticipated prolonged neutropenia (<100 cells/μL for >7 days)
ECOG 0–1	Multiple myeloma	Allogenic HCT
No hepatic insufficiency	Purine analog treatment	AST/ALT >5 times the upper limit of normal
No renal insufficiency	Anticipated neutropenia of 7–10 days	Creatinine clearance <30
MASCC score ≥21		MASCC score <21
		Severe infections such as pneumonia
		Treatment with alemtuzumab within 60 days
		Mucositis grade 3 or 4 Uncontrolled progressive cancer defined as patients with leukemia, not in complete remission or patients without leukemia with evidence of disease progression after more than two cycles of chemotherapy

ALT, Alanine Aminotransferase; *AST,* Aspart Aminotransferase; *ECOG,* Eastern Cooperative Oncology Group; *HCT,* Hematopoetic stem cell transplant; *MASCC,* Multinational Association for Supportive Care in Cancer.

Workup of Neutropenic Fever

Neutropenic fever is a medical emergency and requires prompt evaluation. The following steps, detailed in Fig. 2.1, should be taken when neutropenic fever is diagnosed.

Pharmacological Approaches for Management and Treatment

1. **Neutropenia without fever:** Patients with neutropenia without fever can be managed by delaying the next cycle of chemotherapy.
   - **Antibacterial prophylaxis:** It is recommended that patients with high risk of neutropenia receive prophylactic oral antibiotics. Fluoroquinolones such as levofloxacin (500 mg QD) and ciprofloxacin (500 mg BID) are often used. Antifungal drugs, antiviral drugs, and vaccines can also be used in some high-risk patients.
   - **Granulocyte colony stimulating factor (G-CSF):** A risk benefit analysis for G-CSF should be considered for patients. In some cases, the cost of therapy limits its utility. As per the NCCN guidelines, myeloid growth factors should be given to patients at high risk of neutropenia. Although prevention is not always possible because of the nature of chemotherapy in some patients, therapy with growth factors can reduce

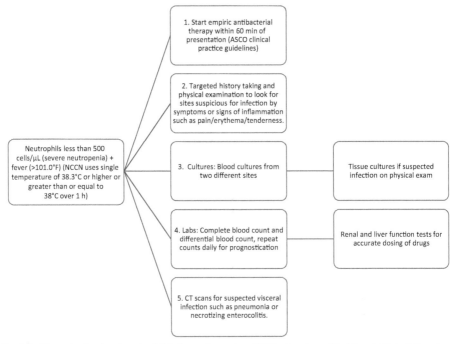

Fig. 2.1 Steps in the treatment of febrile neutropenia. *ASCO,* American Society of Clinical Oncology; *CT,* computed tomography; *NCCN,* National Comprehensive Cancer Network.

complications associated with neutropenia and reduce the duration of chemotherapy-induced neutropenia (Table 2.4).

2. **Febrile neutropenia:** Patients with febrile neutropenia are at risk of various complications, including death. Thus febrile neutropenia is an oncologic emergency and should be treated with broad spectrum antibiotics. Table 2.5 describes the types of antibiotics that should be administered given the risk categorization of patients.

   ■ **Coverage for resistant bacteria:** Empiric antibiotics should be adjusted as soon as bacterial susceptibility is determined.

   ◦ **Methicillin-resistant staphylococcus aureus (MRSA):** Vancomycin, linezolid, daptomycin

   ◦ **Vancomycin-resistant enterococcus (VRE):** Linezolid, daptomycin

   ◦ **Extended-spectrum β-lactamase producing gram-negative bacteria (ESBL):** carbapenems

   ◦ **Carbapenemase-producing organisms (CPO):** polymyxin-colistin or tigecycline

TABLE 2.4 ■ **Categories of Risks of Neutropenia**

High Risk (>20% risk of developing febrile neutropenia)	**Intermediate Risk** (10%–20% risk of developing febrile neutropenia)	**Low Risk** (<10% risk of developing febrile neutropenia)
G-CSF recommended	Individualized approach	G-CSF not recommended

G-CSF, Granulocyte colony-stimulating factor.

TABLE 2.5 ■ Empiric Therapy: Adequate Gram-Positive and Gram-Negative Coverage

Low-Risk Patients	High-Risk Patients
FQ (ciprofloxacin 750 mg orally BD/ levofloxacin 750 mg orally OD) + β-lactam agent (amoxicillin-clavulanic acid 500 mg/125 mg orally TDS). FQ in this setting should not be given to patients taking FQ-based prophylaxis	Antipseudomonal β-lactam should be added. Treatment should be based on presentation. In patients with central venous catheter–related infection or skin or soft tissue infection-gram positive coverage should be added however, for those with complicated presentation, gram-negative coverage should be added. For persistent infections: antifungals should be added
Treat in an outpatient setting with readily available and proximity to medical care	Treat in an inpatient setting
Antibacterial prophylaxis is not recommended	Antibacterial prophylaxis is recommended

BD, Two times a day; *FQ,* fluoroquinolone; *OD,* once a day; *TDS,* three times a day.

Nonpharmacological Approaches for Management and Treatment

■ Neutropenia leading to infections can be a distressing complication for patients. Given that neutropenia often follows the first cycle of chemotherapy, patients are likely to be demotivated to continue therapy. Thus adequate counseling can help patients prepare for this common complication and can improve compliance with treatment.

■ Nonpharmacological management of neutropenia seems to be more critical in patients with hematological malignancies and bone marrow transplants as compared to patients with solid malignancies as the duration of neutropenia is usually much longer in patients with hematological malignancies. Table 2.6 outlines guidelines for neutropenic infection prevention in patients with malignancies.

TABLE 2.6 ■ Nonpharmacological Approaches to Prevent Infections in Neutropenic Patients

Following hand hygiene procedures

Avoiding rectal temperature measurements and rectal examinations or rectal suppositories

Administering stool softeners for constipation

Minimizing exposure to pets

Minimizing exposure to crowded areas

Minimizing exposure to sick contacts

Maintaining hygiene of central catheter and checking daily for signs of infection

Avoiding live vaccines

Avoiding sharps and skin lacerations

Maintaining good oral hygiene)

Avoiding tampons due to the risk of toxic shock syndrome

Avoiding sexual intercourse

Washing fresh fruits and vegetables, cooking poultry to safe temperatures, using pasteurized dairy products

References

1. Todd KH, Thomas CR Jr. Oncologic Emergency Medicine 2016 (**978-3-319-26387-8**). Springer International Publishing.
2. Dale DC. Tracers for tracing neutrophils. *Blood*. 2016;127(26):3300–3302.
3. Coates TD. Overview of neutropenia in children and adolescents; 2015. https://www.uptodate.com/contents/overview-of-neutropenia-in-children-and-adolescents/print#.
4. Lustberg MB. Management of neutropenia in cancer patients. *Clin Adv Hematol Oncol*. 2012;10(12):825–826.
5. Lyman GH, Lyman CH, Agboola O. Risk models for predicting chemotherapy-induced neutropenia. *Oncologist*. 2005;10(6):427–437.
6. Oberoi S, Das A, Trehan A, Ray P, Bansal D. Can complications in febrile neutropenia be predicted? Report from a developing country. *Support Care Cancer*. 2017;25(11):3523–3528.
7. Lopez-Pousa A, Rifa J, Casas de Tejerina A, et al. Risk assessment model for first-cycle chemotherapy-induced neutropenia in patients with solid tumours. *Eur J Cancer Care (Engl)*. 2010;19(5):648–655.
8. Blay JY, Chauvin F, Le Cesne A, et al. Early lymphopenia after cytotoxic chemotherapy as a risk factor for febrile neutropenia. *J Clin Oncol*. 1996;14(2):636–643.
9. Ray-Coquard I, Borg C, Bachelot T, et al. Baseline and early lymphopenia predict for the risk of febrile neutropenia after chemotherapy. *Br J Cancer*. 2003;88(2):181–186.
10. Schwenkglenks M, Pettengell R, Jackisch C, et al. Risk factors for chemotherapy-induced neutropenia occurrence in breast cancer patients: data from the INC-EU Prospective Observational European Neutropenia Study. *Support Care Cancer*. 2011;19(4):483–490.
11. Choi YW, Jeong SH, Ahn MS, et al. Patterns of neutropenia and risk factors for febrile neutropenia of diffuse large B-cell lymphoma patients treated with rituximab-CHOP. *J Korean Med Sci*. 2014;29(11):1493–1500.
12. Intragumtornchai T, Sutheesophon J, Sutcharitchan P, Swasdikul D. A predictive model for life-threatening neutropenia and febrile neutropenia after the first course of CHOP chemotherapy in patients with aggressive non-Hodgkin's lymphoma. *Leuk Lymphoma*. 2000;37(3-4):351–360.
13. Klastersky J, Paesmans M, Rubenstein EB, et al. The multinational Association for Supportive Care in Cancer risk index: a multinational scoring system for identifying low-risk febrile neutropenic cancer patients. *J Clin Oncol*. 2000;18(16):3038–3051.
14. *National Comprehensive Cancer Network (NCCN) Clinical Practice Guidelines in Oncology*Prevention and treatment of cancer-related infections; 2014 Version 2.
15. Keng MK, Thallner EA, Elson P, et al. Reducing time to antibiotic administration for febrile neutropenia in the emergency department. *J Oncol Pract*. 2015;11:450–455.
16. Carmona-Bayonas A, Gomez J, Gonzalez-Billalabeitia E, et al. Prognostic evaluation of febrile neutropenia in apparently stable adult cancer patients. *Br J Cancer*. 2011;105(5):612–617.
17. Freifeld AG, Bow EJ, Sepkowitz KA, et al. Clinical practice guideline for the use of antimicrobial agents in neutropenic patients with cancer: 2010 update by the Infectious Diseases Society of America. *Clin Infect Dis*. 2011;52(4):e56–e93.

CHAPTER 3

Chemotherapy-Induced Anemia

Alankrita Taneja, MBBS ▪ Dale Shepard, MD, PhD

Introduction

- Anemia is caused by the deficiency of red blood cells or hemoglobin, resulting in a reduction in the oxygen-carrying capacity of blood and is commonly associated with cancer-directed therapies. Chemotherapy, radiotherapy, and cancer-related surgery can all contribute to anemia. Despite being common, anemia associated with chemotherapy (CIA) is often underreported and is often only documented when severe, necessitating transfusion. There are several reasons for this; however, the most important is the lack of treatment options for mild anemia. There is also a lower perceived clinical importance of CIA compared with neutropenia or thrombocytopenia.[1]

- CIA results in functional impairment and reduction of quality of life. Fatigue associated with anemia can have considerable implications on the physical, psychosocial, and economic and occupational aspects of patients' and their families' lives.[2] Studies have demonstrated a clear correlation between hemoglobin levels and the severity of cancer-related fatigue, and quality of life.[3-5] Some studies have reported an incidence of 80% to 100% for fatigue in patients undergoing chemotherapeutic treatment for their malignancy.[6,7] Fatigue associated with anemia due to chemotherapy regimens can cause some patients to discontinue treatment altogether.[8] Despite its prevalence and complications, fatigue is often left undiscussed and untreated in cancer patients.

- Anemia is an adverse prognostic marker in patients with several malignancies. Radiotherapy and some forms of chemotherapy depend on adequate tissue oxygen levels for their action, and their efficacy can be impaired by anemia.[9] Anemia is also associated with increased susceptibility to thrombocytopenic bleeding and decreased overall survival. Symptoms of anemia can be manifold with effects in virtually all organ systems.[10]

- Some cancers are associated more with anemia than others (Table 3.1). For example, lung, breast, and ovarian cancers are associated with some of the highest incidences of anemia. More advanced stages and longer durations of cancer are also associated with more severe anemia.

Grading of Anemia

- The grading scheme of anemia is generally rated on a scale from 0 to 4, from normal hemoglobin to life-threatening anemia. In clinical trials, the Common Terminology Criteria for Adverse Events (CTCAE) is commonly used, and is described in Table 3.2.

- The grading of anemia based on the hemoglobin level is useful because it helps determine if patients require transfusions. However, a major drawback of these grading systems is that they do not correlate anemia with clinical presentation, such as fatigue.

TABLE 3.1 ■ Prevalence of Anemia by Cancer Type[12]

Type of Cancer	Studies (n)	Prevalence (%)
Lung	5	8–84
Colon	8	30–67
Breast	3	41–82
Prostate	3	5–32
Head and Neck	4	16–65
Larynx	1	21
Kidney	1	39
Ovary	2	26–85
Cervix/Uterus	3	67–82

TABLE 3.2 ■ Common Terminology Criteria for Adverse Events (CTCAE) Grading System

CTCAE Grade	1	2	3	4	5
Criteria	Hgb > 10 g/dL	Hgb 8–10 g/dL	Hgb < 8 g/dL; transfusion may be indicated	Life-threatening consequences; urgent intervention indicated	Death

Agents Causative of Anemia

■ There are many agents associated with anemia. In terms of malignancy, the type, stage, and duration of malignancy all play a role. Similarly, in terms of chemotherapy, the type, intensity, and duration of chemotherapy are all correlated with the level of anemia (Table 3.3). Specifically, among therapies, platinum-based therapies are notorious for causing anemia.

■ Repeated cycles of chemotherapy also have a cumulative effect on erythropoiesis. Langer et al. evaluated the effects of CIA in patients with advanced non–small-cell lung cancer (NSCLC); grade 2 anemia was cumulative and increased from 30% after the first cycle of treatment to 59% by the fourth cycle.[11]

Mechanisms of anemia: Several mechanisms of anemia in cancer patients have been suggested.

1. **Myelosuppression** associated with chemotherapy can be both long-term and short-term due to the direct toxic effects of these agents on stem cells and progenitor cells.
   a. **Long-term myelosuppression** is associated with non–cell-cycle dependent drugs, such as methotrexate (alkylating agents).
   b. **Short-term myelosuppression** is associated with the use of non-myeloablative doses of chemotherapy agents. Because it is short-term, this type of myelosuppression is associated with the duration and frequency of chemotherapy. Examples of agents include cytarabine, methotrexate, and hydroxyurea.[13]
2. **Therapy-related myelodysplastic syndromes** are associated with chemotherapy, especially with alkylating agents and topoisomerase II inhibitors.[14,15]
3. **Nephrotoxicity** caused by agents such as cisplatin can cause erythropoietin deficiency. Anemia from this cause can be prevented and treated by replacement of erythropoietin.[16]
4. **Hemolytic anemia:** Three types have been observed in patients undergoing chemotherapy: microangiopathic hemolytic anemia, immune hemolytic anemia (positive direct antibody test), and oxidative hemolysis.[17] Cisplatin and oxaliplatin have been particularly

TABLE 3.3 ■ Incidence of Anemia With Different Chemotherapeutic Agents and Regimens[1]

Chemotherapy Drug/Regimen	Grades 1–2 (%)[a]	Grades 3–4 (%)[a]
Cisplatin	–	11
Docetaxel	73–85	2–42
5-FU	50–54	5–11
Paclitaxel	93	7
Topotecan	67	32
Vinorelbine	67–71	5–14
Cisplatin–cyclophosphamide	43	9
Cisplatin–etoposide	59	16–55
Etoposide–ifosfamide–cisplatin	–	52
5-FU–carboplatin	42	14
CHOP	49	17
Paclitaxel–doxorubicin	78–84	8–11
Paclitaxel–carboplatin	10–59	5–34
Imatinib	80	10
Sunitinib	26	–
Sirolimus	–	9

[a]Toxicity was graded using various toxicity grading systems such as the NCI common toxicity criteria, WHO toxicity grading system, Gynecologic Oncology Group criteria, and Eastern Cooperative Oncology Group criteria.
CHOP, Cyclophosphamide, doxorubicin, Oncovin (vincristine), and prednisone; *FU,* fluorouracil.

implicated.[18,19] As another example, in chronic lymphocytic leukemia patients treated with fludarabine, exacerbation of preexisting hemolytic anemia has been observed.[20]

5. **Bone marrow stromal damage** from high-dose chemotherapy.[13]
6. **Other causes of anemia** may coexist and in varying degrees and may contribute to anemia, examples of these include hemorrhage, iron, folate, and vitamin B12 deficiency.
7. **Anemia of chronic disease** as seen in other inflammatory conditions may also be a contributing factor to anemia in cancer patients.

Supportive Care

The mainstay of treatment options for CIA are supportive care, and center largely around RBC transfusions and fluid resuscitation.

■ **RBC transfusions:** RBC transfusions are generally indicated in patients with the characteristics described below. It is worth noting, however, that administration of transfusions should be individualized clinical decisions, for which clear guidelines do not exist.
  ■ Anemia following acute blood loss unresponsive to crystalloid infusions
  ■ Acute symptomatic anemia
  ■ Chronic symptomatic anemia unresponsive to iron replacement
  ■ Select group of patients for whom medical necessity does not allow adequate time for erythropoiesis-stimulating agents (ESAs) to be effective[21]
  ■ Patients with cardiac risk factors putting them at risk of cardiac events in the presence of anemia[22]
  ■ Patients with a hemoglobin of less than 7 g/dL

- Risks associated with RBC transfusions should be considered while making a decision regarding transfusion of blood products.[22]
  - Transmission of blood borne infectious diseases
  - Alloimmunization
  - Transfusion reactions including fever, allergy (urticaria), anaphylaxis (especially in patients with immunoglobulin A [IgA] deficiency), or hemolytic reactions (acute and delayed)
  - Iron overload
  - Transfusion-associated cardiopulmonary overload (TACO)
  - Transfusion-associated acute lung injury (TRALI)
- **Crystalloid infusion:** Crystalloids should be given to patients with symptomatic anemia not considered eligible for RBC transfusion. These are used to replace intravascular volume in patients with transient anemia from acute blood loss or those with symptomatic chronic anemia.[21]

Pharmacologic Approaches to Anemia

- **ESAs,** such as epoetin and darbepoetin, have been studied in the treatment of CIA. The appeal of ESAs is centered around the concept that ESAs can potentially have longer lasting effects while avoiding the costs and risks associated with frequent transfusions. ESA use, however, is not without controversy, and therefore should be used only after careful consideration. Clinicians must consider the potential risks and benefits of ESAs prior to administration. Some important risks include thromboembolism (special caution should be exercised when using ESAs along with chemotherapeutic agents associated with increased risk of thromboembolic complications) and the potential of reduced overall survival (OS). Although some speculate that this could be due to increased risk of venous thromboembolism, others believe that ESAs may potentiate the progression of malignancy.[9] Notably, patients who were treated with curative intent for breast, head and neck, and cervical cancer, and given ESAs to achieve a hemoglobin goal of 12 g/dL appeared to have worse outcomes.
- The American Society of Hematology (ASH) and the American Society of Clinical Oncology (ASCO) have issued practice guidelines on the use of epoetin (EPO) and darbepoetin in adult patients with cancer[23]:
  - ESAs can be considered in patients undergoing myelosuppressive chemotherapy who have a hemoglobin level less than 10 g/dL and are not being treated with curative intent.
  - ESAs should not be given for anemia not related to chemotherapy except in the case of low EPO states or myelodysplastic syndrome (MDS).
  - Patients who have leukemia or lymphoma should be given a chance for their disease to respond to treatment prior to initiation of therapy for anemia.
  - ESAs should be discontinued after 6 to 8 weeks in nonresponders.
  - Iron replacement can be used concomitantly with ESAs to boost responses even in patients without iron deficiency.
  - Careful consideration must be given regarding the risk of thromboembolism with the use of ESAs.
- **Iron and nutrient repletion:** Patients with chronic symptomatic anemia should be assessed for iron, folate, and vitamin B12 deficiency, and should receive replacement therapy as appropriate. Ideal transferrin saturation should be greater than 20% and serum ferritin should be greater than 100 ng/mL. Iron can be given either orally or parenterally.

References

1. Yellen SB, Cella DF, Webster K, Blendowski C, Kaplan E. Measuring fatigue and other anemia-related symptoms with the Functional Assessment of Cancer Therapy (FACT) measurement system. *J Pain Symptom Manage*. 1997;13:63–74.
2. Groopman JE, Itri LM. Chemotherapy-induced anemia in adults: incidence and treatment. *J Natl Cancer Inst*. 1999;91:1616–1634.
3. Gupta D, Lis CG, Grutsch JF. The relationship between cancer-related fatigue and patient satisfaction with quality of life in cancer. *J Pain Symptom Manage*. 2007;34:40–47.
4. Cella D. The Functional Assessment of Cancer Therapy-Anemia (FACT-An) scale: a new tool for the assessment of outcomes in cancer anemia and fatigue. *Semin Hematol*. 1997;34:13–19.
5. Irvine D, Vincent L, Graydon JE, Bubela N, Thompson L. The prevalence and correlates of fatigue in patients receiving treatment with chemotherapy and radiotherapy. A comparison with the fatigue experienced by healthy individuals. *Cancer Nurs*. 1994;17:367–378.
6. Groopman JE. Fatigue in cancer and HIV/AIDS. *Oncology (Williston Park)*. 1998;12:335–344.
7. Winningham ML, Nail LM, Burke MB, et al. Fatigue and the cancer experience: the state of the knowledge. *Oncol Nurs Forum*. 1994;21:23–36.
8. Schrier SL, Steensma DP, Loprinzi CL. Role of erythropoiesis-stimulating agents in the treatment of anemia in patients with cancer. In: Drews RE, ed. *Uptodate.com*. Waltham, MA: UpToDate Inc.; 2018.
9. Ludwig H, Fritz E. Anemia in cancer patients. *Semin Oncol*. 1998;25:2–6.
10. Cella DF, Bonomi AE, Lloyd SR, Tulsky DS, Kaplan E, Bonomi P. Reliability and validity of the Functional Assessment of Cancer Therapy-Lung (FACT-L) quality of life instrument. *Lung Cancer*. 1995;12:199–220.
11. Langer C, Barsevick A, Bruner D, et al. Correlation of quality of life (QOL) with survival, treatment response, and anemia in patients with advanced non-small cell lung cancer (NSCLC) treated with carboplatin and paclitaxel. *Lung Cancer*. 1997;18:23.
12. Knight K, Wade S, Balducci L. Prevalence and outcomes of anemia in cancer: a systematic review of the literature. *Am J Med*. 2004;116(suppl 7A):11s–26s.
13. Drews RE. Hematologic complications of malignancy. In: Schrier SL, ed. *Anemia and Bleeding*. Waltham, MA: UpToDate; 2017.
14. Pedersen-Bjergaard J. Radiotherapy- and chemotherapy-induced myelodysplasia and acute myeloid leukemia. A review. *Leuk Res*. 1992;16:61–65.
15. Cremin P, Flattery M, McCann SR, Daly PA. Myelodysplasia and acute myeloid leukaemia following adjuvant chemotherapy for breast cancer using mitoxantrone and methotrexate with or without mitomycin. *Ann Oncol*. 1996;7:745–746.
16. Wood PA, Hrushesky WJ. Cisplatin-associated anemia: an erythropoietin deficiency syndrome. *J Clin Invest*. 1995;95:1650–1659.
17. Doll DC, Weiss RB. Hemolytic anemia associated with antineoplastic agents. *Cancer Treat Rep*. 1985;69:777–782.
18. Marani TM, Trich MB, Armstrong KS, et al. Carboplatin-induced immune hemolytic anemia. *Transfusion*. 1996;36:1016–1018.
19. Noronha V, Burtness B, Murren J, Duffy TP. Oxaliplatin induces a delayed immune-mediated hemolytic anemia: a case report and review of the literature. *Clin Colorectal Cancer*. 2005;5:283–286.
20. Myint H, Copplestone JA, Orchard J, et al. Fludarabine-related autoimmune haemolytic anaemia in patients with chronic lymphocytic leukaemia. *Br J Haematol*. 1995;91:341–344.
21. Koeller JM. Clinical guidelines for the treatment of cancer-related anemia. *Pharmacotherapy*. 1998;18:156–169.
22. Rizzo JD, Brouwers M, Hurley P, et al. American Society of Hematology/American Society of Clinical Oncology clinical practice guideline update on the use of epoetin and darbepoetin in adult patients with cancer. *Blood*. 2010;116:4045–4059.
23. Rieger PT, Haeuber D. A new approach to managing chemotherapy-related anemia: nursing implications of epoetin alfa. *Oncol Nurs Forum*. 1995;22:71–81.

CHAPTER 4

Cancer Treatment-Related Thrombocytopenia

Salman R. Punekar, MD

Introduction

- A multitude of cancer treatments are known to cause thrombocytopenia (TCP), termed treatment-related thrombocytopenia. Chemotherapy-induced thrombocytopenia (CIT) is a term that refers specifically to thrombocytopenia caused by chemotherapy drugs. Notably, many nonchemotherapy cancer treatments may also cause thrombocytopenia.
- The normal platelet range is 150,000 to 450,000/μL.[1] The National Cancer Institute Common Terminology Criteria for Adverse Events (NCI CTCAE) defines TCP according to grade. Grade 1 is 75,000 to 150,000/μL, Grade 2 is 50,000 to 75,000/μL, Grade 3 is 25,000 to 50,000/μL, and Grade 4 is less than 25,000/μL.[2] Although the risk of bleeding with TCP is difficult to ascertain fully, general practice is to avoid surgical procedures for platelets less than 50,000/μL (100,000–75,000/μL for central nervous system [CNS] procedures). Furthermore, spontaneous bleeding is possible at platelet counts less than 20,000/μL, but more consistently at levels of less than 5000 to 10,000/μL.[3,4]

Mechanisms of Thrombocytopenia

- **Chemotherapy-induced thrombocytopenia:** CIT comprises the bulk of treatment-related TCP. Chemotherapy causes TCP by altering the megakaryocyte to platelet production pathway, either at the stem cell level or at later stages in platelet maturation. Some of the more commonly implicated chemotherapeutic agents are gemcitabine and carboplatin. Regimens such as ICE (ifosfamide, carboplatin, and etoposide) for non-Hodgkin's lymphoma and MAID (*m*esna, *d*oxorubicin, *i*fosfamide, and *d*acarbazine) for sarcoma are associated with particularly high rates of TCP. Aside from cytotoxic effects on the platelet production line, some chemotherapeutic agents are associated with immune-mediated TCP, such as fludarabine.[5,6]
- **Drug-induced thrombotic microangiopathy (DITMA):** DITMA often presents with hemolytic anemia and thrombocytopenia and has been associated with several cancer-directed therapeutic agents such as gemcitabine, bortezomib, carfilzomib, bevacizumab, sunitinib, and others.[7–10] DITMA is a potentially serious condition and is first managed by discontinuation of the offending drug followed by supportive care.
- **Targeted therapy-related thrombocytopenia:** Targeted therapies, such as tyrosine kinase inhibitors (TKIs), can have off-target effects that can be problematic for patients taking them. These TKIs can have platelet decreasing effects and cause a decrease in platelet function, thus require special consideration.[11]
- **Immunotherapy-related thrombocytopenia:** Although rare, checkpoint inhibitors are known to cause immune-related thrombocytopenia (irTCP) in some patients. Aside from a history of autoimmune conditions, risk factors for irTCP are not well known. Patients, whose TCP has a temporal relationship with treatment with immunotherapy, have no

alternate explanations for TCP, are found to have positive antiplatelet antibodies, and do not respond to platelet transfusions, should be considered to have irTCP. These patients can be treated with immunosuppressive drugs (steroids will be first line) if the TCP is severe.[12]

Diagnostic Workup of Thrombocytopenia

■ The diagnostic workup of cancer treatment–related thrombocytopenia is similar to that of thrombocytopenia from other causes. All patients receiving cancer-directed therapy should undergo evaluation with a complete blood count and examination of the peripheral smear (to evaluate for the presence of abnormal cells such as schistocytes), and metabolic testing including determination of liver enzyme levels of lactate dehydrogenase (LDH), and haptoglobin. This testing is important to rule out other confounding etiologies which also need to be considered in these patients.

Treatment of Thrombocytopenia

In general, treatment-related thrombocytopenia is managed identically to other causes of thrombocytopenia:

■ **Remove the offending agent:** In this case, it is often as simple as delaying future chemotherapy or holding oral-targeted therapy. Patients who experience DITMA should be treated with supportive therapy and discontinuation of the offending drug. Plasma exchange or plasmapheresis (PLEX) and anticomplement therapy are not recommended for DITMA because the pathophysiology differs from that of thrombotic thrombocytopenic purpura (TTP).

■ **Manage risk of complications:** The risk of life-threatening bleeding increases as platelet concentration decreases. The American Society of Clinical Oncologists (ASCO) guidelines from 2018 suggest offering platelet transfusions when platelet counts drop below 10,000/μL. Higher platelet goals can be maintained for certain situations, such as for procedures and surgeries.[13] Patients who experience active bleeding should have a minimum platelet goal of 50,000/μL.

■ **Consider risk of repeated thrombocytopenia:** Future treatment may expose the patient to repeated TCP; consideration must be given to either dose-reduction of the likely offending agent(s) or choosing an alternative agent.

Thrombopoietin receptor agonists (TPO-RAs) have garnered much press for the prevention and treatment of CIT. However, studies have shown mixed results and, their utility has not been proven in large clinical trials, thus their use has not become standard of care.[14–16]

References

1. Buckley MF, James JW, Brown DE, et al. A novel approach to the assessment of variations in the human platelet count. *Thromb Haemost*. 2000;83(3):480–484.
2. National Cancer Institute. Common Terminology Criteria for Adverse Events (CTCAE) v5.0; 2017. https://ctep.cancer.gov/protocoldevelopment/electronic_applications/docs/CTCAE_v5_Quick_Reference_8.5x11.pdf.
3. Slichter SJ, Kaufman RM, Assmann SF, et al. Dose of prophylactic platelet transfusions and prevention of hemorrhage. *N Engl J Med*. 2010;362(7):600–613.
4. Avvisati G, Tirindelli MC, Annibali O. Thrombocytopenia and hemorrhagic risk in cancer patients. *Crit Rev Oncol Hematol*. 2003;48(suppl):S13–S16. http://www.ncbi.nlm.nih.gov/pubmed/14563516.
5. Stasi R. How to approach thrombocytopenia. *Hematol Am Soc Hematol Educ Progr*. 2012;2012:191–197.
6. Kuter DJ. Managing thrombocytopenia associated with cancer chemotherapy. *Oncology (Williston Park)*. 2015;29(4):282–294.

7. Saleem R, Reese JA, George JN. Drug-induced thrombotic microangiopathy: an updated systematic review, 2014–2018. *Am J Hematol*. 2018;93(9):E241–E243.
8. Al-Nouri ZL, Reese JA, Terrell DR, Vesely SK, George JN. Drug-induced thrombotic microangiopathy: a systematic review of published reports. *Blood*. 2015;125(4):616–618.
9. Yui JC, Van Keer J, Weiss BM, et al. Proteasome inhibitor associated thrombotic microangiopathy. *Am J Hematol*. 2016;91(9):E348–E352.
10. Eremina V, Jefferson JA, Kowalewska J, et al. VEGF inhibition and renal thrombotic microangiopathy. *N Engl J Med*. 2008;358(11):1129–1136.
11. Tullemans BME, Heemskerk JWM, Kuijpers MJE. Acquired platelet antagonism: off-target antiplatelet effects of malignancy treatment with tyrosine kinase inhibitors. *J Thromb Haemost*. 2018;16(9):1686–1699.
12. Calvo R. Hematological side effects of immune checkpoint inhibitors: the example of immune-related thrombocytopenia. *Front Pharmacol*. 2019;10:454.
13. Schiffer CA, Bohlke K, Delaney M, et al. Platelet transfusion for patients with cancer: American Society of Clinical Oncology clinical practice guideline update. *J Clin Oncol*. 2018;36(3):283–299.
14. Iuliano F, Perricelli A, Iuliano E, et al. Safety and efficacy of metronomic eltrombopag prophylaxis (MEP) in the prevention of chemotherapy-induced thrombocytopenia (CIT) in cancer patients. *J Clin Oncol*. 2018;36(15 suppl):e14566.
15. Parameswaran R, Lunning M, Mantha S, et al. Romiplostim for management of chemotherapy-induced thrombocytopenia. *Support Care Cancer*. 2014;22(5):1217–1222.
16. Zhang X, Chuai Y, Nie W, Wang A, Dai G. Thrombopoietin receptor agonists for prevention and treatment of chemotherapy-induced thrombocytopenia in patients with solid tumours. *Cochrane Database Syst Rev*. 2017;11:CD012035.

CHAPTER 5

Oral Mucositis

Melissa King, MSN, APRN, FNP-C   Alison Carulli, PharmD, BCOP
  Bassam Estfan, MD

Introduction

- Mucositis is defined as inflammation of the mucous membranes lining the alimentary tract, causing mucosal injury. Mucositis can occur in response to systemic chemotherapy or other etiologies (e.g., infection, radiation).[1] Mucositis generally begins approximately 3 to 4 days following administration of chemotherapy.[2,3] Mucosal injury beyond the oropharynx is discussed in Chapter 6.
- Initial stages of oral mucositis are generally mild, with notable soft tissue erythema and may be associated with burning or mucosal irritation.[2,4] Over the following 3 to 5 days, oral mucositis can progress into visible, painful, white desquamative patches advancing to shallow ulcerations due to epithelial sloughing and formation of large painful lesions; most frequently located on buccal tissue, floor of mouth, tongue and soft palate.[2] The severity of oral mucositis ranges from mild to severe, depending on the chemotherapy regimen, and will generally continue for another 3 to 5 days before resolving.[3] Patients receiving concurrent chemoradiotherapy regimens usually develop mucosal soreness by the end of the first week, with ulcerations appearing at the end of the second week. The mucosal ulcerations consolidate to form larger ulcers by the end of the third week and persist for approximately 2 to 4 weeks after completion of radiotherapy, with most ulcers spontaneously resolving without scarring.[3] The more serious forms of oral mucositis are associated with dysphagia and reduced oral intake, and may provoke secondary infections or sepsis, especially in neutropenic patients.[4,5]

Incidence of Oral Mucositis

- Mucositis is one of the most common toxicities of chemotherapy, especially with combination radiation therapy to the mouth or oropharynx. However, the incidence of oral mucositis is generally underreported because toxicity scales are not consistent and oral mucositis is often only reported when considered severe.[3] Table 5.1 describes the incidence of oral mucositis, Table 5.2 describes risk factors for the development of oral mucositis, and Table 5.3 describes the epidemiology of patients with oral mucositis. Notably, targeted therapies, discussed in detail in Part 2, are also complicit in the development of oral mucositis and may compound toxicity when chemotherapy is given in conjunction with radiotherapy.

Differential Diagnoses

- Fungal (candidiasis) or viral (herpes simplex virus) infection should be considered, especially when heavily keratinized mucosa such as the hard palate, gingiva, or dorsal surface of the tongue is involved.[2]

TABLE 5.1 ■ Incidence of Oral Mucositis

Clinically Significant Oral Mucositis in Solid Tumor Patients[a]	Clinically Significant Oral Mucositis in Patients Receiving Chemoradiation and Radiation Therapy[b]
WHO grade 1: 40% 2: 5% 3, 4: 1%	Mean incidence: 80%

[a]Prospective study of 298 patients.[2,30]
[b]Review of 33 studies involving 6000 patients.[2,31]
WHO, World Health Organization.

TABLE 5.2 ■ Risk Factors Influencing the Frequency or Severity of Oral Mucositis[2,7,9,32,33]

Patient related risk factors	Age (young patients) Gender (female) Tumor type (hematological diseases) Oral health (poor oral hygiene, periodontal disease, dental caries) Smoking or alcohol use Nutritional status (malnutrition) Genetic susceptibility (may play a role) Kidney and liver function
Chemotherapeutic agents	Drugs that affect DNA synthesis High doses Route of administration Alkylating agents (cyclophosphamide, ifosfamide, bendamustine, melphalan) Anthracyclines (doxorubicin, daunorubicin) Antimetabolites (methotrexate, pralatrexate, 5-fluorouracil) Antitumor antibiotics (bleomycin, mitomycin) Purine analogues (cytarabine) Taxanes (paclitaxel, docetaxel) Topoisomerase inhibitors (irinotecan, topotecan, etoposide) Secretion into saliva (methotrexate, etoposide)
Other risk factors	Frequency of administration of chemotherapy Concomitant treatment with radiotherapy Radiation to head and neck Bone marrow transplantation

Etiology and Mechanism of Action of Mucositis

■ Animal models have greatly improved our understanding of the mechanism behind cytotoxic therapy-related mucositis. This has been described in a five-phase model by Sonis: initiation, primary damage response, signal amplification, ulceration, and healing.[6]

■ The initiation phase of mucositis occurs when chemotherapy damages DNA, causing breaks, and generating reactive oxygen species (ROS).[7] This results in the activation of the nuclear factor kappa B (NF-κB) transcription factor.[1] Over 200 genes are managed by NF-κB, including cyclooxygenase-2 (COX-2), and proinflammatory cytokines such as TNF, IL-1β, and IL-6, which have been implicated in the primary damage response phase.[2,4] The signal amplification phase occurs as the proinflammatory cytokines accumulate and cause positive feedback loops that continuously activate NF-κB and amplify the response.[2] Ulcerations

TABLE 5.3 ■ Epidemiology of Patients Developing Clinically Significant Oral Mucositis[3]

Treatment or Patient Characteristic	Mucositis Risk
Malignancies of the mouth, oropharynx, hypopharynx, larynx, nasopharynx, and salivary glands	70%
Conditioning regimens of high dose melphalan or carmustine, etoposide, cytarabine, melphalan (BEAM) in multiple myeloma or non-Hodgkin's lymphoma	42%–46% (grades 3–4)
Cyclophosphamide and etoposide	98% (grades 3–4)
Doxorubicin, cyclophosphamide, paclitaxel, or docetaxel in breast cancer	20% (first cycle) 70% (second cycle)
Docetaxel and capecitabine in metastatic breast cancer	60% (grades 1–2) 15% (grades 3–4)
5-Fluorouracil (5-FU) based regimens in colorectal cancer	70% (all grades) 15%–28% (grades 3–4)
Pralatrexate	70% (all grades) 21% (grades 3–4)
Vinflunine for non–small-cell lung cancer	21% (all grades)

form as the result of these processes and may be aggravated by oral flora colonization.[2] When there is proliferation of the epithelium around the ulcer, the healing phase has begun, and lesions will spontaneously resolve within 2 weeks of chemotherapy.[6,8]

Grading of Mucositis

■ Several grading systems for mucositis have been developed, the most common of which are from the World Health Organization (WHO) and the National Cancer Institute (NCI) (Table 5.4).

Mucositis Management

A number of strategies have been used to prevent or minimize chemotherapy-induced mucositis, although the quality of evidence is limited. Although there are no data to suggest basic oral care has an effect on the pathophysiology of oral mucositis, it has largely been considered standard of care for all patients undergoing chemotherapy or radiotherapy based on medical practitioner

TABLE 5.4 ■ WHO and NCI Mucositis Grading Systems

Grade	WHO[7,34]	NCI CTCAE Version 5[35]
1	Soreness and erythema	Asymptomatic or mild symptoms; no intervention indicated
2	Oral erythema, ulcers; can swallow food	Moderate pain or ulcer that does not interfere with oral intake; modified diet indicated
3	Ulcers with extensive erythema; cannot swallow food	Severe pain; interfering with oral intake
4	Oral alimentation impossible	Life-threatening consequences; urgent intervention indicated

CTCAE, Common Terminology Criteria for Adverse Events; NCI, National Cancer Institute; WHO, World Health Organization.

consensus and several small studies reporting reduced incidence of mucositis with aggressive oral care.[9,10] An interdisciplinary health care team that includes dental professionals is important for all patients, particularly those undergoing head and neck cancer treatments. When possible, these patients should be assessed prior to treatment initiation to identify potential dental treatment requirements such as infection prevention, caries treatment, and tooth extraction.[11] To decrease the risk of infection, consistent brushing with a soft toothbrush and flossing is recommended.[7] Avoiding rough-textured and acidic foods and maintaining adequate food and liquid intake of approximately 3 L/day may help prevent mucosal trauma and complications.[11,12]

- **Mouthwashes**, such as normal saline and sodium bicarbonate, have been studied for prevention and treatment of mucositis, with conflicting results. There are no guidelines recommending the use of either, but given their benign nature they are often used for both treatment and prevention.[10] Chlorhexidine mouthwash has also been studied, with conflicting results, in several cancers and no reported benefit in patients with head and neck cancer.[13–15] Based on these results, the Multinational Association of Supportive Care in Cancer/International Society of Oral Oncology (MASCC/ISOO) recommends against the use of chlorhexidine for mucositis prevention.[10,13] "Magic mouthwash" is an option composed of a variety of ingredients, but, without a standard formula. These formulations contain analgesics or local anesthetics, antifungals or antibiotics, corticosteroids (to decrease inflammation), and antacids (to allow for mouth coating).[4] Although normally recommended every 4 hours as needed, they can be used more frequently in special circumstances; patients should avoid eating or drinking for 15 to 30 minutes to allow for maximal effect. There have been limited trials studying the prevention and treatment of mucositis with magic mouthwash, with conflicting efficacy reported.[16] As a result, there is no mouthwash that is recommended over another, and the choice between them should be made based on patient and physician preference.[10,16]

- **Oral cryotherapy** has been studied with fluorouracil and melphalan to decrease mucositis development and severity.[17] Cryotherapy involves swishing ice chips several minutes prior to chemotherapy administration and continuing for a short time after the chemotherapy has been completed. By inducing local vasoconstriction and decreasing oral mucosal blood flow, less chemotherapy is theoretically delivered to that area.[17,18] Based on several studies that reported a decrease in mucositis severity and incidence, cryotherapy is recommended when receiving bolus fluorouracil. There are no definitive data suggesting cryotherapy is effective with infusional fluorouracil, and it is not routinely used. Cryotherapy should be avoided when fluorouracil and oxaliplatin are used in combination due to oxaliplatin cold-induced dysesthesia.[10,17,19,20] Cryotherapy has also been shown to reduce the severity of mucositis in patients receiving high dose melphalan for hematopoietic stem cell transplantation. However, there are limited studies supporting its use so cryotherapy with melphalan is suggested, rather than recommended, by the MASCC guidelines.[10,18,21]

- **Prophylactic low-level laser therapy (LLLT)** is the noninvasive, local application of high-density monochromatic narrow-band light densities (red or infrared) with variations of soft power levels, dose, wavelengths, and duration of treatment.[22] LLLT can have beneficial effects at the molecular, cellular, and tissue levels by increasing adenosine triphosphate (ATP) production in the mitochondria, and activating ROS and transcription factors (ref-1, AP-1, NF-κB, p53, cyclic adenosine monophosphate [cAMP]), which triggers increased cellular proliferation, modulation of cytokines, growth factors and inflammatory mediators, and increases tissue oxygenation.[23] Additionally, immune cells are strongly affected by LLLT causing mast cell degranulation resulting in the release of cytokines that promote leukocyte infiltration of the tissue and increase fibroblast production and epithelial cell motility, promoting wound healing.[23] Several studies have shown efficacy in reducing the frequency and severity of oral mucositis with the use of LLLT, and the incidence of oral complications has decreased from 43% to 6% with significant reduction in pain.[5,22] MASCC/ISOO Clinical Practice Guidelines for Oral Mucositis recommend the use of LLLT (wavelength, 650 nm; power, 40 mW; treated for time required to produce a tissue energy dose of 2 J/cm^2) for the prevention of oral mucositis in patients receiving high-dose chemotherapy for hematopoietic stem cell transplantation with or without total body irradiation.[15,24]

- **Palifermin** is a recombinant keratinocyte growth factor (KGF). KGF is produced in cells when there is epithelial tissue injury to stimulate the proliferation and differentiation of epithelial cells. Currently, palifermin is the only US Food and Drug Administration (FDA)–approved agent for mucositis in patients with hematologic malignancies undergoing autologous hematopoietic stem cell transplantation. Three doses are given prior to the conditioning regimen, with the third dose being administered 24 to 48 hours prior to the start of the conditioning regimen. Three more doses are administered after completion of the conditioning regimen, with the first dose being administered after the stem cell infusion. In patients receiving total body irradiation and high-dose chemotherapy conditioning regimens for allogeneic hematopoietic stem cell transplant, significantly fewer patients receiving IV palifermin had grade 3 or 4 oral mucositis (63%) when compared with placebo (98%) and reported less mouth and throat soreness, opioid use, and total parenteral nutrition use.[25] As there are no studies with hematopoietic stem cell transplant conditioning regimens of chemotherapy alone or in solid tumors, palifermin is currently not recommended in those settings.[10]

- **Ketamine** oral mouth rinse may be used for the symptomatic treatment and palliation of severe mucositis (WHO grades 3–4) in adults who have otherwise been refractory to standard of care treatments. Ketamine is an N-methyl-D-aspartate (NMDA) receptor antagonist that works by selectively depressing the thalamo-neocortical system. Ketamine is a noncompetitive NMDA receptor antagonist that blocks glutamate, leading to decreased nociception and thus inhibiting the inflammatory cascade. Ketamine selectively interrupts pathways (Mu opioid receptor, serotonin reuptake, calcium and sodium channels, and cholinergic transmission) that may contribute to pain. Additionally, ketamine has modest anti-inflammatory properties, which can be beneficial in treating mucositis pain. Dosing of ketamine oral mouth rinse is 20 mg/5 mL every 4 hours as needed; patient should swish for 30 seconds and spit, may gargle, but should not swallow. Several small trials have reported clinically meaningful and statistically significant reductions in oral mucositis pain scores, with an acceptable safety profile. Thus ketamine mouth rinse can be a useful adjunctive treatment in the management of severe mucositis.[26,27]

- **Opioids** are often used in patients with severe mucositis-related pain. Studies on treatment-related mucositis and stomatitis have primarily been in head and neck cancer patients receiving radiation or hematopoietic stem cell transplantation patients receiving total body irradiation, but data have been extrapolated to other forms of treatment-related mucositis.[10,17] Oral morphine 2% mouthwash has been studied in head and neck radiation patients and is recommended by the MASCC guidelines.[10,28] Systemic opioids administered through patient-controlled analgesia pumps, such as morphine and fentanyl, are also considered acceptable pain management strategies in patients undergoing hematopoietic stem cell transplantation conditioning regimens and have been used in patients with chemotherapy-induced mucositis.[10,17,28] The primary difficulty is balancing pain relief with side effects such as nausea, vomiting, confusion, constipation, and sedation. As a result, mouthwashes and nonsystemic treatments are often used prior to opioids to minimize potential side effects.

- **Methylene blue** oral rinse therapy has been shown to be beneficial in the management of intractable oral mucosal pain; however, larger studies are needed to assess efficacy, side effects, and complications.[29] Other trials with sucralfate, prostaglandins, chamomile mouthwash, amifostine, and antimicrobial lozenges have failed to confirm benefit and should not be considered useful for the prevention of chemotherapy-induced mucositis.

References

1. Reyes-Gibby C, Melkonian S, Wang J, et al. Identifying novel genes and biological processes relevant to the development of cancer therapy-induced mucositis: an informative gene network analysis. *PLoS ONE.* 2017;12(7):e0180396.
2. Shankar A, Roy S, Bhandari M, et al. Current trends in management of oral mucositis in cancer treatment. *Asian Pac J Cancer Prev.* 2017;18(8):2019–2026.
3. Sonis S. *Oral Mucositis.* New York: Springer Healthcare Communications; 2012.
4. Moneim A, Guerra-Librero A, Florido J, et al. Oral mucositis: melatonin gel an effective new treatment. *Int J Mol Sci.* 2017;18:1003.
5. Salvador DRN, Soave DF, Sacono NT, et al. Effect of photobiomodulation therapy on reducing the chemo-induced oral mucositis severity and on salivary levels of CXCL8/interleukin 8, nitrite and myeloperoxidase in patients undergoing hematopoietic stem cell transplantation: a randomized clinical trial. *Laser Med Sci.* 2017;32:1801–1810.
6. Sonis ST. Mucositis: the impact, biology and therapeutic opportunities of oral mucositis. *Oral Oncol.* 2009;45:1015–1020.
7. Moslemi D, Nokhandani AM, Otaghsaraei MT, Moghadamnia Y, Kazemi S, Moghadamnia AA. Management of chemo/radiation-induced oral mucositis in patients with head and neck cancer: review of the current literature. *Radiothera Oncol.* 2016;120:13–20.
8. Al-Dasooqu N, Sonis S, Bowen J, et al. Emerging evidence on the pathobiology of mucositis. *Support Care Cancer.* 2013;21:3233–3241.
9. Kishimoto M, Akashi M, Tsuji K, et al. Intensity and duration of neutropenia relates to the development of oral mucositis but not odontogenic infection during chemotherapy for hematological malignancy. *PLoS ONE.* 2017;12(7):e0182021.
10. Lalla R, Bowen J, Barasch A, et al. MASCC/ISOO clinical practice guidelines for the management of mucositis secondary to cancer therapy. *Cancer.* 2014;120:1453–1461.
11. Saito H, Watanabe Y, Sato K, et al. Effects of professional oral health care on reducing the risk of chemotherapy-induced oral mucositis. *Support Care Cancer.* 2014;22:2935–2940.
12. McGuire D, Fulton J, Park J, et al. Systematic review of basic oral care for the management of oral mucositis in cancer patients. *Support Care Cancer.* 2013;21:3165–3177.
13. Cardona A, Balouch A, Abdul M, Sedghizadeh PP, Enciso R. Efficacy of chlorhexidine for the prevention and treatment of oral mucositis in cancer patients: a systematic review with meta-analyses. *J Oral Pathol Med.* 2017;46:680–688.
14. Epstein JB, Vickars L, Spinelli J, Reece D. Efficacy of chlorhexidine and nystatin rinses in prevention of oral complications in leukemia and bone marrow transplantation. *Surg Oral Med Oral Pathol.* 1992;73:682–689.
15. Nagi R, Patil D, Rakesh N, Jain S, Sahu S. Natural agents in the management of oral mucositis in cancer patients—systematic review. *J Oral Biol Craniofac Res.* 2018;8(3):245–254.
16. Dodd M, Dibble S, Miaskowski C. Randomized clinical trial of the effectiveness of 3 commonly used mouthwashes to treat chemotherapy-induced mucositis. *Oral Surg Oral Med Oral Pathol Oral Radiol Endod.* 2000;90:39–47.
17. Bensinger W, Schubert M, Ang KK, et al. NCCN task force report. Prevention and management of mucositis in cancer. *J Natl Compr Cancer Netw.* 2008;6(suppl 1):S1–S21.
18. Aisa Y, Mori T, Kudo M, et al. Oral cryotherapy for the prevention of high-dose melphalan-induced stomatitis in allogeneic hematopoietic stem cell transplant recipients. *Support Care Cancer.* 2005;13(4):266–269.
19. Majood D, Dose A, Loprinzi C, et al. Inhibition of fluorouracil-induced stomatitis by oral cryotherapy. *J Clin Oncol.* 1999;9(3):449–452.
20. Rocke LF, Loprinzi CL, Lee JK, et al. A randomized clinical trial of two different durations of oral cryotherapy for prevention of 5-fluorouracil-related stomatitis. *Cancer.* 1193;72(7):2234–2238.
21. Riley P, Glenny AM, Worthington HV, Littlewood A, Clarkson JE, McCabe MG. Interventions for preventing oral mucositis in patients with cancer receiving treatment: oral cryotherapy. *Cochrane Database Syst Rev.* 2015;23(12):CD011552.
22. Jadaud E, Bensadoun RJ. Low-level laser therapy: a standard of supportive care for cancer therapy-induced oral mucositis in head and neck cancer patients? *Laser Therapy.* 2012;21(4):297–303.

23. Chung H, Dai T, Sharma SK, Huang YY, Carroll JD, Hamblin MR. The nuts and bolts of low-level laser (light) therapy. *Ann Biomed Eng.* 2012;40(2):516–533.
24. Schubert MM, Eduardo FP, Guthrie KA, et al. A phase III randomized double-blind placebo-controlled clinical trial to determine the efficacy of low level laser therapy for prevention of oral mucositis in patients undergoing hematopoietic cell transplant. *Support Care Cancer.* 2007;15:1145–1154.
25. Spielberge R, Bensinger W, Gentile T, et al. Palifermin for oral mucositis after intensive therapy for hematologic cancers. *N Engl J Med.* 2004;351:2590–2598.
26. Ryan AJ, Lin F, Atayee RS. Ketamine mouthwash for mucositis pain. *J Palliative Med.* 2009;12(11):989–991.
27. Shillingburg A, Kanate A, Hamadani M, Wen S, Craig M, Cumpston A. Treatment of severe mucositis pain with oral ketamine mouthwash. *Support Care Cancer.* 2017;25:2215–2219.
28. Cerchiette L, Navigante A, Körte MW, et al. Potential utility of the peripheral analgesic properties of morphine in stomatitis-related pain: a pilot study. *Pain.* 2003;105:265–273.
29. Roldan C, Nouri K, Chai T, Huh B. Methylene blue for the treatment of intractable pain associated with oral mucositis. *Pain Pract.* 2017;17(8):1115–1121.
30. Andreassen C. The biological basis for differences in normal tissue response to radiation therapy and strategies to establish predictive assays for individual complication risk. In: Sonis ST, Keefe DM, eds. *Pathobiology of Cancer Regimen-Related Toxicities.* New York: Springer; 2013:19–33.
31. Barasch A, Peterson DE. Risk factors for ulcerative oral mucositis in cancer patients: unanswered questions. *Oral Oncol.* 2003;39:91–100.
32. Chaveli-Lopez B, Bagan-Sebastian JV. Treatment of oral mucositis due to chemotherapy. *Oral Med Pathol.* 2016;8(2):e201–e209.
33. Yuce U, Yurtsever S. Effect of education about oral mucositis given to the cancer patients having chemotherapy on life quality. *J Canc Educ.* 2019;34(1):35–40.
34. World Health Organization. *Handbook for Reporting Results of Cancer Treatment.* Geneva, Switzerland: World Health Organization; 1979:15–22.
35. National Cancer Institute. *Common Terminology Criteria for Adverse Events (CTCAE), v 5.* Washington, DC: National Institutes of Health, National Cancer Institute; 2017.

CHAPTER 6

Gastrointestinal Complications of Chemotherapy

Arjun Khunger, MD ▪ Bassam Estfan, MD

Introduction

Gastrointestinal (GI) toxicities are common side effects of most chemotherapy agents. Their effect on rapidly dividing GI tract cells can lead to mucosal inflammation, ulceration, and perforation. The most common GI toxicities include oral mucositis (see Chapter 5), dysphagia, odynophagia, esophagitis, gastritis, nausea and vomiting, enterocolitis, diarrhea, constipation, and hepatotoxicity. Other less common manifestations include GI hemorrhage, bowel perforation, pancreatitis, malabsorption, and infections of the GI tract as a result of chemotherapy-induced immunosuppression. This chapter highlights the mechanisms of chemotherapy-induced GI toxicities and important pharmacological and nonpharmacological management strategies.

Esophageal Complications of Chemotherapy

Clinical esophagitis is observed in 1% to 3% of cancer patients undergoing anticancer treatment and is most commonly due to direct toxicity of chemotherapy or radiation therapy.[1] Patients who are on corticosteroids or are immunosuppressed may develop esophagitis caused by a bacterial, fungal, or viral infection. *Candida* species, herpes simplex virus (HSV), cytomegalovirus (CMV), and varicella zoster virus (VZV) comprise the majority of pathogens. Gastric acid suppressants (e.g., proton pump inhibitors) can contribute to fungal and bacterial colonization of the upper GI tract, predisposing to infectious esophagitis.[2] Other risk factors include gastroesophageal reflux disease (GERD) and pill-induced esophagitis.

Chemotherapy implicated in esophagitis: A number of chemotherapy agents, including doxorubicin, vinblastine, 5-fluorouracil (5-FU), methotrexate, and dactinomycin, have been associated with esophagitis.[3–5] However, the incidence of chemotherapy-induced esophagitis is low and is more commonly observed in combination with thoracic radiation therapy. The pathophysiology of esophagitis due to concurrent chemoradiotherapy is complex and multifactorial, but is believed to involve direct cytotoxic injury followed by secondary insult due to the release of proinflammatory cytokines.[6] Agents such as cyclophosphamide, 5-FU, doxorubicin, and dactinomycin also act as radiosensitizers and can exacerbate the cytotoxic effects of radiation.[7–9]

Esophagitis frequently presents with retrosternal burning, dysphagia, and odynophagia. Subsequent reduced oral intake can lead to dehydration, weakness, need for alternate feeding routes, and treatment interruption. A grading system for esophagitis is described in Table 6.1.

Management of esophagitis: Management depends on the degree of clinical impact, etiology, and other patient-related factors. Most cases are treated with conservative measures such as

TABLE 6.1 ■ **Common Terminology Criteria for Adverse Events (CTCAE) for Common Gastrointestinal (GI) Toxicity**

Adverse Event	Grade 1	Grade 2	Grade 3	Grade 4	Grade 5
Enterocolitis	Asymptomatic; clinical or diagnostic observations only; intervention not indicated	Abdominal pain; mucus or blood in stool	Severe abdominal pain; change in bowel habits; medical intervention indicated; peritoneal signs	Life-threatening consequences; urgent intervention indicated	Death
Constipation	Occasional or intermittent symptoms; occasional use of stool softeners, laxatives, dietary modification, or enema	Persistent symptoms with regular use of laxatives or enemas; limiting instrumental ADL	Obstipation with manual evacuation indicated; limiting self-care ADL	Life-threatening consequences; urgent intervention indicated	Death
Diarrhea	Increase of <4 stools per day over baseline; mild increase in ostomy output compared with baseline	Increase of 4–6 stools per day over baseline; moderate increase in ostomy output compared with baseline	Increase of ≥7 stools per day over baseline; incontinence; hospitalization indicated; severe increase in ostomy output compared with baseline; limiting self-care ADL	Life-threatening consequences; urgent intervention indicated	Death
Esophagitis	Asymptomatic; clinical or diagnostic observations only; intervention not indicated	Symptomatic; altered eating/swallowing; oral supplements indicated	Severely altered eating/swallowing; tube feeding, TPN, or hospitalization indicated	Life-threatening consequences; urgent operative intervention indicated	Death
Nausea	Loss of appetite without alteration in eating habits	Oral intake decreased without significant weight loss, dehydration, or malnutrition	Inadequate oral caloric or fluid intake; tube feeding, TPN, or hospitalization indicated	-	-
Vomiting	1–2 episodes (separated by 5 min) in 24 h	3–5 episodes (separated by 5 min) in 24 h	≥6 episodes (separated by 5 min) in 24 h; tube feeding, TPN, or hospitalization indicated	Life-threatening consequences; urgent intervention indicated	Death

ADL, Activities of daily living; *TPN*, total parenteral nutrition.

hydration; soft, bland diet; and adequate pain control. Patients should be instructed to avoid hot beverages, spicy foods, citrus, alcohol, and tobacco. Use of antacid therapy such as proton pump inhibitors, topical lidocaine, or topical soothing agents such as "Magic Mouthwash" is also recommended before meals to facilitate swallowing. Sucralfate can be used as an adjunct medication in the treatment of pill-induced esophagitis because it can hasten the healing rate by adhering to esophageal ulcers. More severe cases may require switching to a liquid diet with high-calorie supplements for nutritional support, and analgesics such as narcotics. Hospitalization may be necessary to provide nutrition via the percutaneous or parenteral route in these cases. Endoscopic evaluation is not commonly indicated and can be complicated by perforation. However, endoscopy may be therapeutic in patients with known or suspected esophageal strictures because the surgical dilation of esophageal strictures is usually associated with excellent results, and can be diagnostic in providing etiology of infectious esophagitis.

Evaluation of esophagitis: Workup of a patient with suspected esophagitis should include a good oral examination and consideration for a smear and culture of oral mucosa for *Candida*.[10] Candidal infection is more common in immunocompromised patients and may or may not be associated with oropharyngeal thrush. The hallmark of esophageal candidiasis is odynophagia, although many patients may be asymptomatic. Treatment involves azole derivatives, such as fluconazole. If definitive diagnosis is not possible or inconclusive, empiric antifungal therapy should be considered due to the risk of esophageal mucosa sloughing and stricture or fistulae formation.[11]

Viral esophagitis: HSV esophagitis usually arises from reactivation of latent virus during treatment-induced immunosuppression.[12] Patients with oral lesions suggestive for HSV infection along with dysphagia or odynophagia are likely to have HSV esophagitis, and culture and histological examination of the oral mucosa are recommended. The treatment of choice is acyclovir. For patients who are able to take oral medications, acyclovir 400 mg PO 5 times a day for 14 to 21 days is effective. For patients who cannot tolerate oral therapy, intravenous acyclovir can be given 5 mg/kg every 8 hours for 7 to 14 days and as soon as their symptoms improve, they can be switched to oral therapy for completion of the therapeutic course. Foscarnet can be used with caution in patients with acyclovir resistance.

Chemotherapy-Induced Nausea and Vomiting

Chemotherapy-induced nausea and vomiting (CINV) remains one of the most distressing and dreaded adverse events associated with chemotherapy. Up to 80% of patients receiving chemotherapy have CINV; however, the incidence and severity depend on the chemotherapy regimen, dosage, duration, and patient risk factors. CINV has been associated with poor adherence to chemotherapy, disruption of treatment schedules, impairment of functional activity, and significant negative impact on quality of life. Uncontrolled or poorly controlled CINV is associated with dehydration, metabolic imbalances, malnutrition, and weight loss leading to frequent hospitalizations and increased use of healthcare resources. Early prevention and active management are essential to reduce the incidence and consequences of CINV and enhance the care of cancer patients.

Significant progress has been made in our understanding of the pathophysiology of CINV, facilitating the development of effective targeted pharmacotherapies including 5-hydroxytryptamine-3 (5-HT3) receptor antagonists and neurokinin-1 (NK-1) receptor antagonists. As many as 70% to 80% of CINV cases can be prevented with appropriate administration of evidence-based antiemetic regimens.[13]

Classification of Chemotherapy-Induced Nausea and Vomiting

CINV is classified into three major categories according to the time of onset: acute, delayed, and anticipatory. In addition, two further categories describe uncontrolled symptoms: breakthrough and refractory CINV.

- **Acute emesis** occurs within 24 hours of initial administration of chemotherapy with a peak incidence seen at 4 to 6 hours.
- **Delayed emesis** occurs more than 24 hours to several days after the initial administration of chemotherapy with a peak incidence at 2 to 3 days. Delayed CINV is typically associated with cisplatin; however, the phenomenon has also been noted with cyclophosphamide, carboplatin, doxorubicin, and ifosfamide administration at higher doses.[14]
- **Anticipatory emesis** precedes drug administration and is believed to be a conditioned response in patients who have experienced significant CINV during previous cycles of treatment. Common triggers for anticipatory CINV include the environment (physician's office or infusion room), foods, smells, or even cognitive stimuli.
- **Breakthrough CINV** is nausea and/or vomiting occurring within 120 hours of chemotherapy administration, despite optimal antiemetic prophylaxis based on CINV guidelines. The incidence of breakthrough CINV is 30% to 50% in patients receiving chemotherapy.[15]
- **Refractory CINV** is the failure to respond to guideline-directed prophylactic antiemetic agents during a previous cycle of treatment, with nausea and vomiting occurring in subsequent chemotherapy cycles.

Risk Factors for the Development of Chemotherapy-Induced Nausea and Vomiting

There are multiple risk factors for the development of CINV. Younger and female patients both have an increased risk of more frequent and severe CINV, whereas patients who are older, male, and those with a history of chronic alcohol consumption tend to be less affected by CINV.[16–18] Patients with a history of motion sickness and/or pregnancy-related nausea and vomiting have a higher risk of developing CINV.[19] The emetogenicity of the chemotherapeutic agent is the single most important risk factor for development of CINV and is the major criterion for determining the optimal antiemetic prophylaxis regimen.[20] Emetogenicity is a measure of how likely a chemotherapy agent is to cause emesis without antiemetic premedication.

Antineoplastic agents are classified as:

- highly emetogenic (>90% of patients experience CINV)
- moderately emetogenic (30%–90% of patients experience CINV)
- lowly emetogenic (10%–30% of patients experience CINV)
- minimally emetogenic (<10% of patients experience CINV)

Table 6.2 lists important IV and oral chemotherapeutic agents by emetic risk. For certain agents such as cyclophosphamide and doxorubicin, emetogenicity depends on the dose. The risk of developing CINV can also be influenced by the route and frequency of chemotherapy administration. For combination regimens, emetogenic levels are determined by identifying the most emetogenic agent in the combination and then assessing the relative contribution of the other agents.

TABLE 6.2 ■ **Emetic Risk of Common Cytotoxic Agents in Adults**

Degree of Emetic Risk	Intravenous Agents	Oral Agents
High (>90%)	Anthracycline + cyclophosphamide Cisplatin Cyclophosphamide >1500 mg/m^2 Dacarbazine	Procarbazine
Moderate (30%–90%)	Azacitidine Bendamustine Busulfan Carboplatin Clofarabine Cyclophosphamide <1500 mg/m^2 Cytarabine >1000 mg/m^2 Anthracyclines Ifosfamide Irinotecan Oxaliplatin	Cyclophosphamide Temozolomide Vinorelbine
Low (10%–30%)	Cabazitaxel Cytarabine <1000 mg/m^2 Docetaxel Eribulin Etoposide Fluorouracil Gemcitabine Methotrexate Mitomycin Mitoxantrone Paclitaxel Pemetrexed Topotecan Vinflunine	Capecitabine Etoposide Fludarabine Lenalidomide Tegafur-uracil Thalidomide
Minimal (<10 %)	Bleomycin Cladribine Fludarabine Pralatrexate Vinca alkaloids	Busulfan Chlorambucil Hydroxyurea Melphalan Methotrexate Pomalidomide 6-Thioguanine

Pathophysiology of Chemotherapy-Induced Nausea and Vomiting

The pathophysiology of CINV is complex and multifactorial. It involves multiple neurotransmitters, neuroreceptors, and neuronal pathways in the central nervous system (CNS) and peripheral structures. The three main neurotransmitters are serotonin, substance P, and dopamine and the receptors associated with them are 5-HT3, NK-1, and dopamine-2 (D2) receptors, respectively. Other receptors involved include corticosteroid, histamine, cannabinoid, acetylcholine, and opiate receptors, although their roles are not precisely defined.

CINV mainly occurs via activation of peripheral and central pathways. The peripheral pathway is mediated via binding of serotonin to 5-HT3 receptors located in the GI tract and is activated within the first 24 hours after chemotherapy administration; it is primarily associated with acute emesis. The central pathway is activated via binding of substance P to NK-1 receptors in the brain and is thought to be predominantly involved in delayed CINV. A simplified illustration of the pathways involved in the pathophysiology of CINV has been depicted in Fig. 6.1. Chemotherapy can stimulate the enterochromaffin cells lining the digestive tract to release serotonin in response to cell damage. Serotonin binds to 5-HT3 receptors on the nearby vagal afferents in the gut, which in turn causes the transmission of sensory input from the GI tract to the vomiting center in the brain, located in the dorsolateral border of medulla. The vomiting center receives signals from

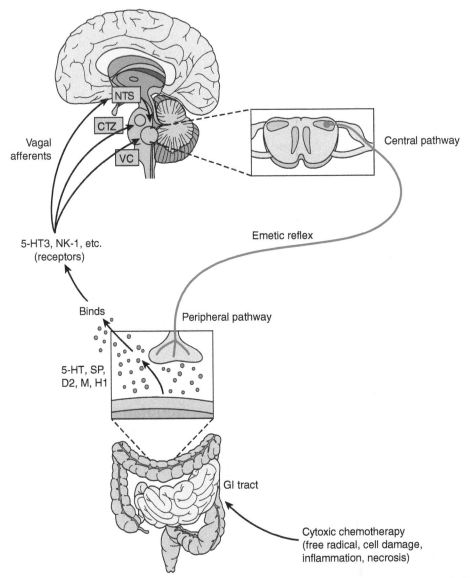

Fig. 6.1 Pathophysiology of chemotherapy induced nausea and vomiting. *5-HT*, 5-Hydroxytryptamine; *CTZ*, chemoreceptor trigger zone; *D2*, dopamine-type 2; *H1*, histamine 1; *M*, muscarinic; *NTS*, nucleus tractus solitarii; *SP*, substance P; *VC*, vomiting center.

other structures, including the chemotherapy trigger zone (CTZ) in the area postrema, which is lined by 5-HT3 and D2 receptors. Chemotherapy can directly activate the CTZ chemoreceptors because they lack an effective blood–brain barrier. All the sensory signals are consolidated in the vomiting center, resulting in the generation of efferent signals that lead to contraction of the abdominal muscles, the stomach, and the diaphragm, causing subsequent emesis. Each of these neurotransmitters and their corresponding receptors are of primary interest and therapeutic targets for development of antiemetic drugs.

Management and Prevention of Chemotherapy-Induced Nausea and Vomiting

PHARMACOLOGICAL THERAPY FOR CHEMOTHERAPY-INDUCED NAUSEA AND VOMITING

CINV is treated by four major classes of medications: 5-HT3 receptor antagonists, NK-1 receptor antagonists, corticosteroids, D2 receptor antagonists, and Olanzapine has been added to the standard antiemetic guidelines due to its effectiveness in managing CINV.

1. **5-HT3 receptor antagonists:** These agents act both centrally and peripherally by antagonizing the action of serotonin at 5-HT3 receptors present in the CTZ and the GI tract. Their efficacy in preventing nausea and vomiting induced by moderately emetogenic chemotherapy (MEC) and highly emetogenic chemotherapy (HEC), coupled with a mild side-effect profile, have made them a key component of prophylactic treatment for acute CINV. Ondansetron, granisetron, and palonosetron are US Food and Drug Administration (FDA)–approved for CINV. Palonosetron is the only second-generation 5-HT3 receptor antagonist and has a stronger binding affinity for serotonin receptors and a longer half-life (about 40 hours) compared with first-generation compounds.[21] Initial trials recorded superior efficacy of palonosetron over other 5-HT3 receptor antagonists in terms of complete response, and rates of acute and delayed CINV in patients receiving MEC.[22,23] However, subsequent studies demonstrated that all 5-HT3 antagonists have comparable efficacy in preventing CINV and therefore, current guidelines recommend use of any of the available 5-HT3 receptor antagonists, tailored to individual needs.[24] The main side effects of 5-HT3 receptor antagonists are constipation, mild headache, and dizziness.[25] Almost all 5-HT3 receptor antagonists have been associated with asymptomatic electrocardiogram changes, such as prolongation of the PR and QTc intervals and benign ventricular arrhythmias,[26] and they should be used in caution in patients with long QT syndrome. Periodic electrocardiographic monitoring is recommended for patients at high risk such as those with congestive heart failure, electrolyte abnormalities, or bradyarrhythmias, and those treated with concomitant medications that can prolong the QTc interval. Palonosetron is the only 5-HT3 receptor antagonist that does not cause clinically significant QT interval prolongation.[27]

2. **NK-1 receptor antagonists:** These agents work by blocking substance P activity at NK-1 receptors in the CNS. Examples include the oral NK-1 receptor antagonist, aprepitant, and the IV prodrug fosaprepitant. These drugs have significantly improved the ability to prevent acute and delayed CINV when used in conjunction with both 5-HT3 receptor antagonists and corticosteroids. The efficacy of combining an NK-1 receptor antagonist with a 5-HT3 receptor antagonist and corticosteroid for the prevention of CINV was initially addressed in a meta-analysis of 17 trials, with a total of 8740 patients who received highly or moderately emetogenic chemotherapeutic agents. The three-drug regimen significantly improved rates of complete response (absence of emesis and no need for rescue antiemetics) compared with a two-drug regimen (72% vs. 54%).[28] This led to newer NK-1 antagonists being incorporated into antiemetic guidelines. NEPA is a fixed-dose oral combination of netupitant (highly selective NK-1 receptor antagonist) and palonosetron which is approved

for patients receiving highly and moderately emetogenic chemotherapy.[29] Another, NK-1 receptor antagonist, rolapitant, is approved in combination with other antiemetic agents in adults for preventing delayed CINV based on promising results of three phase III trials evaluating rolapitant in patients receiving HEC or MEC.[30,31] A number of NK-1 receptor antagonists (aprepitant and fosaprepitant) are inhibitors of the cytochrome P450 3A4 enzyme (CYP3A4), which metabolizes approximately half of all drugs currently on the market and thus caution should be used when coadministering them with oral contraceptives, dexamethasone, warfarin, and other CYP3A4 inducers and inhibitors.[32] Rolapitatant does not inhibit or induce CYP3A4; however, it does have CYP2D6 inhibitory activity. Adverse events associated with NK-1 receptor antagonists include dizziness, anorexia, and diarrhea.

3. **Corticosteroids:** Corticosteroids are a mainstay of any CINV prophylaxis regimen, but their mechanism of action is not well understood. Several hypotheses have been formulated, such as alteration of cell permeability, inhibition of prostaglandin activity, and activation of glucocorticoid receptors in the nucleus of the solitary tract in the medulla.[33] Dexamethasone and methylprednisolone are the most commonly administered antiemetics. Corticosteroids can be effective when administered as a single agent in patients receiving low emetogenic chemotherapy; however, they are most beneficial when used in combination with 5-HT3 and NK1 receptor antagonists. They have demonstrated effectiveness for both acute and delayed emesis caused by MEC and HEC.[34] Side effects from single or short-term dexamethasone usage are infrequent, but their toxicities for repeated use should not be underestimated. Because NK-1 receptor antagonists, such as aprepitant and netupitant, are moderate inhibitors of CYP3A4, the oral dose of dexamethasone should be reduced by 50% when it is coadministered with NK-1 receptor antagonists.

4. **D2 receptor antagonists:** D2 receptor antagonists work by competitive blockade of dopamine receptors centrally in the CTZ and vomiting center. A number of different drugs, including droperidol, prochlorperazine, promethazine, and metoclopramide, have demonstrated antiemetic activity. Metoclopramide blocks dopamine receptors centrally in the CTZ, and peripherally in the GI tract, and also has prokinetic effects, thereby increasing gut motility. However, D2 receptor antagonists, can cause extrapyramidal symptoms, restlessness, hypotension, and CNS depression, limiting the use of these drugs, and thus they have been largely replaced by 5-HT3 receptor antagonists due to their superior efficacy and safety. Currently, use of D2 receptor antagonists has been limited to the prevention of nausea from MEC, treatment of breakthrough nausea and vomiting, and in patients with refractory CINV to serotonin blockers.

5. **Olanzapine:** Olanzapine is a 5-HT2, 5-HT3, and dopamine receptor antagonist and was initially approved as an antipsychotic for use in the treatment of schizophrenia, bipolar disorder, and depression. Various randomized trials have suggested a promising role of olanzapine in the prevention and treatment of acute and delayed CINV. In a phase III study in patients receiving HEC or MEC, olanzapine/5-HT3 receptor antagonist/dexamethasone regimen resulted in superior delayed and overall complete response rates as compared with a 5-HT3 receptor antagonist/dexamethasone regimen. In another phase III trial comparing an olanzapine-based regimen with an aprepitant-based regimen in chemotherapy-naive patients receiving HEC, complete response was observed in 117 patients (97%) in the olanzapine group and 104 patients (87%) in the aprepitant group ($P > .05$).[35] The olanzapine regimen resulted in higher complete response rates during the delayed and overall phases (87% acute, 69% delayed/overall) compared with the aprepitant regimen (87% acute, 38% delayed/overall). In the most recent trial, the benefit of adding olanzapine to a triplet 5-HT3 receptor antagonist/aprepitant/dexamethasone regimen was evaluated. The percentage of patients with no nausea reported was significantly higher in the olanzapine arm compared with the placebo arm in the acute (74% vs. 45%; $P = .002$), delayed (42% vs. 25%; $P = .002$), and overall periods (37% vs. 22%; $P = .002$).[36] A systematic review of randomized trials has supported the use of olanzapine as a single agent for the treatment of breakthrough CINV for patients who did not

receive it prophylactically. In a randomized clinical trial, olanzapine demonstrated superiority over metoclopramide in preventing breakthrough nausea (68% vs. 23%; $P < .01$) and vomiting (60% vs. 23%; $P < .01$) for patients receiving HEC who received prior prophylaxis with palonosetron, fosaprepitant, and dexamethasone.[37] Major side effects of olanzapine include drowsiness, fatigue, disturbed sleep, and dry mouth. Olanzapine should not be coadministered with other dopamine receptor antagonists due to increased risk of extrapyramidal symptoms. Overall, the olanzapine-containing regimens appear to be safe, well tolerated, and cost-effective and have efficacy equivalent to that of aprepitant-based regimens. The National Comprehensive Cancer Network (NCCN) and American Society of Clinical Oncology (ASCO) guidelines have been updated to recommend the use of olanzapine together with 5-HT3 receptor antagonists, dexamethasone, and aprepitant for adults receiving HEC.[38,39]

Antiemetic Regimens Based on Emetogenicity of Chemotherapy

- **Antiemetic regimens for highly emetogenic chemotherapy:** Patients treated with cisplatin or other highly emetogenic single chemotherapeutic agents should be offered a four-drug combination of a NK1 receptor antagonist, a 5-HT3 receptor antagonist, dexamethasone, and olanzapine on day 1 of treatment. Dexamethasone and olanzapine are recommended to be continued on days 2 to 4 (Table 6.3). Alternatively, three-drug regimens including single doses of a 5-HT3 receptor antagonist, dexamethasone, and an NK1 receptor antagonist can also be given for prevention of CINV for HEC. For patients receiving anthracycline/cyclophosphamide (AC) combination chemotherapy, a four-drug combination of NK-1 receptor antagonist, 5-HT receptor antagonist, dexamethasone, and olanzapine is recommended prior to the start of cytotoxic treatment (day 1) and only olanzapine is continued on days 2 to 4. Dexamethasone is not recommended on days 2 to 4 due to limited data supporting its benefit beyond day 1. Alternatively, a three-drug regimen including single doses of a 5-HT3 receptor antagonist, dexamethasone, and an NK1 receptor antagonist can also be given for prevention of CINV in patients receiving AC combination chemotherapy.
- **Antiemetic regimens for moderately emetogenic chemotherapy:** For patients treated with carboplatin-based regimens, three-drug combinations of an NK1 receptor antagonist, 5-HT3 receptor antagonist and dexamethasone on day 1, with no additional prophylaxis beyond day 1, is recommended. If aprepitant is given on day 1 it should be continued on days 2 and 3, as well (see Table 6.3). For patients treated with moderately emetogenic non–carboplatin-based regimens, a two-drug combination of a 5-HT3 receptor antagonist and dexamethasone is recommended on day 1; dexamethasone is only recommended on days 2 and 3 if the chemotherapy treatment contains agents known to induce delayed emesis (e.g., oxaliplatin). In comparison with recommendations for HEC, it remains controversial whether the addition of an NK-1 receptor antagonist to the two-drug combination of 5-HT3 receptor antagonist and dexamethasone is beneficial to patients receiving MEC due to a lack of large homogenous studies. NCCN guidelines recommend addition of NK1 receptor antagonist to 5-HT3 receptor antagonist and dexamethasone-containing regimens for select patients with additional risk factors or failure of previous therapy with a steroid and 5-HT3 receptor antagonist alone.
- **Antiemetic regimen for low emetogenic chemotherapy:** Current guidelines recommend the administration of a single 8-mg dose of dexamethasone or a single dose of 5-HT3 receptor antagonist on the day of chemotherapy for patients receiving low emetic risk agents (see Table 6.3). If contraindicated, a single dose of a dopamine receptor antagonist such as metoclopramide or prochlorperazine can be used. Benzodiazepines, H2 blockers, or proton pump inhibitors can be added (alone or in any combination) to all these agents. Additionally, this patient population generally does not require routine prophylaxis against delayed emesis
- **Antiemetic regimen for minimally emetogenic chemotherapy:** Guidelines do not recommend any routine prophylactic antiemetics for agents with a minimal risk of causing emesis.

TABLE 6.3 ■ **Antiemetic Dosing for Adults Receiving Chemotherapy**

Regimen	Drugs	Dose on Day 1	Dose on Days 2, 3, 4
Highly Emetogenic Chemotherapy			
4-Drug combination regimen (NK-1 RA, 5-HT3 RA, dexamethasone, olanzapine)	NK-1 RA (choose one): Aprepitant Fosaprepitant Rolapitant NEPA	125 mg PO 150 mg IV once 180 mg PO once (300 mg netupitant/0.5 mg palonosetron PO combination) once	80 mg oral on days 2, 3
	5-HT3 RA (choose one): Granisetron Ondansetron Palonosetron	2 mg PO or 1 mg or 0.01 mg/kg IV or 1 transdermal patch or 10 mg sc 8 mg PO twice daily or 8 mg or 0.15 mg/kg IV once 0.50 mg oral or 0.25 mg IV once	
	Dexamethasone	12 mg PO/IV once	8 mg PO/IV daily on days 2, 3, 4
	Olanzapine	10 mg PO	10 mg PO daily on days 2, 3, 4
3-Drug NK-1 RA based combination regimen	NK-1 RA (choose one): Aprepitant Fosaprepitant Rolapitant NEPA	125 mg PO once 150 mg IV once 180 mg PO once (300 mg netupitant/0.5 mg palonosetron PO combination) once	80 mg PO daily on days 2, 3
	5-HT3 RA (choose one): Granisetron Ondansetron Palonosetron	2 mg PO or 1 mg or 0.01 mg/kg IV or 1 transdermal patch or 10 mg sc 8 mg PO twice daily or 8 mg or 0.15 mg/kg IV once 0.50 mg oral or 0.25 mg IV once	
	Dexamethasone	12 mg PO/IV once	8 mg PO/IV daily on days 2, 3, 4
Moderately Emetogenic Chemotherapy			
Carboplatin based: 3-drug combination regimen (NK-1 RA + 5-HT3 RA + dexamethasone)	NK-1 RA (choose one): Aprepitant Fosaprepitant Rolapitant NEPA	125 mg PO 150 mg IV once 180 mg PO once (300 mg netupitant/0.5 mg palonosetron PO combination) once	80 mg PO daily on days 2, 3
	5-HT3 RA (choose one): Granisetron Ondansetron Palonosetron	2 mg PO or 1 mg or 0.01 mg/kg IV or 1 transdermal patch or 10 mg sc 8 mg PO twice daily or 8 mg or 0.15 mg/kg IV once 0.50 mg oral or 0.25 mg IV once	
	Dexamethasone	12 mg PO/IV once	

TABLE 6.3 ■ Antiemetic Dosing for Adults Receiving Chemotherapy (Continued)

Regimen	Drugs	Dose on Day 1	Dose on Days 2, 3, 4
Non-carboplatin based: 2-drug combination regimen (5-HT3 RA + dexamethasone)	5-HT3 RA (choose one): Granisetron Ondansetron Palonosetron	2 mg PO or 1 mg or 0.01 mg/kg IV or 1 transdermal patch or 10 mg sc 8 mg PO twice daily or 8 mg or 0.15 mg/kg IV once 0.25 mg IV once	
	Dexamethasone	8 mg PO/IV once	8 mg PO/IV on day 3
Low Emetogenic Chemotherapy			
Single agent dexamethasone	Dexamethasone	8 mg PO/IV once	
Single agent 5-HT3 RA	5-HT3 RA (choose one): Granisetron Ondansetron Palonosetron	2 mg PO or 1 mg or 0.01 mg/kg IV or 1 transdermal patch or 10 mg sc 8 mg PO twice daily or 8 mg or 0.15 mg/kg IV once 0.25 mg IV once	
Single agent dopamine RA	Dopamine RA (choose one): Metoclopramide Prochlorperazine	10–20 mg PO/IV once 10 mg PO/IV once	
Minimally Emetogenic Chemotherapy			
No routine prophylactic antiemetics			

_5-HT3_, 5-Hydroxytryptamine-3; _IV_, intravenous; _NK-1_, neurokinin-1; _PO_, orally; _RA_, receptor antagonist; _sc_, subcutaneous.

Management of Anticipatory Emesis

The primary approach for the prevention of anticipatory emesis is the best possible control of acute and delayed CINV. In select high-risk patients, upfront intensification of the standard antiemetic regimen according to the risk of the treatment may need to be considered. For patients who develop anticipatory emesis, behavioral therapy (e.g., progressive muscle relaxation training) with systematic desensitization can be offered. Anxiolytic agents such as lorazepam and alprazolam can also be considered. With the availability of more effective antiemetic regimens, there has been a decline in the incidence of anticipatory emesis.

Management of Breakthrough and Refractory Emesis

Breakthrough and refractory emesis are clinical challenges in oncology because, once triggered, they are often difficult to reverse. Adequate patient instruction is the preliminary step to help patients understand the importance of treatment compliance, especially when using oral medications that need to be taken at home. Once established, the first step in patient management should be a comprehensive work-up to recognize any particular disease- or medication-related factor that may be responsible for continued emesis such as opiate analgesics, or concurrent illness (e.g., metastases to CNS, bowel obstruction, and vestibular dysfunction). It is important to confirm that patients are receiving the most appropriate antiemetic regimen and dosage. International guidelines recommend treatment of breakthrough CINV with an agent from a class with a different mechanism of action than that of antiemetics given for prophylaxis. There have been very few formal studies addressing the management of breakthrough CINV. Agents that can be added include D2 receptor antagonists such as metoclopramide or prochlorperazine or steroids if not used previously. A randomized, phase III study has demonstrated that olanzapine is superior to metoclopramide for the treatment of breakthrough CINV in patients receiving HEC.[37] The available evidence suggests the use of olanzapine 10 mg PO for 3 days. It may be helpful to give breakthrough medication at regularly scheduled intervals rather than as needed.

Patients who develop refractory CINV should be considered for step-up therapy or a change in their prophylactic antiemetic regimen. If significant anxiety symptoms are present, a benzodiazepine (e.g., lorazepam or alprazolam) may be added to the prophylactic regimen. Alternate drugs known to exert antiemetic effects such as cannabinoids (e.g., dronabinol and nabilone) can also be offered to the patients. If refractory CINV symptoms persist, the additional agents should be given on a continuous basis, and the patient's nutritional status should be monitored carefully and assessed for the need for IV hydration or for electrolyte supplementation.

Nonpharmacological Approaches for Management of CINV

Considering that it is very difficult to control CINV completely using antiemetic drugs alone, it is common for patients to seek alternate methods of treatment. There are limited data from randomized trials of reasonable quality to support the use of complementary or alternative therapies in the prevention and management of CINV. International guidelines do not recommend for or against the use of any complementary therapies.

Ginger has been evaluated for the prevention CINV in various trials because it has been hypothesized that ginger contains many bioactive compounds that can act on different signaling pathways involved in the pathophysiology of CINV. In a large study of 744 breast cancer patients, it was shown that ginger added to standard prophylactic antiemetic regimen of 5-HT3 receptor antagonist and dexamethasone significantly reduced the incidence of acute CINV compared with placebo.[40] However, a meta-analysis report did not show any significant benefit of ginger on the incidence of acute or delayed vomiting and acute nausea.[41]

Acupuncture-point stimulation is another popular approach used for managing CINV. A study comparing acupuncture with ondansetron in patients receiving moderate emetic risk agents demonstrated comparable effectiveness in management of acute CINV, though acupuncture seemed more effective in prevention of delayed CINV.[42] However, more randomized trials are needed to justify its routine use in the prevention of CINV. Various bio-psychobehavioral interventions such as progressive muscle relaxation, guided imagery, hypnosis, and exercise have also been evaluated and have yielded positive and negative results in reducing the incidence of CINV.[43,44]

Enterocolitis

Chemotherapy-associated enterocolitis is a rare but serious adverse event associated with cytotoxic chemotherapy. Patients receiving chemotherapy may experience severe types of colitis with infectious and noninfectious etiology. Infectious colitis is mostly due to *Clostridium difficile* infection, commonly encountered as a result of immunosuppression, and antibiotic use. Although prior antibiotic therapy is the single most common risk factor for *C. difficile* colitis, several reports have documented *C. difficile* colitis with or without concurrent or recent use of antibiotics at a rate of 6%.[45–47] Treatment usually involves administration of oral metronidazole or vancomycin per usual standards of care. Noninfectious enterocolitis typically manifests as neutropenic enterocolitis (typhlitis) or ischemic enterocolitis.

■ **Neutropenic enterocolitis:** Chemotherapy-induced neutropenia is common in patients receiving it. Neutropenic enterocolitis is a clinicopathological syndrome occurring primarily in neutropenic patients, characterized by necrotizing inflammation of the lower GI tract (typically the cecum). The affected gut becomes edematous and thick-walled, with mucosal ulceration, progressing to partial- to full-thickness hemorrhagic necrosis. It is potentially a life-threatening condition, most often associated with leukemia or lymphoma. Neutropenic enterocolitis was initially described in children following induction chemotherapy for acute leukemia.[48,49] However, it has been reported in adults with hematologic malignancies and other immunosuppressive causes resulting in profound neutropenia, including therapy for solid tumors, AIDS, and organ transplantation.[50] It is most commonly reported with the use of taxanes for the treatment of various solid tumors, though various other agents, including cisplatin, cytosine arabinoside, gemcitabine, vincristine, doxorubicin, gemcitabine, cyclophosphamide, 5-FU have also been implicated.[51–53]

The initial presentation is nonspecific and often overlooked by the symptomatology of primary malignant disease and neutropenia-associated complications. It usually manifests 1 to 2 weeks after chemotherapy administration corresponding to the neutrophil count nadir[54] and presents with fever and abdominal pain particularly in the right lower quadrant. Other presenting symptoms can include nausea, vomiting, diarrhea, and gastrointestinal bleeding. The diagnosis is usually made by computed tomography (CT) scan, when findings include bowel wall thickening, fluid-filled and dilated cecum, right lower quadrant inflammatory mass, and pericolonic inflammation.[49] *C. difficile* infection should be ruled out. Endoscopy to obtain biopsies is usually discouraged due to increased risk of bowel wall perforation.

Initial treatment is usually supportive and consists of bowel rest, intravenous fluids, analgesics, and broad-spectrum antibiotics. Correction of cytopenia and coagulopathy should be encouraged because neutropenia contributes to the pathogenesis of the disease, and coagulopathy can be associated with blood loss from hemorrhage. Recombinant granulocyte colony-stimulating factor can be used to hasten neutrophil recovery.[55] Surgical intervention is recommended for patients having persistent GI bleeding, despite treatment of cytopenia and coagulopathy, and for patients with bowel wall perforation.[54]

- **Ischemic colitis:** Ischemic colitis is a rare complication of cancer chemotherapy. Initially, few cases were reported in patients treated with docetaxel and carboplatin-paclitaxel regimens.[56–60] Ischemic colitis is characterized by symptom presentation of acute onset abdominal pain with or without neutropenia, fever and diarrhea, and associated direct or rebound tenderness on physical examination. Patients may also present with bloody diarrhea. Ischemic colitis differs from neutropenic colitis with respect to the early occurrence of symptoms within 1 week after the initiation of chemotherapy treatment and inconsistent findings of neutropenia and/or fever. As with other clinical colitis syndromes, *C. difficile* infection should be ruled out. Colonoscopy is the preferred method for diagnosis of ischemic colitis and pathological examination of a biopsy specimen may clinch the diagnosis. Supportive management and surgery are frequently employed, although the disease is associated with significant mortality.

Constipation

Constipation is a common complaint in patients undergoing chemotherapy. However, the true incidence of chemotherapy-induced constipation is difficult to estimate due to secondary constipation as a consequence of multiple factors, including poor oral intake, decreased physical activity, and other medications such as opioid analgesics or antiemetic agents.[61] However, high rates of chemotherapy-induced constipation have been reported following the administration of cisplatin, thalidomide, and vinca alkaloids (e.g., vincristine, vinblastine, and vinorelbine) (Table 6.4).[62,63] Constipation is often dose-dependent and is most prominently observed after 3 to 10 days of chemotherapy initiation.[64] Thalidomide and its analogs, including lenalidomide and pomalidomide, can cause severe constipation in older adults and in those receiving concomitant opioid therapy.[65]

TABLE 6.4 ■ **Chemotherapy Drugs Causing Alteration in Bowel Habits**

Agents Likely to Cause Diarrhea	Agents Likely to Cause Constipation
5-Fluorouracil	Vinca alkaloids (e.g., vincristine, vinblastine)
Irinotecan	Platinum compounds (e.g., cisplatin, carboplatin)
Methotrexate	Thalidomide
Capecitabine	
Oxaliplatin	
Taxanes	
Lenalidomide	

Constipation can lead to abdominal discomfort, loss of appetite, and severe impairment of quality of life (see Table 6.1 for toxicity grading). Severe constipation can result in abdominal pain, abdominal distention, hemorrhoids, bleeding, and rectal fissures when passing dry hard stool. Complications of severe, untreated constipation include life-threatening conditions such as bowel obstruction, perforation, ischemia, and necrosis.[66] Therefore, it is important to take early steps for prevention of constipation in cancer patients.

Constipation in cancer patients can be managed with diet, lifestyle intervention, and pharmacological therapy. Nonpharmacological approaches include increasing fiber and liquid intake, and physical activity. Constipating medications should be discontinued when possible. Stool softeners such as docusate can be used initially for treatment of mild constipation. More significant constipation requires intervention with laxatives such as senna, bisacodyl, or polyethylene glycol. Osmotic agents such as lactulose or sorbitol may need to be used in severe cases.[67] Rectal laxatives such as bisacodyl, sodium phosphate, or glycerin, although not commonly used, may be given along with digital stimulation for treating fecal impaction or constipation due to neurogenic bowel dysfunction, but should be avoided in neutropenic patients.

Chemotherapy-Induced Diarrhea (CID)

Diarrhea is a common side effect of cytotoxic chemotherapy and usually occurs in patients treated with fluoropyrimidines (particularly 5-FU and capecitabine), irinotecan, methotrexate, or cisplatin.[68] Antimetabolites, such as pemetrexed and methotrexate, and taxanes are associated with diarrhea to a lesser degree (see Table 6.4).[69] This needs to be differentiated from diarrhea due to concurrent radiation therapy, targeted therapy, neutropenic enterocolitis, *C. difficile* colitis, and graft-versus-host disease, which are described in other sections.

The severity of CID can be described using the National Cancer Institute Common Toxicity Criteria (NCI CTC; see Table 6.1). The overall incidence of CID has been reported to be as high as 50% to 80% (≥30% CTC grades 3–5).[70,71] The mechanism of CID is thought to be multifactorial due to acute damage to the intestinal mucosa, including loss of proliferating intestinal epithelium, disruption of the mucosal barrier, and impaired absorption of water and electrolytes from the luminal wall, resulting in diarrhea.[68,71]

Diarrhea is reported in up to 50% of patients receiving weekly 5-FU/leucovorin combined treatment.[68] The frequency and severity of diarrhea worsens when 5-FU is administered by bolus injection as opposed to continuous intravenous infusion.[72,73] Other factors associated with increased risk of 5-FU–induced diarrhea include female gender, presence of an unresected primary tumor, previous episodes of chemotherapy-induced diarrhea, and treatment during the summer.[74,75] Capecitabine has been associated with up to a 46% incidence of diarrhea in colon cancer patients.[76]

Irinotecan hydrochloride is known to cause early-onset diarrhea (developing within 24 hours after treatment initiation) and delayed-onset diarrhea (occurring 24 hours or more after treatment initiation). Early-onset diarrhea is attributed to structural characteristics of irinotecan causing cholinergic syndrome (inhibition of cholinesterase activity) and is accompanied by abdominal cramping, lacrimation, salivation, and other cholinergic symptoms. These symptoms can be effectively prevented and controlled with anticholinergics (e.g., atropine) and loperamide. However, late-onset diarrhea associated with irinotecan is unpredictable and can be severe in up to 40% of patients. Diarrhea can be worse in combination with fluorouracil.[77,78] In severe cases, fluids and electrolytes depletion, dehydration, and malnutrition may occur, necessitating hospitalization.

Evaluation and Management of Chemotherapy-Induced Diarrhea

The treatment of CID involves aggressive rehydration and electrolyte replacement and the use of pharmacologic agents to reduce fluid loss and decrease intestinal motility. A general approach for the evaluation and management of CID is outlined in Fig. 6.2. Evaluation should begin with a good history and physical examination to assess the severity of diarrhea. Patients should be evaluated for signs of dehydration, infection, or bowel obstruction. Laboratory testing should include a complete blood count, determination of serum urea and creatinine and electrolyte levels, and if indicated, stool testing to rule out infectious etiologies such as *C. difficile*.

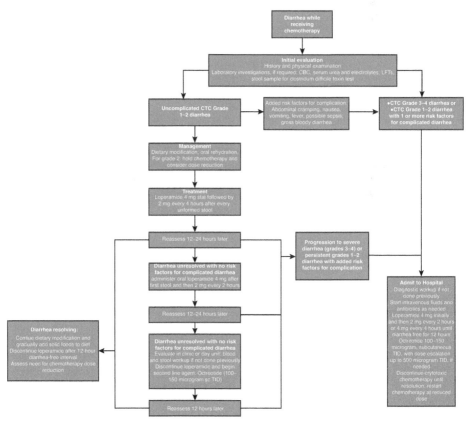

Fig. 6.2 Assessment and management of diarrhea complicating chemotherapy. *CBC,* Complete blood count; *CTC,* Common toxicity criteria; *LFT,* liver function tests; *sc,* subcutaneous; *TID,* three times a day.

Nonpharmacological measures for treatment of diarrhea include dietary measures such as avoiding dairy products, alcohol, caffeine, spicy food, high-fiber diet, and fat. Oral rehydration should be initiated promptly, based on severity of dehydration. Intravenous hydration and electrolyte replacement may be indicated in severe cases. Loperamide is an opioid agonist that is effective in reducing fecal incontinence, frequency of bowel movements, and stool weight.[79] For mild-to-moderate diarrhea, an initial dose of 4 mg loperamide should be given, followed by a further 2 mg every 4 hours or after every unformed stool. Severe cases of diarrhea may require a more aggressive regimen, with an initial dose of 4 mg loperamide followed by a further 2 mg every 2 hours or 4 mg every 4 hours continued around the clock until the patient is diarrhea-free for 12 hours.[80] A diphenoxylate/atropine combination is another option for treatment that can be used around the clock in addition to loperamide if the latter is ineffective, but it has not been well studied in cancer patients.

Octreotide is a synthetic, long-acting, somatostatin analog that acts via numerous mechanisms, including decreased secretion of vasoactive intestinal peptide (VIP), prolongation of intestinal transit time, and reduced secretion of fluid and electrolytes in the gut. Although a clinical trial in patients undergoing treatment with 5-FU demonstrated greater efficacy of octreotide over standard-dose loperamide (90% vs. 15% resolution of diarrhea by day 3),[81] octreotide is generally used as second-line therapy in patients who do not respond to opioids, mainly due to its high cost and need for repeated parenteral administration. The recommended starting dose of octreotide is 100 to 150 µg given subcutaneously three times a day, or 25 to 50 µg every hour if given by intravenous infusion.

Other agents that can be used as adjunctive therapy for the treatment of mild-to-moderate CID include tincture of opium, absorbents such as kaolin and charcoal, and codeine phosphate. Administration of causative chemotherapy agents should be withheld for grade 2 or worse diarrhea and should be restarted only after diarrhea resolves.

Hepatotoxicity

Chemotherapy-related hepatic complications are relatively common and are associated with significant morbidity. Patients undergoing oncologic therapy require comprehensive evaluation of their liver function before initiation and during therapy, and abnormal liver function test results must be investigated. Most hepatotoxicity secondary to oncology therapy is idiosyncratic and, therefore, neither dose dependent nor predictable.[82] However, chemotherapeutic drugs that are dependent upon liver metabolism for clearance require dose adjustment in the presence of considerable liver dysfunction. Hepatotoxicity from chemotherapy may have different clinical outcomes, ranging from an asymptomatic elevation of liver enzymes which may resolve without treatment, to cirrhosis, which may develop despite discontinuation of the chemotherapeutic agent. Patterns of hepatotoxicity associated with oncologic drug classes are listed in Table 6.5.

- **Viral hepatitis:** Patients with preexisting liver disease can be more susceptible to drug-induced hepatotoxicity. Chemotherapy can lead to reactivation of hepatitis B virus (HBV) and its associated disease due to immunosuppression, and screening for HBV should be done in patients at risk.[83,84] Risk factors associated with reactivation include HBV surface antigen seropositivity, detectable HBV DNA before chemotherapy, male gender, diagnosis of breast cancer or lymphoma, and concomitant use of glucocorticoids.[83,85,86] Prophylactic treatment with lamivudine appears to be beneficial in preventing HBV reactivation, or reducing the severity of HBV-related disease in patients undergoing cytotoxic chemotherapy.[87] Newer antiviral drugs, including entecavir, tenofovir, adefovir, and telbivudine, are also recommended based on the duration of treatment.[88] Hepatitis C virus (HCV) reactivation appears to be less common than HBV reactivation and is generally associated

TABLE 6.5 ■ **Chemotherapy Drugs Associated With Hepatotoxicity**

Drug Name	Hepatitis	Cholestasis	Veno-Occlusive Disease	Other Features	Dose Reduction
5-Fluorouracil	Rare	Common	Rare		Not required
6-Mercaptopurine	Rare	Rare	Rare		
Capecitabine	Rare	Common			Not required
Cyclophosphamide	Rare				Not required
Cytarabine	Rare, at high doses	Rare, at high doses		Biliary stricture formation	Reduce dose by 50%; increase if tolerated
Dacarbazine	Rare		Rare		
Doxorubicin	Rare	Rare	rare		Dose adjustment with elevated enzyme levels
Etoposide	Rare	Rare			Dose adjustment with elevated bilirubin levels
Floxuridine	Common	Significant, irreversible sclerosing cholangitis			Dose adjustment with elevated bilirubin levels
Gemcitabine	Rare	Rare			Not required
Irinotecan				Steatosis	Dose adjustment with elevated bilirubin levels
Methotrexate	Common, dose dependent			Rare cases of hepatic fibrosis and cirrhosis	Reduce dose by 25% if bilirubin levels > 3 mg/dL
Oxaliplatin	Rare		Common		Not required
Paclitaxel		Rare			Dose reduction with elevated bilirubin levels

with less complications and better outcomes. It has been documented that the presence of HCV infection increases the risk of having abnormal liver function test results; however, severe episodes of clinical hepatitis are extremely rare.[89]

■ **Hepatic veno-occlusive disease (HVOD):** HVOD or sinusoidal obstruction syndrome is a rare but life-threatening complication reported in patients treated with oxaliplatin for colorectal cancer.[90] It is characterized by nonthrombotic obliteration of small intrahepatic veins by collagenous and reticular intimal thickening.[91] The clinical spectrum of HVOD includes jaundice, tender hepatomegaly, fluid retention, unexplained weight gain, and abnormal liver function. Persistent thrombocytopenia, refractory to transfusion may be an early sign of HVOD.[92] Doppler ultrasonographic findings associated with HVOD include decreased or reversal of flow in the portal vein or increased mean hepatic artery resistive index.[93] CT scan of the abdomen may demonstrate ascites, periportal edema, and a narrowed right hepatic vein.[94] Although diagnosis can be made on clinical grounds, definitive diagnosis can be established by a random liver biopsy. There is no effective standard therapy for HVOD; hence, early detection is important. Mild cases of HVOD are associated with bilirubin levels below 3 mg/dL, and the disease is often self-limiting with expected spontaneous recovery. When suspected, the offending chemotherapy should be suspended. Supportive care mainly includes salt and fluid restriction, and the use of anticoagulants such as low-molecular-weight heparin. However, severe HVOD has a rapidly progressive course, with or without multiorgan failure, and is associated with significant morbidity and mortality.

■ **Steatosis and steatohepatitis:** Steatosis is the accumulation of lipids within the hepatocytes. In later stages of the disease, steatosis is accompanied by an inflammatory response that can lead to hepatic necrosis and fibrosis, called steatohepatitis. Irinotecan and 5-FU are usually associated with steatosis.[95,96] Steatosis is commonly associated with preoperative chemotherapy in patients undergoing hepatic surgery for colorectal metastases. Patients with elevated body mass index, type 2 diabetes mellitus, or metabolic syndrome have an increased risk for the development of steatosis.[96] Patients with baseline nonalcoholic fatty liver disease are at higher risk for chemotherapy-associated steatosis. Steatohepatitis is a distinct entity from steatosis and is observed less frequently than steatosis in patients receiving preoperative chemotherapy, in whom steatohepatitis has only been linked to irinotecan.[90] Steatohepatitis is a severe form of steatosis and is a risk factor for silent progression to liver fibrosis. In addition, severe steatohepatitis can affect the ability to perform large liver resections and increase the risk of hepatic failure after major hepatic surgery.[97] Thus caution is advised for the use of irinotecan in patients with potentially resectable liver metastases, particularly in obese patients. For patients who have neoadjuvant therapy with irinotecan, consideration should be given to obtain a percutaneous liver biopsy and evaluate the histology of the liver parenchyma before undertaking a resection. Liver-function tests are generally not helpful in diagnosis because many patients may have normal laboratory values despite substantial hepatic injury. Imaging modalities are also not useful in identifying patients with steatohepatitis preoperatively because they cannot adequately distinguish between simple steatosis and more advanced steatohepatitis. To prevent adverse outcomes from chemotherapy-associated steatosis and steatohepatitis, extended preoperative chemotherapy should be avoided. A longer interval between chemotherapy and hepatic resection can also potentially reduce hepatotoxicity and surgical complications; however, this interval should be balanced to abrogate the risk of tumor progression during the treatment-free interval.

Conclusion

Although chemotherapy plays a critical role in the management of various malignancies, many of them can cause adverse effects frequently involving the GI tract and can sometimes be life-threatening. The treatment approach of GI complications should be individualized, and consideration should be given to disease pathophysiology that may be contributing.

References

1. Ellenhorn JD, Lambroza A, Lindsley KL, LaQuaglia MP. Treatment-related esophageal stricture in pediatric patients with cancer. *Cancer.* 1993;71(12):4084–4090.
2. Baehr PH, McDonald GB. Esophageal infections: risk factors, presentation, diagnosis, and treatment. *Gastroenterology.* 1994;106(2):509–532.
3. Slee GR, Wagner SM, McCullough FS. Odynophagia in patients with malignant disorders. *Cancer.* 1985;55(12):2877–2879.
4. Kim HK. Acute esophageal stricture after induction chemotherapy for acute leukemia. *Am J Hematol.* 1996;52(4):335–336.
5. Dahms BB, Greco MA, Strandjord SE, Rothstein FC. Barrett's esophagus in three children after antileukemia chemotherapy. *Cancer.* 1987;60(12):2896–2900.
6. Sonis ST. Mucositis: the impact, biology and therapeutic opportunities of oral mucositis. *Oral Oncol.* 2009;45(12):1015–1020.

7. Phillips TL, Wharam MD, Margolis LW. Modification of radiation injury to normal tissues by chemo-therapeutic agents. *Cancer*. 1975;35(6):1678–1684.
8. Horwich A, Lokich J, Bloomer W. Doxorubicin, radiotherapy, and oesophageal stricture. *Lancet*. 1975;306(7934):561–562.
9. Boal D, Newburger PE, Teele RL. Esophagitis induced by combined radiation and adriamycin. *Am J Hematol*. 1979;132(4):567–570.
10. Lal DR, Foroutan HR, Su WT, et al. The management of treatment-related esophageal complications in children and adolescents with cancer. *J Pediatr Surg*. 2006;41(3):495–499.
11. Ismail A, Abdulla S. Post-monilial extensive esophageal stricture. *Ped Hematol Oncol*. 1993;10(1):111–113.
12. Tajiri T, Ikeue T, Sugita T, et al. Two cases of herpes simplex esophagitis during treatment for lung cancer. *Nihon Kokyuki Gakkai Zasshi*. 2007;45(7):546–550.
13. Perwitasari DA, Gelderblom H, Atthobari J, et al. Anti-emetic drugs in oncology: pharmacology and individualization by pharmacogenetics. *Int J Clin Pharm*. 2011;33(1):33–43.
14. Roila F, Donati D, Tamberi S, Margutti G. Delayed emesis: incidence, pattern, prognostic factors and optimal treatment. *Support Care Cancer*. 2002;10(2):88–95.
15. Navari RM. Treatment of breakthrough and refractory chemotherapy-induced nausea and vomiting. *Biomed Res Int*. 2015;2015:595894.
16. Pollera CF, Giannarelli D. Prognostic factors influencing cisplatin-induced emesis. Definition and vali-dation of a predictive logistic model. *Cancer*. 1989;64(5):1117–1122.
17. Hesketh P, Navari R, Grote T, et al. Double-blind, randomized comparison of the antiemetic efficacy of intravenous dolasetron mesylate and intravenous ondansetron in the prevention of acute cisplatin-induced emesis in patients with cancer. Dolasetron Comparative Chemotherapy-induced Emesis Pre-vention Group. *J Clin Oncol*. 1996;14(8):2242–2249.
18. Osoba D, Zee B, Pater J, Warr D, Latreille J, Kaizer L. Determinants of postchemotherapy nausea and vomiting in patients with cancer. Quality of Life and Symptom Control Committees of the National Cancer Institute of Canada Clinical Trials Group. *J Clin Oncol*. 1997;15(1):116–123.
19. Shankar A, Roy S, Malik A, Julka PK, Rath GK. Prevention of chemotherapy-induced nausea and vom-iting in cancer patients. *Asian Pac J Cancer Prev*. 2015;16(15):6207–6213.
20. Hesketh PJ. Defining the emetogenicity of cancer chemotherapy regimens: relevance to clinical practice. *Oncologist*. 1999;4(3):191–196.
21. Tonini G, Vincenzi B, Santini D. New drugs for chemotherapy-induced nausea and vomiting: focus on palonosetron. *Expert Opin Drug Metab Toxicol*. 2005;1(1):143–149.
22. Gralla R, Lichinitser M, Van Der Vegt S, et al. Palonosetron improves prevention of chemotherapy-induced nausea and vomiting following moderately emetogenic chemotherapy: results of a double-blind randomized phase III trial comparing single doses of palonosetron with ondansetron. *Ann Oncol*. 2003;14(10):1570–1577.
23. Eisenberg P, Figueroa-Vadillo J, Zamora R, et al. Improved prevention of moderately emetogenic che-motherapy-induced nausea and vomiting with palonosetron, a pharmacologically novel 5-HT3 receptor antagonist: results of a phase III, single-dose trial versus dolasetron. *Cancer*. 2003;98(11):2473–2482.
24. Kolesar JM, Eickhoff J, Vermeulen LC. Serotonin type 3–receptor antagonists for chemotherapy-induced nausea and vomiting: therapeutically equivalent or meaningfully different? *Am J Health Syst Pharm*. 2014;71(6):507–510.
25. Geling O, Eichler HG. Should 5-hydroxytryptamine-3 receptor antagonists be administered beyond 24 hours after chemotherapy to prevent delayed emesis? Systematic re-evaluation of clinical evidence and drug cost implications. *J Clin Oncol*. 2005;23(6):1289–1294.
26. Benedict CR, Arbogast R, Martin L, Patton L, Morrill B, Hahne W. Single-blind study of the effects of intravenous dolasetron mesylate versus ondansetron on electrocardiographic parameters in normal volunteers. *J Cardiovasc Pharmacol*. 1996;28(1):53–59.
27. Morganroth J, Parisi S, Moresino C, Thorn M, Cullen M. 1156 POSTER High dose palonosetron does not alter ECG parameters including QTc interval in healthy subjects: results of a dose-response, double blind, randomized, parallel E14 study of palonosetron vs. moxifloxacin or placebo. *EJC Supple-ments*. 2007;5(4):158–159.
28. dos Santos LV, Souza FH, Brunetto AT, Sasse AD, da Silveira Nogueira Lima JP. Neurokinin-1 recep-tor antagonists for chemotherapy-induced nausea and vomiting: a systematic review. *J Natl Cancer Inst*. 2012;104(17):1280–1292.

29. Aapro M, Karthaus M, Schwartzberg L, et al. NEPA, a fixed oral combination of netupitant and palonosetron, improves control of chemotherapy-induced nausea and vomiting (CINV) over multiple cycles of chemotherapy: results of a randomized, double-blind, phase 3 trial versus oral palonosetron. *Support Care Cancer*. 2017;25(4):1127–1135.

30. Rapoport BL, Chasen MR, Gridelli C, et al. Safety and efficacy of rolapitant for prevention of chemotherapy-induced nausea and vomiting after administration of cisplatin-based highly emetogenic chemotherapy in patients with cancer: two randomised, active-controlled, double-blind, phase 3 trials. *Lancet Oncol*. 2015;16(9):1079–1089.

31. Schwartzberg LS, Modiano MR, Rapoport BL, et al. Safety and efficacy of rolapitant for prevention of chemotherapy-induced nausea and vomiting after administration of moderately emetogenic chemotherapy or anthracycline and cyclophosphamide regimens in patients with cancer: a randomised, active-controlled, double-blind, phase 3 trial. *Lancet Oncol*. 2015;16(9):1071–1078.

32. McCrea JB, Majumdar AK, Goldberg MR, et al. Effects of the neurokinin1 receptor antagonist aprepitant on the pharmacokinetics of dexamethasone and methylprednisolone. *Clin Pharmacol Ther*. 2003;74(1):17–24.

33. Ho CM, Ho ST, Wang JJ, Tsai SK, Chai CY. Dexamethasone has a central antiemetic mechanism in decerebrated cats. *Anesth Analg*. 2004;99(3):734–739.

34. Ioannidis JP, Hesketh PJ, Lau J. Contribution of dexamethasone to control of chemotherapy-induced nausea and vomiting: a meta-analysis of randomized evidence. *J Clin Oncol*. 2000;18(19):3409–3422.

35. Navari RM, Gray SE, Kerr AC. Olanzapine versus aprepitant for the prevention of chemotherapy-induced nausea and vomiting: a randomized phase III trial. *J Support Oncol*. 2011;9(5):188–195.

36. Navari RM. Olanzapine for the prevention of chemotherapy-induced nausea and vomiting. In: *Management of Chemotherapy-Induced Nausea and Vomiting*. Springer; 2016:107–120.

37. Navari RM, Nagy CK, Gray SE. The use of olanzapine versus metoclopramide for the treatment of breakthrough chemotherapy-induced nausea and vomiting in patients receiving highly emetogenic chemotherapy. *Support Care Cancer*. 2013;21(6):1655–1663.

38. National Comprehensive Cancer Network. Antiemetics; 2018. cited 2018. Available from https://www.nccn.org/professionals/physician_gls/pdf/antiemesis.pdf.

39. Basch E, Hesketh PJ, Kris MG, et al. Antiemetics: American Society of Clinical Oncology clinical practice guideline update. *J Oncol Pract*. 2011;7(6):395–398.

40. Ryan JL, Heckler CE, Roscoe JA, et al. Ginger (*Zingiber officinale*) reduces acute chemotherapy-induced nausea: a URCC CCOP study of 576 patients. *Support Care Cancer*. 2012;20(7):1479–1489.

41. Lee J, Oh H. Ginger as an antiemetic modality for chemotherapy-induced nausea and vomiting: a systematic review and meta-analysis. *Oncol Nurs Forum*. 2013;40(2):163–170.

42. Rithirangsriroj K, Manchana T, Akkayagorn L. Efficacy of acupuncture in prevention of delayed chemotherapy induced nausea and vomiting in gynecologic cancer patients. *Gynecol Oncol*. 2015;136(1):82–86.

43. DuHamel Katherine N, Redd WH, Vickberg SM. Behavioral interventions in the diagnosis, treatment and rehabilitation of children with cancer. *Acta Oncol*. 1999;38(6):719–734.

44. Marchioro G, Azzarello G, Viviani F, et al. Hypnosis in the treatment of anticipatory nausea and vomiting in patients receiving cancer chemotherapy. *Oncology*. 2000;59(2):100–104.

45. Husain A, Aptaker L, Spriggs DR, et al. Gastrointestinal toxicity and *Clostridium difficile* diarrhea in patients treated with paclitaxel-containing chemotherapy regimens. *Gynecol Oncol*. 1998;71(1):104–107.

46. Emoto A, Aptaker L, Spriggs DR, Barakat RR. *Clostridium difficile* colitis associated with cisplatin-based chemotherapy in ovarian cancer patients. *Gynecol Oncol*. 1996;61(3):369–372.

47. Chopra T, Alangaden GJ, Chandrasekar P. *Clostridium difficile* infection in cancer patients and hematopoietic stem cell transplant recipients. *Expert Rev Anti Infect Ther*. 2010;8(10):1113–1119.

48. Cooke JV. Acute leukemia in children. *J Am Med Assoc*. 1933;101(6):432–435.

49. Sloas MM, Flynn PM, Kaste SC, Patrick CC. Typhlitis in children with cancer: a 30-year experience. *Clin Infect Dis*. 1993;17(3):484–490.

50. Davila ML. Neutropenic enterocolitis. *Curr Opin Gastroenterol*. 2006;22(1):44–47.

51. Gomez L, Martino R, Rolston K. Neutropenic enterocolitis: spectrum of the disease and comparison of definite and possible cases. *Clin Infect Dis*. 1998;27(4):695–699.

52. Bremer CT, Monahan BP. Necrotizing enterocolitis in neutropenia and chemotherapy: a clinical update and old lessons relearned. *Curr Gastroenterol Rep*. 2006;8(4):333–341.

53. Kronawitter U, Kemeny NE, Blumgart L. Neutropenic enterocolitis in a patient with colorectal carcinoma: unusual course after treatment with 5-fluorouracil and leucovorin—a case report. *Interdiscipl Int J Am Cancer Soc.* 1997;80(4):656–660.
54. Wade DS, Nava HR, Douglass HO Jr. Neutropenic enterocolitis. Clinical diagnosis and treatment. *Cancer.* 1992;69(1):17–23.
55. Kouroussis C, Samonis G, Androulakis N, et al. Successful conservative treatment of neutropenic enterocolitis complicating taxane-based chemotherapy: a report of five cases. *Am J Clin Oncol.* 2000;23(3):309–313.
56. Ibrahim NK, Sahin AA, Dubrow RA, et al. Colitis associated with docetaxel-based chemotherapy in patients with metastatic breast cancer. *Lancet.* 2000;355(9200):281–283.
57. Kreis W, Petrylak D, Savarese D, Budman D. Colitis and docetaxel-based chemotherapy. *Lancet.* 2000;355(9221):2164.
58. Daniele B, Rossi GB, Losito S, Gridelli C, de Bellis M. Ischemic colitis associated with paclitaxel. *J Clin Gastroenterol.* 2001;33(2):159–160.
59. Tashiro M, Yoshikawa I, Kume K, Otsuki M. Ischemic colitis associated with paclitaxel and carboplatin chemotherapy. *Am J Gastroenterol.* 2003;98(1):231.
60. Elsayed AG, Srivastava R, Pacioles T, Limjoco T, Tirona MT. Ischemic colitis associated with paclitaxel and carboplatin combination. *Case Rep Oncol.* 2017;10(2):689–693.
61. Droney J, Ross J, Gretton S, Welsh K, Sato H, Riley J. Constipation in cancer patients on morphine. *Support Care Cancer.* 2008;16(5):453–459.
62. Anderson H, Scarffe JH, Lambert M, et al. VAD chemotherapy—toxicity and efficacy—in patients with multiple myeloma and other lymphoid malignancies. *Hematol Oncol.* 1987;5(3):213–222.
63. Singhal S, Mehta J, Desikan R, et al. Antitumor activity of thalidomide in refractory multiple myeloma. *N Engl J Med.* 1999;341(21):1565–1571.
64. Legha SS. Vincristine neurotoxicity. Pathophysiology and management. *Med Toxicol.* 1986;1(6):421–427.
65. Dimopoulos MA, Eleutherakis-Papaiakovou V. Adverse effects of thalidomide administration in patients with neoplastic diseases. *Am J Med.* 2004;117(7):508–515.
66. Leung Riutta T, Kotecha J, Rosser W. Chronic constipation: an evidence-based review. *J Am Board Fam Med.* 2011;24(4):436–451.
67. Brandt LJ, Prather CM, Quigley EM, et al. Systematic review on the management of chronic constipation in North America. *Am J Gastroenterol.* 2005;100(s1):S5.
68. Stein A, Voigt W, Jordan K. Chemotherapy-induced diarrhea: pathophysiology, frequency and guideline-based management. *Ther Adv Med Oncol.* 2010;2(1):51–63.
69. Boussios S, Pentheroudakis G, Katsanos K, Pavlidis N. Systemic treatment-induced gastrointestinal toxicity: incidence, clinical presentation and management. *Ann Gastroenterol.* 2012;25(2):106.
70. Kabbinavar F, Hurwitz HI, Fehrenbacher L, et al. Phase II, randomized trial comparing bevacizumab plus fluorouracil (FU)/leucovorin (LV) with FU/LV alone in patients with metastatic colorectal cancer. *J Clin Oncol.* 2003;21(1):60–65.
71. Gibson RJ, Stringer AM. Chemotherapy-induced diarrhoea. *Curr Opin Support Palliat Care.* 2009;3(1):31–35.
72. Grem JL, Shoemaker DD, Petrelli NJ, Douglass HO Jr. Severe life-threatening toxicities observed in study using leucovorin with 5-fluorouracil. *J Clin Oncol.* 1987;5(10):1704-1704.
73. Leichman CG, Fleming TR, Muggia FM, et al. Phase II study of fluorouracil and its modulation in advanced colorectal cancer: a Southwest Oncology Group study. *J Clin Oncol.* 1995;13(6):1303–1311.
74. Sloan JA, Goldberg RM, Sargent DJ, et al. Women experience greater toxicity with fluorouracil-based chemotherapy for colorectal cancer. *J Clin Oncol.* 2002;20(6):1491–1498.
75. Cascinu S, Barni S, Labianca R, et al. Evaluation of factors influencing 5-fluorouracil-induced diarrhea in colorectal cancer patients. *Support Care Cancer.* 1997;5(4):314–317.
76. Twelves C, Wong A, Nowacki MP, et al. Capecitabine as adjuvant treatment for stage III colon cancer. *N Engl J Med.* 2005;352(26):2696–2704.
77. Saltz LB, Cox JV, Blanke C, et al. Irinotecan plus fluorouracil and leucovorin for metastatic colorectal cancer. *N Engl J Med.* 2000;343(13):905–914.
78. Sargent DJ, Niedzwiecki D, O'Connell MJ, Schilsky RL. Recommendation for caution with irinotecan, fluorouracil, and leucovorin for colorectal cancer. *N Engl J Med.* 2001;345(2):144–145, author reply 146.
79. Abigerges D, Armand JP, Chabot GG, et al. Irinotecan (CPT-11) high-dose escalation using intensive high-dose loperamide to control diarrhea. *J Natl Cancer Inst.* 1994;86(6):446–449.

80. Benson AB III, Ajani JA, Catalano RB, et al. Recommended guidelines for the treatment of cancer treatment-induced diarrhea. *J Clin Oncol.* 2004;22(14):2918–2926.
81. Cascinu S, Fedeli A, Fedeli SL, Catalano G. Octreotide versus loperamide in the treatment of fluorouracil-induced diarrhea: a randomized trial. *J Clin Oncol.* 1993;11(1):148–151.
82. Lee WM. Drug-induced hepatotoxicity. *N Engl J Med.* 1995;333(17):1118–1127.
83. Lok AS, Liang RH, Chiu EK, et al. Reactivation of hepatitis B virus replication in patients receiving cytotoxic therapy: report of a prospective study. *Gastroenterology.* 1991;100(1):182–188.
84. Liang R, Lau GK, Kwong Y. Chemotherapy and bone marrow transplantation for cancer patients who are also chronic hepatitis B carriers: a review of the problem. *J Clin Oncol.* 1999;17(1) 394–394.
85. Yeo W, Chan PK, Zhong S, et al. Frequency of hepatitis B virus reactivation in cancer patients undergoing cytotoxic chemotherapy: a prospective study of 626 patients with identification of risk factors. *J Med Virol.* 2000;62(3):299–307.
86. Yeo W, Zee B, Zhong S, et al. Comprehensive analysis of risk factors associating with Hepatitis B virus (HBV) reactivation in cancer patients undergoing cytotoxic chemotherapy. *Br J Cancer.* 2004;90(7):1306.
87. Yeo W, Chan PK, Ho WM, et al. Lamivudine for the prevention of hepatitis B virus reactivation in hepatitis B s-antigen seropositive cancer patients undergoing cytotoxic chemotherapy. *J Clin Oncol.* 2004;22(5):927–934.
88. Bozza C, Cinausero M, Iacono D, Puglisi F. Hepatitis B and cancer: a practical guide for the oncologist. *Crit Rev Oncol Hematol.* 2016;98:137–146.
89. Kawatani T, Suou T, Tajima F, et al. Incidence of hepatitis virus infection and severe liver dysfunction in patients receiving chemotherapy for hematologic malignancies. *Eur J Haematol.* 2001;67(1):45–50.
90. Vauthey JN, Pawlik TM, Ribero D, et al. Chemotherapy regimen predicts steatohepatitis and an increase in 90-day mortality after surgery for hepatic colorectal metastases. *J Clin Oncol.* 2006;24(13):2065–2072.
91. Rollins BJ. Hepatic veno-occlusive disease. *Am J Med.* 1986;81(2):297–306.
92. Rio B, Andreu G, Nicod A, et al. Thrombocytopenia in venocclusive disease after bone marrow transplantation or chemotherapy. *Blood.* 1986;67(6):1773–1776.
93. Bearman SI. The syndrome of hepatic veno-occlusive disease after marrow transplantation. *Blood.* 1995;85(11):3005–3020.
94. Mahgerefteh SY, Sosna J, Bogot N, Shapira MY, Pappo O, Bloom AI. Radiologic imaging and intervention for gastrointestinal and hepatic complications of hematopoietic stem cell transplantation. *Radiology.* 2011;258(3):660–671.
95. Pawlik TM, Olino K, Gleisner AL, et al. Preoperative chemotherapy for colorectal liver metastases: impact on hepatic histology and postoperative outcome. *J Gastrointest Surg.* 2007;11(7):860–868.
96. Robinson SM, Wilson CH, Burt AD, Manas DM, White SA. Chemotherapy-associated liver injury in patients with colorectal liver metastases: a systematic review and meta-analysis. *Ann Surg Oncol.* 2012;19(13):4287–4299.
97. Behrns KE, Tsiotos GG, DeSouza NF, Krishna MK, Ludwig J, Nagorney DM. Hepatic steatosis as a potential risk factor for major hepatic resection. *J Gastrointest Surg.* 1998;2(3):292–298.

CHAPTER 7

Neurological Complications of Chemotherapy

Alison Carulli, PharmD, BCOP ■ Melissa King, MSN, APRN, FNP-C
■ Bassam Estfan, MD

Introduction

Chemotherapy-related neurotoxicity is a frequently observed side effect that has become more prevalent with the increasing number of long-term cancer survivors. These toxicities can be peripheral or central and can range from minor cognitive issues to encephalopathy or dementia. Toxicities are often dose-limiting, resulting in dose reduction or treatment discontinuation, potentially compromising the therapeutic efficacy. This chapter will discuss the incidence, mechanism, symptoms, and management of chemotherapy-related neurotoxicity with a focus on the more common chemotherapeutic agents. The Common Terminology Criteria for Adverse Events (CTCAE) is widely used in the evaluation of chemotherapy-induced peripheral neuropathy. (Table 7.1[1]) Fig. 7.1 illustrates an algorithm for the evaluation and treatment of chemotherapy-related peripheral neuropathy.[2–5]

Chemotherapy-Related Neurotoxicity

- **Taxane chemotherapy:** Taxane-induced peripheral neuropathy is a class effect of toxicity, but is more commonly reported with paclitaxel (57%–83%) compared to docetaxel (11%–64%).[6–10] Although the exact mechanism is not well understood, the most widely accepted hypothesis of taxane-induced neuropathy is the disruption of the axonal microtubule structure. Taxanes inhibit tubulin depolymerization and disrupt the formation of microtubules, including the axon of neurons. Intact microtubules are essential for axonal transport and neuronal survival, and alteration of their structure can lead to peripheral neuropathy.
  - **Presentation:** Taxane-induced neuropathy generally presents with sensory loss in the hands and/or feet in a *glove-and-stocking* type of distribution. Symptoms include numbness, paresthesias, dysesthesias, unsteadiness, and loss of balance, which can impede quality of life and functional status. Motor impairment is unusual, but muscle aches and loss of strength have occurred.[6,9]

TABLE 7.1 ■ **Common Terminology Criteria for Adverse Events (CTCAE) Chemotherapy-Induced Peripheral Neuropathy**[1]

Grade	Definition
1	Asymptomatic; clinical or diagnostic observations only
2	Moderate symptoms; limiting instrumental ADL
3	Severe symptoms; limiting self-care ADL
4	Life-threatening consequences; urgent intervention indicated

ADL, Activities of daily living.

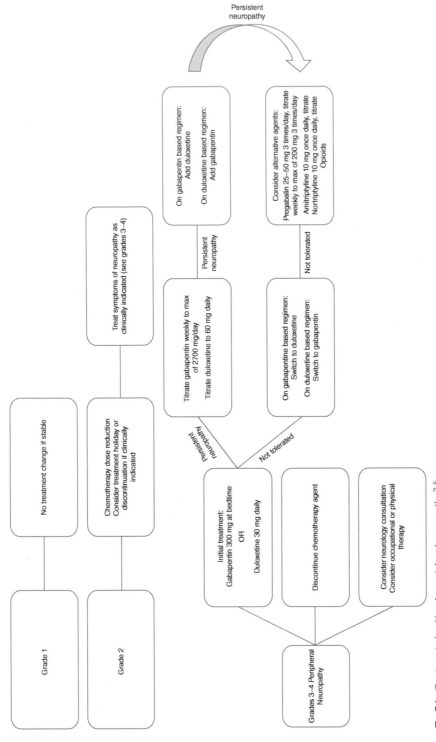

Fig. 7.1　Treatment algorithm for peripheral neuropathy.[2–5]

TABLE 7.2 ■ **Agent, Dose, and Duration of Therapies for Chemotherapy-Related Peripheral Neuropathy**

Drug	Dose	Notes
Duloxetine[a]	Initial: 30 mg once daily Escalation: 30 mg/week to target 60 mg	• Serotonin syndrome monitoring required with concomitant medications • Risk of withdrawal syndrome when discontinued abruptly • Similar dosing to treat mood disorders
Gabapentin	Initial: 300 mg once daily Escalation: 300 mg/week to target dose of 2700 mg/day in divided doses	• Initial dosing at bedtime to decrease sedation • Adjust in renal insufficiency
Lamotrigine	Initial: 25 mg once daily Escalation: 25 mg twice daily, 50 mg twice daily, 100 mg twice daily, 150 mg twice daily every 2 weeks	• Slow titration to decrease risk of Steven Johnson Syndrome (SJS)
Nortriptyline	Initial: 10–25 mg once daily Escalation: Weekly to target of 50–100 mg once daily	• Serotonin syndrome monitoring required with concomitant medications • Initial dosing at bedtime to decrease sedation • Higher doses than used in peripheral neuropathy normally required for treatment mood disorders
Amitriptyline	Starting: 10 mg once daily Escalation: 10 mg/week to target 50 mg	• Serotonin syndrome monitoring required with concomitant medications • Initial dosing at bedtime to decrease sedation • Higher doses than used in peripheral neuropathy normally required for treatment mood disorders

[a]Several agents have been studied in randomized trials but only duloxetine had positive outcomes when used as a preventive measure.[2–4]

■ **Relationship to dose:** Taxane-induced peripheral neuropathy can occur with high cumulative doses, with onset of symptoms typically occurring with doses greater than 300 mg/m² of paclitaxel. Severe symptoms of peripheral neuropathy are generally not seen until doses exceed 400 mg/m² of docetaxel. High single doses of paclitaxel are also associated with an increased risk—up to 75% of patients who receive 175 mg/m² once weekly develop severe peripheral neuropathy. Studies have had conflicting observations regarding the optimal dosing interval of paclitaxel to minimize neurotoxicity. The infusion rate has also been shown to be a risk factor for paclitaxel-induced neuropathy, with shorter infusions (1 or 3 hours) associated with higher rates of peripheral neuropathy when compared with 24-hour infusions.[6,10]

■ **Treatment:** There are no known prophylactic agents and treatment options are limited. Table 7.1 describes treatment options for neuropathy. Most patients experience at least a partial resolution of symptoms within 3 to 6 months of drug discontinuation. Many patients, however, do not experience complete symptom resolution. Up to 40% of patients can have symptoms years after treatment completion.[3] Several agents have been evaluated for the treatment of peripheral neuropathy (Table 7.2).

- **Platinum based chemotherapy**
- **Cisplatin:** Cisplatin can cause peripheral neuropathy, with symptoms such as numbness, paresthesias, and dysesthesias, especially with cumulative doses.
  - **Mechanism:** The development of platinum-induced peripheral neuropathy is attributed to damage of the dorsal root ganglion (DRG) caused by the formation of intrastrand adducts and interstrand crosslinks.
  - **Relationship to dose:** Symptoms are reported at doses greater than 300 mg/m^2 of cisplatin, and 90% of patients have evidence of neuropathy at cumulative doses of greater than 600 mg/m^2. Although peripheral neuropathy caused by other chemotherapeutic agents normally improves with treatment completion, 30% of patients with platinum-induced neuropathy can experience a *coasting effect* where neuropathy worsens several months after drug discontinuation, before any improvement is noted. Symptom improvement is seen in the majority of patients but in several long-term survival studies, 10% to 30% of patients reported mild symptoms of neuropathy up to 15 years after treatment.[7,8,10]
  - **Encephalopathy:** Cisplatin has limited blood–brain barrier penetration and reports of encephalopathy are rare with intravenous administration. Neurotoxicity, however, has occurred after intraarterial cisplatin administration, with headaches, encephalopathy, seizures, and cortical blindness all having been reported.
  - **Ototoxicity:** Cisplatin-induced ototoxicity with high-frequency hearing loss has been described in patients receiving cisplatin. This toxicity is commonly attributed to sensory hair cell death in the cochlea, and develops with increasing cumulative doses. The incidence varies, with reports ranging from 17% to 80% in clinical trials. The primary risk factor is cumulative dosing of cisplatin. Other risk factors include younger age, concurrent radiation to the cochlea or cranial nerves, and renal dysfunction. There are no known effective treatment or prophylactic options for cisplatin-induced ototoxicity in adults.[11] Prophylaxis with vitamin E and amifostine have failed to show benefit in randomized controlled trials and are not recommended.[12] Sodium thiosulfate has been studied as an otoprotective agent that acts by inactivating cisplatin and preventing sensory hair cell death in the cochlea. Historically, it has not been recommended as a standard of care due to concern that the inactivation of cisplatin may negate the efficacy of the chemotherapy treatment. A trial in 109 children younger than 18 years suggested that there is no difference in treatment efficacy if sodium thiosulfate administration is delayed by several hours. In this trial, 57 children received cisplatin 80 mg/m^2 plus sodium thiosulfate, and 52 children received cisplatin alone. Sodium thiosulfate 20 g/m^2 was given 6 hours after cisplatin administration. Grade 1 hearing loss or greater was reported in 33% of patients in the sodium thiosulfate group versus 65% in the cisplatin alone group ($P = .002$). Three-year event free survival and overall survival were similar in both groups. Further studies in the adult population are needed to determine sodium thiosulfate's place in the prevention of ototoxicity.[12,13]
- **Carboplatin:** Carboplatin is a second-generation platinum agent that is less neurotoxic than cisplatin. Peripheral neuropathy and ototoxicity have been reported, but generally only with high doses.[7,8]
- **Oxaliplatin:** Oxaliplatin produces two types of neurotoxicity, an acute cold-triggered neurotoxicity that is usually transient and a chronic dose-limiting peripheral neuropathy.[14]
  - **Acute cold-triggered neuropathy** occurs in 90% of people receiving oxaliplatin and is characterized by distal paresthesias, jaw pain, hand and foot muscle contractions, and dysesthesias. It is exacerbated by cold temperatures and normally reverses within 1 week, although unresolved symptoms between treatments can occur with increasing numbers of cycles. Although the mechanism of oxaliplatin-induced acute neurotoxicity is not fully understood, the leading hypothesis is that oxalate, an oxaliplatin metabolite, chelates calcium causing changes to voltage-dependent sodium channels and hyperexcitability of peripheral nerves.[15]

■ **Chronic dose-limiting peripheral neuropathy** is attributed to damage of the DRG caused by the formation of intrastrand adducts and interstrand crosslinks, which is similar to cisplatin, except that cisplatin produces three times more adducts in the DRG and is associated with more neurotoxicity then oxaliplatin. Peripheral neuropathy is seen in 45% of patients with cumulative doses of oxaliplatin. Like other platinum agents, patients can experience a coasting effect where neuropathy temporarily worsens several months after drug discontinuation. However, several long-term studies have reported that neuropathy is reversible in the majority of patients, with only 13% reporting mild symptoms 4 years after treatment with oxaliplatin.[8,16]

■ **Preventative options** are limited for oxaliplatin-induced neuropathy. Lengthening the infusion duration from 2 to 6 hours has failed to decrease the incidence of neurotoxicity.[14] Prophylaxis with vitamin E, acetyl-L-carnitine, glutamine, α-lipoic acid, magnesium, calcium, and sodium thiosulfate have not shown benefit in randomized controlled trials and are thus not recommended.[12,17] The only proven option to reduce the incidence of neuropathy comes from the OPTIMOX-1 and CONcePT trials. These trials reported that alternating non–oxaliplatin-containing regimens in patients receiving palliative chemotherapy for metastatic colorectal cancer may decrease the risk of severe neuropathy while not compromising efficacy. In certain clinical situations, it may be appropriate to substitute or hold oxaliplatin until the progression of disease in patients responding to oxaliplatin-based therapy to prevent the development of neurotoxicity.[18,19]

■ **Vinca alkaloids:** Vinca alkaloids are associated with a variety of neurological toxicities, including peripheral neuropathy and autonomic neuropathies. Of the vinca alkaloids, vincristine is the most neurotoxic compared to vinblastine and vinorelbine. Vincristine also has a dose-limiting toxicity of axonal neuropathy. Vincristine binds to tubulin to prevent the formation of microtubules, altering their structure and interfering with axonal transport. This damage results in paresthesias in the fingers and toes, gait disturbances, loss of ankle reflexes, distal weakness, and foot drop in 57% of patients treated.[5]

  ■ **Risk factors:** Several risk factors increase the incidence and severity of neuropathy. High single doses or cumulative doses between 30 and 50 mg are correlated with increasing neuropathy. Due to this, most treatment regimens cap a single dose of vincristine at 2 mg. Those with underlying neuropathy disorders are at higher risk and vincristine is contraindicated in patients with Charcot-Marie-Tooth disease. Other risk factors include hepatic impairment, older age, concomitant radiation, and administration with CYP3A4 inhibitor medications.[5,8]

  ■ **Prophylaxis:** There are no known prophylactic options for vincristine-induced neuropathy. Studies are inconclusive on whether neurotoxicity decreases when vincristine is administered as a continuous infusion instead of a bolus and this is not routinely recommended. An adrenocorticotropic hormone (ACTH) analog called Org 2766 was found to prevent cisplatin- and vincristine-based neuropathy in several small trials but failed to show benefit in larger trials. Small trials suggested a decrease in the incidence of neuropathy using glutamic acid, but larger trials are still investigating the long-term outcomes.[12]

  ■ **Outcomes:** Although some patients experience temporary worsening of their neuropathy several months after treatment discontinuation, most long-term studies report resolution of symptoms several months to years later. See Table 7.2 for preventive strategies for peripheral neuropathy.[20]

  ■ **Autonomic neuropathies,** such as constipation or abdominal pain, occur in up to 40% of patients, requiring the initiation of appropriate bowel regimens in all patients receiving vinca alkaloids. Rarely, this can lead to paralytic ileus or megacolon.[8]

- **Focal mononeuropathies** that involve cranial nerves may occur with vincristine, and rare reports of facial atrophy, ptosis, hearing loss, and retinal damage have occurred.[8]
- **CNS toxicity** is uncommon with vincristine unless an overdose has occurred. Rarely inappropriate secretion of antidiuretic hormone (SIADH) may develop, resulting in hyponatremia, confusion, and seizures.[8]
- **Antimetabolites**
- **Methotrexate:** The development of acute, subacute, and delayed neurotoxicity with methotrexate (MTX) is dependent on the dose and route of administration.
  - **Mechanism:** The mechanism of action is uncertain but is likely caused by inhibition of folate and methionine metabolism, resulting in disruption of folate homeostasis in the central nervous system (CNS).[7,8]
  - **Aseptic meningitis** has been described in 10% of patients who receive intrathecal MTX. Literature reports up to 50% of patients have been affected, but this rate has decreased significantly due to the introduction of microfiltration of MTX. Symptoms, such as headaches, stiff neck, fevers, nausea/vomiting, and back pain occur 2 to 4 hours after intrathecal MTX administration and resolve within 72 hours. These symptoms are normally self-limiting and do not require treatment. If additional doses are required, administering intrathecal MTX with intrathecal hydrocortisone has been reported to be protective against some symptoms of aseptic meningitis.[7,8]
  - **Transverse myelopathy** has been rarely reported after intrathecal MTX administrations. Symptoms begin with back or leg pain and can rapidly progress to paraplegia and sensory loss. The onset is between 1 and 48 hours, although there are reports several weeks after administration. Although there is commonly improvement in symptoms, recovery rates vary, and most patients do not return to baseline. There is no standard of care treatment, but a case report on using S-adenosylmethionine (SAM) 200 mg three times daily, folinate 20 mg four times daily, cyanocobalamin 100 μg once daily, and methionine 5 g daily recorded complete resolution of symptoms in Europe. However, further studies are needed before this treatment can be routinely recommended.[21]
  - **Subacute neurotoxicity** can manifest as encephalopathy, seizures, aphasia, or stroke-like symptoms. The median onset is 2 to 10 days after systemic high-dose MTX administration. Symptoms normally resolve within 72 hours and do not require treatment.
  - **Leukoencephalopathy** can occur months to years after therapy and is often considered the most significant delayed toxicity of MTX, with trials reporting an incidence as high as 20%. Leukoencephalopathy most commonly manifests as progressive cognitive dysfunction that can result in dementia, somnolence, and seizures. Symptoms can stabilize or improve after MTX discontinuation, but the clinical course is variable. The mechanism is unknown, but it often occurs after repeated doses of IV high-dose MTX with or without recent cranial radiation. With the exception of avoiding concurrent cranial radiation and high-dose MTX when possible, there are no treatment or prophylaxis strategies available to prevent leukoencephalopathy.[22]
  - **Monitoring of methotrexate:** MTX is almost exclusively excreted in the urine and can precipitate in acidic urine (pH < 7), thus maintaining alkaline urine is important to prevent toxicity. Furthermore, the risk of these toxicities is influenced by clearance of the drug. For this reason, MTX levels should be monitored at least daily until plasma levels drop below 0.1 μM. It is generally expected to reach these levels 72 hours after high-dose MTX administration. Leucovorin, a form of folic acid, can be used for *leucovorin rescue* after high dose MTX administration.
- **Fluorouracil:** Fluorouracil crosses the blood–brain barrier and there are rare reports of cerebellar ataxia, extrapyramidal syndromes, nystagmus, and dysarthria weeks to months after treatment. Neurotoxicity can occur much more commonly in patients who are

dihydropyrimidine dehydrogenase (DPD) deficient and are unable to metabolize fluoro-uracil or capecitabine. Despite this, routine testing for DPD deficiency prior to treatment is not recommended.[8]

■ **Fludarabine:** Neurotoxicity caused by fludarabine at conventional doses is uncommon, with most large trials reporting an incidence of less than 1%. In these rare cases, symptoms are normally mild, consisting of headaches, somnolence, and confusion, and resolve after treatment cessation. At doses greater than 90 mg/m^2/day, more severe encephalopathy, cortical blindness, seizures, and ataxia can occur in up to 36% of patients. There are no known treatment or preventive measures.[7,23–25]

■ **Cytarabine:** High doses of cytarabine greater than 1 g/m^2/day have been reported to cause acute cerebellar syndrome, with a reported incidence up to 25% in patients who receive in excess of 3 g/m^2/day. Symptoms occur within 2 to 5 days of treatment and can range from somnolence and ataxia to dysarthria and nystagmus. In rare cases, seizures have been reported. Patients are at higher risk if they have received cumulative doses greater than 36 g, have renal dysfunction, hepatic dysfunction, elevated alkaline phosphatase levels, or are older. There are no known treatment or preventive measures, but most patients have complete recovery within 2 weeks when cytarabine is discontinued immediately on symptom onset.[7,26,27] Similar to intrathecal MTX, intrathecal cytarabine can rarely cause aseptic meningitis and myelopathy.

■ **Nelarabine:** Central and peripheral neurotoxicity have been reported as dose-limiting side effects in phase I and II trials, with 65% of patients experiencing some form of neurotoxicity. The most common manifestations included fatigue, somnolence, and confusion that occur within the first few weeks of treatment initiation. More severe toxicities, such as seizures and hallucinations, have been reported infrequently. With the exception of peripheral neuropathy, there does not appear to be a correlation between dose and toxicity severity.[7,28,29] Although peripheral neuropathy has been reported after the first course of treatment in some patients, it usually developed after cumulative cycles of therapy. There are no known prophylactic agents for nelarabine-induced neurotoxicity, and treatment options are limited to symptom management; 90% of patients experienced resolution of their symptoms with drug discontinuation. See Table 7.2 for options for peripheral neuropathy.

■ **Ifosfamide:** Ifosfamide-induced encephalopathy has been reported in 10% to 30% of patients receiving ifosfamide within 12 to 146 hours of administration, and normally resolves within 48 to 72 hours of onset.
  ▪ **Symptoms:** The most common manifestations include confusion, decreased level of arousal, stupor, and somnolence. Rarely, extrapyramidal symptoms, seizures, hallucinations, personality changes, and comas have been reported.
  ▪ **Mechanism:** There are several proposed mechanisms of ifosfamide-induced neurotoxicity. Ifosfamide is a prodrug that is activated by CYP3A4 into 2- and 3-dichloroethylifos-famide and chloroacetylaldehyde. Chloroacetylaldehyde causes the depletion of glutathi-one which has been linked to ifosfamide neurotoxicity. Alternatively, subsequent studies linked chloroacetylaldehyde's effect on inhibition of long-chain fatty acid metabolism to ifosfamide encephalopathy.[30]
  ▪ **Risk factors:** Higher incidences of encephalopathy have been reported with bolus or short infusion administrations, renal impairment, low serum albumin levels, concomitant aprepitant, hepatic impairment, prior ifosfamide-induced encephalopathy, prior cisplatin administration, and poor performance status.
  ▪ **Prophylaxis:** There are limited data on the use of methylene blue as prophylaxis for encephalopathy and use based on institutional preference. Methylene blue is believed to act as an alternative electron acceptor that inhibits the transformation of chloroethyl-amine into chloroacetylaldehyde and stimulates long-chain fatty acid oxidation. Several

case reports and small trials have looked at its use for prophylaxis. Based on that data, methylene blue, 50 mg every 6 hours, can be considered for the duration of the ifosfamide infusion if patients have risk factors such as previous ifosfamide neurotoxicity, renal dysfunction, or low serum albumin levels.[7,30]

- **Ifosfamide-induced encephalopathy** is self-limiting and resolves within 72 hours after drug discontinuation. There are case reports using methylene blue, thiamine 100 mg every 4 hours, or dexmedetomidine for treatment.[10]

Chemotherapy-Induced Neurocognitive Deficit (Chemo-Brain)

Improvements in cancer treatment have resulted in an increasing number of cancer survivors worldwide with an emphasis on late effects, including treatment-related cognitive impairment, colloquially known as *chemo-brain*.

- **Presentation:** Symptoms include difficulties with word finding, memory, concentration, processing speed, and multitasking.[31,32] This can occur during treatment or shortly after treatment discontinuation, with variable recoveries. Some report cognitive recovery within 6 months to 2 years, whereas others report lifelong difficulties. The incidence differs among malignancies, with reports between 15% and 60% in trials. There are no definitive risk factors identified in clinical trials but most report baseline fatigue, depression, and decreased cognitive reserve to increase risk.
- **Mechanism:** Although the mechanism is not fully understood, there are likely multiple factors contributing to cognitive decline, including neurotoxicity treatments, inflammation, disruption of brain structural networks, and comorbidities.[33,34]
- **Treatment and Prophylaxis:** There are no known pharmacologic treatment or preventive options for chemo-brain. Case reports using modafinil and methylphenidate to improve cognitive function have been published with limited results, but randomized trials are needed to determine their place in treatment.[32,35]

References

1. *Common Terminology Criteria for Adverse Events (CTCAE), Version 5*, National Institutes of Health, National Cancer Institute; 2017.
2. Hershman D, Lacchetti C, Dworkin R, et al. Prevention and management of chemotherapy-induced peripheral neuropathy in survivors of adult cancers: American Society of Clinical Oncology clinical practice guideline. *J Clin Oncol.* 2014;32(18):1941–1967.
3. Stubblefield M, Burstein H, Burton A, et al. NCCN task force report: management of neuropathy in cancer. *J Natl Compr Canc Netw.* 2009;7(suppl 5):S1–S26.
4. Trivedi M, Hershman D, Crew K, et al. Management of chemotherapy-induced peripheral neuropathy. *Am J Hematol Oncol.* 2015;11(1):4–10.
5. Park S, Goldstein D, Krishnan A, et al. Chemotherapy-induced peripheral neurotoxicity: a critical analysis. *CA Cancer J Clin.* 2013;63:419–437.
6. Brewer J, Morrison G, Dolan E, et al. Chemotherapy-induced peripheral neuropathy: currrent status and progress. *Gynecol Oncol.* 2016;140:176–183.
7. Magge R, DeAngelis L. The double-edged sword: neurotoxicity of chemotherapy. *Blood Reviews.* 2015;29:93–100.
8. Taillibert S, Rhun E, Chamberlain M. Chemotherapy-related neurotoxicity. *Curr Neurol Neurosci Rep.* 2016;16(81).
9. Velasco R, Bruna J. Taxane-induced peripheral neurotoxicity. *Toxics.* 2015;3:152–169.
10. Verstappen C, Heimans J, Hoekman K, et al. Neurotoxic complications of chemotherapy in patients with cancer. *Drugs.* 2003;63(15):1549–1563.
11. Karasawa T, Steyger P. An integrated view of cisplatin-induced nephrotoxicity and ototoxicity. *Toxicol Lett.* 2015;237:219–227.

12. Beijers AJM, Jongen JLM, Vreugdenhil G. Chemotherapy-induced neurotoxicity: the value of neuropro-tective strategies. *Neth J Med.* 2012;70(1):18–25.
13. Brock PR, Maibach R, Childs M, et al. Sodium thiosulfate for protection from cisplatin-induced hearing loss. *N Engl J Med.* 2018;378:2376–2385.
14. Beijers AJM, Vreugdenhil G. A systematic review on chronic oxaliplatin-induced peripheral neuropathy and the relation with oxaliplatin administration. *Support Care Cancer.* 2014;22:1999–2007.
15. McWhinney S, Goldberg R, McLeod H. Platinum neurotoxicity pharmacogenetics. *Mol Cancer Ther.* 2009;8(1):10–16.
16. Pachman D, Qin R, Seisler D, et al. Clinical course of oxaliplatin-induced neuropathy: results from the randomized phase III trial N08CB (Alliance). *J Clin Oncol.* 2015;33(30):3416–3422.
17. Salehi Z, Roayaei M. Effect of vitamin E on oxaliplatin-induced peripheral neuropathy prevention: a randomized controlled trial. *Int J Prev Med.* 2015;6:104.
18. Hochster HS, Grothey A, Hart L, et al. Improved time to treatment failure with an intermittent oxali-platin strategy: results of CONcePT. *Ann Oncol.* 2014;25(6):1172–1178.
19. Tournigand C, Cervantes A, Figer A, et al. OPTIMOX1: a randomized study of FOLFOX4 or FOLFOX7 with oxaliplatin in a stop-and-go fashion in advanced colorectal cancer—a GERCOR study. *J Clin Oncol.* 2006;24(3):394–400.
20. Postma TJ, Benard BA, Huijgens PC, et al. Long term effects of vincristine on the peripheral nervous system. *J Neurooncol.* 1993;15:23–27.
21. Ackermann R, Semmler A, Maurer G. Methotrexate-induced myelopathy responsive to substitution of multiple folate metabolites. *J Neurooncol.* 2010;97:425–427.
22. Bhojwani D, Sabin N, Pei D, et al. Methotrexate-induced neurotoxicity and leukoencephalopathy in childhood acute lymphoblastic leukemia. *J Clin Oncol.* 2014;32(9):949–959.
23. Adkins J, Peters D, Markham A. Fludarabine an update of its pharmacology and use in the treatment of haematological malignancies. *Drugs.* 1997;53(6):1005–1037.
24. Annaloro C, Costa A, Fracchiolla N, et al. Severe fludarabine neurotoxicity after reduced intensity con-ditioning regimen to allogeneic hematopoietic stem cell transplantation: a case report. *Clin Case Rep.* 2015;3(7):650–655.
25. Lee M, McKinney A, Brace J, et al. Clinical and imaging features of fludarabine neurotoxicity. *J Neuro-ophthalmol.* 2010;30:37–41.
26. Hasle H. Cerebellar toxicity during cytarabine therapy associated with renal insufficiency. *Cancer Chemother Pharmacol.* 1990;27:76–78.
27. Tran P, Xiao-Tang K. Cytarabine induced acute cerebellar syndrome during Hyper-CVAD treatment for B-cell acute lymphoblastic leukemia. *Case Rep Neurol.* 2017;9:114–120.
28. Berg S, Blaney S, Devidas M. Phase II study of nelarabine (compound 506U78) in children and young adults with refractory T-cell malignancies: a report from the Children's Oncology Group. *J Clin Oncol.* 205;23(15):3376-3382.
29. Buie L, Epstein S, Lindley C. Nelarabine: a novel purine antimetabolite antineoplastic agent. *Clin Ther.* 2007;29(9):1887–1899.
30. Nicolao P, Giometto B. Neurological toxicity of ifosfamide. *Oncology.* 2003;65(suppl 2):11–16.
31. Ahles TA, Root JC, Ryan EL. Cancer- and cancer treatment-associated cognitive change: an update on the state of the science. *J Clin Oncol.* 2012;30:3675.
32. Hermelink K. Chemotherapy and cognitive function in breast cancer patients: the so-called chemo brain. *J Natl Cancer Inst Monogr.* 2015;51:67–69.
33. Janelsins MC, Heckler CE, Peppone LJ, et al. Cognitive complaints in survivors of breast cancer after chemotherapy compared with age-matched controls: an analysis from a nationwide, multicenter, prospec-tive longitudinal study. *J Clin Oncol.* 2017;35(5):506–514.
34. Jim HD, Philips KM, Chait S, et al. Meta-analysis of cognitive functioning in breast cancer survivors previously treated with standard-dose chemotherapy. *J Clinc Oncol.* 2012;30(29):3578.
35. Hislop J. Yes, Virginia, chemo brain is real. *Clinical Breast Cancer.* 2015;15(2):87–89.

CHAPTER 8

Pulmonary Toxicities of Chemotherapy

Pradnya D. Patil, MD, FACP ▪ Tanmay S. Panchabhai, MD, FACP, FCCP

Introduction

Respiratory insufficiency in patients receiving systemic chemotherapy often is a diagnostic dilemma for clinicians. Patients receiving chemotherapy are frequently immunosuppressed and may have concurrent bone marrow suppression, or pulmonary involvement from underlying malignancy, making the differential diagnosis of respiratory failure quite broad. It is imperative that common etiologies such as respiratory infections, congestive heart failure, venous thromboembolism, alveolar hemorrhage, radiation-induced lung injury, and toxicities from chemotherapeutic drugs be investigated in cancer patients presenting with respiratory failure. As drug toxicity is a diagnosis of exclusion and cannot be defined by uniform diagnostic criteria, an extensive workup, sometimes including a lung biopsy, is required to make a diagnosis. Although the exact incidence of lung injury from chemotherapeutic agents is unknown, some authors suggest that it may be as high as 10% to 20%.[1,2] It is important to recognize the clinicopathologic features that are characteristically associated with different antineoplastic agents and have a high degree of suspicion to allow for early intervention and avoidance of any further exposure to the offending agent.

Pulmonary toxicities of chemotherapeutic agents are mediated through many different mechanisms and can have varied clinical manifestations. In addition, novel targeted agents and immunotherapeutic agents are associated with very distinct pulmonary toxicities in comparison with traditional chemotherapeutic drugs. In this chapter, we will be focusing on pulmonary toxicities of cytotoxic chemotherapy.

- **Pathophysiology:** Several mechanisms have been suggested for lung injury from cytotoxic agents; however, the majority of these are poorly understood. Cytotoxic chemotherapy can result in direct injury to alveolar pneumocytes resulting in a chemical pneumonitis-like pattern. Cytokines appear to play a prominent role in mediating pulmonary toxicities of these agents. Damage to endothelial cells in the lungs can lead to the release of cytokines, which in turn leads to activation and infiltration of inflammatory cells such as lymphocytes and, occasionally, eosinophils. Preclinical mouse models receiving gemcitabine and radiation (a known risk factor for gemcitabine-induced pneumonitis), have shown elevated levels of proinflammatory cytokines such as TNF-α and IL-1α.[3] A similar increase in TNF-α and IL-1β has been noted in preclinical animal models as well as in humans who receive bleomycin.[4] Fibroblast activation by both bleomycin itself and associated cytokine production can lead to collagen deposition.[5-7] A systemic cytokine-mediated capillary leak syndrome resulting in noncardiogenic pulmonary edema has been described with gemcitabine and docetaxel. Free radical–mediated endothelial injury appears to play a prominent role in bleomycin-induced lung injury and has led to the investigation of the therapeutic utility of agents such as dexrazoxane and amifostine in mitigating the damage caused by bleomycin.[8] In addition, other medications or radiation may have synergistic mechanisms which lead to augmented lung damage when used in combination. One such example is the increased incidence of pneumonitis in patients who are treated with gemcitabine and who have previously received radiation.

- **Risk factors:** Patients who have underlying lung disease such as interstitial lung disease, chronic obstructive pulmonary disease (COPD), or other conditions, or those who are receiving a combination of cytotoxic agents or other drugs that can be associated with pulmonary toxicities, appear to be at an increased risk of developing pulmonary toxicities. In addition, prior or concurrent thoracic radiation puts patients at an increased risk for pneumonitis with certain agents such as gemcitabine. Exposure to high fractions of inspired oxygen (FiO_2) has also been well-known to amplify the risk of pneumonitis from bleomycin.[4]
- **Clinical presentation:** Although clinical trials often report pulmonary toxicities of chemotherapeutic agents, the exact clinicopathological presentations are often not described. Whereas some agents are associated with certain classic clinical findings such as bleomycin-induced pneumonitis, others can be associated with nonspecific signs and symptoms at presentation. Clinical manifestations are often nonspecific and include cough, dyspnea, hypoxia, and, occasionally, fever. Other specific signs and symptoms associated with the different clinical syndromes have been described below. Although most of these reactions occur within hours to weeks of initiating therapy, some drugs, such as bleomycin and nitrosureas, have been associated with delayed lung toxicity.[9,10]

Subtypes of Chemotherapy-Associated Pulmonary Toxicity

- **Mast cell-mediated toxicity:** Some agents, such as platinum drugs, taxanes, rituximab, cytarabine, and etoposide, have been associated with acute bronchoconstriction leading to dyspnea and hypoxia either during infusion or shortly thereafter. These infusion reactions are likely mediated by mast cell or basophil activation and can be associated with other systemic signs such as angioedema, hypotension, flushing, pruritis, and urticaria. These patients have prominent wheezing on examination and spirometry reveals severe reversible airflow obstruction.
- **Hypersensitivity pneumonitis:** Towards the other end of the spectrum of allergic reactions are eosinophilic pneumonitis and hypersensitivity pneumonitis. Hypersensitivity pneumonitis is usually a cell-mediated process similar to delayed type IV hypersensitivity reactions. Patients with hypersensitivity pneumonitis develop dyspnea hours to days after receiving the cytotoxic drug. Thoracic imaging reveals new pulmonary infiltrates which may be associated with peripheral eosinophilia. Eosinophilic pneumonia often has diffuse alveolar or mixed alveolar-interstitial opacities on imaging and is characterized by greater than 20% eosinophils on analysis of bronchoalveolar lavage (BAL) samples. Peripheral eosinophilia is often present.
- **Interstitial pneumonitis:** Interstitial pneumonitis often presents with diffuse or focal ground glass opacities (Fig. 8.1) on imaging and septal thickening. Patients may have systemic symptoms such as fever. BAL findings in these patients can be nonspecific.

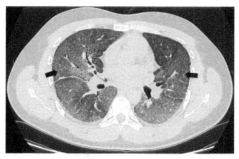

Fig. 8.1   Diffuse ground glass opacities noted on computerized tomogram of the chest *(black arrows)* in a patient receiving bleomycin.

- **Alveolar hemorrhage:** Patients with alveolar hemorrhage present with dyspnea, occasionally associated with hemoptysis and diffuse pulmonary opacities on imaging. Diagnosis can be confirmed by performing a bronchoscopy and BAL, which will reveal a hemorrhagic sample.
- **Noncardiogenic pulmonary edema:** Noncardiogenic causes of pulmonary edema such as capillary leak syndrome (associated with peripheral edema and, occasionally, intravascular volume depletion) should be considered in patients presenting with respiratory compromise who are receiving certain drugs such as cytarabine, gemcitabine, and docetaxel, among others.
- **Differentiation syndrome:** Up to a quarter of patients with acute promyelocytic leukemia (APL) who are treated with either all-trans retinoic acid (ATRA) or arsenic trioxide (ATO) can develop a potentially fatal differentiation syndrome, due to the release of inflammatory cytokines as a result of differentiation of the promyelocytes to more mature neutrophils. These patients usually develop acute respiratory failure, fever, peripheral edema, pulmonary opacities, hypoxemia, hypotension, renal and hepatic dysfunction, rash, and serositis resulting in pleural and pericardial effusions.
- **Radiation recall pneumonitis:** In patients who have received prior thoracic radiation, radiation recall pneumonitis (RRP) in the form of infiltrates in the region of previous radiation exposure has been noted. Drugs that have been associated with this phenomenon include doxorubicin, gemcitabine, paclitaxel, carmustine, etoposide, and trastuzumab.
- **Veno-occlusive disease:** Pulmonary veno-occlusive disease (VOD) is another rare clinical presentation in which patients develop pulmonary hypertension, centrilobular ground glass opacities, septal lines, and lymphadenopathy on imaging.
- **Acute respiratory distress syndrome:** Acute lung injury or acute respiratory distress syndrome (ARDS) has been observed with bleomycin, cytarabine, gemcitabine, mitomycin, and dactinomycin. Patients present with moderate to severe hypoxemia associated, on occasion, with systemic signs such as fever. BAL often shows a predominance of neutrophils.

Diagnostic Workup of Suspected Chemotherapy-Associated Pulmonary Toxicity

The diagnosis of cytotoxic chemotherapy–related pulmonary toxicity is one of exclusion. Careful attention must be paid to medical history, concomitant medications, prior or current thoracic radiation, and accompanying signs and symptoms, in order to rule out other etiologies such as infection, cardiogenic pulmonary edema, alveolar hemorrhage, pulmonary embolism, or a reaction to another medication. Often the diagnosis of drug-induced pneumonitiis is made when other diagnoes are excluded an there is an improvement in the clinical status of the patient after discontinuation of the drug with or without additional treatment such as corticosteroids.

- **Imaging:** Chest imaging in the form of a chest X-ray or high-resolution computed tomography (CT) scans, although not specific, can be informative in recognizing the patterns of pulmonary toxicity, and to rule out other etiologies such as venous thromboembolism. A variety of abnormalities such as diffuse or focal ground glass opacities (see Fig. 8.1) or reticular markings, consolidations, centrilobular nodules, septal thickening, or pleural effusions associated with serositis may be seen.[11] A classic radiographic pattern associated with methotrexate is the appearance of hilar lymphadenopathy.[12]
- **Laboratory analysis:** Laboratory values for the white blood cell count (neutrophilia, lymphocytosis, or eosinophilia) and inflammatory markers such as the erythrocyte sedimentation rate or C-reactive protein may be elevated in some patients. Other testing, which may be considered, based on clinical presentation include a B-type natriuretic peptide (BNP), coagulation studies, and echocardiogram, along with blood and sputum cultures. Although not used in routine clinical practice yet, elevated serum levels of Krebs von den Lunge-6

(KL-6), which is expressed by type II pneumocytes, may be seen in patients with drug induced pneumonitis.[9]

- **Bronchoscopy:** Bronchoscopy and BAL can play an important role in excluding other etiologies such as infection, involvement with malignancy, and hemorrhage. In some patients, a predominantly neutrophilic or eosinophilic BAL specimen may aide in the diagnosis of drug-induced pneumonitis. A lung biopsy can provide more information about the pathophysiology in a patient with respiratory failure; however, the histologic findings are often nonspecific and the risk versus benefit of the biopsy must be considered in each patient. Patterns observed on histopathology may point towards a diagnosis of drug-induced organizing pneumonia, nonspecific interstitial pneumonia, eosinophilic pneumonia, or pulmonary fibrosis.
- **Pulmonary function testing:** Pulmonary function tests can be used to determine the degree of respiratory compromise; however, they are not useful in making a diagnosis.

Cytotoxic Chemotherapy Agents and Mechanisms of Action

ANTINEOPLASTIC ANTIBIOTICS

- **Bleomycin:** Since it was first isolated in 1966, bleomycin has gained widespread application in the management of many malignancies including Hodgkin's lymphoma and germ cell tumors. However, an estimated 10% of treated patients develop pulmonary toxicities, which often limits the clinical utility of the drug.[13] Fatal pulmonary toxicity has been noted in up to 3% of patients.[14,15] Long-term toxicities have been reported in 8% of patients who received three courses of BEP (bleomycin, etoposide, cisplatin)[16] and in 15% to 18% of patients treated for Hodgkin's lymphoma.[17–19] With early discontinuation of bleomycin determined by decline in diffusing capacity of the lungs for carbon monoxide (DLCO), more recent data from the Danish Testicular Cancer database have reported much lower rates of pulmonary toxicity.[20]
  - **Risk factors:** Bleomycin lung toxicity appears to be more common with advanced age,[21,22] although some studies have not found an association.[20] Cumulative drug dose above 400 units has been associated with higher rates of pulmonary toxicity and is generally avoided.[23] Since bleomycin is mostly renally eliminated, patients with renal impairment are at an increased risk of drug accumulation and toxicity. Other factors that have been associated with higher pulmonary toxicity, albeit not consistently, include faster infusion rates,[24] other concomitant chemotherapeutic agents such as cisplatin and gemcitabine,[25,26] thoracic radiation,[18,27] smoking,[4,28] and administration of granulocyte colony stimulating factors.[29–31] The association between bleomycin lung toxicity and high FiO_2 has been shown in animal models; however, the data in humans is limited to retrospective case series and studies.[32–34]
  - **Mechanism:** Bleomycin induces cytotoxicity by causing single and double stranded breaks in DNA by forming a complex with ferrous ions and molecular oxygen.[35–37] After administration, it is rapidly inactivated in tissues by bleomycin hydrolase, especially in the liver and kidney. Cells in the lungs and skin are relatively deficient in this enzyme and are therefore more susceptible to bleomycin toxicity. Pulmonary toxicity by bleomycin is thought to be mediated by various pathways. In murine models, lower bleomycin hydrolase activity has been associated with higher susceptibility to bleomycin and chronic fibrosis.[37,38] Genetic variations may play a role in determining sensitivity to lung toxicity of bleomycin as exemplified by studies that have shown variable susceptibility in murine strains with different genetic variants.[37] Inflammatory response mediated by T cells and cytokines appears to be central to the pathogenesis, suggested by the finding that athymic mice appear to be resistant to bleomycin lung toxicity.[39] The fact that soluble Fas antigen and anti-FasL antibodies have been successful in preventing the progression of

bleomycin-induced pulmonary fibrosis supports the role of these in the pathogenesis of this entity.[40] Animal models have demonstrated increased intrapulmonary TNF-α and IL-1β after bleomycin exposure.[41,42] Free radicals and oxidative damage also appear to play a role in bleomycin toxicity.[43] In addition, bleomycin activates fibroblasts both directly and indirectly due to cytokines such as TNFα, leading to increased collagen deposition and fibrosis. This process is mediated at least in part by transforming growth factor β (TGF β).[4]

- **Presentation:** Patients often present with dyspnea, cough, or asymptomatic reduction in DLCO within 1 to 6 months of initiating therapy. Bleomycin has been reported to present with eosinophilic or hypersensitivity pneumonitis, interstitial pneumonitis, acute lung injury or ARDS, and even pulmonary veno-occlusive disease and, on rare occasions, delayed pulmonary manifestations in the form of pulmonary fibrosis (see Fig. 8.1). Additionally, some authors have reported episodes of chest pain during infusion of bleomycin which was self-limiting.[44]
- **Mitomycin-C:** Mitomycin-C is an antineoplastic antibiotic and a cell cycle specific alkylating agent derived from *Streptomyces caespitosus*. Due to availability of more efficacious regimens, the clinical utility of mitomycin-C in the United States is mostly limited to the treatment of anal cancer. An estimated 2% to 12% of patients exposed to this agent develop pulmonary toxicity. Toxicity associated with mitomycin-C increases with higher doses, especially above 20 mg/m^2.[45,46] Other factors that may lead to a higher risk of lung toxicity include supplemental oxygen, other medications with pulmonary toxicity, and thoracic radiation. Acute bronchospasm, which is usually self-limited, can occur in less than 6% of patients. There appears to be an association between the risk of lung toxicity and coadministration of vinca alkaloids even weeks after receiving mitomycin-C.[47,48] A similar association with vinca alkaloids has also been noted in patients who develop acute lung injury or ARDS.[49] Chronic interstitial pneumonitis and rarely pleural disease and pulmonary veno-occlusive disease have been noted.
- **Doxorubicin:** Doxorubicin is an anthracycline antitumor antibiotic. It has widespread applications in multiple tumor types including breast cancer, acute lymphoblastic leukemia, Hodgkin's lymphoma, and non-Hodgkin's lymphoma, among others. Patients may notice dyspnea during the infusion of the pegylated liposomal doxorubicin. Other lung toxicities that have been reported include interstitial pneumonitis, organizing pneumonia, and radiation recall pneumonitis.[50]
- **Epirubicin and mitoxantrone:** Some topoisomerase II inhibitors such as epirubicin and mitoxantrone have also been associated with pneumonitis; however, the reported cases were usually also receiving concomitant chemotherapy with other agents that could have potentially contributed to the toxicity.[9]

ALKYLATING AGENTS

- **Busulfan:** Busulfan is commonly used for conditioning prior to stem cell transplantation. Prior to the availability of tyrosine kinase inhibitors, it was also used for the treatment of chronic myelogenous leukemia (CML). Overall, less than 8% of patients who receive the drug develop pulmonary toxicity. Busulfan is associated with increased risk of pulmonary complications because it is often coadministered with other drugs such as cyclophosphamide. Other risk factors include radiation exposure, prolonged exposure, or a cumulative dose above 500 mg.[51,52] A variety of histopathologic findings have been noted in patients with busulfan toxicity including degeneration of type 1 pneumocytes and atypical hyperplasia of type II pneumocytes, mononuclear cellular infiltrates, diffuse alveolar damage, and alveolar hemorrhage.[53] Clinically, most lung toxicities manifest between 1 month to 1 year after stem cell transplantation and manifest as acute lung injury, chronic interstitial fibrosis, or alveolar hemorrhage.

■ **Melphalan:** Melphalan is also a drug used for stem cell transplantation conditioning. On rare occasions, acute bronchoconstriction and pneumonitis have been reported with melphalan use.

■ **Cyclophosphamide:** Although pulmonary toxicity from cyclophosphamide is rare (<1%), due to its widespread clinical application and potential for severe lung involvement, clinicians should be aware of the possibility of these toxicities. Some patients present with reversible pneumonitis within 1 to 6 months of receiving the drug, whereas others present with delayed pneumonitis or fibrosis even years after therapy. Late onset pneumonitis and fibrosis are usually resistant to treatment with steroids and eventually lead to terminal lung fibrosis.[54,55] Risk factors for these toxicities are increased FiO_2 exposure, radiation, and concomitant drugs with the potential for pulmonary toxicity.

■ **Ifosfamide:** Ifosfamide can cause pneumonitis similar to that observed with cyclophosphamide. Additionally, ifosfamide uniquely can cause methemoglobinemia. The mechanism for this is via a metabolite of ifosfamide which reacts with glutathione, resulting in the depletion of the red blood cell antioxidant reserve and leading to methemoglobinemia.

■ **Chlorambucil:** Chlorambucil is used mainly for the therapy of chronic lymphocytic leukemia. Pulmonary toxicity has been rarely observed with this drug but can occur during, or even after, discontinuation. In addition, there does not appear to be a correlation between the dose or duration of therapy.[56] Patterns of lung involvement include chronic interstitial pneumonitis, pulmonary fibrosis, organizing pneumonia, and acute interstitial pneumonia.

ANTIMETABOLITES

■ **Methotrexate:** Methotrexate inhibits dihydrofolate reductase and leads to impaired DNA synthesis. Risk factors for pulmonary toxicity include age older than 60 years, involvement of the lungs or pleura with rheumatoid disease, prior therapy with disease-modifying antirheumatic drugs, and diabetes mellitus (hyperinsulinemia in treated diabetes can lead to increased polyglutamation of methotrexate).[57] The most common pattern of toxicity observed is hypersensitivity pneumonitis, which usually occurs days to weeks into treatment, although delayed reactions have been observed. Other forms of toxicity include organizing pneumonia, pleural effusions, and pulmonary fibrosis (Fig. 8.2). Methotrexate-associated pneumonitis has a few

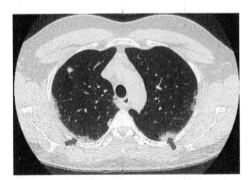

Fig. 8.2 Bilateral peripheral pleural-based consolidations *(red arrows)* in a patient ultimately diagnosed with organizing pneumonia by video-assisted thoracoscopic biopsy. They were receiving methotrexate as a part of their chemotherapy regimen. The consolidations resolved after the drug was withheld and an extended prednisone taper was prescribed.

classic features that set it apart from other reactions—it is usually reversible, accompanied by mild eosinophilia in over half of the cases, associated with weakly formed granulomas in the lung, and has a low chance of recurrence with methotrexate rechallenge after resolution of symptoms.[12] In addition, hilar lymphadenopathy can be seen in close to 10% of patients. Proposed mechanisms for toxicity include activation of the mitogen-activated protein kinase pathway, altered cytokine milieu, alveolar epithelial injury, and host reaction to latent viral infections, such as cytomegalovirus or Epstein-Barr virus.[58,59]

- **Cytarabine:** Cytarabine is a pyrimidine analog that inhibits DNA polymerase resulting in cytotoxicity. It is used in the treatment of acute myeloblastic leukemia and is often used prior to stem cell transplantation. A unique pulmonary toxicity of cytarabine is the development of noncardiogenic pulmonary edema which usually occurs 1 to 2 weeks into therapy. Patients usually develop dyspnea, cough, and increased oxygen requirements, often accompanied by low-grade fever. Histologic findings include excessive alveolar proteinaceous material without any cellular atypia or mononuclear infiltrate.
- **Gemcitabine:** Gemcitabine is a pyrimidine analog with clinical applications in several malignancies including pancreatic cancer, non–small-cell lung cancer, and bladder cancer. Gemcitabine-induced severe pulmonary toxicity is rare (estimated incidence 0%–5%).[60] However, when used in combination with other agents such as bleomycin or taxanes, the incidence is much higher. In addition, because gemcitabine is a radiosensitizer, prior or concurrent radiation increases the risk of pulmonary toxicity. Manifestations include bronchoconstriction, interstitial pneumonitis, acute eosinophilic pneumonia, alveolar hemorrhage, capillary leak syndrome, and noncardiogenic pulmonary edema (Fig. 8.3).
- **Fludarabine:** Fludarabine is a purine analog most commonly used for stem cell transplantation conditioning and for the treatment of chronic lymphocytic leukemia. Up to 10% of patients treated with this agent can develop pulmonary toxicity, with the most common presentation being interstitial pneumonitis. Reactions can either occur in the first few weeks of therapy or be delayed.[61] Because fludarabine leads to severe immunosuppression, it is imperative that an extensive workup to rule out infectious etiologies be performed before attributing respiratory symptoms to a drug toxicity.

NITROSUREAS

- **Carmustine and lomustine:** Nitrosurea agents such as carmustine (BCNU) and lomustine (CCNU) are used in the treatment of brain tumors, lymphoma, and in regimens prior to stem cell transplantation. Three distinct lung toxicities have been noted with these agents:

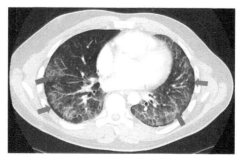

Fig. 8.3 Bilateral lower lobe predominant ground glass opacities and reticulation *(red arrows)* with classic subpleural sparing *(blue arrows)* indicating a nonspecific interstitial pneumonia (NSIP) pattern in a patient receiving gemcitabine.

an idiopathic pneumonia syndrome, interstitial pneumonitis, and, finally, a late onset pleuroparenchymal fibroelastosis (PPFE).

- **Idiopathic pneumonia syndrome (IPS)** is characterized by acute onset of dyspnea, hypoxia, symptoms of pneumonia, and widespread alveolar injury accompanied by multilobar involvement on imaging, all usually within 12 to 19 days after allogeneic or autologous hematopoietic cell transplantation. Although many mechanisms for IPS have been suggested, an association with prior therapy with carmustine has been noted.[62,63]
- **Interstitial pneumonitis:** In the absence of stem cell transplantation, a less aggressive acute and subacute interstitial pneumonitis has been reported in 10% to 30% of patients receiving these agents.[64] The onset is usually within weeks to months of treatment.
- **Pleuroparenchymal fibroelastosis:** Delayed fibrosis known as PPFE has been described in some patients up to 17 years after therapy. Younger patients and those treated with higher doses may be at an increased risk for PPFE. Furthermore, it is worth noting that patients may be asymptomatic with unremarkable radiographic imaging until significant fibrosis has set in.[10]

PODOPHYLLOTOXINS

- **Etoposide:** Hypersensitivity reactions can occur in 1% to 3% of patients treated with intravenous etoposide (due to the drug vehicle) and can be accompanied by dyspnea and bronchoconstriction. Diffuse alveolar damage is otherwise rare and mostly observed with oral etoposide. Etoposide is a radiosensitizer and increases the risk of radiation recall pneumonitis.

TAXANES

- **Paclitaxel, Docetaxel, Nab-paclitaxel:** Acute or subacute interstitial lung disease or pneumonitis has been described in patients receiving paclitaxel and docetaxel. The reported incidence with nab-paclitaxel is lower, however. These are thought to represent a delayed type IV hypersensitivity to the drug and occur within hours to weeks of initiating therapy. Risk factors for pneumonitis include preexisting lung disease, combination with agents such as gemcitabine or radiation, and higher doses, especially for docetaxel. Patients treated with docetaxel can also develop a capillary leak syndrome characterized by noncardiogenic pulmonary edema, peripheral edema, and pleural effusions. This can be ameliorated to a certain extent by pretreatment with dexamethasone and early initiation of diuretics.

DIFFERENTIATION THERAPY: ALL-TRANS RETINOIC ACID (ATRA) AND ARSENIC TRIOXIDE (ATO)

A unique syndrome associated with the use of dual differentiation therapy (ATRA and ATO) for APL is differentiation syndrome, which can occur in up to 25% of patients. In patients with APL, the aberrant PML/RARA protein prevents myeloid differentiation beyond the promyelocytic stage. This is reversed by ATRA leading to rapid differentiation of the malignant cells into mature myelocytes and neutrophils. During this process, many cytokines are released resulting in capillary leak syndrome. In addition, migration of mature leukocytes to the lungs and kidneys also causes organ dysfunction.[65,66] Higher white blood cell count at the time of initiation of ATRA is a risk factor for subsequent differentiation syndrome. Patients usually develop fever, peripheral edema, dyspnea, hypotension, and renal failure within 4 weeks of starting therapy.

PROTEOSOME INHIBITORS

- **Bortezomib:** Bortezomib has been approved for use in multiple myeloma and mantle cell lymphoma. Although pulmonary toxicity is not very common, severe and occasionally fatal pneumonitis, lung infiltrates, ARDS, and rare pulmonary hypertension have been described with its use.[67,68]

- **Carfilzomib:** Carfilzomib is a second-generation proteasome inhibitor that has been associated with transient dyspnea in up to 29% of patients.[69,70] In addition, rare cases of pulmonary hypertension following therapy have also occurred.

Approach to Management

- **Discontinuation of offending agent:** After an extensive workup to rule out other etiologies for respiratory failure as outlined previously, the offending drug causing pulmonary toxicity should be discontinued. A thorough diagnostic evaluation ensures that therapy is not withheld from patients who have respiratory failure from an alternate cause and who may benefit from continued therapy. In some patients, resolution of symptoms after discontinuation of the drug can be diagnostic for drug toxicity. In patients with APL who develop differentiation syndrome and hypoxia, ATRA or ATO may be continued unless clinical manifestations are severe enough to require high-flow oxygen or invasive ventilatory support.
- **Glucocorticoids:** Because inflammation appears to play a pivotal role in the development of pulmonary toxicity with cytotoxic chemotherapy, glucocorticoids are often utilized to mitigate the inflammation in such patients. For patients with mild to moderate pulmonary toxicity in whom symptoms persist despite discontinuation of cytotoxic chemotherapy, steroids should be initiated. On the other hand, patients who are critically ill should receive high doses of steroids immediately. Although there are no clinical trials to determine the optimal dosage for corticosteroids, doses should be based upon severity of lung involvement. For patients in frank respiratory failure, pulse dose methylprednisolone at 1 g/day for up to 3 days may be considered.[9] For less severe cases, lower doses of methylprednisolone or prednisone may be used. For differentiation syndrome in patients with APL, dexamethasone 10 mg twice a day should be used. Certain patterns of lung involvement, such as eosinophilic pneumonia, hypersensitivity pneumonitis, and organizing pneumonia, appear to be more steroid responsive than delayed reactions with a prominent fibrotic component. After resolution of acute symptoms, a gradual tapering course of steroids accompanied by the appropriate prophylactic antibiotics should be prescribed.
- **Rechallenge with cytotoxic agent:** In general, rechallenge with the offending agent may carry a risk of precipitating a more severe reaction. Certain drugs such as methotrexate have been successfully rechallenged without additional toxicity; however, rechallenge with any agent should only be done with careful consideration of risks, benefits, and alternatives.
- **Supportive care:** For patients with acute bronchoconstriction or infusion reactions, withholding further infusion and initiating treatment with bronchodilators, supplemental oxygen, and occasionally short courses of steroids is advised. Although supplemental oxygen plays an important role in the management of pulmonary toxicities of cytotoxic agents, higher FiO_2 may also place patients at higher risk for subsequent pneumonitis (such as with bleomycin) and should be avoided. While on treatment with corticosteroids, appropriate prophylaxis for *Pneumocystis jiroveci* and monitoring for infectious complications is essential. Patients with noncardiogenic pulmonary edema or capillary leak syndrome require diuresis.

Monitoring and Preventative Strategies

For most cytotoxic agents, routine screening and evaluation for pulmonary toxicity is not recommended. There are, however, some exceptions for drugs that are associated with a higher incidence or severity of lung toxicities. In patients receiving bleomycin, routine use of spirometry and DLCO for early detection of respiratory impairment is controversial. Most institutions, however, will perform baseline pulmonary function tests and DLCO and monitor these at regular intervals, particularly with cumulative doses greater than 400 units. Even if the patient is asymptomatic, a drop in the DLCO or pulmonary function tests (PFTs) by over 15% should prompt discontinuation of further therapy.[71] Retrospective data and a single-arm prospective study in patients with APL did not show any significant improvement in survival outcomes with prophylactic steroids to prevent differentiation syndrome.[72,73] Judicious oxygen supplementation with inspired oxygen and avoidance of radiosensitizing agents in patients with prior or ongoing thoracic radiation, as well as close monitoring for patients who are receiving drugs with a dose dependent, cumulative toxicity, are other strategies to prevent pulmonary toxicity.

References

1. Rosenow EC 3rd, Limper AH. Drug-induced pulmonary disease. *Semin Respir Infect*. 1995;10:86.
2. Snyder LS, Hertz MI. Cytotoxic drug-induced lung injury. *Semin Respir Infect*. 1988;3:217.
3. Rübe CE, Wilfert F, Uthe D, et al. Increased expression of pro-inflammatory cytokines as a cause of lung toxicity after combined treatment with gemcitabine and thoracic irradiation. *Radiother Oncol*. 2004;72(2):231–241.
4. Sleijfer S. Bleomycin-induced pneumonitis. *Chest*. 2001;120(2):617–624.
5. Moseley PL, Hemken C, Hunninghake GW. Augmentation of fibroblast proliferation by bleomycin. *J Clin Invest*. 1986;78:1150–1154.
6. Sugarman BJ, Aggarwal BB, Figari IS, et al. Recombinant human tumor necrosis factor-alpha: effects on proliferation of normal and transformed cells in vitro. *Science*. 1985;230:943–945.
7. Schmidt JA, Mizel SB, Cohen D, et al. Interleukin-1: a potential regulator of fibroblast proliferation. *J Immunol*. 1982;128:2177–2182.
8. Moseley PL, Shasby DM, Brady M, et al. Lung parenchymal injury induced by bleomycin. *Am Rev Respir Dis*. 1984;130:1082–1086.
9. Vahid B, Marik PE. Pulmonary complications of novel antineoplastic agents for solid tumors. *Chest*. 2008;133:528.
10. O'Driscoll BR, Hasleton PS, Taylor PM, et al. Active lung fibrosis up to 17 years after chemotherapy with carmustine (BCNU) in childhood. *N Engl J Med*. 1990;323:378.
11. Torrisi JM, Schwartz LH, Gollub MJ, et al. CT findings of chemotherapy-induced toxicity: what radiologists need to know about the clinical and radiologic manifestations of chemotherapy toxicity. *Radiology*. 2011;258:41.
12. Limper AH. Chemotherapy-induced lung disease. *Clin Chest Med*. 2004;25:53.
13. Jules-Elysee K, White DA. Bleomycin-induced pulmonary toxicity. *Clin Chest Med*. 1990;11:1.
14. Levi JA, Raghaven D, Harvey V, et al. The importance of bleomycin in combination chemotherapy for good-prognosis germ cell carcinoma. *J Clin Oncol*. 1993;11:1300–1305.
15. Simpson AB, Paul J, Graham J, et al. Fatal bleomycin pulmonary toxicity in the west of Scotland 1991–95; a review of patients with germ cell tumours. *Br J Cancer*. 1998;78:1061–1066.
16. de Wit R, Roberts JT, Wilkinson PM, et al. Equivalence of three or four cycles of bleomycin, etoposide, and cisplatin chemotherapy and of a 3- or 5-day schedule in good-prognosis germ cell cancer: a randomized study of the European Organization for Research and Treatment of Cancer Genitourinary Tract Cancer Cooperative Group and the Medical Research Council. *J Clin Oncol*. 2001;19:1629.
17. Hirsch A, van der Els N, Straus DJ, et al. Effect of ABVD chemotherapy with and without mantle or mediastinal irradiation on pulmonary function and symptoms in early-stage Hodgkin's disease. *J Clin Oncol*. 1996;14:1297.
18. Jóna Á, Miltényi Z, Ujj Z, et al. Late pulmonary complications of treating Hodgkin lymphoma: bleomycin-induced toxicity. *Expert Opin Drug Saf*. 2014;13:1291.
19. Avivi I, Hardak E, Shaham B, et al. Low incidence of long-term respiratory impairment in Hodgkin lymphoma survivors. *Ann Hematol*. 2012;91:215.
20. Lauritsen J, Kier MG, Bandak M, et al. Pulmonary function in patients with germ cell cancer treated with bleomycin, etoposide, and cisplatin. *J Clin Oncol*. 2016;34:1492.
21. Martin WG, Ristow KM, Habermann TM, et al. Bleomycin pulmonary toxicity has a negative impact on the outcome of patients with Hodgkin's lymphoma. *J Clin Oncol*. 2005;23:7614.
22. O'Sullivan JM, Huddart RA, Norman AR, et al. Predicting the risk of bleomycin lung toxicity in patients with germ-cell tumours. *Ann Oncol*. 2003;14:91.

23. Blum RH, Carter SK, Agre K. A clinical review of bleomycin–a new antineoplastic agent. *Cancer.* 1973;31:903.

24. Cooper KR, Hong WK. Prospective study of the pulmonary toxicity of continuously infused bleomycin. *Cancer Treat Rep.* 1981;65:419.

25. Haugnes HS, Aass N, Fosså SD, et al. Pulmonary function in long-term survivors of testicular cancer. *J Clin Oncol.* 2009;27:2779.

26. Macann A, Bredenfeld H, Müller RP, et al. Radiotherapy does not influence the severe pulmonary toxicity observed with the administration of gemcitabine and bleomycin in patients with advanced-stage Hodgkin's lymphoma treated with the BAGCOPP regimen: a report by the German Hodgkin's Lymphoma Study Group. *Int J Radiat Oncol Biol Phys.* 2008;70:161.

27. Stamatoullas A, Brice P, Bouabdallah R, et al. Outcome of patients older than 60 years with classical Hodgkin lymphoma treated with front line ABVD chemotherapy: frequent pulmonary events suggest limiting the use of bleomycin in the elderly. *Br J Haematol.* 2015;170:179.

28. Lower EE, Strohofer S, Baughman RP. Bleomycin causes alveolar macrophages from cigarette smokers to release hydrogen peroxide. *Am J Med Sci.* 1988;295:193.

29. Fosså SD, Kaye SB, Mead GM, et al. Filgrastim during combination chemotherapy of patients with poor-prognosis metastatic germ cell malignancy. European Organization for Research and Treatment of Cancer, Genito-Urinary Group, and the Medical Research Council Testicular Cancer Working Party, Cambridge, United Kingdom. *J Clin Oncol.* 1998;16:716.

30. Saxman SB, Nichols CR, Einhorn LH. Pulmonary toxicity in patients with advanced-stage germ cell tumors receiving bleomycin with and without granulocyte colony stimulating factor. *Chest.* 1997;111:657.

31. Younes A, Fayad L, Romaguera J, et al. Safety and efficacy of once-per-cycle pegfilgrastim in support of ABVD chemotherapy in patients with Hodgkin lymphoma. *Eur J Cancer.* 2006;42:2976.

32. Goldiner PL, Carlon GC, Cvitkovic E, et al. Factors influencing postoperative morbidity and mortality in patients treated with bleomycin. *Br Med J.* 1978;1:1664.

33. Nygaard K, Smith-Erichsen N, Hatlevoll R, Refsum SB. Pulmonary complications after bleomycin, irradiation and surgery for esophageal cancer. *Cancer.* 1978;41:17.

34. Gilson AJ, Sahn SA. Reactivation of bleomycin lung toxicity following oxygen administration. A second response to corticosteroids. *Chest.* 1985;88:304.

35. Chandler DB. Possible mechanisms of bleomycin-induced fibrosis. *Clin Chest Med.* 1990;11:21.

36. Sikic BI. Biochemical and cellular determinants of bleomycin cytotoxicity. *Cancer Surv.* 1986;5:81.

37. Harrison JH Jr, Hoyt DG, Lazo JS. Acute pulmonary toxicity of bleomycin: DNA scission and matrix protein mRNA levels in bleomycin-sensitive and -resistant strains of mice. *Mol Pharmacol.* 1989;36:231.

38. Harrison Jr JH, Lazo JS. Plasma and pulmonary pharmacokinetics of bleomycin in murine strains that are sensitive and resistant to bleomycin-induced pulmonary fibrosis. *J Pharmacol Exp Ther.* 1988;247:1052.

39. Schrier DJ, Phan SH, McGarry BM. The effects of the nude (nu/nu) mutation on bleomycin-induced pulmonary fibrosis. A biochemical evaluation. *Am Rev Respir Dis.* 1983;127:614.

40. Kuwano K, Hagimoto N, Kawasaki M, et al. Essential roles of the Fas/Fas ligand pathway in the development of pulmonary fibrosis. *J Clin Invest.* 1999;104:13–19.

41. Phan SH, Kunkel SL. Lung cytokine production in bleomycin-induced pulmonary fibrosis. *Exp Lung Res.* 1992;18:29–43.

42. Santana A, Saxena B, Noble NA, et al. Increased expression of transforming growth factor beta isoforms (beta 1, beta 2, beta 3) in bleomycin-induced pulmonary fibrosis. *Am J Respir Cell Mol Biol.* 1995;13:34–44.

43. Fantone JC, Phan SH. Oxygen metabolite detoxifying enzyme levels in bleomycin-induced fibrotic lungs. *Free Radic Biol Med.* 1988;4:399.

44. White DA, Schwartzberg LS, Kris MG, Bosl GJ. Acute chest pain syndrome during bleomycin infusions. *Cancer.* 1987;59:1582.

45. Verweij J, van Zanten T, Souren T, et al. Prospective study on the dose relationship of mitomycin C-induced interstitial pneumonitis. *Cancer.* 1987;60:756.

46. Okuno SH, Frytak S. Mitomycin lung toxicity. Acute and chronic phases. *Am J Clin Oncol.* 1997;20:282.

47. Luedke D, McLaughlin TT, Daughaday C, et al. Mitomycin C and vindesine associated pulmonary toxicity with variable clinical expression. *Cancer.* 1985;55:542.

48. Thomas P, Pradal M, Le Caer H, et al. [Acute bronchospasm due to periwinkle alkaloid and mitomycin association]. *Rev Mal Respir.* 1993;10:268.

49. Kris MG, Pablo D, Gralla RJ, et al. Dyspnea following vinblastine or vindesine administration in patients receiving mitomycin plus vinca alkaloid combination therapy. *Cancer Treat Rep.* 1984;68:1029.

50. Jacobs C, Slade M, Lavery B. Doxorubicin and BOOP. A possible near fatal association. *Clin Oncol (R Coll Radiol)*. 2002;14:262.
51. Ginsberg SJ, Comis RL. The pulmonary toxicity of antineoplastic agents. *Semin Oncol*. 1982;9:34.
52. Sostman HD, Matthay RA, Putman CE. Cytotoxic drug-induced lung disease. *Am J Med*. 1977;62:608.
53. Vergnon JM, Boucheron S, Riffat J, et al. [Interstitial pneumopathies caused by busulfan. Histologic, developmental and bronchoalveolar lavage analysis of 3 cases]. *Rev Med Interne*. 1988;9:377.
54. Malik SW, Myers JL, DeRemee RA, Specks U. Lung toxicity associated with cyclophosphamide use. Two distinct patterns. *Am J Respir Crit Care Med*. 1996;154:1851.
55. Hamada K, Nagai S, Kitaichi M, et al. Cyclophosphamide-induced late-onset lung disease. *Intern Med*. 2003;42:82.
56. Khong HT, McCarthy J. Chlorambucil-induced pulmonary disease: a case report and review of the literature. *Ann Hematol*. 1998;77:85.
57 Alarcón GS, Kremer JM, Macaluso M, et al. Risk factors for methotrexate-induced lung injury in patients with rheumatoid arthritis. A multicenter, case-control study. Methotrexate-Lung Study Group. *Ann Intern Med*. 1997;127:356.
58. Kim YJ, Song M, Ryu JC. Inflammation in methotrexate-induced pulmonary toxicity occurs via the p38 MAPK pathway. *Toxicology*. 2009;256:183.
59. Kim YJ, Song M, Ryu JC. Mechanisms underlying methotrexate-induced pulmonary toxicity. *Expert Opin Drug Saf*. 2009;8:451.
60. Barlési F, Villani P, Doddoli C, et al. Gemcitabine-induced severe pulmonary toxicity. *Fundam Clin Pharmacol*. 2004;18:85.
61. Helman DL Jr, Byrd JC, Ales NC, Shorr AF. Fludarabine-related pulmonary toxicity: a distinct clinical entity in chronic lymphoproliferative syndromes. *Chest*. 2002;122:785.
62. Chen YB, Lane AA, Logan BR, et al. Impact of conditioning regimen on outcomes for patients with lymphoma undergoing high-dose therapy with autologous hematopoietic cell transplantation. *Biol Blood Marrow Transplant*. 2015;21:1046.
63. Rubio C, Hill ME, Milan S, et al. Idiopathic pneumonia syndrome after high-dose chemotherapy for relapsed Hodgkin's disease. *Br J Cancer*. 1997;75:1044.
64. Weinstein AS, Diener-West M, Nelson DF, Pakuris E. Pulmonary toxicity of carmustine in patients treated for malignant glioma. *Cancer Treat Rep*. 1986;70:943.
65. Gordon M, Jakubowski A, Frankel S, et al. Neutrophil (PMN) function in patients with acute promyelocytic leukemia (APL) treated with all-trans retinoic acid (ATRA) (abstract). *Proc Annu Meet Am Soc Clin Oncol*. 1991;10:A761.
66. Frankel SR, Eardley A, Heller G, et al. All-trans retinoic acid for acute promyelocytic leukemia. Results of the New York Study. *Ann Intern Med*. 1994;120:278.
67. Miyakoshi S, Kami M, Yuji K, et al. Severe pulmonary complications in Japanese patients after bortezomib treatment for refractory multiple myeloma. *Blood*. 2006;107:3492.
68. Zappasodi P, Dore R, Castagnola C, et al. Rapid response to high-dose steroids of severe bortezomib-related pulmonary complication in multiple myeloma. *J Clin Oncol*. 2007;25:3380.
69. Siegel DS, Martin T, Wang M, et al. A phase 2 study of single-agent carfilzomib (PX-171-003-A1) in patients with relapsed and refractory multiple myeloma. *Blood*. 2012;120:2817.
70. Vij R, Wang M, Kaufman JL, et al. An open-label, single-arm, phase 2 (PX-171-004) study of single-agent carfilzomib in bortezomib-naive patients with relapsed and/or refractory multiple myeloma. *Blood*. 2012;119:5661.
71. Chu E, DeVita V Jr. *Physician's Cancer Chemotherapy Drug Manual 2018*. 18th ed. Burlington, MA: Jones & Bartlett Learning; 2018.
72. Sanz MA, Martín G, González M, et al. Risk-adapted treatment of acute promyelocytic leukemia with all-trans-retinoic acid and anthracycline monochemotherapy: a multicenter study by the PETHEMA group. *Blood*. 2004;103:1237.
73. Wiley JS, Firkin FC. Reduction of pulmonary toxicity by prednisolone prophylaxis during all-trans retinoic acid treatment of acute promyelocytic leukemia. Australian Leukaemia Study Group. *Leukemia*. 1995;9:774.

CHAPTER 9

Dermatological Toxicities of Chemotherapy

Arjun Khunger, MD   Bassam Estfan, MD

Introduction

Chemotherapy can affect skin in various ways, and several chemotherapeutic agents have been linked to distinctive cutaneous side effects. Although these side effects are rarely life-threatening, they can cause considerable distress and discomfort to patients (alopecia, hyperpigmentation), negatively impacting their quality of life and sometimes leading to interruptions of treatment. Occasionally, cutaneous reactions may be associated with more serious systemic toxicity. Characteristics of these adverse events vary, depending on the chemotherapeutic drug and type of cancer. Some dermatological adverse effects, such as phototoxicity, can occur when chemotherapy drugs are combined with radiotherapy. Recognition of these reactions is important to both dermatologists and oncologists to allow for prompt initiation of appropriate management and for maintaining uninterrupted administration of chemotherapy. In this chapter, we discuss the specific dermatological complications associated with various chemotherapeutic agents and describe the general principles for the diagnosis and treatment of these complications.

Chemotherapy-Induced Alopecia

- **Hair growth cycle:** The hair growth cycle consists of three distinct phases: the growth phase (anagen phase), the deconstruction phase (catagen phase) and the resting phase (telogen phase).[1] Chemotherapy treatment can often result in alopecia affecting the scalp and other body hair attributed to the fact that most hair follicles are in the anagen phase, and chemotherapy can damage these actively dividing cells.[2]
- **Chemotherapy-induced alopecia (CIA):** CIA is a distressing side effect common to numerous treatment regimens in oncology. It has a negative influence on body image, psychosocial well-being, and may sometimes influence treatment decisions. A number of chemotherapy agents have been reported to cause CIA, as listed in Table 9.1. Various classes of drugs, including alkylating agents, anthracyclines, antimetabolites, antitumor antibiotics, vinca alkaloids, and taxanes are known to cause alopecia more readily.[3] Alopecia following chemotherapy occurs in two distinct patterns: anagen effluvium and telegenic effluvium.
  - **Anagen effluvium:** Anagen effluvium is the most commonly observed pattern. It occurs due to chemotherapeutic drugs targeting the active hair follicle in the anagen phase, inducing premature catagen transformation. This results in weakening of the hair shaft, making it prone to breakage and stops hair shaft formation. It presents as complete destruction of hair, thinning of hair, or hair becoming brittle. Because approximately 70% to 85% of hairs of an adult scalp are in anagen phase of hair growth, anagen effluvium can be quite distressing to patients.
  - **Telegen effluvium:** Telegen effluvium occurs due to malnutrition, fever, stress, and emotional distress following chemotherapy and presents as global hair loss.

TABLE 9.1 ■ **Chemotherapy Agents That Cause Alopecia and Their Severity**

Occurrence	Severe Alopecia	Moderate Alopecia	Mild Alopecia
Frequent	Doxorubicin Daunorubicin Cyclophosphamide Ifosfamide Docetaxel Paclitaxel Etoposide	Busulphan Methotrexate Mechlorethamine	Bleomycin Cisplatin
Infrequent	Vincristine Vinblastine Vinorelbine	Mitomycin Actinomycin	5-Fluorouracil Hydroxyurea

- CIA usually begins 2 to 4 weeks after the start of therapy, commonly at 7 to 10 days and peaks at around 1 to 2 months.[4] Hair loss occurs in a diffuse or patchy pattern, depending on the distribution of hairs in the active anagen growth phase. Diffuse or patching alopecia is noticeable when 25% to 40% of scalp hairs are shed. It may be sometimes associated with symptoms of pruritus or pain but is usually asymptomatic. Generally scalp hair is affected, but axillary, pubic hair, eyebrows, and body hair can also be affected. Near complete hair loss is often present by 2 to 3 months and continues for the duration of chemotherapy. A fraction of hairs may be spared that were in the telogen phase at the time of treatment. After chemotherapy is discontinued, the vast majority of patients will naturally regrow hair within 1 to 3 months.

- The severity or degree of alopecia depends on several factors, including the specific agent(s) used, chemotherapy dose, duration of therapy, and serum half-life of the drug. In general, CIA is more severe in patients on multi-agent regimens.[5] In addition, intravenous administration of chemotherapy is generally more deleterious than oral administration at an equivalent dose.

- Hair loss caused by chemotherapy is almost always reversible, although there have been reports of permanent alopecia after treatment with cyclophosphamide and busulfan before bone marrow transplantation.[6,7] More recently, cases of severe and irreversible alopecia following chemotherapy with taxanes have been reported in patients with breast cancer.[8,9] Although hair regrowth is generally the rule, it is important to counsel patients that regrowth is unpredictable and the thickness, color, or texture of their new hair may be different.[10,11]

- **Prevention and treatment of CIA:** So far, there has been limited success in the prevention and treatment of CIA. Use of a scarf or a wig seems to be the best practice adopted by patients. The use of scalp-cooling methods has been investigated for the past few decades in an attempt to lessen the severity of alopecia.[12,13] Scalp cooling is hypothesized to prevent chemotherapy-related alopecia by limiting blood flow to hair follicles during anticancer treatment, thus decreasing exposure to the chemotherapy. It is also hypothesized to decrease the metabolic rate of hair follicles, which may help reduce their susceptibility to the cytotoxic effects of chemotherapy. The primary concern that had limited the use of scalp hypothermia was the risk of scalp micro-metastases and it is generally advised that scalp hypothermia should not be used for patients with circulating malignant cells, such as leukemia or lymphoma, who are undergoing chemotherapy with curative intent.[14] More recently, two prospective studies of scalp-cooling systems have added evidence supporting the efficacy and safety of scalp cooling in the prevention of CIA, leading to US Food and Drug Administration (FDA) clearance of two scalp-cooling devices to prevent chemotherapy-related alopecia in patients with solid malignancies.[15,16] In both studies, patients with

TABLE 9.2 ■ Common Chemotherapeutic Agents Associated With Hypersensitivity Reactions

Drug	Hypersensitivity Reaction
L-Asparaginase	Type I
Bleomycin	Type I
Carboplatin	Type I
Cisplatin	Type I, II
Chlorambucil	Type I, II
Cyclophosphamide	Type I
Cytarabine	Type I
Docetaxel	Type I
Daunorubicin	Type I
Doxorubicin	Type I
Dacarbazine	Type I
Etoposide	Type I, III
5-Fluorouracil	Type I
Ifosfamide	Type I
Mechlorethamine (topical)	Type IV
Methotrexate	Type I, III
Mitomycin	Type I, III, IV
Paclitaxel	Type I
Procarbazine	Type III

breast cancer undergoing treatment with taxanes-based therapy were randomized to receive scalp cooling or placebo; scalp cooling was associated with prevention of significant hair loss in approximately 50% of patients. The adverse effect profile of scalp-cooling devices includes discomfort, headache, scalp pain, and chills, but these are generally tolerable for most patients, as observed in clinical trials.

■ **Pharmacologic interventions:** Multiple pharmacologic interventions for the prevention of CIA have been tested, including minoxidil, bimatoprost, and calcitriol. Minoxidil has been shown to decrease the duration of CIA and may be of some benefit in certain patients.[17,18] Further research is needed to determine significant improvements with the use of pharmacological agents for the treatment of CIA.

Hypersensitivity Reactions

Essentially all chemotherapy drugs have the potential to cause allergic or hypersensitivity reactions. However, in general, cutaneous hypersensitivity reactions occur infrequently and have been documented in approximately 5% of patients.[19] Certain chemotherapy agents such as L-asparaginase, paclitaxel, and mitomycin-C exhibit a high incidence of hypersensitivity reactions and may be severe enough to cause dose-limiting toxicity.[20] Table 9.2 lists chemotherapeutic agents associated with hypersensitivity reactions.

■ **Clinical presentation and treatment:** Hypersensitivity reactions are typically immune-mediated and have been divided into type I, II, III, and IV reactions. Most chemotherapy reactions are thought to be type I, immunoglobulin E (IgE)–mediated reactions. Clinically, patients with type I hypersensitivity reactions can present with a local reaction of erythema or pruritus that may or may not proceed to a life-threatening systemic, anaphylactic reaction. This type of reaction most often occurs within 1 hour of chemotherapy administration, but can occur up to 24 hours after exposure.[20] Patients may also complain of nausea, tightness of the chest, respiratory distress, urticaria or rash, and sometimes erythematous streaks along the affected vein. Type III hypersensitivity reactions, in contrast, are mediated by the formation of circulating antigen–antibody immune complexes and are delayed drug reactions. L-Asparaginase and procarbazine have been noted to cause urticarial reactions via a type III–mediated reaction pattern.[21] Allergic contact dermatitis represents a well-known type IV cell-mediated reaction. Mechlorethamine ranks as one of the major causes of type IV hypersensitivity reactions.[22] In the case of paclitaxel and several other chemotherapeutic agents, the diluent or solvent used to enhance the stability or solubility of the drug for intravenous administration may be responsible for the hypersensitivity reaction rather than the drug itself.[23] These reactions are anticipated and standard prophylaxis with corticosteroids, H2 antagonists, and antihistamines is generally required.[24]

- **Skin testing:** An intradermal skin test should be performed before the initial administration of certain chemotherapy drugs such as bleomycin or asparaginase because hypersensitivity reactions are frequently observed with these agents. However, it should be noted that a negative skin test reaction does not preclude the possibility of development of a hypersensitivity reaction. If reactions occur frequently enough, the agent may require routine prophylaxis using H1-antihistamines, H2-antihistamines, and systemic corticosteroids.
- **Continuation or cessation of therapy:** Once a hypersensitivity reaction is recognized, the issue of continuation and completion of therapy is raised. In the case of mild reactions, readministration by lowering the infusion rate and using premedication therapy can be considered. If equally efficacious non–cross-reacting alternative agents are available, they should be used. For example, replacement of carboplatin with cisplatin has been shown to allow for an efficacious continuation of platinum-containing chemotherapy after intradermal skin testing elicited positive and negative reactions to carboplatin and cisplatin, respectively.[25,26]

Acral Erythema

Acral erythema, palmoplantar erythrodysesthesia (PPE), or hand-foot syndrome is an adverse event caused by many classic chemotherapy agents and molecular targeted therapies. Doxorubicin, capecitabine, cytarabine, docetaxel, and 5-fluorouracil are the most commonly implicated agents.[27-30] Liposomal doxorubicin has also been associated with PPE, and as many as 48% of patients receiving the drug may be affected.[31] It is reported that this syndrome develops more often in patients *when* these agents *are* administered as continuous infusions compared with administration as bolus infusions. Other drugs causing acral erythema include bleomycin, cisplatin, cyclophosphamide, etoposide, gemcitabine, fludarabine, idarubicin, methotrexate, paclitaxel, and vinorelbine.[32-36] Table 9.3 lists the chemotherapy agents most commonly associated with acral erythema. The frequency varies from 6% to 42% of patients, and occurs almost exclusively in adults, but may also occur in children receiving high-dose methotrexate therapy.[37]

- **Pathophysiology:** It has been postulated that the pathophysiology of acral erythema is related to the small capillaries in the palms of the hands and the soles of feet that rupture due to significant exposure to friction and trauma from walking or use, resulting in an inflammatory reaction. PPE seems to be dose-dependent, and both the peak drug concentration and cumulative dose correlate with occurrence and severity. Lesions may develop 1 to 90 days after chemotherapy, and onset of symptoms is typically within 2 to 3 weeks of drug initiation.[38]
- **Clinical presentation:** The patient typically complains of a tingling, numbness, or burning sensation of the palms and soles after initiation of chemotherapy, followed by intense tenderness and/or pruritus and swelling. Subsequently, discrete red plaques develop on the

TABLE 9.3 ■ **Chemotherapy Drugs Most Commonly Associated With Acral Erythema**

Type	Drug
Alkylating agents	Cyclophosphamide
	Melphalan
	Thiotepa
Anthracyclines	Daunorubicin
	Doxorubicin (including liposomal doxorubicin)
	Idarubicin
Antimetabolites	5-Fluorouracil
	Capecitabine
	Methotrexate
	Cytarabine
	Hydroxyurea
	Mercaptopurine
Vinca alkaloids	Vincristine
	Vinblastine
Platinum compounds	Cisplatin
Taxanes	Docetaxel
	Paclitaxel
Other mitotic inhibitors	Bleomycin
	Etoposide
	Mitomycin

thenar and hypothenar eminences and on the distil fat pads, which may spread to the dorsum of the hands and feet (Fig. 9.1).[39] Periungual erythema and erythematous bands over the joint surfaces may occur. In severe cases, it may be followed by the formation of desquamative vesicles or bullae.[40] The palms are typically affected more than the feet and may be the only location of the syndrome in some cases. Re-epithelization can occur as part of the healing process, after withdrawal of the offending agent.

■ **Differential diagnosis:** Early graft-versus-host disease of the hands and feet should be considered in the differential diagnosis and is sometimes difficult to distinguish, especially in patients who have undergone bone marrow transplantation. Serial biopsies performed 3 to 5 days apart may help in differentiating the two disorders, allowing for appropriate management.

■ **Treatment:** The management of acral erythema is largely symptomatic with reduction of drug doses where appropriate. Administration of analgesics, elevation of the extremities, and regional cooling with ice packs, may help ease symptoms. Cold immersion of the hands and feet may also decrease the severity of the syndrome, presumably secondary to vasoconstriction resulting in a lower peak drug concentration being delivered to the extremities.[41] The use of emollients, creams containing lanolin, or urea, or protective gloves may also be helpful in prevention and treatment of acral erythema.[42] The use of pyridoxine and corticosteroids has been reported to be beneficial anecdotally in relieving the associated dysesthesia.[43–45] Patients should be encouraged to communicate all signs of PPE because early recognition and intervention are essential. In addition, patients should be advised to avoid activities that may increase pressure on the soles and palms.[46] Some patients may resume their chemotherapy regimen after symptom improvement, potentially with chemotherapy dose reduction. There are usually no long-term effects of acral erythema.

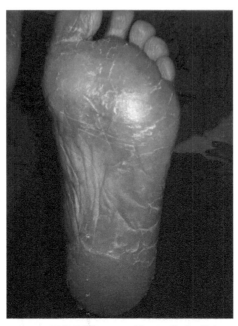

Fig. 9.1 Hand-foot syndrome as a result of 5-fluorouracil in a patient with breast cancer. (From Miller KK, Gorcey L, McLellan BN. Chemotherapy-induced hand-foot syndrome and nail changes: a review of clinical presentation, etiology, pathogenesis, and management. *J Am Acad Dermatol*. 2014;71[4]:787–794.)

Extravasation

Extravasation refers to the escape of a chemotherapeutic drug from a blood vessel to the surrounding tissues, either by leakage or by direct infiltration, causing significant damage to the skin.[47] The true incidence of chemotherapy extravasation varies greatly due to underestimation, but the prevalence of such events is estimated to be 0.1% to 6%, with a higher frequency in children.[48] The severity of tissue injury is dependent on the chemotherapeutic agent used and the concentration of the administered drug.[49] Cytotoxic agents can be classified based on their potential for local toxicity as irritants or vesicants.

- **Irritants:** An irritant is defined as an agent that produces a local inflammatory reaction, aching, tightness, pain, or phlebitis, at the injection site or along the vein.[50] Clinical signs and symptoms include local sclerosis and hyperpigmentation as well as burning, warmth, erythema, and tenderness in the extravasated area. Necrosis is rare. These symptoms are usually short-lived and self-limited, and most resolve without any long-lasting sequelae.[21] The drugs most frequently associated with this complication are bleomycin, carboplatin, docetaxel, etoposide, topotecan, and dexrasoxane.[51]
- **Vesicants:** Vesicants are chemotherapeutic agents that have the potential to cause more severe and lasting tissue injury, including the ability to induce tissue necrosis. A number of chemotherapy agents such as actinomycin D, daunorubicin, doxorubicin, mitomycin C, vinca alkaloids, cisplatin, and paclitaxel are classified as vesicants.[51] The early manifestations are often subtle and the full effect of the extravasation injury may be delayed for several days to weeks.[52] The initial signs and symptoms may resemble

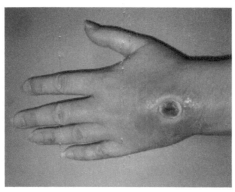

Fig. 9.2 Full-thickness skin necrosis presenting 48 hours following chemotherapy extravasation. (From Goutos I, Cogswell LK, Giele H. Extravasation injuries: a review. *J Hand Surg Eur*. 2014;39:808–818.)

those of an irritant extravasation injury, including local burning, mild erythema, pruritus, and swelling. An alteration in the rate of infusion or cessation of blood return on aspiration are additional indications of potential extravasation injury.[53] Within 2 to 3 days, increased erythema, pain, induration, dry desquamation, or blistering may appear. If the amount of extravasated material is small, these symptoms may disappear over the ensuing weeks.[54] If the extravasation is significant, necrosis, eschar formation, and ulceration with raised, red, painful edges and a necrotic yellow base may appear (Fig. 9.2). Studies have estimated that about one third of vesicant extravasation injuries may eventually progress to tissue ulceration.[55] Ulceration after vesicant extravasation is typically marked by delayed healing. In severe cases, necrosis may involve underlying tissues such as tendons, nerves, and vessels, with the possibility of serious complications, including nerve compression syndromes, contractures, permanent joint stiffness, and residual sympathetic dystrophies.[50] Other rare manifestations include cellulitis, abscess formation, and squamous cell carcinoma.[54,56]

- **Evaluation and treatment:** Extravasation injury should be presumed in any patient with persistent swelling, erythema, or pain and prompt recognition and treatment of extravasation injury are necessary to prevent the development of delayed complications. Evidence of extravasation injury requires immediate cessation of the infusion. The site should be aspirated for the residual drug before removing the intravenous catheter.[54] Additionally, attempts at aspiration of the extravasated agent in the surrounding tissue should be made to limit the extent of tissue damage. Elevation of the affected limb and local application of hot or cold packs have been shown to be helpful in limiting the extent of tissue damage.[57] The application of hot packs is hypothesized to cause local vasodilation, leading to dilution of the extravasated drug. Conversely, cold packs may cause increased degradation of toxic metabolites through vasoconstriction and localization of the drug, in addition to reducing local inflammation and providing pain relief. In the event of extravasation of vinca alkaloids heat should be applied to the affected site. Cold packs should not be administered because cold has been found to increase ulceration after vinca alkaloid extravasation in animal models.[58]

- **Antidotes:** Many studies have investigated the usefulness of antidotes to different chemotherapeutic agents for the prevention of necrosis and ulceration at the site of extravasation.[59] These include topical dimethylsulfoxide (DMSO) for anthracycline extravasation, hyaluronidase for vinca alkaloid and etoposide extravasation, and sodium thiosulfate for mechlorethamine, concentrated dacarbazine, and concentrated cisplatin extravasation.[58,60–62] Currently, dexrazoxane hydrochloride is an FDA–approved treatment for anthracycline extravasation and has been reported to produce significant wound healing activity.[63] High-dose steroids can be used for the extravasation of oxaliplatin but are contraindicated for etoposide and vinca alkaloids, because steroids can worsen skin damage associated with these agents.
- **Surgical intervention:** For persistent or progressive local symptoms, a surgical consult should be obtained because the treatment of unresolved tissue necrosis or pain lasting more than 10 days is surgical debridement. Such a procedure should consist of wide excision of all necrotic tissue until bleeding occurs and only healthy tissue is left for would coverage. Once the wound is clean, immediate or delayed surgical reconstruction and skin grafting can be employed.

Hyperpigmentation

Hyperpigmentation of the skin, hair, mucous membranes, and nails is another common cutaneous manifestation of chemotherapy. It may occur in various anatomic locations and increased pigmentation may be present locally, such as at the site of drug infusion, or diffusely.

- **Mechanism:** The mechanism of this adverse effect has not been fully elucidated, but is believed to be a result of direct toxic effects on melanocytes, stimulating increased melanin secretion.[64]
- **Patterns of hyperpigmentation:** A variety of patterns of hyperpigmentation have been described in association with different chemotherapy agents (Table 9.4).
- **Irregular hyperpigmentation:** Irregular and patchy cutaneous hyperpigmentation is seen following the use of 5-fluorouracil. Cyclophosphamide may be associated with the development of generalized hyperpigmentation of the face and extremities[65] and nail pigmentation.[66]
- **Supravenous hyperpigmentation:** Docetaxel induces a peculiar serpentine supravenous hyperpigmentation, possibly as a result of postinflammatory hyperpigmentation over the vein through which it is infused.[67,68] Unlike clot-forming thrombophlebitis, supravenous hyperpigmentation is characterized by patent underlying vessels. Other chemotherapy agents, including 5-fluoruracil, vinorelbine, and fotemustine, have also been associated with the development of serpentine supravenous hyperpigmentation.[69,70]
- **Nail hyperpigmentation:** Nail hyperpigmentation in the form of longitudinal, transverse or diffuse melanonychia have been observed with the use of hydroxyurea.[71,72] Anthracyclines have also been associated with hyperpigmentation of nails in a diffuse pattern of transverse bands,[73] and in mucocutaneous hyperpigmentation.[74]
- **Flagellate hyperpigmentation:** Perhaps the most unique pattern, *flagellate* hyperpigmentation, which is accompanied by intense pruritus, is induced by bleomycin (Fig. 9.3).[75,76] The most common areas of pigmentation include pressure points such as fingers, elbows, or knees, although generalized hyperpigmentation is also observed. Transverse bands and linear streaks on the nails have been reported with bleomycin. A more diffuse darkening of the skin is seen in patients receiving busulfan that may resemble Addison's disease and is informally referred to as the *busulfan tan*.[77]
- **Other forms of hyperpigmentation:** Methotrexate administered weekly can cause *flag sign*, the hyperpigmented bands alternating with the normal color of the patient's hair.[78] Other drugs that can cause different patterns of hyperpigmentation include cisplatin, ifosfamide, mithramycin, etoposide, paclitaxel, and vinca alkaloids.[79–82]

TABLE 9.4 ■ **Chemotherapeutic Agents Associated With Hyperpigmentation**

Drug	Presentation	Course
Alkylating Agents		
Busulfan	Generalized brown or dusky hyperpigmentation; may resemble Addison's disease	May fade or persist after discontinuation of drug
Cyclophosphamide	Generalized skin hyperpigmentation or patchy involvement of nails (transverse, longitudinal or diffuse), palms/soles, or teeth; Rare bands of permanent pigmentation of gingival margin	Fades after 6 months to 1 year after discontinuation of drug
Ifosfamide	Pigment changes on acral surfaces such as dorsal and plantar surfaces of hands and feet, extensor surfaces of toes and finger	Variable course: hyperpigmentation may fade despite continuation of treatment or may persist despite cessation of therapy
Cisplatin	Localized hyperpigmentation; hyperpigmentation at sites of pressure including elbows, knees, neck, sites of trauma	Thought to be permanent but may decrease in intensity with time
Antimetabolites		
5-Fluorouracil	Hyperpigmentation in sub-exposed areas; serpentine supravenous hyperpigmentation after repeated transfusions; hyperpigmented brown, serpentine streaks on back and buttocks; acral pigmentation; transverse banding of the nails	Immediate reaction after sun exposure; hyperpigmentation may persist for few months; no recurrence of lesions with continued treatment
Methotrexate (MTX)	Horizontal hair banding (flag sign)	Corresponds with weekly MTX therapy; normal hair reappears during drug-free intervals
Antitumor Antibiotics		
Bleomycin	Flagellate hyperpigmentation: linear bandlike, or flagellate streaks, associated with minor trauma	Pigmentation fades soon after discontinuation of therapy but can persist as long as 6 months
Dactinomycin	Diffuse hyperpigmentation or sometimes intertriginous, trauma-induced hyperpigmentation	Resolves few months after discontinuation of therapy
Daunorubicin	Diffuse hyperpigmentation; transverse pigmented nail bands; polycyclic pigmentation of scalp (rare)	Completely disappears after 6–8 weeks of discontinuation of therapy. Hyperpigmentation may reappear after rechallenge of the drug
Doxorubicin	Localized hyperpigmentation of the nails, palms and soles, dorsal hands, face, and interphalangeal and palmar creases; diffuse blue-gray pigmentation (less common); horizontal or longitudinal nail bands	Resolves after discontinuation of drug
Mithramycin	Postinflammatory facial hyperpigmentation after flushing and facial edema	Gradually clears with mild desquamation
Mitotic Inhibitors		
Paclitaxel	Localized reticulate hyperpigmentation	Pigmentation fades after 2–3 months of discontinuation of therapy
Docetaxel	Serpentine, supravenous hyperpigmentation	Resolves after few months of drug discontinuation
Etoposide	Hyperpigmentation in occluded areas	
Miscellaneouos Agents		
Hydroxyurea	Generalized hyperpigmentation; longitudinal nail bands (less common); macular hyperpigmentation of tongue and buccal mucosa	
Vinorelbine	Serpentine, supravenous hyperpigmentation	

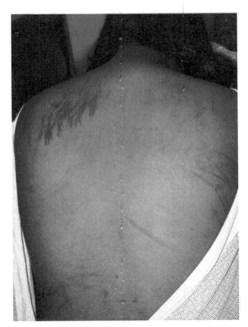

Fig. 9.3   Flagellate hyperpigmentation from bleomycin. (From Huang V, Anadkat M. Dermatologic manifestations of cytotoxic therapy. *Dermatol Ther*. 2011;24[4]:401–410.)

- **Treatment and resolution:** Although hyperpigmentation may be psychologically distressing for some patients, it begins to fade slowly over several months after the chemotherapy drug is discontinued. Generally, no additional intervention is required following onset of hyperpigmentation and administration of chemotherapy regimens should not be affected. 5-Fluorouracil–associated hyperpigmentation has been reported to resolve after 2 to 3 months following completion of treatment.[82] Postinflammatory hyperpigmentation is expected to resolve over a few months to years. Patients may be advised about sun avoidance and photo-protection using sunscreens to minimize progression of pigmentation. Topical retinoids may sometimes be beneficial to stimulate rapid turnover of keratinocytes, with subsequent loss of melanin. Supravenous hyperpigmentation resolves with time but may induce a flare with repeated treatments. No intervention is generally required, and topical bleaching agents such as hydroquinone may not provide any significant benefit. In case of nail hyperpigmentation, the pattern of pigmentation is noted to resolve with nail growth after a few months.

Photosensitivity

Increased sensitivity to sun exposure may be manifested in patients receiving chemotherapy, following intentional or unintentional ultraviolet (UV) exposure. Most of these photosensitivity reactions resemble an exaggerated sunburn, with findings of erythema, edema, pruritus, and/or pain at the site of exposure. Superficial desquamation, and occasionally, blister formation may occur in more severe cases. Subsequent hyperpigmentation may be observed following the disappearance of eruptions.

Photosensitive eruptions can be triggered by a variety of chemotherapeutic agents. Phototoxicity caused by dacarbazine, doxorubicin, fluorouracil (systemic and topical), tegafur, and vinblastine are well documented.[83,84]

- **Fluorouracil** can cause enhanced sunburn, photodistributed hyperpigmentation, and subacute cutaneous lupus erythematosus.[85,86]
- **Tegafur,** a fluorouracil derivative, may cause lichenoid and eczematous photodistributed eruptions.[87]
- **Capecitabine** is implicated to cause a photodistributed lichenoid eruption, though it is considered less photosensitizing than fluorouracil and may be used alternatively for patients unable to tolerate fluorouracil due to photosensitivity.[88]
- **Paclitaxel** has been implicated to cause photodistributed erythema multiforme, photo-oncolysis, and elevated protoporphyrin levels.[89]
- **Hydroxyurea** is reported to cause a photodistributed granulomatous reaction.[90]
- **Diagnosis:** The diagnosis of photosensitivity is aided when the eruptions are noted primarily in sun-exposed areas such as the face, posterior neck, anterior "V" of the chest (upper medial region), dorsum of the arms, and anterior portions of the legs, with a sharp demarcation between involved and uninvolved sites. However, in case of doubt, diagnostic tests such as phototesting, photopatch testing, clinical rechallenge, or rechallenge phototesting can also be performed.
- **Treatment:** Treatment includes discontinuation of the chemotherapy agent and complete avoidance of direct sunlight for at least 2 weeks. Patients receiving the aforementioned drugs should be advised to avoid sunlight exposure and use broad-spectrum sunscreens with protection against both UVA and UVB. Other measures that may be helpful in the treatment of eruptions includes cold compresses, systemic antihistamines, topical or systemic corticosteroids, and calcineurin inhibitors (e.g., tacrolimus, pimecrolimus), depending on the severity of the eruptions. As such, treatment of the eruption should be initiated promptly.
- **Porphyrins:** Porphyrins are photosensitizing agents used for photodynamic therapy in the treatment of solid tumors. Patients undergoing treatment with porphyrins are at great risk for photoxicity, even after taking precautions to prevent UV exposure, including bright lights. In addition, photosensitivity due to porphyrins is of longer duration, and may last up to 6 weeks following discontinuation of therapy.
- **Photo-onycholysis:** Nails can be affected by exposure to UV light in a process called *photo-onycholysis* in which the distal third of the nail plate gets separated from the nail bed. This effect has been reported with the use of mercaptopurine.[91]

Radiation Recall

Radiation recall (radiation dermatitis) refers to the phenomenon in which the initiation of chemotherapy incites an inflammatory reaction confined to previously irradiated areas. The reaction can be cutaneous (more commonly) or systemic. Involved organs may include the skin and mucous membranes, heart, lungs, esophagus, gastrointestinal tract, bladder, and central nervous system. The exact incidence of radiation recall is not well documented; however, it is estimated to affect 2% to 12% of patients receiving chemotherapy after radiotherapy.[92,93]

- **Implicated agents:** The classic culprits associated with radiation recall are doxorubicin[94] and dactinomycin[95]; however, recall dermatitis has been documented after the use of several chemotherapeutic agents, including dacarbazine, paclitaxel, docetaxel, pemetrexed, and methotrexate (Table 9.5).[96–99]

TABLE 9.5 ■ Chemotherapeutic Agents Implicated With Radiation Recall Phenomenon

Type	Drug
Alkylating agents	Cyclophosphamide
	Melphalan
Anthracyclines	Daunorubicin
	Doxorubicin
Antimetabolites	5-Fluorouracil
	Cytarabine
	Gemcitabine
	Hydroxyurea
Taxanes	Docetaxel
	Paclitaxel
Vinca alkaloids	Vinblastine
Other mitotic inhibitors	Bleomycin
	Etoposide
	Mitomycin

- **Presentation:** Radiation recall dermatitis may occur anywhere from 8 days to even 15 years after radiation therapy, and symptoms may manifest within hours to days after chemotherapy administration.[93,100] With intravenous administration, symptoms can precipitate during or immediately after the first dose of drug administration. In contrast, radiation recall may not become evident until months or years after oral administration of the chemotherapeutic agent.[101] Mild reactions are typically characterized by a painless or painful erythema. Desquamation, edema, or pruritus similar to first-degree burns may or may not occur. Severe reactions are associated with painful blistering, necrosis, or ulceration.[101] The surrounding skin appears normal without any redness or tenderness. The severity of the reaction appears to be associated with the interval between radiation therapy and initiation of chemotherapy, with shorter time intervals resulting in more severe reactions.[102] Previous use of higher doses of radiation also appears to correlate with a greater severity of recall dermatitis.
- **Mechanism:** The exact mechanism of the reaction remains unknown but may be linked to altered inflammatory pathways. Radiation may lower the inflammatory response threshold, whereas chemotherapy may upregulate the production of inflammatory cytokines, leading to severe reactions.[92]
- **Management:** Management is usually supportive, and mild cases of dermatitis generally clear without treatment. Cold or ice packs and ointments may provide relief of symptoms. Topical or systemic corticosteroids may significantly improve symptoms of dermatitis, potentially allowing for continuation of the chemotherapy treatment. In severe cases, the chemotherapeutic agent should be discontinued while the skin recovers from the reaction. Radiation-induced necrotic ulcers are slow to heal. Although radiation recall will improve once the offending agent is discontinued, a rechallenge with the same drug may induce a recurrence of the symptoms; hence it is not recommended to readminister the chemotherapeutic agent unless absolutely necessary.[92]

Nail Changes

Nail changes are often observed with the same frequency as other mucocutaneous side effects with the administration of numerous chemotherapeutic agents. The epithelium of the nail matrix is made up of rapidly proliferating cells that differentiate to generate the nail plate and is acutely sensitive to the cytotoxic effects of chemotherapy.[103] Damage to the nail matrix from chemotherapy results in defective nail plate production, leading to structural changes in the nail plate.[103] The severity of nail changes varies greatly. They may range from cosmetic concerns such as hyperpigmentation or ridging of the nail plate to serious changes including onycholysis, acute paronychia, and onychomadesis. More serious consequences include pain, which can impair activities of daily living, and secondary infection.

- **Implicated agents:** Taxanes and anthracyclines are the most commonly implicated drugs in chemotherapy-induced nail toxicities.[103] A recent study estimated that the all-grade incidence of taxane-induced nail changes was 43.7% with paclitaxel, and 34.9% with docetaxel.[104] Other drugs known to induce various nail toxicities include 5-fluorouracil, capecitabine, cytarabine, hydroxyurea, and bleomycin.[105] An overview of nail changes associated with chemotherapy is provided in Table 9.6.
- **Nail hyperpigmentation:** Nail hyperpigmentation is the most commonly observed chemotherapy-induced nail toxicity.[106] It generally occurs 3 to 8 weeks after initiation of treatment and may present as longitudinal, horizontal, or diffuse bands.[21] It is usually associated with the use of doxorubicin, 5-fluorouracil, and cyclophosphamide[107–109] and is more commonly seen in patients undergoing combination therapy. Pigmentary changes are seen secondary to the damage to the nail matrix melanocytes by the offending chemotherapeutic agents, which seem to be independent of adrenocorticotropic hormone (ACTH), melanocyte-stimulating hormone (MSH), and UV light.
- **Beau's lines:** Beau's lines are white transverse ridges presenting in the nail. They occur almost as often as pigmentary changes. The furrows arise from toxic damage to the nail matrix and correspond to cycles of chemotherapy, typically spaced 2 to 3 mm apart.[110] The ridges move distally with nail growth and disappear with nail outgrowth after chemotherapy is discontinued. The pathogenesis of transverse ridges is hypothesized to be secondary to a transient arrest in nail plate growth following exposure to chemotherapy. Docetaxel, doxorubicin, vincristine, and cyclophosphamide have all been implicated as common causative agents of transverse white nail banding.[111]
- **Onychomadesis:** If there is complete inhibition of nail growth for about 2 weeks, it leads to disrupted continuity between the nail and nail bed, and ultimately to onychomadesis. This is seen with the use of taxanes[112] and capecitabine.[113,114]
- **Onycholysis:** Onycholysis refers to the distal detachment of the nail plate from the nail bed.[115] Areas of separation appear white or yellow due to air beneath the nail (Fig. 9.4). It

TABLE 9.6 ■ **Chemotherapeutic Agents Associated With Nail Toxicity**

Type	Drug	Presentation
Alkylating agents	Cyclophosphamide	Beau's lines, onychodystrophy
Anthracyclines	Daunorubicin	Mees' lines
	Doxorubicin	Beau lines, onycholysis
Antimetabolites	5-Fluorouracil	Onycholysis
	Capecitabine	Oncholysis
	Cytarabine	Mees' lines
		Onychodystrophy
Taxanes	Docetaxel	Beau's lines, onycholysis, subungual suppuration, subungual hemorrhage
	Paclitaxel	Oncholysis
Other mitotic inhibitors	Bleomycin	Beau's lines, nail loss and shedding, onycholysis

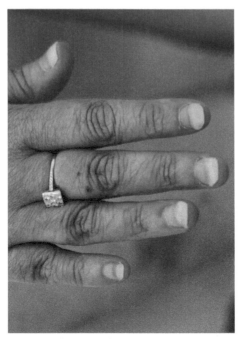

Fig. 9.4 Taxane-induced onycholysis. (From Miller KK, Gorcey L, McLellan BN. Chemotherapy-induced hand-foot syndrome and nail changes: a review of clinical presentation, etiology, pathogenesis, and management. *J Am Acad Dermatol.* 2014;71[4]:787–794.)

tends to occur most commonly on the great toes. It has been associated with the use of mitoxantrone, 5-fluorouracil, doxorubicin, and paclitaxel.[116–118] Both docetaxel and paclitaxel can cause painful or suppurative onycholysis.[119]

- **Differential diagnosis:** Nail changes associated with chemotherapy appear several weeks after drug administration, due to the slow growth rate of the nail plate[117] and can sometimes be mistaken for tinea unguium. Eliciting a history of chemotherapy administration usually establishes the correct diagnosis, but testing nail clippings for potassium-hydroxide, or testing by fungal culture or periodic acid Schiff stain, can help rule out other common nail disorders.
- **Treatment:** There is no established optimal treatment for chemotherapy-induced nail changes. These changes generally reverse within a few months of stopping chemotherapy. There are no recommendations for the prevention of nail changes. Patients must be educated about potential nail toxicities because undue anxiety about nail changes may impact the continuation of chemotherapy and treatment of patients. Foot care should be carried out, and appropriate hygiene measures should be adopted to prevent the chance of secondary infection. In case of pain, pain management is a major goal because nail conditions can be exquisitely painful. Antibiotics may need to be administered when deemed appropriate by culture results. Cryotherapy has been proposed as a means of reducing the incidence of onycholysis, similar to the scalp-cooling systems for prevention of chemotherapy-induced alopecia, and results of the preliminary studies have been encouraging.[120] Previously, frozen glove insertion was tested during docetaxel injection to prevent nail toxicities and results demonstrated significantly reduced and delayed nail toxicity, with onycholysis occurring in only 11% of treated patients as opposed to 51% of untreated subjects.[121]

Conclusion

Dermatological toxicities of chemotherapy are common and distressing side effects and despite their temporary nature, the morbidity of dermatological toxicities continues to be a central issue for patients. Before starting any chemotherapy regimen, it is essential to discuss the impact of various possible cutaneous side effects, and potential alternative approaches with the patient, to avoid any unnecessary interruptions in chemotherapy. Patient handouts and internet site referrals may also be valuable to patients. If dermatological toxicity develops, a multidisciplinary approach to management, with more frequent physician interactions and subspecialty referrals may be beneficial and may help maximize the efficacy of proposed chemotherapy treatment.

References

1. Paus R. Principles of hair cycle control. *J Dermatol*. 1998;25(12):793–802.
2. Paus RG, Cotsarelis G. The biology of hair follicles. *N Engl J Med*. 1999;341(7):491–497.
3. Batchelor D. Hair and cancer chemotherapy: consequences and nursing care—a literature study. *Eur J Cancer Care*. 2001;10(3):147–163.
4. Chon SY, Champion RW, Geddes ER, Rashid RM. Chemotherapy-induced alopecia. *J Am Acad Dermatol*. 2012;67(1),e37–e47.
5. Trueb RM. Chemotherapy-induced hair loss. *Skin Ther Lett*. 2010;15(7):5–7.
6. Ljungman P, Hassan M, Békássy AN, Ringdén O, Oberg G. Busulfan concentration in relation to permanent alopecia in recipients of bone marrow transplants. *Bone Marrow Transplant*. 1995;15(6):869–871.
7. Tran D, Sinclair RD, Schwarer AP, Chow CW. Permanent alopecia following chemotherapy and bone marrow transplantation. *Australas J Dermatol*. 2000;41(2):106–108.
8. Prevezas C, Matard B, Pinquier L, Reygagne P. Irreversible and severe alopecia following docetaxel or paclitaxel cytotoxic therapy for breast cancer. *Br J Dermatol*. 2009;160(4):883–885.
9. Tallon B, Blanchard E, Goldberg LJ. Permanent chemotherapy-induced alopecia: case report and review of the literature. *J Am Acad Dermatol*. 2010;63(2):333–336.
10. Fairlamb DJ. Hair changes following cytotoxic drug induced alopecia. *Postgrad Med J*. 1988;64(757):907.
11. Yun SJ, Kim S-J. Hair loss pattern due to chemotherapy-induced anagen effluvium: a cross-sectional observation. *Dermatology*. 2007;215(1):36–40.
12. Grevelman EG, Breed WPM. Prevention of chemotherapy-induced hair loss by scalp cooling. *Ann Oncol*. 2005;16(3):352–358.
13. Mols F, van den Hurk CJ, Vingerhoets AJ, Breed WP. Scalp cooling to prevent chemotherapy-induced hair loss: practical and clinical considerations. *Support Care Cancer*. 2008;17(2):181–189.
14. Forsberg SA. Scalp cooling therapy and cytotoxic treatment. *Lancet*. 2001;357(9262):1134.
15. Nangia J, Wang T, Osborne C, et al. Effect of a scalp cooling device on alopecia in women undergoing chemotherapy for breast cancer: the SCALP randomized clinical trial. *JAMA*. 2017;317(6):596–605.
16. Rugo HS, et al. Association between use of a scalp cooling device and alopecia after chemotherapy for breast cancer. *JAMA*. 2017;317(6):606–614.
17. Rodriguez R, Machiavelli M, Leone B, et al. Minoxidil (Mx) as a prophylaxis of doxorubicin–induced alopecia. *Ann Oncol*. 1994;5(8):769–770.
18. Duvic M, Lemak NA, Valero V, et al. A randomized trial of minoxidil in chemotherapy-induced alopecia. *J Am Acad Dermatol*. 1996;35(1):74–78.
19. Gobel BH. Chemotherapy-induced hypersensitivity reactions. *Oncol Nurs Forum*. 2005;32(5):1027–1035.
20. Weiss RB, Baker Jr JR. Hypersensitivity reactions from antineoplastic agents. *Cancer Metastasis Rev*. 1987;6(3):413–432.
21. Susser WS, Whitaker-Worth DL, Grant-Kels JM. Mucocutaneous reactions to chemotherapy. *J Am Acad Dermatol*. 1999;40(3):367–398.
22. Coyle T, Bushunow P, Winfield J, Wright J, Graziano S. Hypersensitivity reactions to procarbazine with mechlorethamine, vincristine, and procarbazine chemotherapy in the treatment of glioma. *Cancer*. 1992;69(10):2532–2540.
23. Weiss RB, Donehower RC, Wiernik PH, et al. Hypersensitivity reactions from taxol. *J Clin Oncol*. 1990;8(7):1263–1268.

24. Shepherd GM. Hypersensitivity reactions to chemotherapeutic drugs. *Clin Rev Allergy Immunol.* 2003;24(3):253–262.
25. Porzio G, Marchetti P, Paris I, Narducci F, Ricevuto E, Ficorella C. Hypersensitivity reaction to carboplatin: successful resolution by replacement with cisplatin. *Eur J Gynaecol Oncol.* 2002;23(4):335–336.
26. Libra M, Sorio R, Buonadonna A, et al. Cisplatin may be a valid alternative approach in ovarian carcinoma with carboplatin hypersensitivity. Report of three cases. *Tumori.* 2003;89(3):311–313.
27. Pirisi M, Soardo G. Chemotherapy-induced acral erythema. *N Engl J Med.* 1994;330(18):1279.
28. Cetkovska P, Pizinger K, Cetkovský P. High-dose cytosine arabinoside-induced cutaneous reactions. *J Eur Acad Dermatol Venereol.* 2002;16(5):481–485.
29. Zimmerman GC, Keeling JH, Burris HA, et al. Acute cutaneous reactions to docetaxel, a new chemotherapeutic agent. *Arch Dermatol.* 1995;131(2):202–206.
30. Janusch M, Fischer M, WCh Marsch, Holzhausen HJ, Kegel T, Helmbold P. The hand-foot syndrome—a frequent secondary manifestation in antineoplastic chemotherapy. *Eur J Dermatol.* 2006;16(5):494–499.
31. Lotem M, Hubert A, Lyass O, et al. Skin toxic effects of polyethylene glycol-coated liposomal doxorubicin. *Arch Dermatol.* 2000;136(12):1475–1480.
32. Laack E, Mende T, Knuffmann C, Hossfeld DK. Hand-foot syndrome associated with short infusions of combination chemotherapy with gemcitabine and vinorelbine. *Ann Oncol.* 2001;12(12):1761–1763.
33. Feizy V, Namazi MR, Barikbin B, Ehsani A. Methotrexate-induced acral erythema with bullous reaction. *Dermatol Online J.* 2003;9(1):14.
34. Portal I, Cardenal F, Garcia-del-Muro X. Etoposide-related acral erythema. *Cancer Chemother Pharmacol.* 1994;34(2):181.
35. Vakalis D, Ioannides D, Lazaridou E, Mattheou-Vakali G, Teknetzis A. Acral erythema induced by chemotherapy with cisplatin. *Br J Dermatol.* 1998;139(4):750–751.
36. Hoff PM, Valero V, Ibrahim N, Willey J, Hortobagyi GN. Hand-foot syndrome following prolonged infusion of high doses of vinorelbine. *Cancer.* 1998;82(5):965–969.
37. Hueso L, Sanmartín O, Nagore E, et al. [Chemotherapy-induced acral erythema: a clinical and histopathologic study of 44 cases.] *Actas Dermosifiliogr.* 2008;99(4):281–290.
38. Bastida J. Chemotherapy-induced acral erythema due to Tegafur. *Acta Derm Venereol.* 1997;77:72–73.
39. Demirçay Z, Gürbüz O, Alpdoğan TB, et al. Chemotherapy-induced acral erythema in leukemic patients: a report of 15 cases. *Int J Dermatol.* 1997;36(8):593–598.
40. Waltzer JF, Flowers FP. Bullous variant of chemotherapy-induced acral erythema. *Arch Dermatol.* 1993;129(1):43–45.
41. Zimmerman GC, Keeling JH, Lowry M, Medina J, Von Hoff DD, Burris HA. Prevention of docetaxel-induced erythrodysesthesia with local hypothermia. *J Natl Cancer Inst.* 1994;86(7):557–558.
42. Pendharkar D, Goyal H. Novel and effective management of capecitabine-induced hand-foot syndrome. *J Clin Oncol.* 2004;22(14 suppl):8105.
43. Brown J, Burck K, Black D, Collins C. Treatment of cytarabine acral erythema with corticosteroids. *J Am Acad Dermatol.* 1991;24(6):1023–1025.
44. Vukelja SJ, Baker WJ, Burris HA 3rd, Keeling JH, Von Hoff D. Pyridoxine therapy for palmar-plantar erythrodysesthesia associated with taxotere. *J Natl Cancer Inst.* 1993;85(17):1432–1433.
45. Chen M, Zhang L, Wang Q, Shen J. Pyridoxine for prevention of hand-foot syndrome caused by chemotherapy: a systematic review. *PLoS One.* 2013;8(8):e72245.
46. Webster-Gandy JD, How C, Harrold K. Palmar–plantar erythrodysesthesia (PPE): a literature review with commentary on experience in a cancer centre. *Eur J Oncol Nurs.* 2007;11(3):238–246.
47. Hadaway L. Infiltration and extravasation. *Am J Nurs.* 2007;107(8):64–72.
48. Kreidieh FY, Moukadem HA, El Saghir NS. Overview, prevention and management of chemotherapy extravasation. *World J Clin Oncol.* 2016;7(1):87–97.
49. Davis ME, DeSantis D, Klemm K. A flow sheet for follow-up after chemotherapy extravasation. *Oncology Nurs Forum.* 1995;22(6):979–983.
50. Boyle D, Engelking C. Vesicant extravasation: myths and realities. *Oncol Nurs Forum.* 1995;22(1):57–67.
51. Langer SW. Extravasation of chemotherapy. *Curr Oncol Rep.* 2010;12(4):242–246.
52. Hannon MG, Lee SK. Extravasation injuries. *J Hand Surg Am.* 2011;36(12):2060–2065.
53. Shenaq SM, Abbase E-HA, Friedman JD. Soft-tissue reconstruction following extravasation of chemotherapeutic agents. *Surg Oncol Clin N Am.* 1996;5(4):825–846.

54. Rudolph R, Larson DL. Etiology and treatment of chemotherapeutic agent extravasation injuries: a review. *J Clin Oncol.* 1987;5(7):1116–1126.
55. Bertelli G, Gozza A, Forno GB, et al. Topical dimethylsulfoxide for the prevention of soft tissue injury after extravasation of vesicant cytotoxic drugs: a prospective clinical study. *J Clin Oncol.* 1995;13(11):2851–2855.
56. Picot D, Lauvin R, Hellegouarc'h R. Skin cancer occurring 10 years after the extravasation of doxorubicin. *N Engl J Med.* 1995;332(11):754.
57. Reynolds PM, MacLaren R, Mueller SW, Fish DN, Kiser TH. Management of extravasation injuries: a focused evaluation of noncytotoxic medications. *Pharmacotherapy.* 2014;34(6):617–632.
58. Bertelli G. Prevention and management of extravasation of cytotoxic drugs. *Drug safety.* 1995;12(4):245–255.
59. Dorr R. Antidotes to vesicant chemotherapy extravasations. *Blood Rev.* 1990;4(1):41–60.
60. Ener R, Meglathery S, Styler M. Extravasation of systemic hemato-oncological therapies. *Ann Oncol.* 2004;15(6):858–862.
61. McBride A. Management of chemotherapy extravasations. *Oncology.* 2009;34(suppl 9):3–11.
62. Doellman D, Hadaway L, Bowe-Geddes LA, et al. Infiltration and extravasation: update on prevention and management. *J Infusion Nurs.* 2009;32(4):203–211.
63. El-Saghir N, Otrock Z, Mufarrij A, et al. Dexrazoxane for anthracycline extravasation and GM-CSF for skin ulceration and wound healing. *Lancet Oncol.* 2004;5(5):320–321.
64. Susser WS, Whitaker-Worth DL, Grant-Kels JM. Mucocutaneous reactions to chemotherapy. *J Am Acad Dermatol.* 1999;40(3):367–398.
65. Youssef M, Mokni S, Belhadjali H, et al. Cyclophosphamide-induced generalised reticulated skin pigmentation: a rare presentation. *Int J Clin Pharm.* 2013;35(3):309–312.
66. Srikant M, Van Veen J, Raithatha A, Reilly JT. Cyclophosphamide-induced nail pigmentation. *Br J Haematol.* 2002;117(1):2.
67. Schrijvers D, Van Den Brande J, Vermorken J. Supravenous discoloration of the skin due to docetaxel treatment. *Br J Dermatol.* 2000;142(5):1069–1070.
68. Das A, Kumar Dhiraj, Mohanty Swosti, et al. Serpentine supravenous hyperpigmentation induced by docetaxel. *Indian J Dermatol Venereol Leprol.* 2015;81(4):434.
69. Chan C-C, Lin S-J. Serpentine supravenous hyperpigmentation. *N Engl J Med.* 2010;363(5):e8.
70. Roach EC, Petekkaya I, Gezgen G, Ünlü O, Altundag K. Serpentine supravenous hyperpigmentation resulting from vinorelbine administration. *Breast J.* 2015;21(3):311–312.
71. Aste N, Fumo G, Contu F, Aste N, Biggio P. Nail pigmentation caused by hydroxyurea: report of 9 cases. *J Am Acad Dermatol.* 2002;47(1):146–147.
72. Hernandez-Martin A, Ros-Forteza S, de Unamuno P. Longitudinal, transverse, and diffuse nail hyperpigmentation induced by hydroxyurea. *J Am Acad Dermatol.* 1999;41(2 Pt 2):333–334.
73. Giacobetti R, Esterly NB, Morgan ER. Nail hyperpigmentation secondary to therapy with doxorubicin. *Am J Dis Child.* 1981;135(4):317–318.
74. Rothberg H, Place CH, Shteir O. Adriamycin (NSC-123127) toxicity: unusual melanotic reaction. *Cancer Chemother Rep.* 1974;58(5 Pt 1):749–751.
75. Ibrahimi OA, Anderson RR. Bleomycin-induced flagellate hyperpigmentation. *N Engl J Med.* 2010;363(24):e36.
76. Vennepureddy A, Siddique MN, Odaimi M, Terjanian T. Bleomycin-induced flagellate erythema in a patient with Hodgkin's lymphoma—a case report and review of literature. *J Oncol Pharm Pract.* 2016;22(3):556–560.
77. Harrold B. Syndrome resembling Addison's disease following prolonged treatment with busulphan. *BMJ.* 1966;1(5485):463.
78. Wheeland RG, Burgdorf WH, Humphrey GB. The flag sign of chemotherapy. *Cancer.* 1983;51(8):1356–1358.
79. Al-Lamki Z, Pearson P, Jaffe N. Localized cisplatin hyperpigmentation induced by pressure. A case report. *Cancer.* 1996;77(8):1578–1581.
80. Teresi ME, Murry DJ, Cornelius AS. Ifosfamide-induced hyperpigmentation. *Cancer.* 1993;71(9):2873–2875.
81. Wyatt AJ, Leonard GD, Sachs DL. Cutaneous reactions to chemotherapy and their management. *Am J Clin Dermatol.* 2006;7(1):45–63.
82. Sibaud V, Lebœuf NR, Roche H, et al. Dermatological adverse events with taxane chemotherapy. *Eur J Dermatol.* 2016;26(5):427–443.
83. Serrano G, Aliaga A, Febrer I, Pujol C, Camps C, Godes M. Dacarbazine-induced photosensitivity. *Photodermatol.* 1989;6(3):140–141.

84. Horio T, Murai T, Ikai K. Photosensitivity due to a fluorouracil derivative. *Arch Dermatol.* 1978;114(10): 1498–1500.
85. Falkson G, Schulz EJ. Skin changes in patients treated with 5-fluorouracil. *Br J Dermatol.* 1962;74:229–236.
86. Almagro BM, Steyls MC, Navarro NL, et al. Occurrence of subacute cutaneous lupus erythematosus after treatment with systemic fluorouracil. *J Clin Oncol.* 2011;29(20):e613–e615.
87. Horio T, Yokoyama M. Tegaful photosensitivity—lichenoid and eczematous types. *Photodermatol.* 1986;3(3):192–193.
88. Hasan T, Nyberg F, Stephansson E, et al. Photosensitivity in lupus erythematosus, UV photoprovocation results compared with history of photosensitivity and clinical findings. *Br J Dermatol.* 1997;136(5):699–705.
89. Beutler BD, Cohen PR. Nab-paclitaxel-associated photosensitivity: report in a woman with non-small cell lung cancer and review of taxane-related photodermatoses. *Dermatol Pract Concept.* 2015;5(2):121–124.
90. León-Mateos A, Zulaica A, Caeiro JL, et al. Photo-induced granulomatous eruption by hydroxyurea. *J Eur Acad Dermatol Venereol.* 2007;21(10):1428–1429.
91. Gould JW, Mercurio MG, Elmets CA. Cutaneous photosensitivity diseases induced by exogenous agents. *J Am Acad Dermatol.* 1995;33(4):551–573.
92. Burris HA 3rd, Hurtig J. Radiation recall with anticancer agents. *Oncologist.* 2010;15(11):1227.
93. Camidge R, Price A. Characterizing the phenomenon of radiation recall dermatitis. *Radiother Oncol.* 2001;59(3):237–245.
94. Haffty BG, Vicini FA, Beitsch P, et al. Timing of chemotherapy after MammoSite radiation therapy system breast brachytherapy: analysis of the American Society of Breast Surgeons MammoSite breast brachytherapy registry trial. *Int J Radiat Oncol Biol Phys.* 2008;72(5):1441–1448.
95. Prindaville B, Horii KA, Canty KM. Radiation recall dermatitis secondary to dactinomycin. *Pediatr Dermatol.* 2016;33(5):e278–e279.
96. Kennedy R, McAleer J. Radiation recall dermatitis in a patient treated with dacarbazine. *Clin Oncol.* 2001;13(6):470–472.
97. Ge J, Verma V, Hollander A, et al. Pemetrexed-induced radiation recall dermatitis in a patient with lung adenocarcinoma: case report and literature review. *J Thorac Dis.* 2016;8(12):E1589–E1593.
98. Barlési F, Tummino C, Tasei AM, Astoul P. Unsuccessful rechallenge with pemetrexed after a previous radiation recall dermatitis. *Lung Cancer.* 2006;54(3):423–425.
99. Morkas M, Fleming D, Hahl M. Challenges in oncology: case 2. Radiation recall associated with docetaxel. *J Clin Oncol.* 2002;20(3):867–869.
100. Burdon J, Bell R, Sullivan J, Henderson M, et al. Adriamycin-induced recall phenomenon 15 years after radiotherapy. *JAMA.* 1978;239(10):931.
101. Azria D, Magné N, Zouhair A, et al. Radiation recall: a well-recognized but neglected phenomenon. *Cancer Treat Rev.* 2005;31(7):555–570.
102. D'Angio GJ, Farber S, Maddock CL. Potentiation of X-ray effects by actinomycin D. *Radiology.* 1959;73(2):175–177.
103. Minisini AM, Tosti A, Sobrero AF, et al. Taxane-induced nail changes: incidence, clinical presentation and outcome. *Ann Oncol.* 2003;14(2):333–337.
104. Capriotti K, Capriotti JA, Lessin S, et al. The risk of nail changes with taxane chemotherapy: a systematic review of the literature and meta-analysis. *Br J Dermatol.* 2015;173(3):842–845.
105. Gilbar P, Hain A, Peereboom V-M. Nail toxicity induced by cancer chemotherapy. *J Oncol Pharm Pract.* 2009;15(3):143–155.
106. Reddy PK, Prasad AL, Sumathy TK, Reddy RV. Nail changes in patients undergoing cancer chemotherapy. *Int J Res Dermatol.* 2017;3(1):49–54.
107. Pratt CB, Shanks EC. Hyperpigmentation of nails from doxorubicin. *JAMA.* 1974;228(4):460.
108. Falkson G, Schulz E. Skin changes in patients treated with 5-fluorouracil. *Br J Dermatol.* 1962;74(6):229–236.
109. Dave S, Thappa DM. Peculiar pattern of nail pigmentation following cyclophosphamide therapy. *Dermatol Online J.* 2003;9(3):14.
110. Llombart-Cussac A, Pivot X, Spielmann M. Docetaxel chemotherapy induces transverse superficial loss of the nail plate. *Arch Dermatol.* 1997;133(11):1466–1467.

111. Chapman S, Cohen PR. Transverse leukonychia in patients receiving cancer chemotherapy. *South Med J.* 1997;90(4):395–398.
112. Woo IS, Shim KH, Kim GY, et al. Nail changes during docetaxel containing combination chemotherapy. *Korean J Intern Med.* 2004;19(2):132.
113. Chen GY, Chen YH, Hsu MM, et al. Onychomadesis and onycholysis associated with capecitabine. *Br J Dermatol.* 2001;145(3):521–522.
114. Li A, Li Y, Ge L, Li P, Li W. Onychomadesis associated with chemotherapy: case report and mini literature review. *Drug Des Devel Ther.* 2017;11:2373–2376.
115. Robert C, Sibaud V, Mateus C, et al. Nail toxicities induced by systemic anticancer treatments. *Lancet Oncol.* 2015;16(4):e181–e189.
116. Creamer J, Mortimer P, Powles T. Mitozantrone-induced onycholysis. A series of five cases. *Clin Exp Dermatol.* 1995;20(6):459–461.
117. Hussain S, Anderson DN, Salvatti ME, et al. Onycholysis as a complication of systemic chemotherapy: report of five cases associated with prolonged weekly paclitaxel therapy and review of the literature. *Cancer.* 2000;88(10):2367–2371.
118. Curran CF. Onycholysis in doxorubicin-treated patients. *Arch Dermatol.* 1990;126(9):1244.
119. Roh MR, Cho JY, Lew W. Docetaxel-induced onycholysis: the role of subungual hemorrhage and suppuration. *Yonsei Med J.* 2007;48(1):124–126.
120. Biasotto V, Polesel J, Mazzega Fabbro C, Tabaro G. Efficacy of cryotherapy in paclitaxel-induced nail toxicity: final results from a Phase II clinical study. *Ann Oncol.* 2017;28(suppl 6):VI105.
121. Scotté F, Tourani JM, Banu E, et al. Multicenter study of a frozen glove to prevent docetaxel-induced onycholysis and cutaneous toxicity of the hand. *J Clin Oncol.* 2005;23(19):4424–4429.

CHAPTER 10

Cardiovascular Toxicities of Chemotherapy

Arjun Khunger, MD ▪ Bassam Estfan, MD

Introduction

Cardiotoxic effects of chemotherapy are challenging in nature, since myocardial tissue possesses limited regenerative capacity, which renders the heart susceptible to transient and permanent side effects of chemotherapy agents. Furthermore, with increasing incidence of cardiovascular disease in the general population and improvement in survival of cancer patients as a result of marked advancement in cancer therapy, chemotherapy-induced cardiotoxicity is becoming a more significant issue for clinicians and patients. Cardiovascular toxicities of chemotherapy have a broad clinical spectrum and may manifest as hypertension, myocardial ischemia, arrhythmia, thromboembolism, systolic dysfunction, congestive heart failure (CHF), or other adverse events. Additionally, they may manifest acutely during treatment or years later after treatment has ended. Anthracyclines are perhaps the most notorious offenders and have been linked to cardiomyopathy and CHF. Failure to diagnose and treat cardiotoxic complications early can result in significant cardiac morbidity and treatment delays or suboptimal delivery. Hence, it is imperative that an oncologist has full knowledge of the cardiovascular complications of antineoplastic agents, and the appropriate management steps to be taken after their detection. In this chapter, we review the cardiovascular toxicity associated with chemotherapy by discussing cardiotoxicity profiles of individual antineoplastic agents (Table 10.1) and describing the general principles for diagnosis, prevention, monitoring, and treatment of these toxicities.

TABLE 10.1 ▪ Cardiovascular Toxicities of Commonly Used Chemotherapy Agents

Drug	Left Ventricular Dysfunction	Arrhythmias	Myocardial Ischemia	Hypertension	Thromboembolism
Anthracyclines					
Doxorubicin	+	+	−	−	−
Epirubicin	+	−	−	−	−
Idarubicin	+	+	−	−	−
Liposomal doxorubicin	−	−	+	−	−
Alkylating Agents					
Cyclophosphamide	+	+	−	−	−
Ifosfamide	+	+	−	−	−
Cisplatin	−	+	−	−	+
Antimicrotubule Agents					
Vinca alkaloids	−	−	+	+	−
Paclitaxel	−	+	+	−	−
Docetaxel	+	+	+	−	−
Antimetabolites					
5-Fluorouracil	−	+	+	−	−
Capecitabine	−	+	+	−	−

Antineoplastic Antibiotics

ANTHRACYCLINES

Anthracyclines are a class of antibiotics isolated from pigment-producing bacillus *Streptomyces* and include daunorubicin, doxorubicin, epirubicin, and idarubicin. Anthracyclines are key components of many curative and palliative regimens in combination with other agents for the treatment of various malignancies, including breast cancer, sarcoma, acute leukemia, and lymphoma. They are the class of antineoplastic agents most closely associated with cardiotoxicity. A meta-analysis of published studies has concluded that patients treated with anthracycline-based chemotherapy were five times more likely to develop reduced left ventricular ejection fraction (LVEF) and CHF in comparison with patients treated with nonanthracycline regimens.[1]

- **Mechanism:** There are several hypotheses regarding the mechanism of anthracycline-induced cardiotoxicity, but free-radical formation after binding to iron, which leads to DNA damage, is generally the most accepted hypothesis.[2] It is believed that the myocardium is more susceptible to free-radical damage than other tissues because it has less free-radical scavenging enzymes.[3] Other possible mechanisms that have been postulated include mitochondrial dysfunction leading to reduced adenosine triphosphate (ATP) production in cardiac myocytes and a decrease in glutathione peroxidase concentration.

- **Presentation:** Anthracycline-induced cardiotoxicity has been categorized into three forms: acute, early-onset chronic, and late-onset chronic.[4,5] Each form may be classified further as subclinical (without CHF) or clinical (with CHF).[6] Acute cardiotoxicity is rare, occurring in less than 1% of patients and is observed immediately after infusion. It typically manifests as an acute but transient decrease in LVEF due to decline in myocardial contractibility. This is frequently reversible within weeks after discontinuation of therapy.[7] Arrhythmias can also be an acute presentation, including tachyarrhythmias (supraventricular or ventricular) and bradyarrhythmias (heart block). Other findings including myocardial ischemia, dilation of the left ventricle, and in rare cases, myocarditis and pericarditis may be observed. Myocarditis typically presents as chest discomfort and shortness of breath shortly after intravenous infusion of chemotherapy. The electrophysiological abnormalities may present as an increased QT interval, ST-T changes, and decreased QRS voltage, and are generally observed in 20% to 30% of patients.[8] Abnormalities in cardiac biomarkers, such as increased serum B-type natriuretic peptide (BNP) and cardiac troponin levels, may also occur.[9] Usually, the manifestations of acute toxicity resolve after discontinuation of the causative agent.

- **Incidence:** Early-onset chronic cardiotoxicity occurs in 1.6% to 2.1% of patients during treatment or within 1 year after completion of treatment, with a peak incidence at about 3 months post-treatment. The late-onset chronic form occurs in 1.6% to 5% of patients, at least 1 year after completion of treatment. In a few cases, it may not be clinically evident even 10 to 20 years after the first dose of chemotherapy.[10] Middle-age adults make up a large proportion of cancer-survivors with clinical signs of chronic onset cardiotoxicity who have received anthracycline-based chemotherapeutics as children or young adults.[11] Early-onset and late-onset chronic cardiotoxicity typically present as a progressive decline in the LVEF leading to a dilated cardiomyopathy or, less commonly, a restrictive cardiomyopathy.[5] In the most severe form, they can progress to severe left ventricular (LV) systolic dysfunction and clinical heart failure which may be progressive, and is associated with a poor prognosis.[12]

- **Risk factors:** Many risk factors have been identified for the development of anthracycline-induced cardiotoxicity, but the most important risk factor is the lifetime cumulative dose of anthracycline. Studies that have evaluated the cumulative probability of doxorubicin-induced HF have determined that it occurs in 3% to 5% with 400 mg/m^2, 7% to 26% at 550 mg/m^2, and 18% to 48% at 700 mg/m^2.[12–14] Other risk factors for anthracycline toxicity include intravenous bolus administration, higher single doses, female gender, preexisting cardiac disease, and history of prior mediastinal irradiation.[12] Also, children and older adults (age > 70 years) appear to be more susceptible to anthracycline-induced cytotoxicity.[15,16] Finally, concomitant use of other agents with known cardiotoxic effects, such as cyclophosphamide, actinomycin D, mitomycin, etoposide, trastuzumab, and paclitaxel, may have an additive effect on anthracycline-induced cardiomyopathy.[17]

■ **Pretreatment evaluation:** Given the multitude of cardiovascular toxicities, it is generally warranted that all adult patients scheduled to receive an anthracycline-based therapy should have a comprehensive assessment of their baseline cardiac function before initiation of therapy (Fig. 10.1). For patients with baseline LVEF less than 40% or patients with current CHF or history of CHF with reduced ejection fraction less than 50%, anthracycline-based chemotherapy is generally not recommended. Even for patients with no history of CHF and baseline LVEF greater than 50%, it is recommended to optimize controllable risk factors, especially hypertension, before the initiation of therapy. Routine surveillance imaging using periodic echocardiography should be offered during treatment based on the patient's risk factors for developing cardiac dysfunction. Cardiac magnetic resonance imaging (MRI) or a multigated acquisition (MUGA) scan can be used alternatively if echocardiography is not

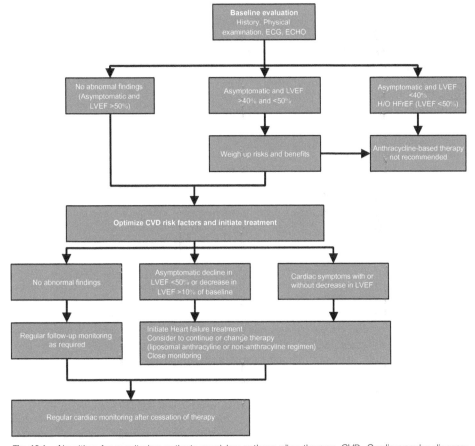

Fig. 10.1 Algorithm for monitoring patients receiving anthracycline therapy. *CVD,* Cardiovascular disease; *ECG,* electrocardiography; *ECHO,* echocardiography; *HFrEF,* heart failure with reduced ejection fraction; *H/O,* history of; *LVEF,* left ventricular ejection fraction.

technically feasible or available.[18] A study by Cardinale and colleagues demonstrated the importance of monitoring cardiac function using echocardiography to detect anthracycline-related cardiotoxicity.[19] It was observed that with repeated cardiac imaging, most cases of cardiotoxicity were detected within 1 year of chemotherapy completion. Some clinicians advocate quantification of LVEF before and after therapy and sometimes after every one to two cycles in select high-risk patient populations. A post-anthracycline LVEF measurement is critically important in breast cancer patients who are scheduled to receive trastuzumab, a monoclonal antibody associated with cardiac dysfunction and clinical CHF. It is recommended that a decrease in LVEF of more than 15% to a level less than 50% of baseline or decline to an LVEF less than 40% should result in considering cessation of anthracycline administration or switching to non–anthracycline-containing regimens. It is also recommended that in patients who require chest radiation therapy, radiation be administered at lower doses and with the use of more precise radiation fields, excluding the heart as much as possible.

- **Biomarkers:** Blood cardiac biomarkers can also be used to identify cardiotoxicity while receiving therapy, especially plasma troponin increase. Increases in cardiac troponins T and I reflect myocardial cell death or injury, while chronic increases in BNP indicate ventricular wall stress.[20] Troponin elevations represent an effective method for monitoring cardiac status as numerous studies have demonstrated correlations between troponin elevations and subsequent LVEF decline.[21–23] Unfortunately, early rises in biomarker levels are difficult to link with final clinical endpoints because clinically apparent signs of heart failure can often arise years after initial therapy. More conclusive studies are needed to establish the utility of these biomarkers for anthracycline-induced cardiotoxicity diagnosis in clinical practice.[24]
- **Treatment of heart failure:** Patients developing CHF due to anthracycline-induced cardiomyopathy should cease anthracycline therapy and should be aggressively managed with current standard of care regimens for CHF using combinations of various medications including angiotensin converting enzyme (ACE) inhibitors, diuretics, β-blockers, and spironolactone.[25,26] Other procedural interventions can be considered on an individual basis and may depend on cancer status.
- **Treatment of asymptomatic LV dysfunction:** Patients who develop asymptomatic decline in LVEF (<50%) due to cardiotoxicity can be managed with guideline-based CHF treatment using ACE inhibitors/angiotensin receptor blockers (ARB) alone or in combination with β-blockers.[16] Studies have shown that early initiation of ACE inhibitors in isolation or in combination with β-blockers is associated with greater LVEF improvement or recovery. Also, clinicians should regularly follow up these patients and evaluate and manage cardiovascular risk factors, including hypertension, diabetes, and dyslipidemia.
- **Prevention:** Multiple approaches have been proposed for the prevention of anthracycline-induced cardiomyopathy. Reducing the cumulative anthracycline dose limits cardiotoxicity, hence various contemporary treatment protocols that use high doses of anthracyclines (>400 mg/m^2) are now less frequently prescribed. It has been observed that slow continuous infusion rather than bolus administration is associated with a lower occurrence of clinical heart failure and subclinical cardiac damage.[27] However, replacing bolus administration with a slow infusion may exacerbate exposure effects including myelotoxicity, mucositis, and alopecia, and may also lead to patient discomfort due to prolonged hospitalization.[28] This strategy did not find merit in children with acute lymphoblastic leukemia.[29] Liposomal encapsulation of anthracycline alters the pharmacokinetics and tissue distribution without affecting antitumor efficacy and has also been shown to reduce cardiotoxicity.[1,30–32] It has been proposed that due to their large size, liposomes are unable to cross the gap junctions of normal endothelium in the heart and other normal tissues, but diffuse more readily through the leaky vasculature of tumors.[30] Liposomal infusions are generally recommended for patients who are likely to receive a lifetime cumulative dose of doxorubicin greater than 450 mg/m^2.

- **Dexrazoxane:** Dexrazoxane is the only US Food and Drug Administration (FDA)–approved cardioprotective agent for anthracycline-induced cardiotoxicity.[33] In various trials, it has been shown to reduce cardiotoxicity by minimizing LVEF decline and reducing cardiac marker release.[31,34] Unfortunately, concerns about the possible compromise of antineoplastic efficacy and increase in secondary tumors, especially in childhood lymphoma and leukemia following dexrazoxane, have led to its restricted use.[35,36] Dexrazoxane has largely been evaluated in women with advanced breast cancer and adults with sarcoma, and it is currently approved for breast cancer patients undergoing treatment with extended anthracycline dosing in excess of 300 mg/m².
- **Cardiac drugs:** β-blockers, ACE inhibitors, ARBs, and statins have been evaluated in randomized controlled trials for the primary prevention of anthracycline-induced cardio-toxicity.[37] Early trials using carvedilol[38] and nebivolol[39] suggested a cardioprotective role of β-blockers to prevent anthracycline-induced LV dysfunction. However, a trial including 192 women with HER2-negative breast cancer, did not demonstrate any benefit of carvedilol monotherapy over placebo with regard to LVEF decline and diastolic function.[40] A combined role of β-blocker and ACE inhibitor in the primary prevention of anthracy-cline-induced cardiotoxicity was evaluated in the OVERCOME trial.[41] The combination of carvedilol with enalapril was beneficial in preventing anthracycline-induced cardiotox-icity with treated patients demonstrating a lower incidence of CHF or death compared with placebo. A randomized trial comparing the cardioprotective effects of candesartan and metoprolol in patients with early breast cancer undergoing adjuvant chemotherapy found that candesartan, and not metoprolol, was effective in preventing anthracycline-induced decline in LVEF.[42] Additionally, a few studies have shown that statins seem to have pro-tective effects during chemotherapy with anthracycline.[43–45] In a retrospective analysis of anthracycline-treated patients with breast cancer, incidental statin prescription was linked with less deterioration of LVEF and lower incident CHF.[43] However, there is not enough evidence to support statin administration to the general population scheduled for anthracy-cline therapy and large multicenter studies are needed.

ANTHRAQUINONES

Mitoxantrone is an anthraquinone derivative used in the treatment of acute leukemias. It was de-veloped in an attempt to produce drugs with a broad spectrum of antitumor activity and devoid of significant cardiotoxicity. However, in the initial phase studies, a few cases of dose-related cardiac dysfunction and arrhythmias were reported.[46,47] Cardiac events associated with mitoxantrone include decreased LVEF, CHF, arrhythmias, and very rarely, myocardial infarction (MI).[47–49] A systemic review of the literature revealed that 0% to 6.7% of patients developed symptomatic mitoxantrone-induced cardiotoxicity and 0% to 80% of patients developed asymptomatic mitoxantrone-related cardiotoxicity.[50] It was reported that cumulative doses greater than 160 mg/m² were associated with a significant increase (>5%) in the incidence of CHF.[51] Currently, most authorities recommend that patients should not receive a cumulative mitoxantrone dose greater than 140 mg/m². CHF caused by mitoxantrone should be treated with current standard of CHF medications including diuretics, ACE inhibitors, and β-blockers, as it has been reported that mitoxantrone-related CHF often responds to standard therapy for CHF.[48]

MITOMYCIN C

Mitomycins are a family of antineoplastic antibiotics that mainly act as alkylating agents. Cardio-toxicity in the form of CHF has been reported in patients receiving multiple doses of mitomycin C.[52,53] A study of anthracycline-induced cardiotoxicity found that there was a 10% incidence of cardiotoxicity with a median cumulative dose of 60 mg/m².[54] In addition, there is evidence to indicate synergistic cardiotoxic effect of mitomycin in combination with anthracyclines.[52,53]

BLEOMYCIN

Bleomycin is used in the treatment of lymphomas, germ cell tumors, and squamous cell tumors. Although there is a well-known association of pulmonary toxicity with bleomycin, pericarditis is an uncommon but potentially fatal cardiotoxicity associated with bleomycin.[55,56] A few episodes of acute chest pain syndrome have also been reported with bleomycin-based therapy.[57] It is generally associated with sudden onset substernal chest pain and treatment is supportive. In addition, a few cases of coronary artery disease (CAD), myocardial ischemia, and MI have been observed in patients during and after treatment with bleomycin-based treatment regimens, although the incidence is less than 1%.[58–60]

Alkylating Agents

- **Cyclophosphamide:** Cyclophosphamide is a non–cell cycle-specific alkylating agent commonly used in combination chemotherapy regimens for the treatment of Hodgkin's and non-Hodgkin's lymphoma, leukemia, multiple myeloma, and breast cancer. It is a mainstay of most pretransplant preparative regimens. At low doses, cyclophosphamide rarely leads to cardiotoxicity. The administered total dose of cyclophosphamide is the main predictive factor for the development of acute cardiotoxicity.[61] A total dose of greater than 200 mg/kg over 2 to 4 days has been reported to cause symptomatic cardiotoxicity.[61] Also, studies have shown a lower incidence of cyclophosphamide-induced cardiotoxicity in children compared with adults.[62]
- **Presentation:** Common manifestations of cyclophosphamide-associated cardiotoxicity include a clinical syndrome of CHF, myocarditis, or both.[63,64] An asymptomatic decrease in LVEF that is generally transient and resolves over 3 to 4 weeks can also been seen. Electrocardiography (ECG) voltage changes, including decreased amplitude of QRS waves and non–specific ST-segment changes, can be seen 5 to 14 days after beginning cyclophosphamide therapy, even in patients without clinical signs of cardiotoxicity.[65] Pericarditis is another complication observed in a few patients that manifests as acute-onset chest pain and pericardial friction rub.[64] Furthermore, acute-onset fulminant CHF has been reported in patients receiving high-dose cyclophosphamide.[65] Fatal episodes of hemorrhagic myo-pericarditis have also been described.[66]
- **Treatment:** Patients developing heart failure should be aggressively treated with current standard of care regimens for CHF. Pericardial effusions may be treated with supportive care or pericardiocentesis, or may require a pericardial window if cardiac tamponade is suspected.
- **Combined therapy with anthracyclines:** Cyclophosphamide and anthracyclines are commonly used in combination in various antineoplastic regimens, and there is mixed evidence for the additive effects of cyclophosphamide and anthracycline-induced cardiomyopathy.[67,68] Therefore, caution should be exercised when prescribing this combination regimen and regular cardiac monitoring should be undertaken to prevent any possible development of CHF, especially in patients older than 50 years.[69] Furthermore, the risk of cardiotoxicity may be minimized by substituting liposomal anthracyclines, and using cardioprotective agents, such as dexrazoxane.
- **Ifosfamide:** Ifosfamide is structurally related to cyclophosphamide and has been associated with ECG changes including ST-wave abnormalities, decreased QRS complexes, and LV dysfunction.[70,71] A dose-dependent incidence of CHF has been reported in patients receiving ifosfamide in doses greater than 12.5 g/m^2.[70] Arrhythmias appear to be reversible after discontinuation of the drug. In addition, it has been observed that signs and symptoms of CHF resolve a few days after the initiation of supportive therapy.
- **Cisplatin:** Cisplatin is a platinum-based alkylating agent with a wide spectrum of antineoplastic activity. Cisplatin is infamous for its nephrotoxicity and neurotoxicity but

cardiotoxicity is an uncommon complication associated with cisplatin chemotherapy. Hence, cardiac monitoring is generally not recommended for its use. Cisplatin has been implicated as a cause of various conduction abnormalities, including supraventricular tachycardia, bradycardia, ST-T wave changes, and left bundle branch block.[72,73] In addition, cisplatin infusions are known to precipitate an acute clinical syndrome causing chest pain, palpitations, and occasionally, elevation of cardiac enzyme levels indicative of an MI.[74] Various incidents of ischemic and nonischemic cardiomyopathy have also been reported with cisplatin chemotherapy.[75,76] Additionally, cisplatin has been implicated in other vascular complications, including Raynaud's phenomenon and cerebral ischemic events. Combinations of cisplatin with other anticancer drugs such as methotrexate, 5-fluorouracil, bleomycin, and doxorubicin are associated with lethal cardiomyopathy and with occlusive thromboembolic events.[77]

Microtubule-Directed Agents

■ **Vinca alkaloids:** The vinca alkaloids, namely: vincristine, vinblastine, and vinorelbine, are integral components of chemotherapy regimens used in the treatment of many hematologic malignancies and solid tumors. The most common cardiovascular events associated with vinca alkaloids include myocardial ischemia, hypertension, and other vaso-occlusive complications.[78–80] Many cases of MI have been reported with the typical onset ranging from a few hours to 3 days after the first dose or subsequent doses of vinca alkaloids. ECG abnormalities are usually consistent with an acute MI, including ST elevation, and T wave inversion.[81] Symptoms may last anywhere from 2 to 24 hours and are usually reversible.[82] Cardiotoxic adverse events have been described most commonly with vinblastine, but a few cases have also been reported with vincristine and vinorelbine. Patients with coexisting myocardial ischemia are more at risk of developing these complications.[83] If patients develop MI symptoms, immediate care with standard medical therapy for MI should be provided.

■ **Paclitaxel:** Paclitaxel is currently used in various oncology protocols for the treatment of ovarian, thyroid, lung, and breast cancers, among others. The most common cardiotoxic adverse event associated with paclitaxel administration is asymptomatic bradycardia. In one phase II study, 29% of patients treated with paclitaxel developed asymptomatic bradycardia, and two patients progressed to higher-grade heart block.[84] In a study of 3400 patients treated with paclitaxel, there was 0.5% incidence of grades 4 and 5 cardiac adverse events (life threatening and death, respectively).[85] Cardiac rhythm disturbances in the form of atrial flutter, atrial fibrillation, supraventricular tachycardia, and ventricular tachyarrhythmias have also been reported with paclitaxel.[86] They may be observed occasionally during the infusion of the first cycle but are usually seen after the second or subsequent cycles. Severe conduction abnormalities can occur in patients with an underlying cardiac disease or electrolyte abnormalities. A few cases of myocardial ischemia and infarction have also been reported with paclitaxel infusion.[87,88] The exact mechanism of paclitaxel-induced myocardial ischemia is unknown, although it is appears to be linked to coronary vasospasm.[89] Paclitaxel is frequently used in combination with anthracyclines and it is hypothesized that cardiotoxic effects of anthracyclines may be increased due to the decreased renal excretion caused by paclitaxel. Of note, CHF induced by anthracyclines may occur at a lower cumulative dose when used in combination with paclitaxel.[90,91] Hence, it has been suggested that the maximum cumulative doxorubicin dose that is administered should be decreased to less than 340 to 380 mg/m[2], when used in combination with paclitaxel. On the other hand, sequential administration of paclitaxel and doxorubicin does not seem to result in an increased risk of cardiac toxicity.[92]

- **Docetaxel:** Similarly to paclitaxel, docetaxel is commonly used both alone and in combination with a number of other agents for the management of various malignant conditions, including breast, gastric, prostate, head and neck, and non–small-cell lung cancers. The most commonly encountered cardiovascular adverse events reported with docetaxel are conduction abnormalities, angina, and cardiovascular collapse.[93–95] Significant elevation of BNP serum concentration has also been reported after docetaxel administration.[96] There is evidence to suggest potentiating effect of anthracycline-induced cardiomyopathy associated with docetaxel administration.[97]

Antimetabolites

- **5-Fluorouracil:** 5-Fluorouracil (5-FU) is a synthetic pyrimidine antimetabolite that is commonly used in the treatment of several malignancies including colorectal, breast, gastric, esophageal, bladder, and breast cancers. The cardiotoxic effects of 5-FU range from anginal chest pain to massive MI, which can progress to cardiogenic shock and death.[98–101] 5-FU is one of the most commonly known antineoplastic agents to cause myocardial ischemia, with the reported incidence ranging from 1% to 18%.[102,103] Ischemic events are more frequent when 5-FU is administered as a long continuous infusion or given in combination with cisplatin.[103,104] Also, patients with preexisting structural heart disease or CAD, or with prior chest radiation therapy, are at higher risk of developing cardiovascular events.[105,106] Hence, it is necessary for clinicians to screen patients for the presence of underlying risk factors that can predispose to the development of 5-FU–induced cardiotoxicity.
  - **Mechanism:** The most accepted mechanism for 5-FU–associated cardiac events is coronary vasospasm leading to ischemia.
  - **Presentation:** Patients exhibiting cardiotoxicity typically present with chest pain, with or without transient ECG changes.[107] Silent ischemia has also been recorded in studies where continuous ambulatory ECG monitoring on patients undergoing 5-FU infusion was performed, and results showed that more than half of patients exhibited ECG changes.[108–110] Cardiac rhythm disturbances, such as atrial fibrillation, ventricular tachycardia, and ventricular fibrillation, have been noted, which may persist for a few days following cessation of 5-FU treatment. 5-FU–mediated adverse effects can progress to symptoms of acute MI, including chest pain, diaphoresis, and shortness of breath, with myocardial injury changes suggested on ECG and LV dysfunction.[100] Ventricular dysfunction can persist for a few days to even a few weeks following cessation of 5-FU therapy. A few cases of cardiogenic shock, cardiac arrest, and sudden death following 5-FU treatment have also been documented.[107,111] The incidence of mortality due to 5-FU–associated cardiotoxicity ranges between 2.2% and 13%.[103,112]
  - **Delivery of 5-FU:** The development of cardiotoxicity symptoms of 5-FU varies according to the delivery mode. 5-FU is administered intravenously either as a bolus, as part of the 5-FU, folinic acid, and oxaliplatin (FLOX) regimen or as a continuous infusion (24–96 h) as part of the folinic acid, fluorouracil, and oxaliplatin (FOLFOX) regimen. The use of bolus 5-FU as a short-term infusion over a few minutes is associated with chest pain that usually occurs during the push or immediately after the first cycle. However, in the case of the absence of symptoms during the initial cycle, it is unusual to occur subsequently. The chest pain description suggests a cardiac origin and is associated with elevation of the ST segment on the ECG suggestive of acute ST-segment elevation MI (*initial bolus pattern*). Chest pain associated with continuous infusion of 5-FU may also occur with the first or sometimes second chemotherapy cycle, and typically occurs 24 to 72 hours after infusion initiation.[113] The pain may be atypical compared with classic angina pain and may occur at rest and resolve spontaneously. These symptoms can also

recur cyclically during subsequent infusions and can even persist following completion of therapy. Unlike bolus infusion, many patients can tolerate these symptoms and are able to complete the planned infusion course. Additionally, because infusions are administered on an outpatient basis, without telemetry monitoring, ECG changes are generally not captured. With subsequent cycles, symptoms can sometimes recur with more intensity and for a longer duration (*continuous exposure pattern*).

- **Treatment:** The acute management of patients with 5-FU–associated chest pain is prompt discontinuation of chemotherapy because 5-FU–related cardiotoxicity can be potentially fatal. Also, symptoms should be treated empirically with antianginal therapy such as short-acting sublingual nitrates and/or calcium channel blockers. This approach has been shown to terminate acute symptoms in up to 69% of affected patients.[114] The pivotal next step is an acute assessment for myocardial injury using ECG monitoring, measurement of cardiac troponin levels, and echocardiography if required.[115] Also, it is necessary to identify if the symptoms are reasonably attributed to 5-FU. This poses a challenging question because further administration of 5-FU can potentially lead to recurrence of symptoms, whereas withholding the chemotherapy regimen can compromise cancer treatment. Unfortunately, there is no definitive test to establish diagnosis of 5-FU–induced cardiotoxicity. When it is likely that cardiotoxicity can be attributed to 5-FU infusion, the safest option is to explore alternative chemotherapy regimens with non–fluoropyrimidine-containing agents. Prophylactic treatment using nitrates and calcium antagonist has been found to be ineffective in preventing ischemia symptoms on rechallenge of the drug.[116,117] If a 5-FU–based regimen is preferable, it would be appropriate first to determine the underlying pathological process that could explain the symptoms and potentially reverse it. Patients with risk factors for cardiovascular disease can be scheduled to undergo coronary angiography and, if angiography reveals clinically significant coronary stenosis, an attempt at revascularization followed by a rechallenge of 5-FU would be reasonable. In addition, if rechallenging with 5-FU is considered, appropriate precautions, including pretreating patients with cardioprotective medication such as aspirin, calcium antagonists, or long-acting nitrates, and careful cardiac monitoring in an inpatient unit should be employed.[118] Additionally, it has been reported that using a bolus regimen is a much safer option than a continuous infusion and should be the method of choice for administration.[119] Further randomized clinical trials using different approaches to manage these patients are essential to determine the optimal strategy.

- **Capecitabine:** Capecitabine is an oral prodrug of 5-FU that is known to generate 5-FU preferentially at the tumor site. Its effectiveness has been studied in cancers such as breast, gastric, and colorectal cancers. Although it has gained popularity because of its ease of administration and milder toxicity profile, multiple case reports have documented significant cardiovascular adverse events associated with capecitabine administration. It is generally suggested that the incidence of cardiotoxicity with capecitabine is 1.5% to 2% lower than that of 5-FU.[120] However, in a retrospective study of patients undergoing chemotherapy treatment for metastatic breast and colon cancer, it was found that the incidence of capecitabine-induced cytotoxicity was comparable to that of 5-FU.[121]

  - **Presentation:** Capecitabine-related cardiac events range from angina and reversible ST-segment deviations to MI, arrhythmias, and even cardiac arrest.[122,123] Chest pain and palpitations are the most common clinical manifestations of capecitabine-induced cardiotoxicity.[124] It is reported that most of the symptoms of cardiotoxicity tend to occur during the first cycle, with a median time for onset of less than 4 days after initiation of therapy.[105,125] The most common ECG abnormalities noted include ST-segment deviation, sinus tachycardia, and prolonged QTc interval.[115,124] Patients developing chest pain should be immediately evaluated using ECG monitoring and measurement of cardiac enzymes. Most patients tend to respond to conservative management with antianginal agents and supportive care. The administration of capecitabine should be immediately discontinued in patients who develop pulmonary edema, MI, or arrhythmias.

■ **Rechallenge:** Once cardiotoxicity has occurred, it is uncertain whether rechallenge with a modified dose of capecitabine or together with a prophylactic antianginal agents can be done safely. A retrospective study of patients with capecitabine cardiac toxicity reported symptom recurrence in 10 of 16 patients on rechallenge and a lack of benefit of dose reduction or medical prophylaxis on rechallenging.[126] Also, it is not advisable to administer capecitabine to patients with a history of 5-FU–induced cardiotoxicity.[120]

Conclusion

Chemotherapy-induced cardiotoxicity is evolving as a ubiquitous complication of cancer treatment due to the ageing of the population and a disproportionate increase in the incidence of cancer among older individuals. With the discovery and approval of new therapies, clinicians should be familiar with the potential of various chemotherapeutic drugs known to cause cardiotoxicity and should promptly evaluate and closely monitor all cardiac events that occur during the course of therapy. In addition, long-term surveillance is warranted with some treatments because certain cardiovascular complications including LV dysfunction or CHF may develop more than a decade after the initial administration.

References

1. Smith LA, et al. Cardiotoxicity of anthracycline agents for the treatment of cancer: systematic review and meta-analysis of randomised controlled trials. *BMC Cancer.* 2010;10(1):337.
2. Giantris A, et al. Anthracycline-induced cardiotoxicity in children and young adults. *Crit Rev Oncol Hematol.* 1998;27(1):53–68.
3. Doroshow JH. Anthracycline antibiotic-stimulated superoxide, hydrogen peroxide, and hydroxyl radical production by NADH dehydrogenase. *Cancer Res.* 1983;43(10):4543–4551.
4. Grenier MA, Lipshultz SE. Epidemiology of anthracycline cardiotoxicity in children and adults. *Semin Oncol.* 1998;25(4 suppl 10):72–85.
5. Lipshultz SE, Alvarez JA, Scully RE. Anthracycline associated cardiotoxicity in survivors of childhood cancer. *Heart.* 2008;94(4):525–533.
6. Yeh ET, Bickford CL. Cardiovascular complications of cancer therapy: incidence, pathogenesis, diagnosis, and management. *J Am Coll Cardiol.* 2009;53(24):2231–2247.
7. Geiger S, et al. Anticancer therapy induced cardiotoxicity: review of the literature. *Anticancer Drugs.* 2010;21(6):578–590.
8. Frishman WH, et al. Cardiovascular toxicity with cancer chemotherapy. *Curr Prob Cancer.* 1997;21(6): 301–360.
9. Cardinale D, et al. Myocardial injury revealed by plasma troponin I in breast cancer treated with high-dose chemotherapy. *Ann Oncol.* 2002;13(5):710–715.
10. Curigliano G, et al. Cardiovascular toxicity induced by chemotherapy, targeted agents and radiotherapy: ESMO Clinical Practice Guidelines. *Ann Oncol.* 2012;23(suppl 7):vii155–vii166.
11. Armstrong GT, et al. Modifiable risk factors and major cardiac events among adult survivors of childhood cancer. *J Clin Oncol.* 2013;31(29):3673.
12. Von Hoff DD, et al. Risk factors for doxorubicin-induced congestive heart failure. *Ann Intern Med.* 1979;91(5):710–717.
13. Swain SM, et al. Cardioprotection with dexrazoxane for doxorubicin-containing therapy in advanced breast cancer. *J Clin Oncol.* 1997;15(4):1318–1332.
14. Wouters KA, et al. Protecting against anthracycline-induced myocardial damage: a review of the most promising strategies. *Br J Haematol.* 2005;131(5):561–578.
15. Kremer LC, Caron HN. Anthracycline cardiotoxicity in children. *N Engl J Med.* 2004;351:120–121.

16. Zamorano JL, et al. 2016 ESC position paper on cancer treatments and cardiovascular toxicity developed under the auspices of the ESC Committee for Practice Guidelines: the task force for cancer treatments and cardiovascular toxicity of the European Society of Cardiology (ESC). *Eu Heart J.* 2016; 37(36):2768–2801.
17. van Dalen EC, et al. Different anthracycline derivates for reducing cardiotoxicity in cancer patients. *Cochrane Database Syst Rev.* 2010;(5):CD005006.
18. de Geus-Oei LF, et al. Scintigraphic techniques for early detection of cancer treatment-induced cardiotoxicity. *J Nucl Med.* 2011;52(4):560–571.
19. Cardinale D, et al. Early detection of anthracycline cardiotoxicity and improvement with heart failure therapy. *Circulation.* 2015;131(22):1981–1988.
20. Todorova VK, et al. Biomarkers for presymptomatic doxorubicin-induced cardiotoxicity in breast cancer patients. *PLoS ONE.* 2016;11(8):e0160224.
21. Auner HW, et al. Prolonged monitoring of troponin T for the detection of anthracycline cardiotoxicity in adults with hematological malignancies. *Ann Hematol.* 2003;82(4):218–222.
22. Specchia G, et al. Monitoring of cardiac function on the basis of serum troponin I levels in patients with acute leukemia treated with anthracyclines. *J Lab Clin Med.* 2005;145(4):212–220.
23. Cardinale D, et al. Prognostic value of troponin I in cardiac risk stratification of cancer patients undergoing high-dose chemotherapy. *Circulation.* 2004;109(22):2749–2754.
24. Singh D, Thakur A, Wilson Tang WH. Utilizing cardiac biomarkers to detect and prevent chemotherapy-induced cardiomyopathy. *Curr Heart Fail Rep.* 2015;12(3):255–262.
25. Cardinale D, et al. Anthracycline-induced cardiomyopathy: clinical relevance and response to pharmacologic therapy. *J Am Coll Cardiol.* 2010;55(3):213–220.
26. Hamo CE, et al. Cancer therapy-related cardiac dysfunction and heart failure. Part 2: prevention, treatment, guidelines, and future directions. *Circ Heart Fail.* 2016;9(2):e002843.
27. van Dalen EC, van der Pal HJ, Kremer L. Different dosage schedules for reducing cardiotoxicity in people with cancer receiving anthracycline chemotherapy. *Cochrane Database Syst Rev.* 2016;3(3):CD005008.28.
28. Chatterjee K, et al. Doxorubicin cardiomyopathy. *Cardiology.* 2010;115(2):155–162.
29. Lipshultz SE, et al. Continuous versus bolus infusion of doxorubicin in children with ALL: long-term cardiac outcomes. *Pediatrics.* 2012;130(6):1003–1011.
30. Gabizon AA. Pegylated liposomal doxorubicin: metamorphosis of an old drug into a new form of chemotherapy. *Cancer Invest.* 2001;19(4):424–436.
31. van Dalen EC, et al. Different anthracycline derivates for reducing cardiotoxicity in cancer patients. *Cochrane Database Syst Rev.* 2006;18(4):CD005006.
32. Cortes J, et al. Nonpegylated liposomal doxorubicin (TLC-D99), paclitaxel, and trastuzumab in HER-2-overexpressing breast cancer: a multicenter phase I/II study. *Clin Cancer Res.* 2009;15(1):307–314.
33. Vejpongsa P, Yeh ET. Prevention of anthracycline-induced cardiotoxicity: challenges and opportunities. *J Am Coll Cardiol.* 2014;64(9):938–945.
34. Chow EJ, et al. Late mortality after dexrazoxane treatment: a report from the Children's Oncology Group. *J Clin Oncol.* 2015;33(24):2639–2645.
35. Tebbi CK, et al. Dexrazoxane-associated risk for acute myeloid leukemia/myelodysplastic syndrome and other secondary malignancies in pediatric Hodgkin's disease. *J Clin Oncol.* 2007;25(5):493–500.
36. Vrooman LM, et al. The low incidence of secondary acute myelogenous leukaemia in children and adolescents treated with dexrazoxane for acute lymphoblastic leukaemia: a report from the Dana-Farber Cancer Institute ALL Consortium. *Eur J Cancer.* 2011;47(9):1373–1379.
37. Abdel-Qadir H, et al. Interventions for preventing cardiomyopathy due to anthracyclines: a Bayesian network meta-analysis. *Ann Oncol.* 2016;28(3):628–633.
38. Kalay N, et al. Protective effects of carvedilol against anthracycline-induced cardiomyopathy. *J Am Coll Cardiol.* 2006;48(11):2258–2262.
39. Kaya MG, et al. Protective effects of nebivolol against anthracycline-induced cardiomyopathy: a randomized control study. *Int J Cardiol.* 2013;167(5):2306–2310.
40. Avila MS, et al. Carvedilol for prevention of chemotherapy related cardiotoxicity. *J Am Coll Cardiol.* 2018:24730.
41. Bosch X, et al. Enalapril and carvedilol for preventing chemotherapy-induced left ventricular systolic dysfunction in patients with malignant hemopathies: the OVERCOME trial (preventiOn of left

Ventricular dysfunction with Enalapril and caRvedilol in patients submitted to intensive ChemOtherapy for the treatment of Malignant hEmopathies). *J Am Coll Cardiol.* 2013;61(23):2355–2362.

42. Gulati G, et al. Prevention of cardiac dysfunction during adjuvant breast cancer therapy (PRADA): a 2 × 2 factorial, randomized, placebo-controlled, double-blind clinical trial of candesartan and metoprolol. *Eur Heart J.* 2016;37(21):1671–1680.

43. Seicean S, et al. Effect of statin therapy on the risk for incident heart failure in patients with breast cancer receiving anthracycline chemotherapy: an observational clinical cohort study. *J Am Coll Cardiol.* 2012;60(23):2384–2390.

44. Acar Z, et al. Efficiency of atorvastatin in the protection of anthracycline-induced cardiomyopathy. *J Am Coll Cardiol.* 2011;58(9):988–989.

45. Chotenimitkhun R, et al. Chronic statin administration may attenuate early anthracycline-associated declines in left ventricular ejection function. *Can J Cardiol.* 2015;31(3):302–307.

46. Saletan S. Mitoxantrone: an active, new antitumor agent with an improved therapeutic index. *Cancer Treat Rev.* 1987;14(3–4):297–303.

47. Unverferth D, et al. Cardiac evaluation of mitoxantrone. *Cancer Treat Rep.* 1983;67(4):343–350.

48. Schell FC, et al. Potential cardiotoxicity with mitoxantrone. *Cancer Treat Rep.* 1982;66(8):1641–1643.

49. Pratt CB, et al. Fatal congestive heart failure following mitoxantrone treatment in two children previously treated with doxorubicin and cisplatin. *Cancer Treat Rep.* 1983;67(1):85–88.

50. Van Dalen E, et al. Cumulative incidence and risk factors of mitoxantrone-induced cardiotoxicity in children: a systematic review. *Eur J Cancer.* 2004;40(5):643–652.

51. Posner LE, et al. Mitoxantrone: an overview of safety and toxicity. *Invest New Drugs.* 1985;3(2):123–132.

52. Villani F, et al. Possible enhancement of the cardiotoxicity of doxorubicin when combined with mitomycin C. *Med Oncol Tumor Pharmacother.* 1985;2(2):93–97.

53. Buzdar AU, et al. Adriamycin and mitomycin C: possible synergistic cardiotoxicity. *Cancer Treat Rep.* 1978;62(7):1005–1008.

54. Verweij J, et al. A prospective study on the dose dependency of cardiotoxicity induced by mitomycin C. *Med Oncol Tumor Pharmacother.* 1988;5(3):159–163.

55. Durkin W, et al. Treatment of advanced lymphomas with bleomycin (NSC-125066). *Oncology.* 1976; 33(3):140–145.

56. Yosef RB, Gez E, Catane R. Acute pericarditis following bleomycin: a case report and literature analysis. *J Chemother.* 1990;2(1):70–71.

57. White DA, et al. Acute chest pain syndrome during bleomycin infusions. *Cancer.* 1987;59(9):1582–1585.

58. Vogelzang N, Frenning D, Kennedy B. Coronary artery disease after treatment with bleomycin and vinblastine. *Cancer Treat Rep.* 1980;64(10-11):1159–1160.

59. Schwarzer S, et al. Non-Q-wave myocardial infarction associated with bleomycin and etoposide chemotherapy. *Eur Heart J.* 1991;12(6):748–750.

60. Dieckmann K-P, et al. Myocardial infarction and other major vascular events during chemotherapy for testicular cancer. *Ann Oncol.* 2010;21(8):1607–1611.

61. Dow E, Schulman H, Agura E. Cyclophosphamide cardiac injury mimicking acute myocardial infarction. *Bone Marrow Transplant.* 1993;12(2):169–172.

62. Goldberg MA, et al. Cyclophosphamide cardiotoxicity: an analysis of dosing as a risk factor. *Blood.* 1986;68(5):1114–1118.

63. Gardner S, et al. High-dose cyclophosphamide-induced myocardial damage during BMT: assessment by positron emission tomography. *Bone Marrow Transplant.* 1993;12(2):139–144.

64. Braverman A, et al. Cyclophosphamide cardiotoxicity in bone marrow transplantation: a prospective evaluation of new dosing regimens. *J Clin Oncol.* 1991;9(7):1215–1223.

65. Gottdiener JS, et al. Cardiotoxicity associated with high-dose cyclophosphamide therapy. *Arch Intern Med.* 1981;141(6):758–763.

66. Appelbaum F, et al. Acute lethal carditis caused by high-dose combination chemotherapy: a unique clinical and pathological entity. *Lancet.* 1976;307(7950):58–62.

67. Cazin B, et al. Cardiac complications after bone marrow transplantation. A report on a series of 63 consecutive transplantations. *Cancer.* 1986;57(10):2061–2069.

68. Steinherz LJ, et al. Cardiac changes with cyclophosphamide. *Med Pediatr Oncol.* 1981;9(5):417–422.

69. Hertenstein B, et al. Cardiac toxicity of bone marrow transplantation: predictive value of cardiologic evaluation before transplant. *J Clin Oncol.* 1994;12(5):998–1004.

70. Quezado ZM, et al. High-dose ifosfamide is associated with severe, reversible cardiac dysfunction. *Ann Intern Med.* 1993;118(1):31–36.
71. Kandylis K, et al. Ifosfamide cardiotoxicity in humans. *Cancer Chemother Pharmacol.* 1989;24(6):395–396.
72. Hashimi LA, Khalyl MF, Salem PA. Supraventricular tachycardia. *Oncology.* 1984;41(3):174–175.
73. Canobbio L, et al. Cardiac arrhythmia: possible complication from treatment with cisplatin. *Tumori.* 1986;72(2):201–204.
74. Berliner S, et al. Acute coronary events following cisplatin-based chemotherapy. *Cancer Invest.* 1990;8(6): 583–586.
75. Tomirotti M, et al. Ischemic cardiopathy from cis-diamminedichloroplatinum (CDDP). *Tumori.* 1984; 70(3):235–236.
76. Gill D, Pattar S, Kan L. Nonischemic cardiomyopathy due to cisplatin therapy. *Am J Ther.* 2018;25(2): e286–e289.
77. Cheriparambil KM, et al. Acute reversible cardiomyopathy and thromboembolism after cisplatin and 5-fluorouracil chemotherapy: a case report. *Angiology.* 2000;51(10):873–878.
78. Subar M, Muggia F. Apparent myocardial ischemia associated with vinblastine administration. *Cancer Treat Rep.* 1986;70(5):690–691.
79. Kantor A, et al. Are vinca alkaloids associated with myocardial infarction? *Lancet.* 1981;317(8229):1111.
80. Bergeron A, Raffy O, Vannetzel J. Myocardial ischemia and infarction associated with vinorelbine. *J Clin Oncol.* 1995;13(2):531–532.
81. Yancey R, Talpaz M. Vindesine-associated angina and ECG changes. *Cancer Treat Rep.* 1982;66(3):587.
82. Cargill R, Boyter A, Lipworth B. Reversible myocardial ischaemia following vincristine containing chemotherapy. *Respir Med.* 1994;88(9):709–710.
83. Samuels BL, Vogelzang NJ, Kennedy B. Severe vascular toxicity associated with vinblastine, bleomycin, and cisplatin chemotherapy. *Cancer Chemother Pharmacol.* 1987;19(3):253–256.
84. McGuire WP, et al. Taxol: a unique antineoplastic agent with significant activity in advanced ovarian epithelial neoplasms. *Ann Intern Med.* 1989;111(4):273–279.
85. Arbuck SG, et al. A reassessment of cardiac toxicity associated with Taxol. *J Natl Cancer Inst Monogr.* 1993;(15):117–130.
86. Rowinsky EK, et al. Cardiac disturbances during the administration of taxol. *J Clin Oncol.* 1991;9(9): 1704–1712.
87. Schrader C, et al. Symptoms and signs of an acute myocardial ischemia caused by chemotherapy with paclitaxel (Taxol) in a patient with metastatic ovarian carcinoma. *Eur J Med Res.* 2005;10(11):498–501.
88. Esber C, et al. Acute myocardial infarction in patient with triple negative breast cancer after paclitaxel infusion: a case report. *Cardiol Res.* 2014;5(3-4):108–111.
89. Nguyen-Ho P, Kleiman NS, Verani MS. Acute myocardial infarction and cardiac arrest in a patient receiving paclitaxel. *Can J Cardiol.* 2003;19(3):300–302.
90. Gianni L, et al. Paclitaxel by 3-hour infusion in combination with bolus doxorubicin in women with untreated metastatic breast cancer: high antitumor efficacy and cardiac effects in a dose-finding and sequence-finding study. *J Clin Oncol.* 1995;13(11):2688–2699.
91. Dombernowsky P, et al. Doxorubicin and paclitaxel, a highly active combination in the treatment of metastatic breast cancer. *Semin Oncol.* 1996;23(5 suppl 11):23–27.
92. Perez EA. Paclitaxel and cardiotoxicity. *J Clin Oncol.* 1998;16(11):3481–3482.
93. Bissett D, et al. Phase I and pharmacokinetic study of taxotere (RP 56976) administered as a 24-hour infusion. *Cancer Res.* 1993;53(3):523–527.
94. Fossella FV, et al. Phase II study of docetaxel for advanced or metastatic platinum-refractory non-small-cell lung cancer. *J Clin Oncol.* 1995;13(3):645–651.
95. Francis P, et al. Phase II trial of docetaxel in patients with platinum-refractory advanced ovarian cancer. *J Clin Oncol.* 1994;12(11):2301–2308.
96. Shimoyama M, et al. Docetaxel induced cardiotoxicity. *Heart.* 2001;86(2):219.
97. Malhotra V, et al. Neoadjuvant and adjuvant chemotherapy with doxorubicin and docetaxel in locally advanced breast cancer. *Clin Breast Cancer.* 2004;5(5):377–384.
98. Labianca R, et al. Cardiac toxicity of 5-fluorouracil: a study on 1083 patients. *Tumori.* 1982;68(6): 505–510.
99. Patel B, et al. 5-Fluorouracil cardiotoxicity: left ventricular dysfunction and effect of coronary vasodilators. *Am J Med Sci.* 1987;294(4):238–243.

100. De Forni M, et al. Cardiotoxicity of high-dose continuous infusion fluorouracil: a prospective clinical study. *J Clin Oncol.* 1992;10(11):1795–1801.

101. Akhtar SS, Salim KP, Bano ZA. Symptomatic cardiotoxicity with high-dose 5-fluorouracil infusion: a prospective study. *Oncology.* 1993;50(6):441–444.

102. Tsibiribi P, et al. Cardiotoxicity of 5-fluorouracil in 1350 patients with no prior history of heart disease. *Bull Cancer.* 2006;93(3):10027–10030.

103. Kosmas C, et al. Cardiotoxicity of fluoropyrimidines in different schedules of administration: a prospective study. *J Cancer Res Clin Oncol.* 2008;134(1):75–82.

104. Jeremic B, et al. Cardiotoxicity during chemotherapy treatment with 5-fluorouracil and cisplatin. *J Chemother.* 1990;2(4):264–267.

105. Jensen SA, Sørensen JB. Risk factors and prevention of cardiotoxicity induced by 5-fluorouracil or capecitabine. *Cancer Chemother Pharmacol.* 2006;58(4):487–493.

106. Meydan N, et al. Cardiotoxicity of de Gramont's regimen: incidence, clinical characteristics and long-term follow-up. *Jpn J Clin Oncol.* 2005;35(5):265–270.

107. Alter P, et al. Cardiotoxicity of 5-fluorouracil. *Cardiovasc Hematol Agents Med Chem.* 2006;4(1):1–5.

108. Rezkalla S, et al. Continuous ambulatory ECG monitoring during fluorouracil therapy: a prospective study. *J Clin Oncol.* 1989;7(4):509–514.

109. Meyer CC, et al. Symptomatic cardiotoxicity associated with 5-fluorouracil. *Pharmacotherapy.* 1997;17(4): 729–736.

110. Lestuzzi C, et al. Effort myocardial ischemia during chemotherapy with 5-fluorouracil: an underestimated risk. *Ann Oncol.* 2014;25(5):1059–1064.

111. Ensley JF, et al. The clinical syndrome of 5-fluorouracil cardiotoxicity. *Invest New Drugs.* 1989;7(1):101–109.

112. Keefe DL, Roistacher N, Pierri MK. Clinical cardiotoxicity of 5-fluorouracil. *J Clin Pharmacol.* 1993;33(11):1060–1070.

113. Jensen SA, et al. Fluorouracil induces myocardial ischemia with increases of plasma brain natriuretic peptide and lactic acid but without dysfunction of left ventricle. *J Clin Oncol.* 2010;28(36):5280–5286.

114. Jensen SA, Sorensen JB. Risk factors and prevention of cardiotoxicity induced by 5-fluorouracil or capecitabine. *Cancer Chemother Pharmacol.* 2006;58(4):487–493.

115. Stewart T, Pavlakis N, Ward M. Cardiotoxicity with 5-fluorouracil and capecitabine: more than just vasospastic angina. *Intern Med J.* 2010;40(4):303–307.

116. Eskilsson J, Albertsson M. Failure of preventing 5-fluorouracil cardiotoxicity by prophylactic treatment with verapamil. *Acta Oncol.* 1990;29(8):1001–1003.

117. Oleksowicz L, Bruckner HW. Prophylaxis of 5-fluorouracil-induced coronary vasospasm with calcium channel blockers. *Am J Med.* 1988;85(5):750–751.

118. Cianci G, et al. Prophylactic options in patients with 5-fluorouracil-associated cardiotoxicity. *Br J Cancer.* 2003;88(10):1507–1509.

119. Saif MW, et al. Bolus 5-fluorouracil as an alternative in patients with cardiotoxicity associated with infusion 5-fluorouracil and capecitabine: a case series. *In Vivo.* 2013;27(4):531–534.

120. Frickhofen N, et al. Capecitabine can induce acute coronary syndrome similar to 5-fluorouracil. *Ann Oncol.* 2002;13(5):797–801.

121. Van Cutsem E, et al. Incidence of cardiotoxicity with the oral fluoropyrimidine capecitabine is typical of that reported with 5-fluorouracil. *Ann Oncol.* 2002;13(3):484–485.

122. Polk A, et al. Cardiotoxicity in cancer patients treated with 5-fluorouracil or capecitabine: a systematic review of incidence, manifestations and predisposing factors. *Cancer Treat Rev.* 2013;39(8):974–984.

123. De Gennaro L, et al. Cardiac arrest and ventricular fibrillation in a young man treated with capecitabine: case report and literature review. *Int J Cardiol.* 2016;220:280–283.

124. Koca D, et al. Clinical and electrocardiography changes in patients treated with capecitabine. *Chemotherapy.* 2011;57(5):381–387.

125. Ng M, Cunningham D, Norman AR. The frequency and pattern of cardiotoxicity observed with capecitabine used in conjunction with oxaliplatin in patients treated for advanced colorectal cancer (CRC). *Eur J Cancer.* 2005;41(11):1542–1546.

126. Manojlovic N, et al. Capecitabine cardiotoxicity–case reports and literature review. *Hepatogastroenterology.* 2008;55(85):1249–1256.

CHAPTER 11

Cancer Treatment Infusion Reactions

Sharanya Vemula, BPharm, PhD

Introduction

Cancer treatments have the potential to cause infusion reactions (IRs). It is important to manage IRs because they may cause treatment disruption and require costly medical interventions.[1, 2] Both cytotoxic and biological agents cause IRs. In general, IRs can be anaphylactic or anaphylactoid.

- **Anaphylactic IRs:** Anaphylactic IRs are allergic in nature and are usually mediated by immunoglobulin E (IgE).[2] Clinical symptoms do not vary widely among the agents, but the time course and severity of IRs differ among chemotherapeutic agents and range from mild to severe reactions. Severe reactions are rare but the incidence of mild to moderate reactions is quite high. IRs may affect any organ system in the body and range in severity from a mild rash to systemic anaphylaxis.[3] Mild-to-moderate IRs usually cause flushing, rash, fever, rigors, chills, dyspnea, and mild hypotension. Severe reactions are typically characterized by hypotension, bronchospasms, cardiac dysfunction, anaphylaxis, and other symptoms.[1]
- **Anaphylactoid IRs:** Anaphylactoid IRs present in a similar fashion as anaphylactic reactions; however, they are not IgE-mediated and are characterized by non–immune-mediated release of cytokines and immune mediators.

IRs from cancer treatments can be due to age-related factors, concomitant diseases, cardiovascular diseases, or concurrent medications.[4,5] Apart from being aware of the potential risk of an IR from a specific drug, it is imperative for clinicians to recognize their symptoms, understand their pathology, and use optimal risk assessment and prophylactic regimens. Inappropriate assessment of the nature and severity of the reaction could negatively affect treatment decisions. This chapter reviews the features and management strategies of severe IRs for some, commonly used chemotherapy drugs and monoclonal antibodies.

Recognition of Infusion Reactions

Prompt recognition and immediate medical attention are needed to reduce the risk from IRs.[3] IRs can have a significant negative impact on both patients and clinicians because these reactions usually occur while treatment is being administered or shortly thereafter.

Based on patient symptoms and status and available emergency resources, management of patients who suffer an IR from an anticancer agent is very individualized and varies with the severity of the reaction.[6] Severe reactions are less frequent and may be fatal without appropriate intervention. IRs can also lead to significant anxiety in patients, distress to staff, and the use of substantial resources.[7] It is important for clinicians to be aware of the possibility of IRs and have protocols in place to prevent and manage these reactions.[5] Mild and moderate infusion reactions are characterized by transient symptoms without any signs or symptoms of anaphylaxis. Severe infusion reactions, by definition, are associated with any features of anaphylaxis such as respiratory compromise, angioedema, hypotension, or generalized urticaria.

Prevention and Treatment of Infusion Reactions

In general, antihistamines, histamine (H)2 blockers, and steroids are used to prevent infusion reactions. The most commonly used drugs are diphenhydramine (50 mg), ranitidine (50 mg), and dexamethasone (4–10 mg). Once an infusion reaction is suspected, consideration should be given to the severity of the reaction. True anaphylactic reactions should be treated just like anaphylaxis of any cause, with prompt airway management, administration of epinephrine, and emergency room evaluation. Tables 11.1 and 11.2 provide detailed recommendations for the prevention and management of IRs caused by various agents. Fig. 11.1 depicts a general treatment algorithm for mild to moderate and severe infusion reactions.

Skin Testing

Some groups have recommended skin testing for patients at risk of developing severe infusion reactions. Given the difficulty with achieving accurate results from skin testing, it is rarely used. A notable exception, however, is for patients at high risk of platinum-based drug-related anaphylaxis, in which skin testing may have some utility.

Infusion Reactions Caused by Monoclonal Antibodies

Monoclonal antibodies are used to treat several types of cancers, as well as nonmalignant disorders. Over the past 2 or 3 decades, the use of monoclonal antibodies has increased dramatically, and several different monoclonal antibodies are currently available.[8] Monoclonal antibodies can cause IRs, with symptoms ranging from mild symptoms to life-threatening anaphylaxis.[2,9] Mild-to-moderate IRs to monoclonal antibodies may generally be managed by slowing the infusion rate, but severe reactions require emergency intervention. Reactions with monoclonal antibodies are less common, but have the potential to become severe and cause fatal outcomes if not managed appropriately.[10] Most acute IRs can be avoided by desensitization in preselected patients.[11,12] The incidence, prevention, and management of IRs with frequently used monoclonal antibodies are presented in Table 11.1.

Infusion Reactions Caused by Chemotherapy Drugs

All chemotherapy drugs have the potential to cause IRs.[13,14] IRs to chemotherapy drugs require prompt recognition and immediate treatment to avoid significant complications. IRs due to chemotherapeutics are infrequent and usually mild, but some drugs still have a significant incidence of IRs.[4] However, should a reaction occur, it is imperative to minimize exposure to the inciting agent and implement appropriate therapeutic and supportive measures by desensitization or treatment with a related compound.[15] The incidence, prevention, and management of IRs with frequently used chemotherapeutic drugs are presented in Table 11.2.

Desensitization

Desensitization measures can be used for patients with repeated moderate infusion reactions or severe infusion reactions. Desensitization procedures are generally complex and are done in intensive care settings with the aid of intensive care physicians, allergy and immunology physicians, and oncologists. Widely accepted protocols do not exist, and thus the specifics of desensitization generally vary by institution.

TABLE 11.1 ■ Infusion Reactions With Frequently Used Humanized and Chimeric Monoclonal Antibodies

INCIDENCE, PREVENTION, AND MANAGEMENT

Drug	Incidence of Severe Infusion Reaction	Symptoms	Prophylaxis	Management
Humanized				
Alemtuzumab[4,16]	3%	Shortness of breath, dizziness, hypotension, fever, headache, bronchospasm, chills, rash.	Premedicate with antihistamines, and corticosteroids.	Stop the infusion. Treatment can be resumed at a slower rate, after resolution of all symptoms. Antihistamines, and corticosteroids can be used to prevent infusion related events.
Bevacizumab[4,9]	<1%	Dyspnea, flushing, rash, chest pain, rigors, nausea, hypertension, wheezing, headaches.	Premedication is not recommended.	Treatment interruption; can be resumed at a slower rate after resolution of all symptoms. Supportive therapy.
Pembrolizumab[4,17]	<1%	Fever, chills	Premedicate with antihistamines.	Discontinue
Trastuzumab[4,18]	<1%	Chills, fever, anaphylaxis, urticaria, bronchospasms, angioedema, and/or hypotension	Premedication is not recommended.	Treatment interruption; can be resumed at a slower rate after resolution of all symptoms.
Chimeric				
Rituximab[2,4,9,16]	~10%	Fever, chills, rash, hypotension, nausea, rhinitis, urticaria, pruritus, asthenia, angioedema, bronchospasm. May be associated with features of tumor lysis syndrome.	Premedication: epinephrine, antihistamines, glucocorticoid. Close monitoring during all infusions for patients with preexisting cardiac and pulmonary conditions. A slow initial rate of infusion.	Treatment interruption; can be resumed at 50% reduction in infusion rate, after resolution of all symptoms.
Cetuximab[4,9,19,20]	3%	Chills, fever, urticaria, bronchospasms, angioedema, and/or hypotension.	Slower infusion rate. Premedication: epinephrine, antihistamines, glucocorticoid.	Treatment interruption; can be resumed at a slower rate after resolution of all symptoms.

TABLE 11.2 ■ Infusion Reactions With Frequently Used Chemotherapy Drugs

INCIDENCE, PREVENTION, AND MANAGEMENT

Drug	Incidence of Severe Infusion Reaction	Description/Symptoms	Prophylaxis	Management
Anthracyclines[4,16]	<1%	Pruritus, rash, tachycardia, hypotension, dyspnea, nausea, vomiting, headache, back pain, chest pain, syncope, flushing, chills, fever, urticaria, angioedema.	Slow infusion rate.	Desensitization; slower infusion rate.
Platinum Compounds				
Carboplatin[2,4,9,16]	12%	Rash, urticaria, abdominal cramps, bronchospasm, hypotension, tachycardia, dyspnea, chest pain, pruritus.	Contraindicated in patients allergic to platinum compounds.	Desensitization; slower infusion rate; treatment interruption and symptomatic therapy.
Oxaloplatin[2,4,9,16]	<1%	Sweating, urticaria, pruritus, rash, back or chest pain, fever, bronchospasm, hypotension.	Contraindicated in patients allergic to platinum compounds.	Treatment interruption; desensitization; slower infusion rate; symptomatic therapy with epinephrine, corticosteroids, and antihistamines.
Taxanes				
Docetaxel[2,4,9,16]	2%	Sweating, urticaria, pruritus, rash, back or chest pain, fever, bronchospasm, hypotension.	Premedicate with corticosteroids.	For severe reaction, immediate discontinuation and aggressive symptomatic therapy; desensitization.
Paclitaxel[2,4,9,16]	2%–4%	Sweating, urticaria, pruritus, rash, back or chest pain, fever, bronchospasm, hypotension.	Contraindicated in patients allergic to paclitaxel or other drugs solubilzed in Kolliphor. Premedicate with dexamethasone.	For severe reaction, immediate discontinuation and aggressive symptomatic therapy; desensitization.

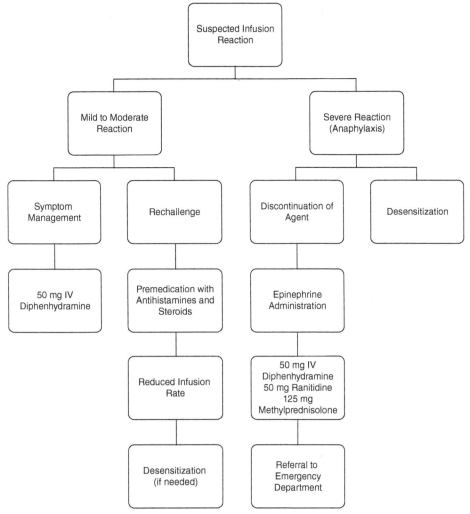

Fig. 11.1 Treatment algorithm for infusion reactions. *IV*, Intravenous.

Conclusion

Oncologic agents are associated with a risk for IRs, which can be unpredictable. Careful patient monitoring, and prompt intervention can reduce the risk for severe IRs. Understanding the basic principles of IRs will allow clinicians to provide optimal prophylactic measures and symptom management.

References

1. Perreault S, Baker J, Medoff E, et al. Infusion reactions are common after high-dose carmustine in BEAM chemotherapy and are not reduced by lengthening the time of administration. *Support Care Cancer.* 2017;25(1):205–208.
2. Vogel WH. Infusion reactions: diagnosis, assessment, and management. *Clin J Oncol Nurs.* 2010; 14(2):E10–E21.

3. Cmelak AJ, Goldberg RM. Infusion reactions associated with monoclonal antibodies in patients with solid tumors. Introduction. *Oncology (Williston Park).* 2009;23(2 suppl 1):5–6.
4. Rosello S, Blasco I, García Fabregat L, Cervantes A, Jordan K. Management of infusion reactions to systemic anticancer therapy: ESMO Clinical Practice Guidelines. *Ann Oncol.* 2017;28(suppl 4):iv100–iv118.
5. Simons FE, Ardusso LR, Bilò MB, et al. World allergy organization guidelines for the assessment and management of anaphylaxis. *World Allergy Organ J.* 2011;4(2):13–37.
6. Cortijo-Cascajares S, Jimenez-Cerezo MJ, Herreros de Tejada A. Review of hypersensitivity reactions to antineoplastic agents. *Farm Hosp.* 2012;36(3):148–158.
7. Chadda S, Larkin M, Jones C, et al. The impact of infusion reactions associated with monoclonal antibodies in metastatic colorectal cancer: a European perspective. *J Oncol Pharm Pract.* 2013;19(1):38–47.
8. Gatto B. Monoclonal antibodies in cancer therapy. *Curr Med Chem Anticancer Agents.* 2004;4(5):411–414.
9. Lenz HJ. Management and preparedness for infusion and hypersensitivity reactions. *Oncologist.* 2007;12(5):601–609.
10. Patel DD, Goldberg RM. Cetuximab-associated infusion reactions: pathology and management. *Oncology (Williston Park).* 2006;20(11):1373–1382; discussion 1382, 1392–1394, 1397.
11. Hong DI, Bankova L, Cahill KN, Kyin T, Castells MC. Allergy to monoclonal antibodies: cutting-edge desensitization methods for cutting-edge therapies. *Expert Rev Clin Immunol.* 2012;8(1):43–52; quiz 53–54.
12. Vultaggio A, Castells MC. Hypersensitivity reactions to biologic agents. *Immunol Allergy Clin North Am.* 2014;34(3):615–632.
13. Syrigou E, Makrilia N, Koti I, Saif MW, Syrigos KN. Hypersensitivity reactions to antineoplastic agents: an overview. *Anticancer Drugs.* 2009;20(1):1–6.
14. Rossi F, Incorvaia C, Mauro M. Hypersensitivity reactions to chemotherapeutic antineoplastic agents. *Recenti Prog Med.* 2004;95(10):476–481.
15. Zanotti KM, Markman M. Prevention and management of antineoplastic-induced hypersensitivity reactions. *Drug Saf.* 2001;24(10):767–779.
16. Joerger M. Prevention and handling of acute allergic and infusion reactions in oncology. *Ann Oncol.* 2012;23(suppl 10):x313–x319.
17. Garon EB, Rizvi NA, Hui R, et al. Pembrolizumab for the treatment of non-small-cell lung cancer. *N Engl J Med.* 2015;372(21):2018–2028.
18. Slamon DJ, Leyland-Jones B, Shak S, et al. Use of chemotherapy plus a monoclonal antibody against HER2 for metastatic breast cancer that overexpresses HER2. *N Engl J Med.* 2001;344(11):783–792.
19. Siena S, Glynne-Jones R, Adenis A, et al. Reduced incidence of infusion-related reactions in metastatic colorectal cancer during treatment with cetuximab plus irinotecan with combined corticosteroid and antihistamine premedication. *Cancer.* 2010;116(7):1827–1837.
20. Chung CH. Managing premedications and the risk for reactions to infusional monoclonal antibody therapy. *Oncologist.* 2008;13(6):725–732.

Mechanisms of Toxicities Associated With Targeted Therapy

Nadine Abdallah, MD ▪ Misako Nagasaka, MD ▪ Ammar Sukari, MD

Introduction

Over the last several years, molecularly targeted therapy has emerged as a new generation of cancer treatment and has been integrated into treatment protocols of many hematologic and solid tumors, either as monotherapy or in combination with chemotherapy. In general, targeted therapies include monoclonal antibodies and small molecule inhibitors that specifically affect the activity of genes or proteins mediating carcinogenesis. As described by Hanahan and Weinberg, cancer cells gain several hallmark features as they develop into invasive tumors.[1] The acquisition of these features is achieved by deregulation of physiologic pathways for proliferation, growth, apoptosis, and angiogenesis. This is achieved mainly by genetic or transcriptional alterations, including chromosomal translocations, somatic mutations, gene amplification, overexpression, and/or downregulation of target proteins or enzymes. Understanding of the molecular events underlying the process of tumorigenesis, coupled with the advent of advanced testing options, has allowed the specific targeting of cancer cells harboring such alterations and the sparing of normal cells lacking them. This has translated into the development of several targeted therapy agents which have become integral parts of cancer treatment. Imatinib inhibits BCR-ABL translocation and is the prototype of successful application of targeted therapy in chronic myelogenous leukemia (CML) (Fig. 12.1). This chapter will introduce molecular targets and their mechanisms of deregulation in cancer as they relate to the development of toxicities.

Receptor Tyrosine Kinases (RTKs)

- **Mechanism:** RTKs are transmembrane proteins that play integral roles in the cellular signaling pathways involved in growth, proliferation, differentiation, metabolism, and motility. Deregulation of these receptors and/or their downstream effectors occurs in many cancers, making them attractive molecular targets in treatment. RTKs share a basic structure composed of an extracellular ligand-binding domain, a transmembrane α-helical domain, and a cytoplasmic domain. The latter includes a juxta-membrane region, a conserved tyrosine kinase domain, and carboxy-terminal region.[2] The kinase domain catalyzes the phosphorylation of tyrosine residues on itself (autophosphorylation) and on other signaling molecules using adenosine triphosphate (ATP) as a substrate.[3] First, extracellular ligands including growth factors, cytokines, and hormones bind specifically to their monomeric receptors, which promotes the formation of receptor dimers (homodimers or heterodimers). Unlike other RTKs, the insulin receptor (IR) preexists in a dimeric state, which is stabilized by ligand binding.[4] The conformational change induced by ligand binding causes release of cis-autoinhibition and allows trans-autophosphorylation of tyrosine residues in the cytoplasmic domains. This induces receptor catalytic activity and generates docking sites for downstream cytoplasmic signaling proteins that possess Src homology-2 (SH2) or phosphotyrosine-binding (PTB) domains.[5] This, in turn, leads to the activation of multiple signal transduction pathways, including the RAS/mitogen activated protein kinase (MAPK), phosphoinositide 3-kinase

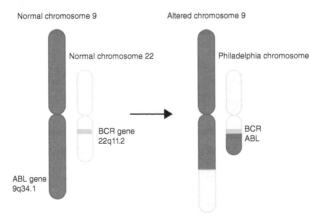

Fig. 12.1 Chromosomal translocation occurs between the long arms of *chromosome 9*, which has the *ABL gene*, and *chromosome 22*, which has the *BCR gene*. This produces the *Philadelphia chromosome* and creates a fusion gene which encodes a constitutively active tyrosine kinase.

(PI3K)/protein kinase B (AKT), and Janus kinase (JAK)/signal transducer and activator of transcription (STAT) pathways, which translates the extracellular signal into gene transcription and cellular response.

- **Alterations in malignancy:** Aberrant activation of RTKs is a key event in the transformation of many tumors. The main mechanisms include gain-of-function mutations, chromosomal translocations resulting in oncogenic fusion genes, gene amplification, protein overexpression, and increased autocrine stimulation.[6] RTKs most commonly implicated in cancers include EGFR (epidermal growth factor receptor), HER2, FGFR (fibroblast growth factor receptor), IGFR (insulin-like growth factor receptor), VEGFR (vascular endothelial growth factor receptor), PDGFR (platelet derived growth factor receptor), MET (hepatocyte growth factor receptor), ALK (anaplastic lymphoma kinase), KIT, and RET (rearranged during transfection).
- **RTK inhibitors:** RTK inhibitors fall under 2 main categories: Monoclonal antibodies (mAbs) and small molecule tyrosine kinase inhibitors (TKIs). MAbs bind to the extracellular domain (ECD) of RTKs by competing with endogenous ligands, preventing ligand-induced receptor activation and inhibition of downstream signaling. This also leads to immune destruction of tumor cells by antibody-mediated and complement-mediated cytotoxicity, and antibody-mediated phagocytosis.[7] TKIs are generally orally administered, low-molecular-weight molecules that cross the plasma membrane and act on the cytoplasmic side to inhibit tyrosine kinase activity, thus preventing autophosphorylation and activation of downstream signaling pathways. There are three types of TKIs; Type I TKIs compete with ATP for binding to the ATP binding site. This is the most common type. Many of these lack specificities and inhibit multiple RTKs owing to conservation of the ATP-binding site. Types II and III TKIs inhibit TKI activity by inducing conformational changes in RTKs independent of ATP competition.[8] RTKs have been developed that have been successfully targeted in cancer therapy. Some of these targets include EGFR, HER2, VEGF/VEGFR, ALK, MET, RET, and KIT. Toxicities associated with these targets are largely due to inhibition of these targets in normal tissues.

RAS/RAF/MEK/ERK Pathway

- **Mechanism:** The RAS/RAF/MEK/ERK pathway is a key pathway involved in growth and proliferation and is deregulated in many cancers.[9] RAS, RAF, MEK, and ERK are the

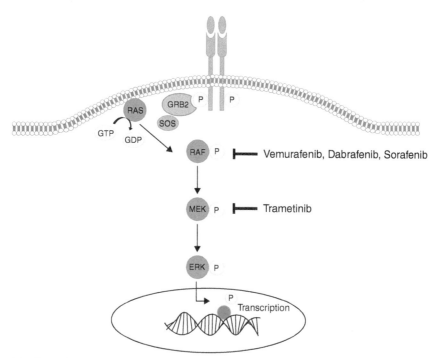

Fig. 12.2   The RAS-RAF-MEK-ERK pathway: Signaling is initiated when growth factors or cytokines bind cell-surface receptors, RTKs, or G-protein coupled receptors. This creates docking sites for *GRB2* which recruits *SOS*. This activates *RAS* by exchanging *GDP* for *GTP*. RAS induces dimerization and activation of *RAF*, which in turn phosphorylates and activates *MEK*. Then, MEK phosphorylates and activates *ERK* leading to activation of transcription factors turning on gene expression. *P,* phosphoric acid.

main players in this pathway. RAS is a guanosine triphosphate (GTP)–binding protein with intrinsic GTPase activity that exists in two states, the inactive GDP-bound state (RAS-GDP), and the active GTP-bound state (RAS-GTP). Cycling between these two states is regulated by guanine nucleotide exchange factors (GEFs) and GTPase activating proteins (GAPs). GEFs, such as SOS (son of sevenless), promote GDP dissociation and GTP binding. GAPs, such as neurofibromin 1 (NF1) augment the GTPase activity of RAS, causing GTP hydrolysis and resulting in the inactive state.[10] Signaling is initiated when growth factors or cytokines bind cell surface receptors such as RTKs or G-protein coupled receptors. This creates docking sites for adaptor proteins such as growth factor receptor-bound protein (GRB2) and SRC homology 2 domain-containing protein (SHC), which recruit GEFs like SOS to the cell membrane, resulting in RAS activation through exchange of GDP for GTP.[11] This process stimulates dimerization and activation of RAF proteins, which are cytoplasmic serine/threonine kinases.[12] RAF phosphorylates and activates MEK1 and MEK2 proteins, which are dual tyrosine and serine/threonine kinases. This in turn leads to phosphorylation and activation of ERK1 and ERK2 kinases, which phosphorylate cytoplasmic substrates and translocate to the nucleus to phosphorylate and activate transcription factors. The end result of this is activation of genes involved in survival, cell cycle progression, differentiation, apoptosis, migration, and feedback control of the pathway (Fig. 12.2).[11,13–15]

- **Role in cancer:** Oncogenic transformation occurs with mutations causing constitutive activation of this pathway. This is achieved by activating mutations in RAS, RAF, MEK or

ERK, RTK overexpression, PI3K and Akt amplification, and loss of negative regulators including PTEN and NF1.[10,16]

- **RAS:** RAS exists in three main isoforms, H-RAS, K-RAS and N-RAS.[17] Mutations in RAS are very common, occurring in 30% of cancers[18] and result in a constitutively activated RAS protein, trapped in a GTP-bound state with loss of GTPase activity.[19] Mutations are found in both solid and hematologic malignancies, with involvement of different isoforms depending on the cell origin.[20] Oncogenic activation is mainly through missense mutations resulting in amino acid substitutions in one of three hotspots, G12, G13, and Q61 in codons 12, 13, and 61, respectively. G12 and Q61 account for most KRAS and NRAS respectively, whereas HRAS has similar mutation frequencies among the three.[21] G12 mutations make RAS insensitive to GAP inactivation. Q61 mutation deceases the rate of RAS GTP hydrolysis.[11] Despite its prominent role in oncogenesis, RAS inhibitors, specifically in the form of KRAS inhibitors, are only recently being evaluated in clinical trials.

- **RAF:** RAF (rapidly accelerated fibrosarcoma) is a family of cytoplasmic serine/threonine protein kinases that includes BRAF, ARAF, and CRAF.[12] BRAF is frequently mutated in human cancers (8%), most commonly in melanoma (~60%). Mutations are also common in colorectal, lung, thyroid, and ovarian cancers, among others.[22,23] Normally, activated RAS binds to BRAF, which undergoes phosphorylation, and adopts an active conformation. Then it forms homodimers or heterodimers with other RAF proteins. This activates its serine/threonine kinase activity, allowing it to phosphorylate downstream signaling molecules, MEK1 and MEK2.[24] Its activity is tightly regulated by negative feedback.[25]

- **BRAF targeted in cancer:** BRAF mutations have been successfully targeted in cancer treatment. Vemurafenib and dabrafenib are reversible inhibitors of BRAF that compete with ATP for binding the kinase domain. Vemurafenib is approved for the treatment of melanoma with BRAF V600E mutation.[26] Dabrafenib is approved as monotherapy for melanoma with V600E mutation.[27] Dabrafenib is also approved for the treatment of melanoma with BRAF V600E/K mutations in combination with trametinib, a MEK inhibitor. The combination of dabrafenib and trametinib has also been US Food and Drug Administration (FDA)–approved for metastatic non–small-cell lung cancer (NSCLC) with BRAF V600E mutation and anaplastic thyroid cancer with BRAF V600E mutation.[28–30]

- **MEK:** Mitogen activated protein kinase (MAPKK), also known as MEK or MAP2K, is a family of protein kinases coded for by seven genes: MEK1–2 and MKK3–7. MEK1 and MEK2 are dual-specificity kinases, that can phosphorylate both tyrosine and serine/threonine residues. Their substrates ERK1 and ERK2, which are serine/threonine kinases, in turn phosphorylate nuclear and cytosolic targets leading to cellular responses.[31] Unlike RAS and BRAF, mutations in MEK are rare in cancer.

- **Targeted therapy:** Acquired resistance to BRAF inhibitors led to the development of downstream inhibitors of MEK. Trametinib is a selective allosteric MEK1 and MEK2 inhibitor that binds to the unphosphorylated form of MEK, preventing its activation by RAF.[32] It is approved as a single-agent treatment of patients with advanced melanoma with BRAF V600E or V600K mutation. Clinical trials have shown that the combination of the BRAF inhibitor dabrafenib with the MEK inhibitor trametinib is more effective than single agents.[33]

Conclusion

As described, targeted therapies interfere with molecular pathways that are deregulated in cancer cells. However, some of these targets may also be expressed in normal cells, albeit at lower levels, and are essential for their survival and functioning. This can account for toxicities related to the affected organ. Small molecule TKIs are less specific than mAbs and often inhibit more than one target, leading to increased risk for toxicity. The next chapters will discuss organ-related toxicities, including mechanisms and culprit drugs.

References

1. Hanahan D, Weinberg RA. The hallmarks of cancer. *Cell*. 2000;100(1):57–70.
2. Hubbard SR. Structural analysis of receptor tyrosine kinases. *Prog Biophys Mol Biol*. 1999;71(3–4): 343–358.
3. Hunter T. The Croonian Lecture 1997. The phosphorylation of proteins on tyrosine: its role in cell growth and disease. *Philos Trans R Soc Lond B Biol Sci*. 1998;353(1368):583–605.
4. Schlessinger J. Cell signaling by receptor tyrosine kinases. *Cell*. 2000;103(2):211–225.
5. Schlessinger J, Lemmon MA. SH2 and PTB domains in tyrosine kinase signaling. *Sci STKE*. 2003;2003(191):RE12.
6. Du Z, Lovly CM. Mechanisms of receptor tyrosine kinase activation in cancer. *Mol Cancer*. 2018;17(1):58.
7. Fauvel B, Yasri A. Antibodies directed against receptor tyrosine kinases: current and future strategies to fight cancer. *MAbs*. 2014;6(4):838–851.
8. Hojjat-Farsangi M. Small-molecule inhibitors of the receptor tyrosine kinases: promising tools for targeted cancer therapies. *Int J Mol Sci*. 2014;15(8):13768–13801.
9. McCubrey JA, Steelman LS, Chappell WH, et al. Roles of the Raf/MEK/ERK pathway in cell growth, malignant transformation and drug resistance. *Biochim Biophys Acta*. 2007;1773(8):1263–1284.
10. Downward J. Targeting RAS signalling pathways in cancer therapy. *Nat Rev Cancer*. 2003;3(1):11–22.
11. Santarpia L, Lippman SM, El-Naggar AK. Targeting the MAPK-RAS-RAF signaling pathway in cancer therapy. *Expert Opin Ther Targets*. 2012;16(1):103–119.
12. Maurer G, Tarkowski B, Baccarini M. Raf kinases in cancer-roles and therapeutic opportunities. *Oncogene*. 2011;30(32):3477–3488.
13. Meloche S, Pouyssegur J. The ERK1/2 mitogen-activated protein kinase pathway as a master regulator of the G1- to S-phase transition. *Oncogene*. 2007;26(22):3227–3239.
14. Mebratu Y, Tesfaigzi Y. How ERK1/2 activation controls cell proliferation and cell death: is subcellular localization the answer? *Cell Cycle*. 2009;8(8):1168–1175.
15. Lito P, Rosen N, Solit DB. Tumor adaptation and resistance to RAF inhibitors. *Nat Med*. 2013;19(11): 1401–1409.
16. Burotto M, Chiou VL, Lee JM, et al. The MAPK pathway across different malignancies: a new perspective. *Cancer*. 2014;120(22):3446–3456.
17. Colicelli J. Human RAS superfamily proteins and related GTPases. *Sci STKE*. 2004;2004(250):RE13.
18. Downward J. Ras signalling and apoptosis. *Curr Opin Genet Dev*. 1998;8(1):49–54.
19. Roberts PJ, Der CJ. Targeting the Raf-MEK-ERK mitogen-activated protein kinase cascade for the treatment of cancer. *Oncogene*. 2007;26(22):3291–3310.
20. Bos JL. Ras oncogenes in human cancer: a review. *Cancer Res*. 1989;49(17):4682–4689.
21. Prior IA, Lewis PD, Mattos C. A comprehensive survey of Ras mutations in cancer. *Cancer Res*. 2012;72(10):2457–2467.
22. Davies H, Bignell GR, Cox C, et al. Mutations of the BRAF gene in human cancer. *Nature*. 2002;417(6892):949–954.
23. Xing M. BRAF mutation in papillary thyroid cancer: pathogenic role, molecular bases, and clinical implications. *Endocr Rev*. 2007;28(7):742–762.
24. Kyriakis JM, App H, Zhang XF, et al. Raf-1 activates MAP kinase-kinase. *Nature*. 1992;358(6385):417–421.
25. Dougherty MK, Muller J, Ritt DA, et al. Regulation of Raf-1 by direct feedback phosphorylation. *Mol Cell*. 2005;17(2):215–224.
26. Chapman PB, Hauschild A, Robert C, et al. Improved survival with vemurafenib in melanoma with BRAF V600E mutation. *N Engl J Med*. 2011;364(26):2507–2516.
27. Hauschild A, Grob JJ, Demidov LV, et al. Dabrafenib in BRAF-mutated metastatic melanoma: a multicentre, open-label, phase 3 randomised controlled trial. *Lancet*. 2012;380(9839):358–365.
28. Flaherty KT, Infante JR, Daud A, et al. Combined BRAF and MEK inhibition in melanoma with BRAF V600 mutations. *N Engl J Med*. 2012;367(18):1694–1703.

29. Planchard D, Besse B, Groen HJM, et al. Dabrafenib plus trametinib in patients with previously treated BRAF(V600E)-mutant metastatic non-small cell lung cancer: an open-label, multicentre phase 2 trial. *Lancet Oncol.* 2016;17(7):984–993.
30. Subbiah V, Kreitman RJ, Wainberg ZA, et al. Dabrafenib and trametinib treatment in patients with locally advanced or metastatic BRAF V600-mutant anaplastic thyroid cancer. *J Clin Oncol.* 2018;36(1):7–13.
31. Roskoski R Jr. MEK1/2 dual-specificity protein kinases: structure and regulation. *Biochem Biophys Res Commun.* 2012;417(1):5–10.
32. Samatar AA, Poulikakos PI. Targeting RAS-ERK signalling in cancer: promises and challenges. *Nat Rev Drug Discov.* 2014;13(12):928–942.
33. Lugowska I, Kosela-Paterczyk H, Kozak K, et al. Trametinib: a MEK inhibitor for management of metastatic melanoma. *Onco Targets Ther.* 2015;8:2251–2259.

CHAPTER 13

Gastrointestinal Toxicities of Targeted Therapy

Tahmida Chowdhury, MD ▪ Ammar Sukari, MD ▪ Misako Nagasaka, MD

Introduction

Targeted therapies are a category of drugs that inhibit cancer by interfering with specific molecules involved in the growth, progression, and spread of malignant cells. Targeted therapies act on specific molecular targets, whereas most standard chemotherapies act on many rapidly dividing normal and cancer cells. Many different targeted therapies have been approved by the US Food and Drug Administration (FDA) to treat specific types of cancer. Targeted therapies are generally less toxic than standard chemotherapy drugs because just as they are sometimes more efficacious because they are designed to act on specific molecular targets, they have less effects on other cells. Some therapies, however, do have substantial side effects. The most common gastrointestinal side effects seen with targeted therapies are discussed in this chapter and include diarrhea, nausea, vomiting, hepatotoxicity, and gastrointestinal perforation.

Diarrhea

Targeted therapy-induced diarrhea: Targeted therapy-induced diarrhea is a challenge in daily clinical practice. The frequency, severity, and causes of symptoms differ based on the agent used and is common in patients receiving tyrosine kinase inhibitors (TKIs). Targeted therapies that are commonly associated with diarrhea include—endothelial growth factor receptor (EGFR)–targeted TKIs (e.g., erlotinib, gefitinib, afatinib, osimertinib), EGFR-targeted monoclonal antibodies (mAbs) (e.g., cetuximab, panitumumab), c-Kit TKIs (e.g., imatinib, sunitinib, regorafenib), multi-TKIs (e.g., sorafenib, sunitinib, axitinib), and mitogen-activated protein kinase (MEK) inhibitors (e.g., trametinib, selumetinib). The most commonly used method for assessing the severity of diarrhea is National Cancer Institute Common Toxicity Criteria (NCI CTC) (Table 13.1).

EGFR–Targeting Agents

- **Diarrhea and the EGFR pathway:** EGFR-TKIs increase chloride secretion and induce secretory diarrhea.[1] This is thought to be mediated by inhibition of wild-type EGFR in the gut. The incidence and severity of diarrhea are higher with EGFR-TKIs than with EGFR-mAbs. The occurrence of diarrhea is up to 60% for all grades, with grade 3 diarrhea developing in 6% to 9% of cases with EGFR-TKIs. EGFR-mAbs cause grade 2 diarrhea in 21% of cases and grade 3 diarrhea in about 1% to 2% of cases.[2–4]
- **Mechanism of action:** The EGFR, also known as Erb1 or HER1, works via activation of intercellular signaling pathways, particularly RAS/MAPK (mitogen-activating protein kinase) and PI3K (phosphoinositide-3 kinase)/AKT pathways,[5,6] and results in the upregulation of mitogenic, anti-apoptotic, angiogenic, and pro-invasive cellular mechanisms. EGFR is overexpressed in many cancers such as breast, colorectal, head and neck, non–small-cell lung, ovarian, and pancreatic cancers, making it a useful target for cancer-directed therapy.[7–15]

TABLE 13.1 ■ National Cancer Institute Common Terminology Criteria for Grading Diarrhea

Grade	Severity of Diarrhea
1	Increase of <4 stools per day over baseline; mild increase in ostomy output compared with baseline
2	Increase of 4–6 stools per day over baseline; IV fluids indicated <24 h; moderate increase in ostomy output compared with baseline
3	Increase of ≥7 stools per day over baseline; incontinence; IV fluids >24 h; hospitalization indicated; severe increase in ostomy output compared with baseline; limiting self-care ADL
4	Life-threatening consequences; urgent intervention indicated
5	Death

ADL, Activities of daily living.

■ **Anti-EGFR TKIs:** Anti-EGFR TKIs compete with adenosine triphosphate (ATP) and inhibit EGFR tyrosine kinase activity. FDA-approved TKIs include gefitinib, erlotinib, afatinib, and osimertinib. Gefitinib and erlotinib are reversible TKIs used for metastatic non–small-cell lung cancer (NSCLC) with EGFR exon 19 deletions or the exon 21-substitution mutation L858R. Erlotinib is also used in pancreatic cancer.[16] Afatinib is an irreversible HER2, EGFR, and HER4 directed TKI used in metastatic NSCLC.[17] Osimertinib is an irreversible TKI approved for metastatic NSCLC with T790M mutation on progression on or after EGFR TKI therapy[18]; it is also approved as first line treatment of NSCLC with sensitizing EGFR mutations.[19] Gefitinib causes diarrhea in 39% to 49.7% of cases, erlotinib in 48%, and afatinib in 22%.

■ **Anti-EGFR mAbs:** Cetuximab and panitumumab are FDA-approved anti-EGFR mAbs. The FDA first approved cetuximab in 2004 for the treatment of advanced colorectal cancer. More recently, cetuximab has also been approved in combination with radiation for head and neck squamous cell carcinoma.[13,14] Panitumumab was approved for the treatment of metastatic colorectal cancer in 2006.[15] Cetuximab is a mouse–human chimeric monoclonal immunoglobulin G1 (IgG1) that binds to the extracellular ligand-binding domain of EGFR and prevents tyrosine kinase activation and downstream EGFR signaling, promoting EGFR internalization and antibody-dependent cell-mediated cytotoxicity (ADCC).[11] Diarrhea occurs more often with cetuximab or panitumumab given in combination with chemotherapy than with monotherapy.[20,21] The overall incidence of diarrhea is about 80% in patients treated with cetuximab and chemotherapy and 70% in patients treated with panitumumab and chemotherapy.[22–24]

c-KIT–Targeting Agents

■ **Diarrhea and the c-KIT pathway:** Diarrhea is one of the most common adverse effects observed during treatment with imatinib. Approximately 20% to 26% of patients experience diarrhea during therapy. Sunitinib and regorafenib cause diarrhea in 44%, and 34% to 40% of patients, respectively. The high expression of KIT in the intestinal cells of Cajal might be a potential mechanism for diarrhea by imatinib or sunitinib.[25]

■ **Mechanism of action:** Stem cell growth factor receptor, c-KIT, or CD117, regulates cell proliferation and differentiation. Stem cell factor dimers interact with KIT, inducing receptor dimerization, leading to auto-inhibition and transphosphorylation of intercellular proteins and activation of intercellular signaling pathways.[26] Normally this pathway plays an important role in mast cell survival and function, pigmentation, gametogenesis, differentiation of hematopoietic stem cells, and development of gastric pacemaker cells. c-KIT deregulation in cancer occurs mainly through c-KIT overexpression and genetic mutation. c-KIT mutations occur in gastrointestinal stromal tumor (GIST),[27] acute myeloid leukemia (AML),[28] germ cell tumors,[29,30] melanoma,[31] mastocytosis,[32] and sinonasal NK/T cell lymphoma.[33]

- **c-KIT TKIs:** FDA-approved agents are imatinib, sunitinib, and regorafenib. Imatinib inhibits BCR-ABL kinase in CML, and also inhibits other receptor tyrosine kinases including c-KIT and PDGF, and is currently approved for c-KIT–positive GIST tumors.[34,35] Sunitinib is a second-generation multi-TKI used for GIST upon disease progression. Regorafenib is also a multikinase inhibitor approved for patients with GIST refractory to both imatinib and sunitinib.[36]

VEGF–Targeting Agents

- **Diarrhea and the vascular endothelial growth factor (VEGF) pathway:** VEGF–targeting TKIs that cause diarrhea include sorafenib, sunitinib (44%), pazopanib (52%, grade 3 diarrhea), axitinib (11%), vandetanib (52% any grade diarrhea, 5.6% high-grade diarrhea), regorafenib (34%–40%), lenvatinib, and cabozatinib (64%).
- **Mechanism of action:** The VEGF family includes 5 glycoproteins: VEGFA, VEGFB, VEGFC, VEGFD, and placental growth factor (PGF), which interact with and activate receptors belonging to the tyrosine kinase family: VEGFR1, VEGFR2, and VEGFR3.[37] Upon interaction with their ligands, VEGFRs activate downstream signaling pathways, leading to endothelial cell effects including proliferation, survival, migration, vasodilation, and increased permeability.[38] VEGFRs are expressed on tumor cells and endothelial cells in NSCLC,[39] gastric cancer,[40] breast cancer,[41] leukemia,[42] prostate cancer,[43] and hepatocellular carcinoma.[44] VEGF signaling also has important effects that promote tumor angiogenesis and distant metastasis.
- **VEGF–targeted therapy:** Inhibitors of the VEGF pathway include TKIs, mAbs against VEGF or VEGFRs, and soluble VEGF receptors. FDA-approved TKIs are sorafenib, sunitinib, pazopanib, axitinib, vandetanib, regorafenib, lenvatinib, cabozantinib, and ponatinib. Sorafenib is approved for the treatment of advanced renal cell carcinoma and is in late stage clinical trials for hepatocellular carcinoma, metastatic melanoma, and NSCLC. Bevacizumab is an mAb against VEGF, and is approved for colorectal cancer,[45] breast cancer,[46] cervical cancer,[47] ovarian cancer,[48] renal cell carcinoma,[49] glioblastoma,[50] and NSCLC.[51]

CDK4/6 Inhibitors

- **Diarrhea and CDK4/6 inhibitors:** Palbociclib and ribociclib often cause low-grade (grades 1 and 2) diarrhea, whereas abemaciclib commonly causes grade 3 diarrhea.[52] Abemaciclib monotherapy for patients with hormone receptor (HR) positive, HER2 negative metastatic breast cancer typically causes diarrhea within 1 week of therapy initiation. Most cases of diarrhea resolve quickly, with a median duration of 7.5 days (grade 2) and 4.5 days (grade 3).
- **Mechanism of action:** The cyclin D-cyclin–dependent kinase 4/6-Rb (CDK4/6) pathway controls the transition from the G1 (first growth phase) to the S phase (DNA replication phase). Mitogenic growth factor signaling activates the RAS/MAPK and PI3K pathways, leading to the upregulation of D-type cyclins (D1, D2 and D3) by increased transcription and decreased proteasomal degradation.[53] D cyclin binds to CDK4 and CDK6 to form a complex required for DNA replication.[54] Cyclin D1 overexpression occurs in breast cancer, head and neck squamous cell carcinoma (HNSCC), NSCLC, colorectal cancer, endometrial cancer, pancreatic cancer, melanoma, and neuroblastoma.[55,56]

- **CDK4/6 targeted–therapy**: CDK4 and CDK6 have been targeted in HR positive, HER2 negative breast cancer. FDA-approved CDK4/6 inhibitors are palbociclib, ribociclib, and abemaciclib.

Mitogen-Activated Protein Kinase Inhibitors

- **Diarrhea and mitogen-activated protein kinase (MEK) inhibitors**: Trametinib and selumetinib are selective inhibitors of MEK1 and MEK2. Approximately 45% to 50% of patients treated with these drugs experience diarrhea of any grade.
- **Mechanism of action**: MEK is a family of protein kinases consisting of seven genes: MEK1–2 and MKK3–7. The MAPK signaling pathway includes the enzymes RAS, RAF, MEK, and extracellular signal-regulated kinase (ERK) and is an important pathway in cellular proliferation. MEK1 and MEK2 have the ability to phosphorylate both tyrosine and serine/threonine residues, and their substrates ERK1 and ERK2, phosphorylate nuclear and cytosolic targets leading to cellular responses.[57]
- **MEK inhibitors**: Trametinib is a selective MEK1 and MEK2 inhibitor, approved as a single agent treatment of patients with advanced melanoma with serine/threonine kinase (BRAF) V600E or V600K mutations.[58]

Management of Diarrhea

There are no specific guidelines available on the management of different grades of targeted therapy-induced diarrhea. Patients must be rehydrated orally or by parenteral infusion based on severity, to prevent diarrhea-related complication such as dehydration, electrolyte imbalances, and hypovolemic shock in extreme scenarios (Table 13.2).

TABLE 13.2 ■ Suggested Management of Diarrhea According to Grade[59]

Grade	Management
1	• Continue kinase inhibitors; prescribe loperamide or codeine • Rule out infective cause • Dietary modification
2	• Withhold kinase inhibitors until symptoms have resolved to grade 1 or baseline; restart at a lower dose • Continue loperamide or codeine • Rule out infectious causes • Dietary modification
3	• Stop kinase inhibitors; scheduled use of loperamide or codeine • Hospitalization for intravenous rehydration and electrolyte replacement • Rule out infectious causes • Give antibiotics including a fluroquinolone if diarrhea persists for over 24 h, patient develops fever, or has grade 3/4 neutropenia • Hold kinase inhibitors until < grade 1 then restart with a lower dose
4	• Permanent discontinuation of kinase inhibitors • Hospitalization for intravenous hydration and electrolyte replacement • Consider colonoscopy to assess for colitis and to exclude infectious causes • Cover with antibiotics if no improvement in 24 h, patient develops fever, or has grade 3/4 neutropenia

Pharmacological Management of Diarrhea

1. **Opioids**: Loperamide is the opioid of choice for the management of diarrhea because it has local activity in the gut. It reduces stool weight, frequency of bowel movements, urgency, and fecal incontinence. Other opioids that are also used include tincture of opium, morphine, and codeine. Loperamide can be started at an initial dose of 4 mg followed by 2 mg every 2 to 4 hours (with a maximum daily dosage of 16 mg). If diarrhea persists over 48 hours, other agents such as diphenoxylate/atropine, octreotide, or tincture of opium should be introduced. Diphenoxylate/atropine, 2.5 mg/0.025 mg tablet, should be started at one to two tablets as needed and the maximum daily dose should not exceed 20 mg/0.2 mg. The recommended dose of tincture of opium is 10 to 15 drops every 3 to 4 hours.[60]
2. **Octreotide**: Octreotide is a somatostatin analog that decreases the secretion of a number of hormones. It suppresses the release of insulin, glucagon, vasoactive intestinal peptide (VIP), and gastric acid. Octreotide also prolongs intestinal transit time, reducing secretion and increasing absorption of fluid and electrolytes. It can be started at an initial dose of 100 to 150 μg every 8 hours intravenously or subcutaneously; the dose can be titrated up to 500 μg every 8 hours.[61]
3. **Steroids:** Treatment with corticosteroids alone or in combination with loperamide is controversial and thus is not currently recommended.
4. **Over the counter:** Over the counter bismuth-containing medications can provide diarrhea and cramping relief.

NONPHARMACOLOGICAL MANAGEMENT OF DIARRHEA

1. Avoidance of dairy
2. Encouragement of low-fiber diet
3. Encouragement of foods high in potassium
4. Avoidance of spicy foods, high-fat foods, and high-fiber foods
5. Avoidance of caffeine and alcohol

Targeted Therapy-Related Nausea and Vomiting

Nausea and vomiting are common adverse effects of targeted therapy. Incidence rates depend on the type of drug used, dose of the drug, and route of administration of the drug (intravenous drugs cause nausea and vomiting more rapidly than drugs given orally). Some other risk factors include female gender, age younger than 50 years, and history of anxiety or motion sickness. Targeted therapies that are well known to cause nausea and vomiting are anaplastic lymphoma kinase (ALK) inhibitors (e.g., crizotinib, alectinib), mesenchymal epithelial transition factor (c-MET) kinase inhibitors (e.g., cabozantinib), CDK4/6 inhibitors (e.g., palbociclib, ribociclib, abemaciclib), and poly ADP-ribose polymerase (PARP) inhibitors (e.g., olaparib).

ALK Targeted–Therapy and Nausea and Vomiting

Grade 1 and 2 nausea or vomiting are commonly seen with crizotinib (39%–56%) and alectinib use.[62] Taking crizotinib with food is a helpful strategy for alleviating nausea. Nausea and vomiting can be prevented using antiemetics such as ondansetron, metoclopramide, or dimenhydrinate. Ondansetron should be avoided in patients with risk of QT prolongation.

■ **Mechanism of action:** ALK is a receptor tyrosine kinase that belongs to the insulin receptor superfamily. The ALK protein, also known as CD246, was first identified in anaplastic large cell lymphoma as a constitutively active fusion gene product.[63] ALK is normally expressed in brain, small intestine, colon, prostate, and testicular cells.[64] The ALK protein is encoded by the ALK gene located on chromosome 2 (2p23 segment). Chromosomal rearrangement resulting in an oncogenic fusion gene is the most common alteration of ALK in human cancer. Multiple fusion partners for ALK have been identified such as nucleophosmin-anaplastic lymphoma kinase (NPM-ALK), an oncogenic protein found in ALK-positive anaplastic large cell lymphoma (ALCL).[65] TPM3-ALK and TPM4-ALK translocations have been found in renal cell cancer[66,67] and esophageal cancer, respectively. EML4-ALK translocations have been found in NSCLC, breast, and colorectal cancers.[68–70] Patients with ALK rearrangements tend to be younger at diagnosis (median age 50 years) and are typically nonsmokers. Amplification of the ALK gene has been observed in neuroblastoma, NSCLC, and inflammatory breast cancer. ALK gene mutations have been observed in familial neuroblastoma,[71] anaplastic thyroid cancer,[72] and NSCLC.[73]

- **ALK–targeted therapy:** The first clinically approved ALK inhibitor was crizotinib, approved by the FDA for use in ALK-positive NSCLC.[74] Crizotinib is an oral TKI that was initially developed as a c-MET inhibitor but was later found to inhibit ALK. It also inhibits Hepatocyte Growth Factor Receptor (HGFR), ROS1 (c-ros), and Recepteur d'Origine Nantais (RON). The therapeutic efficacy of crizotinib is limited by secondary resistance, so more potent second-generation ALK inhibitors were developed. Other FDA-approved ALK inhibitors are ceritinib,[75,76] alectinib,[77,78] and brigatinib.[79]

c-MET Targeted–Therapy and Gastrointestinal Side Effects

The most common gastrointestinal side effects of cabozantinib are nausea and vomiting. Cabozantinib is a substrate of CYP3A4. Clinicians should be aware that drugs that inhibit this enzyme may potentially increase the adverse effects of cabozantinib. Grapefruit should be avoided because it may increase the concentration of drug in the blood.[80]

- **c-MET:** c-MET is also known as hepatocyte growth factor receptor (HGFR). c-MET is a receptor tyrosine kinase encoded by c-MET proto-oncogene.[81] It has a high affinity for hepatocyte growth factor (also known as scatter factor). The precursor protein undergoes proteolytic cleavage to yield a heterodimer, ligand binding then induces receptor dimerization and subsequent activation of intercellular signaling pathways such as RAS/MAPK, PI3k/AKT, SRC, and JAK/STAT pathways. This activation leads to cellular responses, including cellular proliferation, migration, invasion, angiogenesis, protection from apoptosis, and metastasis.[82,83] The c-MET receptor tyrosine kinase can be activated via gene mutation, amplification, protein overexpression, and/or ligand-dependent autocrine/paracrine activation.[84] Overexpression of c-MET has been found in head and neck, lung, gastric, colorectal, breast, and brain cancers.[85] Gene mutations have been observed in NSCLC, gastric, hepatocellular, and papillary renal carcinomas.[86–89] Coexpression of c-MET and HGF has been reported in breast cancer and glioma.[90–92] There is an interaction between c-MET and EGFR pathways, where EGFR signaling leads to ligand-dependent c-MET activation.[90]

- **c-MET–targeted therapy:** Several strategies have been developed to inhibit the c-MET signaling pathway; these include selective c-MET kinase inhibitor such as tivantinib, nonselective c-MET kinase inhibitors such as cabozantinib, anti-c-MET monoclonal antibody, and anti-HGF monoclonal antibodies.[93] Cabozantinib is a multikinase inhibitor used in advanced renal cell carcinoma and medullary thyroid cancer.

Pharmacological Management[94–104]

1. Serotonin (5-HT3) antagonists block the effects of serotonin in the central nervous system (CNS). Serotonin is important in triggering nausea and vomiting in the brain. Examples: ondansetron, granisetron, dolasetron, palonosetron.

2. NK-1 antagonists are usually used in combination with other antiemetics to delay nausea and vomiting. Examples: aprepitant (oral formulation), rolapitant (IV formulation).
3. Dopamine antagonists prevent dopamine from binding to the areas in the brain that trigger nausea and vomiting. Examples: prochlorperazine, metoclopramide.
4. Antianxiety drugs also reduce nausea and vomiting. Examples: lorazepam, alprazolam, olanzapine.
5. Steroids have potent antinausea effects. Examples: dexamethasone, methylprednisone.
6. Cannabinoids, although not universally accepted, have shown promise in the treatment of nausea and vomiting.

Nonpharmacological Treatment[94–104]

There are several nonpharmacological treatment options that may be used alone for mild nausea or can be used in conjunction with antiemetics. Studies are limited and include:
1. Frequent, small meals
2. Clear liquid diet
3. Hard candy
4. Bland foods
5. Avoidance of fatty, fried, or spicy foods
6. Encouragement to sit upright for at least 1 hour after each meal
7. Cognitive behavioral therapy including biofeedback techniques, guided imagery, and self-hypnosis

Hepatotoxicity

Targeted therapy and hepatotoxicity: Liver damage is a clinically significant adverse effect of targeted therapy. Liver damage can occur in the form of necrosis of hepatocytes, cholestatic liver damage, and in severe cases, cirrhosis. The types of targeted therapies that have been known to cause hepatotoxicity include TKIs such as c-KIT TKIs (sunitinib, regorafenib), multi-TKIs (pazopanib), MEK inhibitors (trametinib), anti-HER-2 therapy (lapatinib), and anti-EGFR targeting agents (gefitinib, erlotinib). TKIs are also associated with increased risk of drug-induced liver injury (DILI).

Assessment of Liver Toxicity

Table 13.3 delineates the grading system most commonly used when assessing for liver toxicity caused by cancer-directed therapies.
- **Sunitinib:** Sunitinib is orally available multikinase inhibitor. Its targets include VEGFR-1, VEGFR-2, platelet-derived growth factor receptors (PDGFRs) alpha and beta, c-KIT, and FMS–like tyrosine kinase-3 ligand (FLT3L). Sunitinib is also metabolized by CYP3A4. As a result, sunitinib can cause hepatotoxicity.[106]
- **Regorafenib:** Regorafenib is a diphenylurea-based multikinase inhibitor of VEGFR1, VEGFR2, VEGFR2, TIE2, KIT, RET, RAF1, BRAF, PDGFR, and fibroblast growth factor receptor (FGFR). Similar to sunitinib, regorafenib is metabolized by CYP3A4 and is associated with hepatotoxicity.
- **Pazopanib:** Pazopanib is an angiogenesis inhibitor. It works by targeting PDGFR, VEGFR, and c-KIT. Pazopanib has been associated with increased serum alanine aminotransferase (ALT) and aspartate aminotransferase (AST) levels at least three times higher than the upper limit of normal in 18% of cases. Furthermore, grade 4 toxicity has been reported in up to 25% of patients. An increase in the serum bilirubin level is seen in 36% of patients who are treated with pazotinib.[107]

TABLE 13.3   **Grading Criteria for the Assessment of Liver Toxicity According to the NCI CTCAE**[105]

Grade	Severity of Liver Toxicity
1	Any of the parameters below without evidence of biliary obstruction or progressive disease: • ALP ≥2.5 × ULN • ALT or AST ≥3 × ULN • Bilirubin ≥ ULN – 1.5 × ULN with ≥35% direct bilirubin
2	Any of the parameters below without evidence of biliary obstruction or progressive disease: • ALP ≥2.5 × ULN • ALT or AST ≥3 × ULN Bilirubin ≥ ULN – 1.5 × ULN with ≥35% direct bilirubin • INR ≥1.5
3 or 4	Any of the parameters below without evidence of biliary obstruction or progressive disease: • ALT, AST or ALP ≥ 5 × ULN • Bilirubin ≥3 × ULN with ≥35% direct bilirubin • INR ≥2.5 • Clinical signs of liver failure

ALT, Alanine aminotransferase; *AST*, aspartate aminotransferase; *CTCAE*, Common Terminology Criteria for Adverse Events; *INR*, international normalized ratio; *NCI*, National Cancer Institute; *ULN*, upper limit of normal.

- **Lapatinib:** Lapatinib is a TKI that inhibits ERBB1 (Her1/EGFR) and ERRB2 (Her2/EGFR2). It is associated with ALT and AST increases at least three times higher than the upper limit of normal and bilirubin increases of more than twice the upper limit of normal. It is also metabolized by CYP3A4 and is associated with hepatotoxicity.[108]
- **Trametinib:** Trametinib is a selective MEK1 and MEK2 inhibitor. When used in combination with dabrafenib, it is associated with elevated alkaline phosphatase levels in 60% of patients.

Management

Hepatotoxicity is a common, but rarely fatal, adverse effect of targeted therapy. It is predominantly idiosyncratic and thus impossible to predict. Given this, there are no defined methods for the prevention of targeted therapy–related hepatotoxicity. However, the following recommendations should be considered to mitigate this risk[109]:

1. Avoidance of drug combinations at high risk of negative interactions
2. Prevention of reactivation of viral hepatitis using antiviral drugs
3. Periodic monitoring of liver function
4. For grade 3 or 4 toxicity, discontinuation of the drug is recommended.
5. Patients taking targeted therapy should avoid large doses of other hepatotoxic compounds, such as alcohol and acetaminophen.

Gastrointestinal Perforation

Gastrointestinal perforation, fistula formation, and/or intra-abdominal abscess formation are rare but severe adverse effects of molecular-targeted therapy. Gastrointestinal perforation has been associated with anti-VEGF therapy (bevacizumab in 2.4% of cases), c-Kit targeting TKIs, MEK inhibitors, and sorafenib (<1%). Risk factors for perforation are a tumor at the site of perforation, abdominal carcinomatosis, acute diverticulitis, bowel obstruction, recent history of colonoscopy or sigmoidoscopy, and history of pelvic or abdominal radiation. The mechanism of underlying gastrointestinal perforation is still unknown but appears to be related to small vessel thrombosis and impaired wound healing. Some cases of bowel perforation require bowel resection and anastomosis for management.[110]

References

1. Frieling T, Heise J, Wassilew SW. Multiple colon ulcerations, perforation and death during treatment of malignant melanoma with sorafenib. *Dtsch Med Wochenschr*. 2009;134:1464–1466.
2. Van Cutsem E, Peeters M, Siena S, et al. Open-label phase III trial of panitumumab plus best supportive care compared with best supportive care alone in patients with chemotherapy-refractory metastatic colorectal cancer. *J Clin Oncol*. 2007;25:1658–1664.
3. Davila M, Bresalier RS. Gastrointestinal complications of oncologic therapy. *Nat Clin Pract Gastroenterol Hepatol*. 2008;5:682–696.
4. Vincenzi B, Schiavon G, Pantano F, Santini D, Tonini G. Predictive factors for chemotherapy-related toxic effects in patients with colorectal cancer. *Nat Clin Pract Oncol*. 2008;5:455–465.
5. Hynes NE, Lane HA. ERBB receptors and cancer: the complexity of targeted inhibitors. *Nat Rev Cancer*. 2005;5(5):341–354.
6. Goffin JR, Zbuk K. Epidermal growth factor receptor: pathway, therapies, and pipeline. *Clin Ther*. 2013;35(9):1282–1303.
7. Normanno N, De Luca A, Bianco C, et al. Epidermal growth factor receptor (EGFR) signaling in cancer. *Gene*. 2006;366(1):2–16.
8. Gan HK, Kaye AH, Luwor RB. The EGFRvIII variant in glioblastoma multiforme. *J Clin Neurosci*. 2009;16(6):748–754.
9. Tang CK, Gong XQ, Moscatello DK, et al. Epidermal growth factor receptor vIII enhances tumorigenicity in human breast cancer. *Cancer Res*. 2000;60(11):3081–3087.
10. Moscatello DK, Holgado-Madruga M, Godwin AK, et al. Frequent expression of a mutant epidermal growth factor receptor in multiple human tumors. *Cancer Res*. 1995;55(23):5536–5539.
11. Garcia de Palazzo IE, Adams GP, Sundareshan P, et al. Expression of mutated epidermal growth factor receptor by non-small cell lung carcinomas. *Cancer Res*. 1993;53(14):3217–3220.
12. Kurai J, Chikumi H, Hashimoto K, et al. Antibody-dependent cellular cytotoxicity mediated by cetuximab against lung cancer cell lines. *Clin Cancer Res*. 2007;13(5):1552–1561.
13. Vermorken JB, Mesia R, Rivera F, et al. Platinum-based chemotherapy plus cetuximab in head and neck cancer. *N Engl J Med*. 2008;359(11):1116–1127.
14. Jonker DJ, O'Callaghan CJ, Karapetis CS, et al. Cetuximab for the treatment of colorectal cancer. *N Engl J Med*. 2007;357(20):2040–2048.
15. Van Cutsem E, Peeters M, Siena S, et al. Open-label phase III trial of panitumumab plus best supportive care compared with best supportive care alone in patients with chemotherapy-refractory metastatic colorectal cancer. *J Clin Oncol*. 2007;25(13):1658–1664.
16. Moore MJ, Goldstein D, Hamm J, et al. Erlotinib plus gemcitabine compared with gemcitabine alone in patients with advanced pancreatic cancer: a phase III trial of the National Cancer Institute of Canada Clinical Trials Group. *J Clin Oncol*. 2007;25(15):1960–1966.
17. Miller VA, Hirsh V, Cadranel J, et al. Afatinib versus placebo for patients with advanced, metastatic non-small-cell lung cancer after failure of erlotinib, gefitinib, or both, and one or two lines of chemotherapy (LUX-Lung 1): a phase 2b/3 randomised trial. *Lancet Oncol*. 2012;13(5):528–538.
18. Mok TS, Wu YL, Ahn MJ, et al. Osimertinib or platinum-pemetrexed in EGFR T790M-positive lung cancer. *N Engl J Med*. 2017;376(7):629–640.
19. Soria JC, Ohe Y, Vansteenkiste J, et al. Osimertinib in untreated EGFR-mutated advanced non-small-cell lung cancer. *N Engl J Med*. 2018;378(2):113–125.
20. Sobrero AF, Maurel J, Fehrenbacher L, et al. EPIC: phase III trial of cetuximab plus irinotecan after fluoropyrimidine and oxaliplatin failure in patients with metastatic colorectal cancer. *J Clin Oncol*. 2008;26:2311–2319.

21. Bokemeyer C, Bondarenko I, Makhson A, et al. Fluorouracil, leucovorin, and oxaliplatin with and without cetuximab in the first-line treatment of metastatic colorectal cancer. *J Clin Oncol.* 2008;27:663–671.

22. Reynold N, Wagstaff AJ. Cetuximab in the treatment of metastatic colorectal cancer. *Drugs.* 2004;64: 109–118.

23. Peeters M, Price TJ, Cervantes A, et al. Randomized phase III study of panitumumab with fluorouracil, leucovorin, and irinotecan (FOLFIRI) compared with FOLFIRI alone as second-line treatment in patients with metastatic colorectal cancer. *J Clin Oncol.* 2010;28:4706–4713.

24. Hecht JR, Mitchell E, Chidiac T, et al. A randomized phase IIIb trial of chemotherapy, bevacizumab, and panitumumab compared with chemotherapy and bevacizumab alone for metastatic colorectal cancer. *J Clin Oncol.* 2008;27:672–680.

25. Deininger M, O'Brien SG, Ford JM, Druker BJ. Practical management of patients with chronic myeloid leukemia receiving imatinib. *J Clin Oncol.* 2003;21:1637–1647.

26. Liang J, Wu YL, Chen BJ, et al. The C-kit receptor-mediated signal transduction and tumor-related diseases. *Int J Biol Sci.* 2013;9(5):435–443.

27. Hirota S, Isozaki K, Moriyama Y, et al. Gain-of-function mutations of c-kit in human gastrointestinal stromal tumors. *Science.* 1998;279(5350):577–580.

28. Cammenga J, Horn S, Bergholz U, et al. Extracellular KIT receptor mutants, commonly found in core binding factor AML, are constitutively active and respond to imatinib mesylate. *Blood.* 2005;106(12):3958–3961.

29. Kemmer K, Corless CL, Fletcher JA, et al. KIT mutations are common in testicular seminomas. *Am J Pathol.* 2004;164(1):305–313.

30. Hoei-Hansen CE, Kraggerud SM, Abeler VM, et al. Ovarian dysgerminomas are characterised by frequent KIT mutations and abundant expression of pluripotency markers. *Mol Cancer.* 2007;6:12.

31. Beadling C, Jacobson-Dunlop E, Hodi FS, et al. KIT gene mutations and copy number in melanoma subtypes. *Clin Cancer Res.* 2008;14(21):6821–6828.

32. Chatterjee A, Ghosh J, Kapur R. Mastocytosis: a mutated KIT receptor induced myeloproliferative disorder. *Oncotarget.* 2015;6(21):18250–18264.

33. Hongyo T, Li T, Syaifudin M, et al. Specific c-kit mutations in sinonasal natural killer/T-cell lymphoma in China and Japan. *Cancer Res.* 2000;60(9):2345–2347.

34. Heinrich MC, Griffith DJ, Druker BJ, et al. Inhibition of c-kit receptor tyrosine kinase activity by STI 571, a selective tyrosine kinase inhibitor. *Blood.* 2000;96(3):925–932.

35. FDA grants imatinib (Gleevec) full approval for adjuvant treatment of GIST. *Oncology (Williston Park).* 2012;26(3):264, 309.

36. Demetri GD, Reichardt P, Kang YK, et al. Efficacy and safety of regorafenib for advanced gastrointestinal stromal tumours after failure of imatinib and sunitinib (GRID): an international, multicentre, randomised, placebo-controlled, phase 3 trial. *Lancet.* 2013;381(9863):295–302.

37. Shibuya M. Vascular endothelial growth factor (VEGF) and its receptor (VEGFR) signaling in angiogenesis: a crucial target for anti- and pro-angiogenic therapies. *Genes Cancer.* 2011;2(12):1097–1105.

38. Simons M, Gordon E, Claesson-Welsh L. Mechanisms and regulation of endothelial VEGF receptor signalling. *Nat Rev Mol Cell Biol.* 2016;17(10):611–625.

39. Tanno S, Ohsaki Y, Nakanishi K, et al. Human small cell lung cancer cells express functional VEGF receptors, VEGFR-2 and VEGFR-3. *Lung Cancer.* 2004;46(1):11–19.

40. Wang X, Chen X, Fang J, et al. Overexpression of both VEGF-A and VEGF-C in gastric cancer correlates with prognosis, and silencing of both is effective to inhibit cancer growth. *Int J Clin Exp Pathol.* 2013;6(4):586–597.

41. Liang Y, Brekken RA, Hyder SM. Vascular endothelial growth factor induces proliferation of breast cancer cells and inhibits the anti-proliferative activity of anti-hormones. *Endocr Relat Cancer.* 2006;13(3): 905–919.

42. Song G, Li Y, Jiang G. Role of VEGF/VEGFR in the pathogenesis of leukemias and as treatment targets (Review). *Oncol Rep.* 2012;28(6):1935–1944.

43. Li R, Younes M, Wheeler TM, et al. Expression of vascular endothelial growth factor receptor-3 (VEGFR-3) in human prostate. *Prostate.* 2004;58(2):193–199.

44. Yamaguchi R, Yano H, Nakashima Y, et al. Expression and localization of vascular endothelial growth factor receptors in human hepatocellular carcinoma and non-HCC tissues. *Oncol Rep.* 2000;7(4):725–729.

45. Hurwitz H, Fehrenbacher L, Novotny W, et al. Bevacizumab plus irinotecan, fluorouracil, and leucovorin for metastatic colorectal cancer. *N Engl J Med.* 2004;350(23):2335–2342.

46. Miller K, Wang M, Gralow J, et al. Paclitaxel plus bevacizumab versus paclitaxel alone for metastatic breast cancer. *N Engl J Med*. 2007;357(26):2666–2676.
47. Tewari KS, Sill MW, Penson RT, et al. Bevacizumab for advanced cervical cancer: final overall survival and adverse event analysis of a randomised, controlled, open-label, phase 3 trial (Gynecologic Oncology Group 240). *Lancet*. 2017;390(10103):1654–1663.
48. Garcia A, Singh H. Bevacizumab and ovarian cancer. *Ther Adv Med Oncol*. 2013;5(2):133–141.
49. Yang JC, Haworth L, Sherry RM, et al. A randomized trial of bevacizumab, an anti-vascular endothelial growth factor antibody, for metastatic renal cancer. *N Engl J Med*. 2003;349(5):427–434.
50. Cohen MH, Shen YL, Keegan P, et al. FDA drug approval summary: bevacizumab (Avastin) as treatment of recurrent glioblastoma multiforme. *Oncologist*. 2009;14(11):1131–1138.
51. Planchard D. Bevacizumab in non-small-cell lung cancer: a review. *Expert Rev Anticancer Ther*. 2011;11(8):1163–1179.
52. Williams GH, Stoeber K. Cell cycle, CDKs and cancer: a changing paradigm. *Nat. Rev. Cancer*. 2009;9(3):153–166.
53. Hamilton E, Infante JR. Targeting CDK4/6 in patients with cancer. *Cancer Treat Rev*. 2016;45:129–138.
54. O'Leary B, Finn RS, Turner NC. Treating cancer with selective CDK4/6 inhibitors. *Nat Rev Clin Oncol*. 2016;13(7):417–430.
55. Musgrove EA, Caldon CE, Barraclough J, et al. Cyclin D as a therapeutic target in cancer. *Nat Rev Cancer*. 2011;11(8):558–572.
56. Molenaar JJ, Ebus ME, Koster J, et al. Cyclin D1 and CDK4 activity contribute to the undifferentiated phenotype in neuroblastoma. *Cancer Res*. 2008;68(8):2599–2609.
57. Samatar AA, Poulikakos PI. Targeting RAS-ERK signalling in cancer: promises and challenges. *Nat Rev Drug Discov*. 2014;13(12):928–942.
58. Lugowska I, Kosela-Paterczyk H, Kozak K, et al. Trametinib: a MEK inhibitor for management of metastatic melanoma. *Onco Targets Ther*. 2015;8:2251–2259.
59. *Ther Adv Med Oncol*. 2015;7(2):122–136 Mar.
60. Zidan J, Haim N, Beny A, Stein M, Gez E, Kuten A. Octreotide in the treatment of severe chemotherapy-induced diarrhea. *Ann Oncol*. 2001;12:227–229.
61. Karthaus M, Ballo H, Abenhardt W, et al. Prospective, double-blind, placebo-controlled, multicenter, randomized phase III study with orally administered budesonide for prevention of irinotecan (Cpt-11)-induced diarrhea in patients with advanced colorectal cancer. *Oncology*. 2005;68:326–332.
62. Camidge DR, Bang YJ, Kwak EL, et al. Activity and safety of crizotinib in patient with ALK-positive NSCLC: updated result from a phase 1 study. *Lancet Oncol*. 2012;13:1011–1013.
63. Morris SW, Kirstein MN, Valentine MB, et al. Fusion of a kinase gene, ALK, to a nucleolar protein gene, NPM, in non-Hodgkin's lymphoma. *Science*. 1994;263(5151):1281–1284.
64. Wahara T, Fujimoto J, Wen D, et al. Molecular characterization of ALK, a receptor tyrosine kinase expressed specifically in the nervous system. *Oncogene*. 1997;14(4):439–449.
65. Pulford K, Morris SW, Turturro F. Anaplastic lymphoma kinase proteins in growth control and cancer. *J Cell Physiol*. 2004;199(3):330–358.
66. Sukov WR, Hodge JC, Lohse CM, et al. ALK alterations in adult renal cell carcinoma: frequency, clinicopathologic features and outcome in a large series of consecutively treated patients. *Mod Pathol*. 2012;25(11):1516–1525.
67. Sugawara E, Togashi Y, Kuroda N, et al. Identification of anaplastic lymphoma kinase fusions in renal cancer: large-scale immunohistochemical screening by the intercalated antibody-enhanced polymer method. *Cancer*. 2012;118(18):4427–4436.
68. Soda M, Choi YL, Enomoto M, et al. Identification of the transforming EML4-ALK fusion gene in non-small-cell lung cancer. *Nature*. 2007;448(7153):561–566.
69. Toyokawa G, Seto T. Anaplastic lymphoma kinase rearrangement in lung cancer: its biological and clinical significance. *Respir Investig*. 2014;52(6):330–338.
70. Takahashi T, Sonobe M, Kobayashi M, et al. Clinicopathologic features of non-small-cell lung cancer with EML4-ALK fusion gene. *Ann Surg Oncol*. 2010;17(3):889–897.
71. Mosse YP, Laudenslager M, Longo L, et al. Identification of ALK as a major familial neuroblastoma predisposition gene. *Nature*. 2008;455(7215):930–935.
72. Murugan AK, Xing M. Anaplastic thyroid cancers harbor novel oncogenic mutations of the ALK gene. *Cancer Res*. 2011;71(13):4403–4411.

73. Wang YW, Tu PH, Lin KT, et al. Identification of oncogenic point mutations and hyperphosphorylation of anaplastic lymphoma kinase in lung cancer. *Neoplasia*. 2011;13(8):704–715.

74. Sharma GG, Mota I, Mologni L, et al. Tumor resistance against ALK targeted therapy-where it comes from and where it goes. *Cancers (Basel)*. 2018;10(3):62.

75. Shaw AT, Spigel DR, Tan DS, et al. MINI01.01: whole body and intracranial efficacy of ceritinib in ALK-inhibitor naive patients with ALK+ NSCLC and brain metastases: results of ASCEND 1 and 3: topic: medical oncology. *J Thorac Oncol*. 2016;11(11S):S256.

76. Crino L, Ahn MJ, De Marinis F, et al. Multicenter phase II study of whole-body and intracranial activity with ceritinib in patients with ALK-rearranged non-small-cell lung cancer previously treated with chemotherapy and crizotinib: results from ASCEND-2. *J Clin Oncol*. 2016;34(24):2866–2873.

77. Larkins E, Blumenthal GM, Chen H, et al. FDA approval: alectinib for the treatment of metastatic, ALK-positive non-small cell lung cancer following crizotinib. *Clin Cancer Res*. 2016;22(21):5171–5176.

78. Peters S, Camidge DR, Shaw AT, et al. Alectinib versus crizotinib in untreated ALK-positive non-small-cell lung cancer. *N Engl J Med*. 2017;377(9):829–838.

79. Markham A. Brigatinib: first global approval. *Drugs*. 2017;77(10):1131–1135.

80. Cabozantinib tablet (cabometyx) UK Summary of Product Characteristics, UK Electronic Medicines Compendium, September 2026. https://www.medicines.org.uk/emc/medicine/32431#gref.

81. Bottaro DP, Rubin JS, Faletto DL, et al. Identification of the hepatocyte growth factor receptor as the c-met proto-oncogene product. *Science*. 1991;251(4995):802–804.

82. Blumenschein Jr GR, Mills GB, Gonzalez-Angulo AM. Targeting the hepatocyte growth factor-cMET axis in cancer therapy. *J Clin Oncol*. 2012;30(26):3287–3296.

83. Nakamura T. Structure and function of hepatocyte growth factor. *Prog Growth Factor Res*. 1991;3(1):67–85.

84. Mo HN, Liu P. Targeting MET in cancer therapy. *Chronic Dis Transl Med*. 2017;3(3):148–153.

85. Viticchie G, Muller PAJ. c-MET and other cell surface molecules: interaction, activation and functional consequences. *Biomedicines*. 2015;3(1):46–70.

86. Danilkovitch-Miagkova A, Zbar B. Dysregulation of Met receptor tyrosine kinase activity in invasive tumors. *J Clin Invest*. 2002;109(7):863–867.

87. Lee JH, Han SU, Cho H, et al. A novel germ line juxtamembrane Met mutation in human gastric cancer. *Oncogene*. 2000;19(43):4947–4953.

88. Schmidt L, Duh FM, Chen F, et al. Germline and somatic mutations in the tyrosine kinase domain of the MET proto-oncogene in papillary renal carcinomas. *Nat Genet*. 1997;16(1):68–73.

89. Ma PC, Kijima T, Maulik G, et al. c-MET mutational analysis in small cell lung cancer: novel juxtamembrane domain mutations regulating cytoskeletal functions. *Cancer Res*. 2003;63(19):6272–6281.

90. Tuck AB, Park M, Sterns EE, et al. Coexpression of hepatocyte growth factor and receptor (Met) in human breast carcinoma. *Am J Pathol*. 1996;148(1):225–232.

91. Koochekpour S, Jeffers M, Rulong S, et al. Met and hepatocyte growth factor/scatter factor expression in human gliomas. *Cancer Res*. 1997;57(23):5391–5398.

92. Abounader R, Ranganathan S, Lal B, et al. Reversion of human glioblastoma malignancy by U1 small nuclear RNA/ribozyme targeting of scatter factor/hepatocyte growth factor and c-met expression. *J Natl Cancer Inst*. 1999;91(18):1548–1556.

93. Jo M, Stolz DB, Esplen JE, et al. Cross-talk between epidermal growth factor receptor and c-Met signal pathways in transformed cells. *J Biol Chem*. 2000;275(12):8806–8811.

94. Fauci AS, Braunwald E, Kasper DL, et al. *Harrison's Principles of Internal Medicine*. 17th ed. New York: McGraw-Hill Medical; 2008.

95. Camp-Sorrell D, Hawkins RA. *Clinical Manual for the Oncology Advanced Practice Nurse*. 2nd ed. Pittsburgh: Oncology Nursing Society; 2006.

96. Cope DG, Reb AM. *An Evidence-Based Approach to the Treatment and Care of the Older Adult with Cancer*. Pittsburgh: Oncology Nursing Society; 2006.

97. Houts PS, Bucher JA. *Caregiving*. Rev. ed. Atlanta: American Cancer Society; 2003.

98. Kaplan M. *Understanding and Managing Oncologic Emergencies: A Resource for Nurses*. Pittsburgh: Oncology Nursing Society; 2006.

99. Kuebler KK, Berry PH, Heidrich DE. *End-of-Life Care: Clinical Practice Guidelines*. Philadelphia: W.B. Saunders Co; 2002.

100. National Comprehensive Cancer Network. *Palliative Care.* Version 1.2015. www.nccn.org/profession-als/physician_gls/pdf/palliative.pdf.
101. Oncology Nursing Society. Cancer symptoms. www.cancersymptoms.org.
102. Ripamonti C, Bruera E. *Gastrointestinal Symptoms in Advanced Cancer Patients.* New York: Oxford University Press; 2002.
103. Varricchio CG. *A Cancer Source Book for Nurses.* 8th ed. Sudbury, MA: Jones and Bartlett; 2004.
104. Yarbro CH, Frogge MH, Goodman M. *Cancer Symptom Management.* 3rd ed. Sudbury, MA: Jones and Bartlett; 2004.
105. US Department of Health and Human Services, National Institutes of Health, National Cancer Institute (NCI). *Common Terminology Criteria for Adverse Events (CTCAE).* Ver. 5.0. https://ctep.cancer.gov/protocolDevelopment/electronic_applications/docs/CTCAE_v5_Quick_Reference_5x7.pdf.
106. Mueller E, Rockey M, Rashkin M. Sunitinib-related fulminant hepatic failure: case report and review of literature. *Pharmacotherapy.* 2008;28:1066–1070.
107. Strenberg C, Davis I, Mardiak J, Szczylik C, et al. Pazopanib in locally advanced or metastatic renal cell carcinoma: results of a randomized phase 3 trial. *J Clin oncol.* 2010;28:1061–1068.
108. Teng WC, Oh JW, New LS, et al. Mechanism-based inactivation of cytochrome p450 3A4 lapatinib. *Mol Pharmacol.* 2010;78:693–703.
109. Abou-Alfa GK, et al. Phase 2 study of sorafenib in patient with advance hepatocellular carcinoma. *J Clin Oncol.* 2006;24:4293–4300.
110. Kabbinavar FF, Schulz J, McCleod M, et al. Addition of bevacizumab to bolus fluorouracil and leucovorin in first-line metastatic colorectal cancer: results of a randomized phase II trial. *J Clin Oncol.* 2005;23:3697–3705.

CHAPTER 14

Pulmonary Toxicities of Targeted Therapy

Pradnya D. Patil, MD, FACP ■ Tanmay S. Panchabhai, MD, FACP, FCCP

Introduction

Prior to the 1990s, cytotoxic chemotherapy was used uniformly for all malignancies. This resulted in heterogeneous responses even within a specific tumor type. As insight was gained about the role of driver mutations (key alterations in the oncogenic addiction pathways of malignant cells), the concept of targeted therapies was born. By inhibiting driver pathways for carcinogenesis, these targeted agents were successful in managing cancers that did not have robust responses to cytotoxic chemotherapy. Imatinib, a tyrosine kinase inhibitor targeting the BCR-ABL1 fusion gene seen in chronic myeloid leukemia, and trastuzumab for human epidermal growth factor receptor 2 (HER2)-positive breast cancer, were among the earliest targeted agents discovered. The success of these agents heralded an era of targeted therapies that are now being used in a broad spectrum of solid tumors and hematologic malignancies. With genomic sequencing being used more frequently than in the past, newer therapeutic targets are being discovered. With these discoveries come targeted drug development that will lead to many more targeted therapies in the coming years.

There are some limitations to molecular-targeted therapies. In malignancies that develop in the presence of carcinogen or environmental exposures, often multiple coexisting mutations are observed. In such malignancies, targeting a single pathway either leads to a complete lack of response or development of early resistance by a variety of escape pathways. Some examples of such cancers are non–small-cell lung cancer (NSCLC) related to smoking or melanoma as a result of exposure to ultraviolet (UV) radiation. Even in malignancies that are dependent on a driver mutation for oncogenesis, tumor cells eventually develop resistance to targeted agents via alternate pathways.

In the current era, molecular-targeted therapies play an important role in the treatment of multiple tumor types. Preclinical work has shown that these agents demonstrate clinical efficacy when combined with other therapeutic modalities such as immunotherapy. Ongoing clinical trials are exploring the utility of combining these molecular-targeted therapies with immunotherapies; therefore it is quite likely that the clinical application of targeted agents will continue to rise in the foreseeable future.

As targeted therapies are being widely used, it is imperative that prescribing clinicians are aware of the potential for toxicity and monitor patients closely while on therapy. In this chapter, we will discuss pulmonary toxicities of targeted therapies. Similar to other drugs, lung toxicity with targeted therapy may be idiosyncratic, or may be more predictable when related to cumulative dosing of the drug. By having a low-degree of suspicion in patients on therapy with drugs that have the potential for pulmonary toxicity and early intervention, morbidity and mortality can be significantly reduced. In the next section, we describe the various targeted therapies listed by class and their specific pulmonary toxicities including the pathogenesis, risk factors, and clinical manifestations.

Agents and Mechanism of Action

EPIDERMAL GROWTH FACTOR RECEPTOR (EGFR) TYROSINE KINASE INHIBITORS

- Driver mutations in the EGFR gene are seen in close to 15% of patients with NSCLC in the United States and in over 60% in Asian populations, possibly due to the lower number of smokers.[1,2] Patients with EGFR mutations have a better prognosis than other NSCLC patients and usually have favorable responses to therapy with EGFR tyrosine kinase inhibitors (TKIs). The EGFR TKIs that are currently being used in clinical practice include first-generation reversible TKIs, erlotinib and gefitinib, the second-generation irreversible TKI, afatinib, and the third-generation TKI, osimertinib. Since the results of the FLAURA trial, which compared outcomes with first-line osimertinib versus erlotinib or gefitinib demonstrated superior overall survival, progression-free survival, tolerability, reduction in intracranial metastases, and activity against the T790M resistance-mutated lung cancer, osimertinib has become the agent of choice for frontline therapy for many practitioners.[3,4]
- **Incidence:** In a meta-analysis of 15 trials studying a total of 2201 patients treated with first- and second-generation EGFR TKIs, the most frequent etiology of mortality related to toxicity of the drug was pneumonitis (11 deaths, comprising 65% of the total reported deaths).[5] Overall, the incidence of interstitial lung disease (ILD) with EGFR TKIs is less than 5%, but the associated mortality can range from 0.6% with osimertinib to as high as 31%, which has been reported with gefitinib.[6,7]
- **Risk factors:** Risk factors for pulmonary toxicity include preexisting pulmonary disease, smoking, and radiation exposure.[7–9] A higher incidence of gefitinib-induced ILD was noted in men (6.6%) compared with women (3.3%) in an analysis of over 1900 Japanese patients treated with the agent.[8] Patients usually become symptomatic in the first few months of treatment.
- **Pathophysiology:** EGFR pathways are essential for the turnover and repair of the alveolar wall. They are expressed on type II pneumocytes. By inhibiting the EGFR pathway and impairing the repair mechanism, EGFR TKIs can not only induce alveolar damage themselves, but also increase susceptibility to other injury mediated by infections, radiation, or other drugs.[7,10,11]

Specific EGFR–Targeting Agents

- **Gefitinib:** The incidence of gefitinib-associated ILD has been reported to be slightly different in postmarketing experience in the United States (0.3%) versus Asian populations (2%).[6] Patients usually present with dyspnea, with or without cough, and low-grade fever, with a median onset of symptoms between 24 and 42 days. Endo et al. performed a multi-institutional analysis of the various radiographic manifestations of ILD and classified them into four major patterns: (1) nonspecific ground-glass opacities, (2) multifocal airspace consolidations, (3) patchy ground-glass opacities with septal thickening, and (4) extensive ground-glass opacities or consolidations with traction bronchiectasis[12] (Fig. 14.1). The majority of the patients had areas of ground-glass opacities, or a pattern of extensive parenchymal involvement (fourth pattern), which reflects diffuse alveolar damage. The fourth pattern was associated with the highest mortality. The histological findings on pathology include interstitial pneumonitis or fibrosis and other less common findings such as diffuse alveolar damage, organizing pneumonia, hypersensitivity, or eosinophilic pneumonitis.[13]
- **Erlotinib:** The overall incidence of ILD with erlotinib is approximately 1.1%[14] (Fig. 14.2). In an analysis of 9907 Japanese patients treated with erlotinib in the phase IV POLARSTAR surveillance study, the reported incidence was 3.4% to 5.1%.[15] Risk factors for ILD

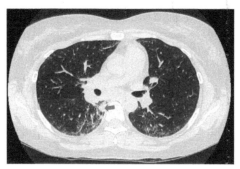

Fig. 14.1   Basilar traction bronchiectasis *(yellow arrows)* with rare ground glass opacities consistent with a nonspecific interstitial pneumonia pattern in a patient treated with gefitinib for non–small-cell lung cancer with an epidermal growth factor receptor (EGFR). The *red arrow* points to the residual tumor.

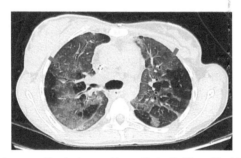

Fig. 14.2   Diffuse ground glass opacities *(red arrows)* in a patient with Stage IV epidermal growth factor receptor (EGFR)-mutated non–small-cell lung cancer treated with erlotinib.

include preexisting pulmonary fibrosis or lung disease, radiation, and use of other drugs with potential for pulmonary toxicity, such as gemcitabine. Clinical presentation and imaging findings are similar to gefitinib-induced lung disease.

- **Afatinib:** Afatinib is an irreversible ErbB family TKI. Three out of 230 patients in the LUX-Lung 3 trial[16] developed ILD. One out of 242 patients in the LUX-Lung 6 trial had fatal ILD secondary to afatinib.[17]
- **Osimertinib:** The overall incidence of pneumonitis has been reported to be around 3.5%.[18] Osimertinib is an irreversible EGFR-TKI that selectively inhibits EGFR sensitizing mutations, as well as the resistance mutation, T790M, but has lesser activity against wild-type EGFR, which could be a potential explanation for the lower grade 3 and 4 adverse events noted in comparison with erlotinib or gefitinib.[4] The clinical manifestations appear to be similar to other EGFR TKIs. A unique pulmonary manifestation of osimertinib, which has been described in literature, is transient asymptomatic pulmonary opacities that occur at a median time of 8.7 weeks (range 1.6–43 weeks) into therapy and last for a median duration of 6 weeks (range 1–11 weeks). Patients with these asymptomatic transient opacities may be continued on therapy with close monitoring.[19]

Anaplastic Lymphoma Kinase (ALK) Inhibitors

- The identification of the role ALK rearrangements in 2% to 7% of patients with NSCLC in 2007 led to the development of ALK inhibitors to target the EML4-ALK fusion oncogene. The ALK inhibitors that have been used in clinical practice since 2011 include crizotinib (a multitargeted small molecule TKI) and second-generation agents including ceritinib, alectinib, and brigatinib. Although crizotinib was the first targeted agent to be approved, in the global ALEX study, alectinib demonstrated superior efficacy in terms of progression-free survival and central nervous system (CNS) progression and had lower toxicity in comparison to crizotinib.[20] Although the overall incidence of pneumonitis with ALK inhibitors is low, many of these can be severe and life threatening. Among patients treated with the earlier ALK inhibitors crizotinib and ceritinib, 1% to 4% develop pneumonitis. Alectinib has been associated with a lower incidence of pneumonitis (0.4%). Brigatinib has a higher incidence of pulmonary toxicity, with 3.7% of patients in the 90 mg group and 9.1% of patients in the 180 mg after a 90-mg lead-in group reported in the ALTA trial. Pneumonitis developed in 6.4% of patients within 9 days of initiation of brigatinib-therapy, with a median onset of 2 days. Therefore patients who are initiated on brigatinib should be monitored very closely for respiratory symptoms in the first few weeks of therapy.[21,22]

BCR-ABL1 Tyrosine Kinase Inhibitors

- **Imatinib:** Imatinib is a TKI that inhibits BCR-ABL, the constitutive abnormal gene product of the Philadelphia chromosome, in addition to other targets in such as platelet-derived growth factor (PDGFR), stem cell factor, and c-Kit. Imatinib has clinical activity in chronic myelogenous leukemia (CML), Philadelphia chromosome positive acute lymphoblastic leukemia (ALL), certain hypereosinophilic syndromes, and gastrointestinal stromal tumors (GISTs). A variety of pulmonary toxicities have been associated with the use of this drug including pleural effusions, interstitial pneumonitis,[23–27] hypersensitivity pneumonitis,[28] and eosinophilic pneumonia.
  - The most common pulmonary complication of imatinib is secondary to the associated fluid retention, which can lead to pleural effusions and pulmonary edema. In patients with CML, 1.3% of newly diagnosed patients and 2% to 6% of other CML patients on imatinib develop severe fluid retention.[29] The incidence of severe fluid retention is higher in patients with GIST at 9% to 13.1%.
  - The median time to onset of interstitial pneumonitis was 49 days (range 10–282 days) in the largest case series of 27 patients with imatinib-induced ILD. Notably, there was no clear correlation between the dose or duration of therapy and development of pneumonitis.[27] Among these patients, 41% had preexisting pulmonary disease, suggesting a predisposition in this patient population. Imaging findings in these patients revealed a hypersensitivity pattern (30%) (Fig. 14.3A–C), interstitial pneumonitis (26%), and cryptogenic organizing pneumonia (15%) (Fig. 14.4), a peribronchovascular bundle pattern (15%), and a nodular pattern in 11% of patients. Transbronchial lung biopsies were performed in five patients which demonstrated varying degrees of inflammatory changes and fibrosis. Peripheral eosinophilia was noted in 5 of 27 patients.
- **Dasatinib:** Dasatinib is a second-generation BCR-ABL TKI that binds to both active and inactive conformations of the ABL gene and is 325 times more potent than imatinib in inhibiting the growth of BCR/ABL cells in vitro. It is predominantly used in the treatment of CML. It has the highest incidence of reported pulmonary adverse events.
  - The most common pulmonary toxicity reported with dasatinib is the development of pleural effusions. The median time to onset of pleural effusions is 11 months (range 3.6–18.6 months).[30] In a 5-year analysis of patients from the DASISION trial comparing dasatinib to imatinib, the overall incidence of pleural effusions was 28% in the dasatinib group versus 0.8% in the imatinib group.[31] Patients who were older than 65 years had a higher incidence of pleural effusions. Some reports suggest that the rate

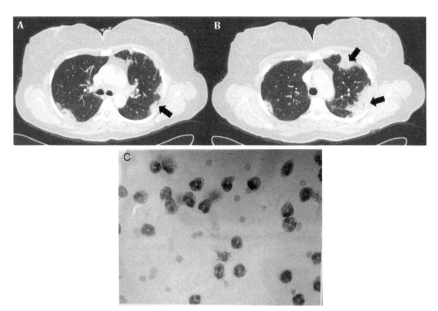

Fig. 14.3 (A, B) Dense peripheral consolidations (*black arrows*) in a patient treated with imatinib. Bronchoalveolar lavage showed 40% eosinophils on differential counts consistent with a diagnosis of chronic eosinophilic pneumonia. (C) Forty percent eosinophils noted on the smear of the bronchoalveolar lavage obtained from the patient consistent with a diagnosis of chronic eosinophilic pneumonia.

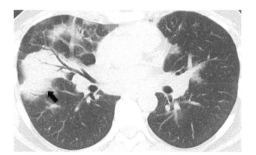

Fig. 14.4 Dense consolidations *(black arrow)* on computerized tomogram of a patient who was treated with imatinib. Transbronchial biopsy findings were consistent with a diagnosis of organizing pneumonia.

of recurrent pleural effusions can be as high as 15%.[30] Other risk factors that have been associated with the development of pleural effusions include prior pulmonary disease in patients treated with higher doses (140 mg).

- Pulmonary hypertension has also been noted with dasatinib in an estimated 5% of treated patients, however, because all reported patients did not have confirmatory right heart catheterizations, the exact incidence is unknown.[31] Based on data from the French Pulmonary Hypertension registry, pulmonary hypertension occurs after 8 to 48 months of exposure. Patients in this registry developed precapillary pulmonary hypertension.[32] Evidence suggests that receptors of tyrosine kinases (RTKs) such as PDGFR, fibroblast growth factor 2, c-KIT, c-Src, and epidermal growth factor, play a role in the pathogenesis of pulmonary hypertension. As an example, the src tyrosine kinase pathway is essential for the activation of K⁺ channels in the pulmonary smooth muscle cells, which results in muscle relaxation. TKIs that inhibit this pathway result in pulmonary vasoconstriction and vascular remodeling over time, resulting in pulmonary hypertension.[33] Unlike imatinib and nilotinib, dasatinib is a potent inhibitor of RTKs that may be responsible for the higher incidence of pulmonary hypertension observed with the drug.[34-36] Whereas in some patients pulmonary hypertension may be reversible, most patients do not recover completely despite discontinuation of the drug.[37]

- The other less common pulmonary toxicity of dasatinib is pneumonitis, which is usually reversible with interruption of therapy.
- **Bosutinib:** Up to 8% of patients treated with bosutinib can develop pleural effusions.[38] Additionally, a case report of worsening preexisting pulmonary hypertension while on bosutinib has been described.[39]
- **Nilotinib:** Pulmonary toxicity is rare and is seen in less than 1% of treated patients.
- **Ponatinib:** For patients with CML who develop the T315I resistance mutation, ponatinib is the drug of choice. Pleural effusions can be seen in 1% of treated patients. Other pulmonary toxicities are rare. A case report of a patient who had been treated with dasatinib in the past and developed pulmonary hypertension while on treatment with ponatinib has been described.[33]

Vascular Endothelial Growth Factor (VEGF) Inhibitors

- **Sunitinib, sorafenib, and pazopanib:** Sunitinib, sorafenib, and pazopanib are oral multikinase inhibitors that are used in the therapy of renal cell cancer, hepatocellular carcinoma, thyroid cancer, and GIST. Similar to other antiangiogenic agents, pulmonary hemorrhage can be seen with sunitinib. In clinical trials, up to 26% of patients who received sunitinib complained of dyspnea, but only 6% had grade 3 or higher toxicity.[40] Other respiratory symptoms include flu-like symptoms or upper respiratory tract infections and nasopharyngitis.
  - Dyspnea, cough, and upper respiratory tract symptoms are less common with sorafenib. In patients who develop sorafenib-induced lung injury (incidence <1%, peak time to onset within 2–4 weeks), the mortality is 41% in those with a diffuse alveolar damage pattern on imaging.[41]
  - A unique pulmonary toxicity observed in patients treated with pazopanib is the development of pneumothoraces, which have been reported in 3% to 14% of treated patients. Patients with lung metastases with pleural or subpleural involvement seem to have a higher incidence of pneumothoraces, possibly due to the formation of pleural fistulas, as a result of tumor necrosis.[42,43]
- **Bevacizumab:** Bevacizumab is a recombinant monoclonal antibody against VEGF, which is used in the treatment of patients with NSCLC, colorectal cancer, and glioblastoma, among other malignancies. In patients with lung cancer, bevacizumab use can lead to central tumor cavitation in 14% to 25% of cases.[44,45] In patients with lung cancer of squamous histology, a high incidence of pulmonary hemorrhage and hemoptysis (4 out of 13) was noted in a phase II clinical trial, and subsequently, the use of bevacizumab for squamous NSCLC has been discouraged.[46] Pulmonary hemorrhage is uncommon with bevacizumab in other tumor types. Another unique side effect of bevacizumab, which occurs in patients who have been exposed to radiation in the past, or are receiving concurrent chemoradiation, is the development of a tracheoesophageal fistula. Because bevacizumab has been associated with an increased risk of venous thromboembolism, pulmonary embolism should be considered in the differential diagnosis of a patient presenting with a new onset dyspnea and hypoxia.

Human Epidermal Growth Factor Receptor 2 (HER2)-Targeting Antibodies

- **Trastuzumab:** Trastuzumab is used in the treatment of HER2-positive breast cancers and gastric malignancies that express HER2. Similar to other monoclonal antibodies, infusion reactions are seen in 20% to 40% of patients receiving the drug. These reactions often present with pulmonary symptoms such as hoarseness and shortness of breath. A higher incidence of infusion reactions may be seen when trastuzumab is given in combination with other chemotherapeutic agents.[47] In a postmarketing analysis, 0.3% of patients who received the drug had severe infusion reactions with an anaphylactoid presentation.[48]
  - Other rare but potentially fatal pulmonary toxicities reported with trastuzumab include interstitial pneumonitis,[49,50] organizing pneumonia,[51] pleural effusions, noncardiogenic pulmonary edema, acute respiratory distress syndrome, and pulmonary fibrosis.[52] Bronchoalveolar lavage in these patients may reveal a predominantly eosinophilic or neutrophilic fluid. In addition to preexisting ILD, patients with extensive lung metastases are also at an increased risk.
- **Ado-trastuzumab emtansine (T-DM1):** Ado-trastuzumab emtansine is an antibody–drug conjugate of trastuzumab that is used in advanced breast cancer patients who have previously received trastuzumab. Infusion reactions are much less frequent than with trastuzumab and are usually very mild. Cases of ILD have been reported in 0.8% of patients treated with T-DM1 and may be severe enough to lead to acute respiratory distress syndrome.
- **Pertuzumab:** Hypersensitivity reactions during infusions are seen in 13% of patients, however, most of them are very mild with less than 1% being grade 3 or higher.

CD20-Targeting Agents

- **Rituximab:** Rituximab is a murine human chimeric monoclonal antibody targeting the CD20 molecule on the surface of B lymphocytes. By binding to CD20, it activates antibody-dependent cellular cytotoxicity and complement-dependent cytotoxicity and is therefore used in the treatment of chronic lymphocytic leukemia (CLL), non-Hodgkin lymphoma, and CNS lymphoma, in addition to many other nonmalignant conditions that require immunosuppression, such as autoimmune hemolytic anemia and rheumatoid arthritis, among others.
  - Infusion reactions occur with the first infusion of this drug in over 50% of patients, however, incidence of severe reactions accompanied by bronchospasm or hypotension are seen in less than 10% of patients. These usually occur within 2 hours of infusion initiation. Some patients may also develop pulmonary infiltrates and acute respiratory distress syndrome with rituximab infusions. These reactions are secondary to cytokines and tumor necrosis factor α that are released as a result of the cytotoxic effect on B lymphocytes by rituximab. Therefore patients with CLL, mantle cell lymphoma, or malignancies with a high tumor burden are more likely to develop a reaction to rituximab. In these patients, using a fractionated regimen of rituximab may be safer. Infusion reactions tend to be less severe with subsequent administrations of the drug.
  - Interstitial pneumonitis is rare but has been reported in patients who received chemotherapeutic regimens containing rituximab for lymphomas.[53,54]

EGFR-Targeting Antibodies

- **Cetuximab:** Cetuximab is a recombinant chimeric monoclonal antibody, which binds to the EGFR and inhibits binding with EGFR ligands, thereby activating the receptor-associated kinases. Cetuximab is predominantly used in KRAS wild-type colorectal cancer and head and neck cancer. Cetuximab has been associated with severe infusion reactions, which may be associated with rapid onset of airway obstructive symptoms such as bronchospasm and hoarseness of voice. These infusion reactions have been reported in 2% to 5% of patients receiving the drug[55] and may occur despite premedication with antihistamines. ILD is a rare but potentially fatal adverse effect of cetuximab. Four out of 1570 patients included in the original clinical trials testing this drug developed ILD, out of which one was fatal. Older patients or those with prior lung disease appear to be at an increased risk.[56]

- **Panitumumab:** Panitumumab is a recombinant human monoclonal antibody targeting the EGFR with clinical application in colorectal cancer. Because it does not have a murine component and lacks galactose 1,3-alpha galactose on the Fab fragment, infusion reactions are less frequent (1%) than with cetuximab. Pulmonary fibrosis has been reported in less than 1% of patients, however, it can be fatal. In a patient with preexisting pulmonary fibrosis, there was significant progression of fibrosis, leading to death after four doses of panitumumab. Therefore patients with preexisting lung disease have, in general, been excluded from clinical trials.

Mitogen-Activated Protein Kinase (MEK) Inhibitors

- **Trametinib:** Trametinib is a reversible inhibitor of the mitogen-activated extracellular kinases (MEK) 1 and 2. It is used in combination with BRAF inhibitors for patients with melanoma whose tumors harbor the BRAF V600 mutation. In the MEKINIST and METRIC clinical trials, the reported incidence of interstitial lung disease was 2% and 2.4%, respectively, with a median time to symptom onset of 5.3 months.[57] Permanent discontinuation of the drug is recommended once ILD develops because there is insufficient data regarding the reversibility of lung damage with this drug.

Polyadenosine Diphosphate-Ribose Polymerase (PARP) Inhibitors

- **Olaparib, niraparib, and rucaparib:** PARP inhibitors are used in the management of patients with BRCA-mutated breast cancer. Pneumonitis has been observed in less than 1% of patients treated with olaparib, but some were associated with fatalities. Niraparib has been associated with nasopharyngitis in 23% of patients, dyspnea in 20%, and cough in 16% of patients.[58] Rucaparib can also have similar respiratory manifestations as those seen with niraparib.

Cyclin-Dependent Kinase (CDK) 4/6 Inhibitors

- **Abemaciclib:** Abemaciclib is used in the treatment of hormone-positive, HER2-negative advanced breast cancer. In the MONARCH 2 trial, up to 5% of patients who received a combination of abemaciclib and fulvestrant developed venous thromboembolism. In addition, cough has been reported in up to 19% of patients receiving this drug in the MONARCH 1 trial, a single-arm, open-label study of abemaciclib in 132 women.[59]

Phosphatidylinositol-3-Kinase (PI3K) Inhibitors

- **Idelalisib:** Idelalisib inhibits the delta isoform of phosphatidylinositol 3-kinase, a molecule that is highly expressed in malignant B lymphocytes and thus has clinical applications in CLL, small lymphocytic lymphoma, and follicular lymphoma. Severe and fatal pneumonitis have been reported in 4% of treated patients, therefore the US Food and Drug Administration (FDA) suggests close monitoring for pulmonary symptoms and thorough evaluation of patients with a decrease in oxygen saturation of over 5%. Other manifestations that have been reported include pneumonia (25%), cough (29%), and dyspnea (17%).

- **Copanlisib:** Copanlisib is used in refractory follicular lymphoma and has also been associated with severe pneumonitis. In addition, up to 17% of patients develop infections with this drug; pneumonia is the most commonly reported. In particular, these patients are at an increased risk of developing pneumocystis jiroveci pneumonia (PJP), and thus it is recommended to initiate PJP prophylaxis prior to treatment in at-risk populations.

mTOR Inhibitors

- **Everolimus:** Everolimus has been used in the treatment of advanced hormone receptor-positive, HER2-negative breast cancer, advanced renal cell carcinoma, and neuroendocrine tumors. Among patients treated with this drug, 8% to 14% were reported to develop pneumonitis, most of which were low grade.[60,61] As with most other drugs, the presence of baseline lung disease predisposes patients to pulmonary toxicity. Bronchoalveolar lavage in these patients have revealed either lymphocytic or eosinophilic samples. The most common radiographic findings in these patients are focal consolidations at the lung bases and ground-glass opacities.[62]
- **Temsirolimus:** Temsirolimus is used in patients with advanced renal cell carcinoma and endometrial cancer and has been reported to cause pneumonitis in up to 5% of patients; however, pulmonary involvement is often mild and may be asymptomatic in close to half of affected patients.[63]

Pharmacological Approaches for the Management of Pulmonary Toxicities

- As described previously, although most targeted therapies have a low incidence of pulmonary toxicities, some of these are potentially fatal and therefore warrant close monitoring and a low-degree of clinical suspicion for such adverse events. If a patient develops dyspnea, cough, hypoxia, or other respiratory symptoms on treatment, it is advisable to perform a thorough workup to determine the etiology of the dyspnea, including chest radiography, tests to rule out infections, cardiovascular etiologies, and venous thromboembolism. On occasion, invasive testing with bronchoscopy and bronchoalveolar lavage with or without transbronchial lung biopsies may provide crucial information to support a diagnosis of therapy-induced pulmonary toxicity.
- **Discontinuation of drug:** If drug-induced pulmonary toxicity is suspected, the suspected culprit drug should be discontinued. In a very small fraction of patients, such as those with asymptomatic or mild symptoms, as is seen commonly in everolimus-associated pneumonitis, the drug may be continued with close monitoring. In continuation of this example, the FDA label for everolimus states that for patients who develop moderate to severe symptoms while on the standard dose of 10 mg daily, the drug may be withheld temporarily but may be reintroduced at a lower dose of 5 mg daily, if clinically indicated, after the resolution of symptoms. In some drug-related lung disease, discontinuation of the drug may lead to the reversal of pulmonary symptoms, whereas others might require further pharmacological interventions with glucocorticoids.
- **Glucocorticoids:** Glucocorticoids form the mainstay of therapy for drug-induced pneumonitis. The optimal dose of steroids depends on the severity of lung involvement and symptoms and degree of hypoxia. Once respiratory symptoms improve, steroids should be tapered gradually over an extended time (at least 4 weeks). Some patients may require a

longer taper of corticosteroids, and the regimen should be tailored to each individual patient's clinical progress. Some patients may have a rapidly deteriorating course despite the use of corticosteroids. ILD associated with EGFR inhibitors such as gefitinib and erlotinib may be resistant to steroids in a fraction of patients.

- **Alternative dosing:** Some situations will allow for alternative dosing schedules. As an example, for dasatinib-associated pleural effusions, an alternative dosing strategy of 100 mg daily instead of 70 mg twice a day has been associated with a reduced risk of further pleural effusions without affecting the efficacy of the drug.[64] Note that for some indications, 140 mg once daily or 180 mg once daily may be appropriate. Diuretics and glucocorticoids may be used for the management of pleural effusions in this population. Endothelin receptor antagonists and calcium channel blockers have been used in the treatment of pulmonary hypertension related to dasatinib, however, their exact role in altering the clinical course of pulmonary arterial hypertension from dasatinib is unknown.[32]
- **Bronchospastic reactions:** For bronchospasm related to a hypersensitivity reaction, beta-2 agonists and steroids should be promptly administered. If the reaction occurs during an infusion, the infusion should be halted. For monoclonal antibodies associated with a high incidence of infusion reactions, premedication with acetaminophen and diphenhydramine should be used prophylactically prior to infusion. Prophylactic steroids prior to rituximab infusions do not reduce the incidence of severe infusion reactions.[65] Fractionated doses of rituximab may also be used to reduce the risk of infusion reactions in at-risk patients. Epinephrine should be administered in any patients experiencing anaphylaxis.

Rechallenge

- For most drug-related pulmonary toxicities, permanent discontinuation of the offending drug is recommended. In the case of certain drugs such as imatinib, a reduced dose has been reintroduced successfully without recurrence of ILD in a few patients.[27] On the other hand, certain toxicities, such as pulmonary arterial hypertension with dasatinib, are an absolute contraindication for rechallenge with the drug. Some authors, however, report successful use of a more selective kinase such as nilotinib after dasatinib-induced pulmonary hypertension.[66] In patients with other lung toxicities from dasatinib, rechallenge with a lower dose of dasatinib may be an option in the absence of alternative therapies.[67] For patients with gefitinib-associated pneumonitis, erlotinib has been used without any major lung adverse events.[68,69] For patients who develop infusion reactions with rituximab, the likelihood of subsequent reactions is lower. For mild reactions, a lower infusion rate is usually well tolerated. However, patients with recurrent infusion reactions should be premedicated with steroids (hydrocortisone 100 mg or dexamethasone 10-12 mg) along with acetaminophen and diphenhydramine. Some patients may require desensitization protocols if they continue to have infusion-reactions with rituximab.

Nonpharmacological Approaches for Management of Pulmonary Toxicities

- Optimal patient selection is important in order to decrease the risk of pulmonary toxicities. For example, pazopanib should be avoided in patients with extensive pulmonary or pleural metastases, and bevacizumab should be avoided in patients with squamous cell lung cancer. Patients who have received radiation should be carefully evaluated for the risk of subsequent pulmonary toxicities. In addition, caution is advised in patients with preexisting pulmonary disease, as they are at increased risk of lung toxicity with treatment.
- Supportive care and symptom management play important roles in the management of pulmonary toxicities. Oxygen and ventilatory support may be prescribed as indicated. For patients with

pleural effusions, such as those seen with dasatinib, therapeutic thoracentesis or even pleurodesis may be required if recurrent. Patients with bleeding secondary to antiangiogenic agents should be supported with blood products as needed. In cases with severe bleeding, bronchoscopic interventions for bleeding, bronchial arterial embolization, radiation, or surgery may be required.

References

1. Kawaguchi T, Koh Y, Ando M, et al. Prospective analysis of oncogenic driver mutations and environmental factors: Japan molecular epidemiology for lung cancer study. *J Clin Oncol.* 2016;34:2247.
2. Shi Y, Au JS, Thongprasert S, et al. A prospective, molecular epidemiology study of EGFR mutations in Asian patients with advanced non-small-cell lung cancer of adenocarcinoma histology (PIONEER). *J Thorac Oncol.* 2014;9:154.
3. Ramalingam SS, Vansteenkiste J, Planchard D, et al. FLAURA Investigators. Overall Survival with Osimertinib in Untreated, *EGFR*-Mutated Advanced NSCLC. *N Engl J Med.* 2020 Jan 2;382(1):41-50. doi: 10.1056/NEJMoa1913662. Epub 2019 Nov 21. PMID: 31751012.
4. Soria JC, Ohe Y, Vansteenkiste J, et al. Osimertinib in untreated EGFR-mutated advanced non-small-cell lung cancer. *N Engl J Med.* 2018;378:113–125.
5. Ding PN, Lord SJ, Gebski V, et al. Risk of treatment-related toxicities from EGFR tyrosine kinase inhibitors: a meta-analysis of clinical trials of gefitinib, erlotinib, and afatinib in advanced EGFR-mutated non-small cell lung cancer. *J Thorac Oncol.* 2017;12(4):633–643.
6. Cohen MH, Williams GA, Sridhara R, et al. FDA drug approval summary: gefitinib (ZD1839) (Iressa) tablets. *Oncologist.* 2003;8:303.
7. Kudoh S, Kato H, Nishiwaki Y, et al. Interstitial lung disease in Japanese patients with lung cancer: a cohort and nested case-control study. *Am J Respir Crit Care Med.* 2008;177:1348.
8. Ando M, Okamoto I, Yamamoto N, et al. Predictive factors for interstitial lung disease, antitumor response, and survival in non-small-cell lung cancer patients treated with gefitinib. *J Clin Oncol.* 2006;24:2549–2556.
9. Chiang CL, Chen YW, Wu MH, Huang HC, Tsai CM, Chiu CH. Radiation recall pneumonitis induced by epidermal growth factor receptor-tyrosine kinase inhibitor in patients with advanced nonsmall-cell lung cancer. *J Chin Med Assoc.* 2016;79(5):248–255.
10. Miettinen PJ, Warburton D, Bu D, et al. Impaired lung branching morphogenesis in the absence of functional EGF receptor. *Dev Biol.* 1997;186:224.
11. Takano T, Ohe Y, Kusumoto M, et al. Risk factors for interstitial lung disease and predictive factors for tumor response in patients with advanced non-small cell lung cancer treated with gefitinib. *Lung Cancer.* 2004;45:93.
12. Endo M, Johkoh T, Kimura K, Yamamoto N. Imaging of gefitinib-related interstitial lung disease: multiinstitutional analysis by the West Japan Thoracic Oncology Group. *Lung Cancer.* 2006;52:135.
13. Cleverley JR, Screaton NJ, Hiorns MP, Flint JD, Müller NL. Drug-induced lung disease: high-resolution CT and histological findings. *Clin Radiol.* 2002;57(4):292–299.
14. https://www.accessdata.fda.gov/drugsatfda_docs/label/2010/021743s14s16lbl.pdf.
15. Yoshioka H, Komuta K, Imamura F, et al. Efficacy and safety of erlotinib in elderly patients in the phase IV POLARSTAR surveillance study of Japanese patients with non-small-cell lung cancer. *Lung Cancer.* 2014;86:201.
16. Sequist LV, Yang JC, Yamamoto N, et al. Phase III study of afatinib or cisplatin plus pemetrexed in patients with metastatic lung adenocarcinoma with EGFR mutations. *J Clin Oncol.* 2013;31:3327.
17. Wu YL, Zhou C, Hu CP, et al. Afatinib versus cisplatin plus gemcitabine for first-line treatment of Asian patients with advanced non-small-cell lung cancer harbouring EGFR mutations (LUX-Lung 6): an open-label, randomised phase 3 trial. *Lancet Oncol.* 2014;15:213.
18. https://www.accessdata.fda.gov/drugsatfda_docs/label/2017/208065s006lbl.pdf.
19. Noonan SA, Sachs PB, Camidge DR. Transient asymptomatic pulmonary opacities occurring during osimertinib treatment. *J Thorac Oncol.* 2016;11(12):2253–2258.
20. Peters S, Camidge DR, Shaw AT, et al. Alectinib versus crizotinib in untreated ALK-positive non-small-cell lung cancer. *N Engl J Med.* 2017;377:829.
21. https://www.accessdata.fda.gov/drugsatfda_docs/label/2017/208772lbl.pdf.

22. Gettinger SN, Bazhenova LA, Langer CJ, et al. Activity and safety of brigatinib in ALK-rearranged non-small-cell lung cancer and other malignancies: a single-arm, open-label, phase 1/2 trial. *Lancet Oncol.* 2016;17:1683.

23. Rosado MF, Donna E, Ahn YS. Challenging problems in advanced malignancy: case 3. imatinib mesylate-induced interstitial pneumonitis. *J Clin Oncol.* 2003;21:3171.

24. Yokoyama T, Miyazawa K, Kurakawa E, et al. Interstitial pneumonia induced by imatinib mesylate: pathologic study demonstrates alveolar destruction and fibrosis with eosinophilic infiltration. *Leukemia.* 2004;18:645.

25. Ma CX, Hobday TJ, Jett JR. Imatinib mesylate-induced interstitial pneumonitis. *Mayo Clin Proc.* 2003;78:1578.

26. Lin JT, Yeh KT, Fang HY, Chang CS. Fulminant, but reversible interstitial pneumonitis associated with imatinib mesylate. *Leuk Lymphoma.* 2006;47:1693.

27. Ohnishi K, Sakai F, Kudoh S, Ohno R. Twenty-seven cases of drug-induced interstitial lung disease associated with imatinib mesylate. *Leukemia.* 2006;20:1162.

28. Bergeron A, Bergot E, Vilela G, et al. Hypersensitivity pneumonitis related to imatinib mesylate. *J Clin Oncol.* 2002;20:4271.

29. https://www.accessdata.fda.gov/drugsatfda_docs/label/2008/021588s024lbl.pdf.

30. Latagliata R, Breccia M, Fava C, et al. Incidence, risk factors and management of pleural effusions during dasatinib treatment in unselected elderly patients with chronic myelogenous leukaemia. *Hematol Oncol.* 2013;31:103.

31. Cortes JE, Saglio G, Kantarjian HM, et al. Final 5-year study results of DASISION: The Dasatinib Versus Imatinib Study in Treatment-Naïve Chronic Myeloid Leukemia Patients trial. *J Clin Oncol.* 2016;34:2333.

32. Montani D, Bergot E, Gunther S, et al. Pulmonary arterial hypertension in patients treated by dasatinib. *Circulation.* 2012;125(17):2128–2137.

33. Quilot FM, Georges M, Favrolt N, et al. Pulmonary hypertension associated with ponatinib therapy. *Eur Respir J.* 2016;47(2):676–679.

34. Nagaraj C, Tang B, Bálint Z, et al. Src tyrosine kinase is crucial for potassium channel function in human pulmonary arteries. *Eur Respir J.* 2013;41(1):85–95.

35. Dahal BK, Cornitescu T, Tretyn A, et al. Role of epidermal growth factor inhibition in experimental pulmonary hypertension. *Am J Respir Crit Care Med.* 2010;181(2):158–167.

36. Tu L, Dewachter L, Gore B, et al. Autocrine fibroblast growth factor-2 signaling contributes to altered endothelial phenotype in pulmonary hypertension. *Am J Respir Cell Mol Biol.* 2011;45(2):311–322.

37. Dumitrescu D, Seck C, ten Freyhaus H, et al. Fully reversible pulmonary arterial hypertension associated with dasatinib treatment for chronic myeloid leukaemia. *Eur Respir J.* 2011;38(1):218–220.

38. Khoury HJ, Cortes JE, Kantarjian HM, et al. Bosutinib is active in chronic phase chronic myeloid leukemia after imatinib and dasatinib and/or nilotinib therapy failure. *Blood.* 2012;119:3403.

39. Hickey PM, Thompson AA, Charalampopoulos A, et al. Bosutinib therapy resulting in severe deterioration of pre-existing pulmonary arterial hypertension. *Eur Respir J.* 2016;48(5):1514–1516.

40. https://www.accessdata.fda.gov/drugsatfda_docs/label/2017/021938s033lbl.pdf.

41. Horiuchi-Yamamoto Y, Gemma A, Taniguchi H, et al. Drug-induced lung injury associated with sorafenib: analysis of all-patient post-marketing surveillance in Japan. *Int J Clin Oncol.* 2013;18:743.

42. van der Graaf WT, Blay JY, Chawla SP, et al. Pazopanib for metastatic soft-tissue sarcoma (PALETTE): a randomised, double-blind, placebo-controlled phase 3 trial. *Lancet.* 2012;379:1879.

43. Verschoor AJ, Gelderblom H. Pneumothorax as adverse event in patients with lung metastases of soft tissue sarcoma treated with pazopanib: a single reference centre case series. *Clin Sarcoma Res.* 2014;4:14.

44. Crabb SJ, Patsios D, Sauerbrei E, et al. Tumor cavitation: impact on objective response evaluation in trials of angiogenesis inhibitors in non-small-cell lung cancer. *J Clin Oncol.* 2009;27:404.

45. Marom EM, Martinez CH, Truong MT, et al. Tumor cavitation during therapy with antiangiogenesis agents in patients with lung cancer. *J Thorac Oncol.* 2008;3:351.

46. Johnson DH, Fehrenbacher L, Novotny WF, et al. Randomized phase II trial comparing bevacizumab plus carboplatin and paclitaxel with carboplatin and paclitaxel alone in previously untreated locally advanced or metastatic non-small-cell lung cancer. *J Clin Oncol.* 2004;22:2184.

47. Fountzilas G, Tsavdaridis D, Kalogera-Fountzila A, et al. Weekly paclitaxel as first-line chemotherapy and trastuzumab in patients with advanced breast cancer. A Hellenic Cooperative Oncology Group phase II study. *Ann Oncol.* 2001;12:1545.

48. Cook-Bruns N. Retrospective analysis of the safety of Herceptin immunotherapy in metastatic breast cancer. *Oncology*. 2001;61(suppl 2):58.
49. Pepels MJ, Boomars KA, van Kimmenade R, Hupperets PS. Life-threatening interstitial lung disease associated with trastuzumab: case report. *Breast Cancer Res Treat*. 2009;113:609.
50. Bettini AC, Tondini C, Poletti P, et al. A case of interstitial pneumonitis associated with Guillain-Barré syndrome during administration of adjuvant trastuzumab. *Tumori*. 2008;94:737.
51. Radzikowska E, Szczepulska E, Chabowski M, Bestry I. Organising pneumonia caused by trastuzumab (Herceptin) therapy for breast cancer. *Eur Respir J*. 2003;21:552.
52. https://www.accessdata.fda.gov/drugsatfda_docs/label/2010/103792s5250lbl.pdf.
53. Burton C, Kaczmarski R, Jan-Mohamed R. Interstitial pneumonitis related to rituximab therapy. *N Engl J Med*. 2003;348:2690.
54. Ennishi D, Terui Y, Yokoyama M, et al. Increased incidence of interstitial pneumonia by CHOP combined with rituximab. *Int J Hematol*. 2008;87:393.
55. https://www.accessdata.fda.gov/drugsatfda_docs/label/2012/125084s0228lbl.pdf.
56. Satoh T, Gemma A, Kudoh S, et al. Incidence and clinical features of drug-induced lung injury in patients with advanced colorectal cancer receiving cetuximab: results of a prospective multicenter registry. *Jpn J Clin Oncol*. 2014;44:1032.
57. https://www.accessdata.fda.gov/drugsatfda_docs/label/2017/204114s005lbl.pdf.
58. https://www.accessdata.fda.gov/drugsatfda_docs/label/2017/208447lbl.pdf.
59. Dickler MN, Tolaney SM, Rugo HS, et al. MONARCH 1, a phase II study of abemaciclib, a CDK4 and CDK6 inhibitor, as a single agent, in patients with refractory HR+/HER2−metastatic breast cancer. *Clin Cancer Res*. 2017;23(17):5218–5224.
60. White DA, Schwartz LH, Dimitrijevic S, et al. Characterization of pneumonitis in patients with advanced non-small cell lung cancer treated with everolimus (RAD001). *J Thorac Oncol*. 2009;4:1357.
61. Motzer RJ, Escudier B, Oudard S, et al. Efficacy of everolimus in advanced renal cell carcinoma: a double-blind, randomised, placebo-controlled phase III trial. *Lancet*. 2008;372:449.
62. White DA, Camus P, Endo M, et al. Noninfectious pneumonitis after everolimus therapy for advanced renal cell carcinoma. *Am J Respir Crit Care Med*. 2010;182:396.
63. Dabydeen DA, Jagannathan JP, Ramaiya N, et al. Pneumonitis associated with mTOR inhibitors therapy in patients with metastatic renal cell carcinoma: incidence, radiographic findings and correlation with clinical outcome. *Eur J Cancer*. 2012;48:1519.
64. Porkka K, Khoury HJ, Paquette RL, et al. Dasatinib 100 mg once daily minimizes the occurrence of pleural effusion in patients with chronic myeloid leukemia in chronic phase and efficacy is unaffected in patients who develop pleural effusion. *Cancer*. 2010;116:377.
65. Coiffier B, Lepage E, Briere J, et al. CHOP chemotherapy plus rituximab compared with CHOP alone in elderly patients with diffuse large-B-cell lymphoma. *N Engl J Med*. 2002;346:235.
66. Orlandi EM, Rocca B, Pazzano AS, Ghio S. Reversible pulmonary arterial hypertension likely related to long-term, low-dose dasatinib treatment for chronic myeloid leukaemia. *Leuk Res*. 2012;36:e4.
67. Bergeron A, Réa D, Levy V, et al. Lung abnormalities after dasatinib treatment for chronic myeloid leukemia: a case series. *Am J Respir Crit Care Med*. 2007;176:814.
68. Fukui T, Otani S, Hataishi R, et al. Successful rechallenge with erlotinib in a patient with EGFR-mutant lung adenocarcinoma who developed gefitinib-related interstitial lung disease. *Cancer Chemother Pharmacol*. 2010;65:803.
69. Chang SC, Chang CY, Chen CY, Yu CJ. Successful erlotinib rechallenge after gefitinib-induced acute interstitial pneumonia. *J Thorac Oncol*. 2010;5:1105.

CHAPTER 15

Dermatological Toxicities of Targeted Therapy

Rahul Pansare, MD ▦ Misako Nagasaka, MD ▦ Ammar Sukari, MD

Introduction

Targeted therapies are a rapidly expanding group of anticancer drugs, which promise to provide better tolerated and higher efficacy medications compared with conventional systemic chemotherapy. Inhibition of novel pathways or molecules brings about some unexpected and unforeseen adverse effects which are similar, yet distinct to those seen with chemotherapy. Cutaneous toxicity is the most common adverse drug reaction seen with targeted therapy. It ranges from benign, easily reversible effects to more life-threatening toxicity, which may even require cessation of therapy. Treatment of these adverse reactions poses different challenges, and thus, it is important to understand their clinical manifestations and mechanisms of action to aid in providing appropriate therapy.

Acneiform Rash

■ **Incidence:** Acneiform rash is the most common side effect of tyrosine kinase inhibitors (TKIs), reportedly seen in 50% to 100% of treated cases.[1] This rash can affect not only the quality of life of patients but can also decrease compliance to therapy. For example, acneiform rash is very common with epidermal growth factor receptor (EGFR)–targeting agents. Both the incidence (81%–100%)[2-4] and the frequency of grade 3 rash (15%) are highest with afatinib[5] when compared with gefitinib or erlotinib. Cetuximab is reported to have a slightly lower incidence of 75% to 91%.[6]

Mechanism of Rash and the EGFR Pathway

■ Proliferating keratinocytes in the epidermis normally express abundant EGFR, which acts as a ligand to a number of molecules such as epidermal growth factor (EGF), transforming growth factor-α (TGF-α), heparin-binding EGF (HB-EGF), amphiregulin (AR), epiregulin (EREG), betacellulin (BTC), epigen (EPG), and neuregulin 1–4 (NRG1–4). This receptor-ligand interaction activates the intracellular tyrosine kinase domain, causing autophosphorylation, which then eventually leads to activation of intracellular signaling pathways, particularly the RAS/mitogen-activated protein kinase (MAPK) and PI3K/AKT pathways, which ultimately promote proliferation, survival, and migration.[7]

■ Anti-EGFR TKIs compete with ATP and inhibit EGFR tyrosine kinase activity, which in turn results in keratinocyte apoptosis, inhibiting cell growth while promoting cell adhesivity and differentiation. This also triggers release of inflammatory chemokines such as chemokine ligand 2, ligand 5, and chemokine 10/interferon gamma-inducible protein 10. These cellular changes within the keratinocytes bring about the skin changes observed clinically.[8]

Approved EGFR–Targeting Therapies

US Food and Drug Administration (FDA)–approved EGFR-TKIs include the first-generation TKIs, gefitinib and erlotinib, the second-generation TKI, afatinib, and the third-generation TKI, osimertinib. Gefitinib and erlotinib are reversible TKIs used for metastatic non–small-cell lung cancer (NSCLC) with the EGFR exon 19 deletion or the exon 21 substitution mutation L858R.[9] Erlotinib is also used in pancreatic cancer.[10] Afatinib is an irreversible HER2, EGFR, and HER4 TKI used in metastatic NSCLC.[11] Osimertinib is an irreversible TKI approved for metastatic NSCLC with T790M mutation upon progression, on or after EGFR TKI therapy.[12] Osimertinib was also recently approved as a first-line treatment of NSCLC with sensitizing EGFR mutations.[13] Osimertinib spares wild-type EGFR and is known to have less skin and gastrointestinal toxicities.[14]

Cetuximab and panitumumab are FDA–approved anti-EGFR monoclonal antibodies (mAbs). Cetuximab is a mouse–human chimeric monoclonal immunoglobulin G1 (IgG1) that binds to the extracellular ligand binding domain of EGFR with higher affinity than endogenous ligands. This prevents tyrosine kinase activation and downstream EGFR signaling, and promotes EGFR internalization. This also promotes antibody-dependent cell-mediated cytotoxicity (ADCC)[15] and induces apoptosis.[16] Cetuximab has a long half-life of 7 days and can bind both wild-type and mutant EGFRvIII. It is used in metastatic colorectal cancer and head and neck squamous cell carcinoma.[17,18] Panitumumab is a fully human immunoglobulin G2 (IgG2) that prevents ligand binding and promotes receptor internalization and degradation. It is used in metastatic colorectal cancer.[19]

- **Clinical description:** The rash associated with EGFR–targeting therapies presents similar to *acne vulgaris* and is described as painful and pruritic follicular-centered papules or pustules.[20] Unlike acne, however, comedones are never present, and the rash has a monotonous morphology. This rash generally involves the face, scalp, upper chest, and upper back but spares the periorbital region and the palms and soles.[21] The rash occurs in a dose-dependent pattern and is noted to disappear after discontinuation of the drug.[22,23] It develops in the first 1 to 2 weeks of treatment, generally peaks at 3 to 4 weeks, and eventually decreases in intensity but has been known to persist for months.[24] It may be preceded by sensory disturbances in the form of paresthesia, erythema, or edema. Unlike Drug Rash with Eosinophilia and Systemic Symptoms (DRESS), the rash typically does not involve the mucosal surfaces although xerophthalmia and xerostomia may be seen in 12% to 35% of cases.[8] In terms of severity, lesions secondary to monoclonal antibodies have been reported to be more severe and extensive when compared with those secondary to small-molecule TKIs.[25]

- **Histopathology:** A biopsy of the rash associated with EGFR–targeting therapies shows a distinct pattern when compared with acne vulgaris. Whereas acne vulgaris is characterized by sebaceous gland hypertrophy and inflammatory infiltrate related to *Propionibacterium acnes* colonization,[26] this rash has been described as a sterile process as demonstrated by the absence of infective etiology. However, affected areas can get secondarily infected with herpes simplex virus or *Staphylococcus aureus*.[27-29] It is broadly described as having two unique patterns: a hyperkeratotic follicular infundibulum surrounded by a superficial dermal inflammatory cell infiltrate or a neutrophilic suppurative folliculitis.[30]

- **Grading:** The National Cancer Institute Common Terminology Criteria for Adverse Events (NCI-CTCAE) version 5.0 grading scale (Table 15.1) is used.[31]

- The clinical grading system is often used as a tool to describe treatment algorithms. Interestingly, the severity of the rash predicts therapy response and is often used as a surrogate marker of response to therapy.[32]

TABLE 15.1 ■ The NCI-CTCAE (Version 5.0) Grading Scale[a]

Grades	Percent BSA Involved	Clinical Presentation
1	<10%	+/− pruritic or tenderness
2	10%–30%	Limiting self-care ADL, psychosocial impact
3	>30%	Limiting self-care ADL, local superinfection, treated with oral antibiotics
4	Any	Severe superinfection, life-threatening, treated with IV antibiotics
5	Any	Death

[a]This is the most commonly used criteria for assessment of dermatological toxicity from cancer directed therapies.[31]
ADL, Activities of daily living; *BSA*, body surface area; *NCI-CTCAE*, National Cancer Institute Common Terminology Criteria for Adverse Events.

- **Management of acneiform rash:** Treatment options are divided based on the intent—preventive versus reactive. Preventive treatments are preemptive in nature and are based on various studies conducted that showed favorable outcomes with regard to severity of the rash, although it did not have a significant impact on the absolute incidence of the rash.
- **Pharmacological treatment:** Pharmacological treatment is classified as topical therapy or oral therapy. Oral treatments primarily consist of antibiotics although other supplementary treatments have also been described. The rash grading system described previously is crucial in decision making to step-up treatment because no intervention is required for the management of mild grade (grade 1) rash, although topical steroid creams may provide potential benefit. Oral antibiotics are typically described for moderate grade (grade 2) rash along with topical steroids.[33,34] Severe grade (grade 3) rash often requires discontinuation[35] of the regimen for 2 to 4 weeks, which can be resumed once the rash improves. Permanent discontinuation can be considered if the rash continues unabated despite temporary cessation.
  - **Steroids:** Topical hydrocortisone 1% is commonly prescribed for grade 1 to 3 rash. There are no randomized clinical trials to support this practice, rather its use is supported by anecdotal and expert opinion.
  - **Antibiotics:** Oral tetracyclines, such as doxycycline and minocycline, have been studied for prophylaxis and treatment of grades 2 to 3 acneiform rash. In the Pan Canadian Rash trial, the overall incidence of rash was similar in the three treatment arms (prophylactic minocycline, minocycline after rash developed, and no treatment), however, minocycline was associated with a higher "mean time to onset of any grade maximum rash."[36] Minocycline 100 mg has been shown to decrease lesion count and the frequency of moderate to severe pruritus in patients treated with cetuximab.[37] Minocycline also has the added benefit of not carrying a risk of photosensitivity, compared with tetracycline and doxycycline. Doxycycline 100 mg and tetracycline 250 mg have both been described to lower the severity of grade 2 or higher rash.[38] Notably, doxycycline in particular, is a suitable option for patients with renal dysfunction.
  - **Supplementary treatments**
    - **Retinoids:** Topical retinoids promote gene transcription and cause subsequent activation of a downstream retinoid signaling pathway,[39,40] and induction of HBEGF and amphiregulin, which are ligands for EGFR.[41] Isotretinoin, tazarotene, and adapalene have been described in this context. Adapalene additionally inhibits proliferation of keratinocytes, reduces leukocyte migration, and has anticyclooxygenase activity, which promotes antiinflammatory effects.[40,42] Tazarotene not only had a low compliance rate due to local skin irritation, but also did not show significant improvement at 4 weeks and is thus not recommended.[37] Isotretinoin and adapalene have been shown to have efficacy, albeit based on case reports rather than large prospective trials.[43–45]

- **Vitamin K:** Vit K3 (menadione) has been recommended for prophylactic use and has been studied in the context of cetuximab-related skin toxicities. A shorter median time for improvement of skin toxicity (8 vs. 18 days) was noted in one particular study.[46]
- **Nonpharmacological treatment:** The high incidence of acneiform rashes makes patient education an important aspect of treatment to ensure continued therapy compliance. Certain instructions should be built into supportive care protocols upon prescription of these agents. These include having a skin care routine including cleanliness and use of moisturizers, application of alcohol-free and perfume-free emollient creams, and avoidance of hot showers and products that cause skin dryness.[35,47] In UVB-mediated skin damage due to inhibition of EGFR-mediated signaling processes lies the rationale to using sunscreen in this population.[25,48] Although there is not much evidence to support the use of sun protectants as a single agent preventive strategy, patients enrolled in some pharmacological trials used skin care as part of their daily care routine. Thus its effectiveness in combination with other methods cannot be discarded.

Hand-Foot Skin Reaction

- **Incidence:** There is considerable variation in the incidence of hand-foot skin reaction (HFSR) among different multikinase inhibitors ranging from up to 61% (regorafinib) to 34% (sorafinib) to as low as 4.5% (pazopanib).[49] Even with the same drug, incidence rates differ depending on the tumor type being treated. This can be explained in part by the different molecular pathways involved and the degree of target inhibition achieved.
- **Mechanism of HFSRs with multikinase inhibitors:** Angiogenesis is essential for the growth and metastasis of tumor cells[50] and is mediated through vascular endothelial growth factor (VEGF) and its receptor (VEGFR). The VEGF family includes five glycoproteins: VEGFA, VEGFB, VEGFC, VEGFD, and placenta growth factor (PGF), which interact with and activate three receptors belonging to the RTK family: VEGFR1, VEGFR2, and VEGFR3.[51] Upon interaction with their ligands, VEGFRs activate downstream signaling pathways, mainly the PLCγ/PKC/RAF/MAPK and PI3K/AKT pathways. This leads to endothelial cell effects including proliferation, survival, migration, vasodilation, and increased permeability.[52] Inhibition of these pathways causes microvascular structural changes and disruption of endothelial and vascular repair mechanisms, which result in damage to vessels in locations where skin is subjected to friction, heat, or recurrent trauma, such as the palms and soles.[53] Antiangiogenic TKIs inhibit additional pathways involving PDGFR, C-Kit, EGFR, FGFR, RET, and RAF kinases. It is postulated that HFSR occurs as a result of blockade of multiple pathways. Thus receptor specific drugs such as bevacizumab, which targets VEGF, only rarely causes HFSR.[54,55]
- **Approved multikinase inhibitors:** Antiangiogenic TKIs are often multikinase inhibitors and inhibit other kinases, as well as VEGFR including PDGFR, c-KIT, EGFR, FGFR, RET, and RAF kinases. FDA–approved agents with activity against VEGFR include sorafenib, sunitinib, pazopanib, axitinib, vandetanib, regorafenib,[56] lenvatinib,[57] cabozatinib,[58] and ponatinib.[59]
- **Clinical description:** HFSR is a dose-limiting cutaneous toxicity described in patients treated with multikinase inhibitors and BRAF inhibitors. It is similar to hand-foot syndrome (HFS) seen with use of traditional cytotoxic chemotherapies,[60] such as capecitabine and anthracyclines. HFSR, however, is clinically and histopathologically distinct from HFS. Its onset after initiation of targeted therapy is generally days to weeks versus weeks to months as seen in HFS. Some symptoms are similar to those of HFS, including dysesthesia, erythema, and scaling. In addition, HFSR is characterized by well-demarcated, significantly edematous, and painful blisters involving pressure points. Heels, metatarsal heads, and areas subject to repeated friction,

TABLE 15.2 ■ NCI-CTCAE Versions 4 and 5 Grading Scales for Hand-Foot Syndrome

Grading	NCI-CTCAE Version 4.0 and 5.0[31,72,73]	Symptoms[74]
Grade 1	• Minimal skin changes or dermatitis (e.g., erythema, edema or hyperkeratosis) without pain	• Numbness, unpleasant sensations when touching ordinary things, a burning or prickly feeling, tingling, painless swelling, redness, or discomfort of hands/feet; symptoms do not affect ADL
Grade 2	• Skin changes (e.g., peeling, blisters, edema, or hyperkeratosis) with pain; limiting instrumental ADL	• One or more of the following: painful redness, swelling, skin thickening of the hands/feet; symptoms create discomfort, but do not affect ADL
Grade 3	• Severe skin changes (e.g., peeling, blisters, bleeding, edema, or hyperkeratosis) with pain; limiting self-care ADL	• One or more of the following: scaling, open sores, blistering, skin thickening, severe pain of the hands/feet, severe discomfort; unable to work or perform ADL
Grade 4	—	—
Grade 5	—	—

ADL, Activities of daily living; *NCI-CTCAE,* National Cancer Institute Common Terminology Criteria for Adverse Events.

and weight bearing sites are commonly involved.[61–65] Several weeks later, thickening of skin and pain at the site of lesions impairs range of motion, function, and quality of life.[66] Acral dysesthesia and paresthesia commonly precede the lesions. Just like acneiform rash, the therapeutic response has been correlated with HFSR occurrence except in the case of regorafenib.[67–70]

■ **Histopathology:** Epidermal hyperplasia, papillomatosis, and parakeratotic hyperkeratosis are detected on histopathology. Dyskeratosis and vacuolar degeneration with intraepidermal blister formation is also seen.[71]

■ **Grading system:** There is no grading specific to HFSR, however, a general consensus exists to use the grading system for HFS (Table 15.2).[72,73]

■ **Management of HFSR:** Management of HFSR requires a multidisciplinary approach involving a team consisting of oncologists, dermatologists, podiatrists, primary care physicians, and nurses.[74–76] Prior to treatment, it is important to recognize and optimally treat risk factors that could predispose to development of HFSR such as diabetes mellitus, fungal infection, peripheral neuropathy, and other related conditions.[77] It is also recommended that an experienced professional assess the quality of life using established tools such as Skindex[78] or the Dermatology Life Quality Index.[79]

■ **Pharmacological treatment:** Pharmacological treatment is determined based on the grade of symptoms. Treatment should be given in addition to continuing supportive measures. For grade 1 symptoms, keratolytics such as 10% to 40% urea or 10% salicylic acid along with topical lidocaine can be used. If progression to grade 2 toxicity is noted, then topical steroids such as clobetasol 0.05% ointment can be used.[71] Dose reduction of targeted therapy can also be considered if symptoms persist despite topical steroid use.[62,80] The use of hydrocolloid dressings containing ceramide with a low-friction external surface has been shown to prolong median time to progression of grade 1 HFSR and can also be considered.[81] Further worsening to grade 3 toxicity generally requires the use of topical antibiotics along with temporary interruption of targeted therapy for at least 7 days to observe for resolution of toxicity.[77] It is important to reinforce patient education at each clinical visit for continued use of supportive and preventive measures to ensure patient compliance.

- **Nonpharmacological treatment:** Supportive measures should be considered prior to the start of treatment with agents that may cause HFSR. This includes close inspection of the hands and feet for preexisting calluses or hyperkeratotic skin lesions, which could predispose to the development of HFSR. Manicure and pedicure or use of pumice stones to remove any calluses along with daily use of non–urea-based moisturizers can be recommended.[82] Although prophylactic use of 10% urea showed a lower occurrence of any-grade rash and improvement in patient quality of life, it has not shown a change in dose reduction, interruption, or cessation of sorafenib therapy.[83] Patient education regarding predisposing factors can mitigate or even reduce the severity of dermatological toxicity. This includes avoidance of triggers like rubbing, pinching or skin friction, vigorous activity, excessive heat, and constrictive footwear. Liberal use of moisturizers and use of thick cotton gloves and socks to prevent injury and friction are other helpful supportive measures that should be considered.[82]

Stomatitis

- **Incidence:** Stomatitis is a common adverse drug effect reported with almost all targeted therapies.[84] All-grade stomatitis in angiogenesis inhibitors ranges from 7% to 29%, varying based on the drug used. A higher incidence is reported with sunitinib, where any-grade stomatitis ranges from 16.5% to 27%, which is higher than other multi-TKIs when compared.[85–87] Of note, the incidence of high grade (≥3) stomatitis is reported to be up to 4% with multitargeted angiogenesis inhibitors. A high relative risk has been documented with CDK 4/6 inhibitors in a systematic meta-analysis ranging from 2.62 to 4.87. Mammalian target of rapamycin (mTor) inhibitor-associated stomatitis (mIAS) is considered a class effect,[88] with an overall incidence of any grade and high grade (≥3) ranging from 33.5% to 52.9% and from 4.1% to 5.4%, respectively, irrespective of the specific mTOR inhibitor used.[89]
- **Clinical presentation:** Although stomatitis is specifically defined as inflammation of the inner lining of the mouth, resulting in swelling and painful sores, it is used more broadly to include any mucosal injuries including mucosal sensitivity, taste alterations, dry mouth, and necrosis of jaw.[90] Symptoms of stomatitis are dose-dependent depending on the type of targeted therapy utilized. Symptoms associated with angiogenesis inhibitors include diffuse mucosal hypersensitivity and dysesthesia,[91] moderate erythema,[92] and painful inflammation of the oral mucosa. Stomatitis may also manifest as a burning sensation in the mouth, particularly triggered by hot or spicy foods.[91] Symptoms have been reported as early as 9 to 16 days after treatment with EGFR inhibitors or several weeks after treatment initiation in the case of angiogenesis inhibitors. Ulcerous lesions are seen more commonly with classical chemotherapy, but ulcerations of the nonkeratinized mucosa have also been noted with sunitinib or sorafenib and are referred to as linear lingual ulcers. Commonly affected areas are nonkeratinized labial and buccal mucosa, the mucosa of the tongue, of the floor of the mouth, and the soft palate.[93]
- **Grading of stomatitis:** The Common Terminology Criteria for Adverse Events grading system sets out five grades of oral mucositis (Table 15.3).[31,94] This grading system helps guide optimal treatments for affected patients.
- **Mechanism of action:** Stomatitis develops by a similar mechanism as does HFSR. EGF plays a major role in the maintenance of mucosal integrity by acting as a mitogen and by inducing mucus and prostaglandin synthesis.[95] EGF promotes cell growth and regular turnover in response to the daily wear and tear. Further, inhibition of squamous epithelium maturation in the gastrointestinal tract promotes ulcer formation.[96] For mIAS, the exact pathobiology has not been determined, however, it is postulated to be secondary to altered downstream effects of the mTOR signaling pathway. The mTOR pathway normally

TABLE 15.3 ■ The NCI-CTCAE Grading System Often Used to Characterize Grade of Oral Mucositis[31,94]

Grade 1	Asymptomatic or mild symptoms; intervention not indicated
Grade 2	Moderate pain not interfering with oral intake, modified diet indicated
Grade 3	Severe pain; interfering with oral intake
Grade 4	Life-threatening consequences; urgent intervention indicated
Grade 5	Death

NCI-CTCAE, National Cancer Institute Common Terminology Criteria for Adverse Events.

functions as a central modulator of extracellular and intracellular signaling of mediators and growth factors, thereby controlling downstream cellular events of translation, metabolism, and ultimately, growth.[97] mTOR inhibition can disengage these extracellular and intracellular events with a resultant decrease in expression of CD4+, CD25+ regulatory T cells, and increase in CD8+ T cell infiltration and upregulation of heat shock protein 27 and interleukin-10, with a resultant recurrent aphthous ulceration.[98,99] There are other possible explanations, however. The oral microbiota mechanism[100] suggests that the predominance of certain species such as bacteroidales[101] may be involved in the pathogenesis of recurrent ulcers. Another proposed mechanism is that specific gene polymorphisms that code for certain proinflammatory cytokines may drive risk for stomatitis development.[102]

■ Antiangiogenic TKIs are often multikinase inhibitors and inhibit other kinases as along with VEGFR, including PDGFR, c-KIT, EGFR, FGFR, RET, and RAF kinases. FDA–approved agents with activity against VEGFR include: sorafenib, sunitinib, pazopanib, axitinib, vandetanib, regorafenib,[103] lenvatinib,[104] cabozatinib,[105] and ponatinib.[106] Sorafenib and sunitinib, in particular, are known for causing mucositis.

■ mTOR inhibitors in combination with endocrine agents (everolimus plus exemestane) have been approved for the treatment of metastatic breast cancer.[107] They have also been approved for different kinds of solid tumors and tuberous sclerosis complex.[108] As described previously, mTOR inhibitors are associated with mIAS.

■ **Management of stomatitis**
  ■ **Nonpharmacological treatment:** Mucosal sensitivity is a common patient complaint that may require dietary modifications, such as avoiding irritating foods and tobacco.[91] Before the start of treatment, a thorough assessment of the patient's oral cavity should be made, not only to assess existing risk factors such as dental caries, dentures, and broken teeth, but also to establish a baseline in order to identify new changes that might occur after therapy.[109] This assessment should be made by a health care professional and must be continued throughout treatment.[110] Patient education regarding maintaining good oral hygiene is essential.[111–113] A good oral routine includes brushing the teeth and tongue with a soft-bristle brush, flossing, and rinsing. Special care should be taken for using softer, nonabrasive materials or a foam swab/gauze to maintain good oral hygiene if ulcers restrict use of a toothbrush. Also, mouthwashes containing alcohol could potentially irritate and dry mucosal membranes and thus should be avoided.[114]
  ■ **Pharmacological treatment:** Treatment is based on the grade of stomatitis. In general, no intervention is recommended for grade 1 lesions. Triamcinolone in dental paste can be applied two to three times daily for pain and inflammation arising from ulcers.[115] In addition to this oral regimen, topical steroids in the form of mouth rinse or magic mouthwashes have been recommended.[116,117] For grade 2 mIAS, which persists or is associated with significant pain, intralesional steroid injections or low-level laser therapy

(wavelength of 633–685 or 780–830 nm, energy density 2–3 J/cm^2 on the tissue surface) has been observed to provide relief.[118] Either oral erythromycin (250–350 mg) or minocycline should be added for grade 2 toxicity. For grade 3 toxicity, clobetasol ointment is used instead of triamcinolone in dental paste, and the erythromycin dose is increased to 500 mg daily or the minocycline dose to 100 mg. Additionally, systemic corticosteroids in the form of high-dose pulse therapy with 30–60 mg or 1 mg/kg oral prednisone for 1 week followed by tapering has been recommended for mIAS.[116] Antifungal agents may be administered depending on individual case assessments.[119] As with acneiform rash, the dose of targeted therapy should be maintained for grades 1 and 2 stomatitis and may require temporary discontinuation for 2 to 4 weeks in case of grade 3 events.[120]

Alopecia

- **Incidence:** Alopecia is a common side effect seen with many targeted therapy drugs. The incidence of all-grade alopecia is much less (14.7%)[121] when compared with cytotoxic chemotherapy (65%).[122] Although not life-threatening, alopecia significantly affects the self-image of patients and overall quality of life. There are reports suggesting poor compliance and even refusal to continue therapy due to the traumatizing nature of this adverse drug reaction.[123,124] The highest incidence of alopecia is reported with vismodegib (59.9%), followed by sorafenib (29%), and vemurafenib (23.7%).[121] Of note, the incidence varies among drugs targeting the same primary molecule, as is observed between sunitinib (6.9%) and sorafenib. This is explained by the fact that these drugs often work on multiple pathways. Among the CDK 4/6 inhibitors, considerable incidence of alopecia (up to 33%) has been reported in a systematic meta-analysis including 2007 patients.[125]

- **Clinical presentation:** The onset and pattern of alopecia associated with targeted therapies is not uniformly reported. The alopecia may be in a frontal, diffuse, or patchy pattern but is usually reversible and is not associated with complete baldness.[126] The alopecia is generally nonscarring[127,128] and may be accompanied by pruritus. Scarring may be seen, however, with alopecia associated with infection such as folliculitis decalvans, as seen with erlotinib.[129,130] The onset after the start of therapy ranges from a few weeks to months and generally resolves in 1 to 6 months after the discontinuation of therapy. The quality of hair (brittle), rate of regrowth, hair structure (thin, curly), and color (brown to orange or red); however, may be affected in the regrowth process.[110,131,132] These changes mainly apply to scalp hair but have also been noted in other areas of the body. Although not common with immunotherapy, significant alopecia involving the scalp, eyebrows, face, pubic region, and trunk has been reported with ipilimumab, in a manner mimicking alopecia areata, clinically and histologically.[133]

- **Grading of alopecia:** Alopecia is assigned two levels of grade depending on the amount of hair loss since the initiation of treatment. Grade 1 alopecia is defined as loss of less than 50% of the initial volume of hair, not requiring wearing a wig. Grade 2 alopecia is defined as loss of more than 50% of the initial volume of hair, requiring wearing a wig, and is associated with psychosocial sequelae.[134] Further, the grade of alopecia was not detailed in most studies of CDK4/6 inhibitors except for the PALOMA-3 trial, where it was mostly grade 1 and only 1% of patients exhibited grade 2 alopecia.[135]

- **Mechanism of action:** Alopecia has been described in two ways.[136] The first is telogen effluvium, which occurs when a large percentage of scalp hair moves from the anagen to the telogen phase of the hair cycle, leading to no more than 50% hair loss. The second is anagen effluvium, which occurs when root sheath cells are damaged, resulting in severe hair weakening and ultimately hair loss. The mechanism of action of alopecia induced by chemotherapy is predominantly secondary to nonselective cytotoxicity,[137] however, this is not the case with targeted therapies. Rather, the pathogenesis of targeted therapy-related alopecia is due to blockage of a wide spectrum of oncogenic molecules and pathways. Inhibitors of the Sonic Hedgehog (Shh), vascular endothelial growth factor receptor (VEGFR), and mitogen-activated protein kinase (MAPK) signaling pathways are among the most commonly associated. EGFR pathways play a pivotal role in hair follicle biology and epidermal homeostasis. EGFR is located in the outer root sheath of a hair follicle[138] and is critical to anagen to catagen transition,[139] and its blockage results in follicular disintegration by pushing the hair follicle to the telogen phase.[140,141] Fibroblast growth factor (FGF) stimulates anagen hair growth[142] and PDGF signaling helps in induction and maintenance of the anagen phase in hair follicles.[143] Shh pathway inhibition in the skin can lead to (reversible) alopecia and arrest of hair growth in the telogen phase,[144] which explains the occurrence of alopecia with vismodegib.

- **CDK 4/6 inhibitors:** CDK 4/6 inhibitors are associated with a considerable incidence of alopecia. CDK4 and CKD6 have been successfully targeted in ER+ HER2–breast cancer. Three agents selective for CDK4 and CDK6 inhibitors that are currently approved for treatment of advanced estrogen receptor–positive (ER+) breast cancer in combination with anti-estrogen therapy are palbociclib, ribociclib, and abemaciclib. Abemaciclib is also approved as monotherapy after progression on chemotherapy and/or hormonal therapy.[145]
- **Management of alopecia**
  - **Pharmacological treatment:** No pharmacological treatment is available to prevent alopecia, however, topical minoxidil 5% twice daily is sometimes used off-label. Minoxidil has been shown to shorten the duration of hair loss but, cannot prevent it.[146,147] Off-label use of clobetasol in shampoo or solution has also been used. Alopecia, irrespective of grade, does not require dose modification or cessation because it is not life-threatening. However, it still requires frequent monitoring and should be assessed periodically. Additionally, adequate workup of alopecia includes evaluation for nutritional deficiencies, as these may cooccur due to chemotherapy- or targeted therapy-induced poor gastrointestinal absorption. This workup should include thyroid function testing, vitamin D levels, iron studies, and assessment for protein deficiency.[131]
  - **Nonpharmacological treatment:** Patients should be counseled regarding alopecia as a potential adverse effect of targeted therapy. This is necessary to maintain compliance and ensure continued therapy.[123,124] Some patients may require support in the form of formal counseling to alleviate distress and trauma associated with alopecia.[148] Furthermore, frequent brushing is recommended, which helps loosen scalp hair kinkiness, making it less brittle.[149] In cases where eyelashes are affected, it might be important to trim them because inward curling may result in keratitis.[150] Use of depilatory treatments, including laser depilation and eflornithine creams, can also be used.[151]

Cutaneous Squamous Cell Carcinoma

- **Incidence:** Individual studies have reported varying incidences of cutaneous squamous cell carcinoma (cuSCC) in patients treated with BRAF inhibitors ranging from a low of 3.92% to as high as 33.33%.[152] In a meta-analysis including 7442 patients from 24 studies, the incidence of BRAF inhibitor–associated squamous cell carcinoma was reported to be about 12.5% for all-grade and 11.6% for high-grade cuSCC.[153] Subgroup analysis revealed no difference in incidence when considering tumor type, particular drug used, or the study design chosen. Interestingly, the use of dual BRAF inhibitors resulted in a lower incidence of cuSCC than single agent use for all-grade and high-grade lesions.[154]
- **Clinical presentation:** cuSCC has been reported to occur between 2 and 6 months after BRAF inhibitor therapy initiation.[155,156] On average, lesions occur within 3 months

of treatment with a median time of diagnosis of 61 to 68 days.[158] Although lesions occur equally in both genders, there is preponderance for older individuals, and as such, lesions are uncommon in individuals less than 40 years.[157,158] At the time of detection, lesions are generally noninvasive, measure 8.7 mm on average, and are described as papular or nodular in appearance.[159] Invasive lesions can be distinguished from noninvasive lesions because they are characterized by centrally located thrombosed vessels, adherent scales, and an erythematous halo. No cases of metastatic cuSCCs resulting from BRAF inhibitor therapy have been reported to date.[154,159]

- **Histopathology:** Most cuSCCs are well-differentiated, but a few cases of unusually aggressive spindle cell variants have been reported.[160–162] Histopathologically, lesions can be grouped as keratoacanthoma-like or wart-like, both of which demonstrate invasive lobules and atypical keratinocytes. These can be differentiated by the presence of papillomatosis, hyperkeratosis, acanthosis, and koilocytosis, which are characteristic of wart-like lesions.[163,164]
- **Mechanism of action of cuSCC and the BRAF pathway:** BRAF alterations are found in about 8% of human cancers including melanomas, thyroid, ovarian, and colorectal cancers.[165,166] The substitution of glutamic acid to valine at position 600 (V600E) is involved in 90% of BRAF mutant melanomas.[167] This results in sustained activation of the mitogen-activated protein kinase (MAPK) and activation of downstream cellular pathways in the absence of growth factor signals,[168] causing unregulated cell growth, proliferation, and differentiation of cancer cells. BRAF inhibitors inhibit the MAPK pathway and inadvertently result in an increased incidence of cuSCC. The exact pathogenesis is not known, but there are two mechanisms that have been proposed. Both hypothesized mechanisms essentially occur in wild-type BRAF cells and those that have oncogenic RAS mutations due to UV damaged skin. The first hypothesis involves RAS-mediated dimerization of BRAF-CRAF and the consequent activation of a pathway through CRAF.[169,170] The second hypothesis involves an activated RAS (activated upstream by EGFR) and transactivation of a BRAF-inhibitor-bound BRAF/BRAF homodimer or a BRAF-inhibitor-bound BRAF/CRAF heterodimer.[169,171] This activation is suggested to be dose dependent, occurring at low concentrations of BRAF inhibitors. Further, it has been elucidated in vitro that mutant RAS cell lines hyperproliferate after treatment with BRAF inhibitors. There is evidence that BRAF inhibitors paradoxically activate MAPK pathways in cells that lack a BRAF mutation.[172]
- **Approved BRAF inhibitors:** Vemurafenib and dabrafenib are reversible inhibitors of BRAF that compete with ATP for binding to the kinase domain. Vemurafenib is approved for the treatment of melanoma with BRAF V600E mutation, where valine is substituted for glutamate at codon 600.[173] Dabrafenib is approved as monotherapy for melanoma with V600E mutation.[174] It is also approved for treatment of melanoma with BRAF V600E/K mutations in combination with trametinib, a MEK inhibitor. The combination of dabrafenib and trametinib has also been FDA–approved for metastatic NSCLC with BRAF V600E mutation and anaplastic thyroid cancer with BRAF V600E mutation.[175–177]
- **Management of cuSCC**
  - **Nonpharmacological treatment:** It is important to educate patients about the known adverse effects of BRAF inhibitor therapy to avoid cessation or interruption of tumor therapy. Preventive methods include avoidance of prolonged sun exposure and avoidance of alcohol-containing skin products. Patients should undergo regular dermatological follow-up for continued evaluation of possible cuSCC. Supportive measures include use of sunscreen to protect against UVB damage, use of daily moisturizers, and a good skin care routine through use of nonalcoholic, nonirritant skin care products.
  - **Pharmacological treatment:** Dual therapy with BRAF inhibitors and MEK inhibitors[154] has been reported to be associated with a much lower incidence of cuSCC compared with BRAF inhibitors alone. Surgical treatment is the current standard of care

for BRAF inhibitor-induced cuSCCs. This approach is appropriate for single, first-time lesions, but the relative inconvenience of excision of multiple or recurrent lesions has made way for the use of pharmacological agents. This includes use of systemic retinoids such as acitretin[178–181] and 5-fluorouracil.[182–184] Both agents have been successful in treating existing lesions, and follow-up studies also indicate a reduction in the rate of cuSCC recurrence.[183] There is growing evidence linking human papilloma virus (HPV)[185,186] and human polyoma virus (HPyV)[187,188] in BRAF inhibitor-associated cuSCCs, and the possible use of antiviral therapy has been raised.

References

1. Fabbrocini G, Panariello L, Caro G, Cacciapuoti S. Acneiform rash induced by EGFR inhibitors: review of the literature and new insights. *Skin Appendage Disorders*. 2015;1:31–37.
2. Kato T, Yoshioka H, Okamoto I, et al. Afatinib versus cisplatin plus pemetrexed in Japanese patients with advanced non-small cell lung cancer harboring activating EGFR mutations: subgroup analysis of LUX-Lung 3. *Cancer Sci*. 2015;106:1202–1211.
3. Sequist LV, Yang JC-H, Yamamoto N, et al. Phase III study of afatinib or cisplatin plus pemetrexed in patients with metastatic lung adenocarcinoma with EGFR mutations. *J Clin Oncol*. 2013;31:3327–3334.
4. Wu Y-L, Zhou C, Hu C-P, et al. Afatinib versus cisplatin plus gemcitabine for first-line treatment of Asian patients with advanced non-small-cell lung cancer harbouring EGFR mutations (LUX-Lung 6): an open-label, randomised phase 3 trial. *Lancet Oncol*. 2014;15:213–222.
5. Takeda M, Nakagawa K. Toxicity profile of epidermal growth factor receptor tyrosine kinase inhibitors in patients with epidermal growth factor receptor gene mutation-positive lung cancer. *Mol Clin Oncology*. 2017;6(1):3–6.
6. Heidary N, Naik H, Burgin S. Chemotherapeutic agents and the skin: an update. *J Am Acad Dermatol*. 2008;58:545–570.
7. Goffin JR, Zbuk K. Epidermal growth factor receptor: pathway, therapies, and pipeline. *Clin Ther*. 2013;35(9):1282–1303.
8. Lichtenberger BM, Gerber PA, Holcmann M, et al. Epidermal EGFR controls cutaneous host defense and prevents inflammation. *Sci Transl Med*. 2013;5:199ra111.
9. Riely GJ, Pao W, Pham D, et al. Clinical course of patients with non-small cell lung cancer and epidermal growth factor receptor exon 19 and exon 21 mutations treated with gefitinib or erlotinib. *Clin Cancer Res*. 2006;12(3 Pt 1):839–844.
10. Moore MJ, Goldstein D, Hamm J, et al. Erlotinib plus gemcitabine compared with gemcitabine alone in patients with advanced pancreatic cancer: a phase III trial of the National Cancer Institute of Canada Clinical Trials Group. *J Clin Oncol*. 2007;25(15):1960–1966.
11. Miller VA, Hirsh V, Cadranel J, et al. Afatinib versus placebo for patients with advanced, metastatic non-small-cell lung cancer after failure of erlotinib, gefitinib, or both, and one or two lines of chemotherapy (LUX-Lung 1): a phase 2b/3 randomised trial. *Lancet Oncol*. 2012;13(5):528–538.
12. Mok TS, Wu YL, Ahn MJ, et al. Osimertinib or platinum-pemetrexed in EGFR T790M-positive lung cancer. *N Engl J Med*. 2017;376(7):629–640.
13. Soria JC, Ohe Y, Vansteenkiste J, et al. Osimertinib in untreated EGFR-mutated advanced non-small-cell lung cancer. *N Engl J Med*. 2018;378(2):113–125.
14. Choo JR, Tan CS, Soo RA. Treatment of EGFR T790M-positive non-small cell lung cancer. *Target Oncol*. 2018;13(2):141–156.
15. Kurai J, Chikumi H, Hashimoto K, et al. Antibody-dependent cellular cytotoxicity mediated by cetuximab against lung cancer cell lines. *Clin Cancer Res*. 2007;13(5):1552–1561.
16. Liu B, Fang M, Schmidt M, et al. Induction of apoptosis and activation of the caspase cascade by anti-EGF receptor monoclonal antibodies in DiFi human colon cancer cells do not involve the c-jun N-terminal kinase activity. *Br J Cancer*. 2000;82(12):1991–1999.
17. Vermorken JB, Mesia R, Rivera F, et al. Platinum-based chemotherapy plus cetuximab in head and neck cancer. *N Engl J Med*. 2008;359(11):1116–1127.
18. Jonker DJ, O'Callaghan CJ, Karapetis CS, et al. Cetuximab for the treatment of colorectal cancer. *N Engl J Med*. 2007;357(20):2040–2048.

19. Van Cutsem E, Peeters M, Siena S, et al. Open-label phase III trial of panitumumab plus best support-
    ive care compared with best supportive care alone in patients with chemotherapy-refractory metastatic
    colorectal cancer. *J Clin Oncol*. 2007;25(13):1658–1664.
20. Lacouture ME, Lai SE. The PRIDE (Papulopustules and/or paronychia, Regulatory abnormalities of
    hair growth, Itching, and Dryness due to Epidermal growth factor receptor inhibitors) syndrome. *Br J
    Dermatol*. 2006;155(4):852–854.
21. Belloni B, Schonewolf N, Rozati S, Goldinger SM, Dummer R. Cutaneous drug eruptions associated
    with the use of new oncological drugs. *Chem Immunol Allergy*. 2012;97:191–202.
22. Harandi A, Zaidi AS, Stocker AM, Laber DA. Clinical efficacy and toxicity of anti-EGFR therapy in
    common cancers. *J Oncol*. 2009;2009:567486.
23. Giovannini M, Gregorc V, Belli C, et al. Clinical significance of skin toxicity due to EGFR-targeted
    therapies. *J Oncol*. 2009;2009:849051.
24. Fukuoka M, Yano S, Giaccone G, et al. Multi-institutional randomized phase II trial of gefitinib for
    previously treated patients with advanced non-small-cell lung cancer (The IDEAL 1 Trial) [corrected].
    J Clin Oncol. 2003;21:2237–2246.
25. Jacot W, Bessis D, Jorda E, et al. Acneiform eruption induced by epidermal growth factor receptor inhibi-
    tors in patients with solid tumours. *Br J Dermatol*. 2004;151(1):238–241.
26. Gridelli C, Maione P, Amoroso D, et al. Clinical significance and treatment of skin rash from erlotinib
    in non-small cell lung cancer patients: results of an Experts Panel Meeting. *Crit Rev Oncol Hematol*.
    2008;66:155–162.
27. Eilers RE, Gandhi M, Patel JD, et al. Dermatologic infections in cancer patients treated with epidermal
    growth factor receptor inhibitor therapy. *J Natl Cancer Inst*. 2010;102(1):47–53.
28. Kardaun SH, van Duinen KF. Erlotinib-induced florid acneiform rash complicated by extensive impe-
    tiginization. *Clin Exp Dermatol*. 2008;33(1):46–49.
29. Lord HK, Junor E, Ironside J. Cetuximab is effective, but more toxic than reported in the Bonner trial.
    Clinical Oncology. 2008;20(1):96.
30. Lacouture ME. Mechanisms of cutaneous toxicities to EGFR inhibitors. *Nat Rev Cancer*. 2006;6:803–812.
31. United States Department of Health and Human Services National Institutes of Health National Can-
    cer Institute (NCI). *Common Terminology Criteria for Adverse Events (CTCAE)*. Bethesda, MD: NCI;
    2017 Ver. 5.0 https://ctep.cancer.gov/protocolDevelopment/electronic_applications/docs/CTCAE_v5_
    Quick_Reference_5x7.pdf.
32. Wacker B, Nagrani T, Weinberg J, Witt K, Clark G, Cagnoni PJ. Correlation between development of
    rash and efficacy in patients treated with the epidermal growth factor receptor tyrosine kinase inhibitor
    erlotinib in two large phase III studies. *Clin Cancer Res*. 2007;13:3913–3921.
33. Micantonio T, Fargnoli MC, Ricevuto E, et al. Efficacy of treatment with tetracyclines to prevent acne-
    iform eruption secondary to cetuximab therapy. *Arch Dermatol*. 2005;141:1173–1174.
34. Sapadin AN, Fleischmajer R. Tetracyclines: nonantibiotic properties and their clinical implications. *J Am
    Acad Dermatol*. 2006;54:258–265.
35. Melosky B. Supportive care treatments for toxicities of anti-EGFR and other targeted agents. *Curr Oncol*.
    2012;19(suppl 1):S59–S63.
36. Melosky B, Anderson H, Burkes RL, et al. Pan Canadian Rash Trial: a randomized phase III trial
    evaluating the impact of a prophylactic skin treatment regimen on epidermal growth factor receptor-
    tyrosine kinase inhibitor-induced skin toxicities in patients with metastatic lung cancer. *J Clin Oncol*.
    2016;34(8):810–815.
37. Scope A, Agero ALC, Dusza SW, et al. Randomized double-blind trial of prophylactic oral minocycline
    and topical tazarotene for cetuximab-associated acne-like eruption. *J Clin Oncol*. 2007;25:5390–5396.
38. Jatoi A, Rowland K, Sloan JA, et al. Tetracycline to prevent epidermal growth factor receptor inhibitor-
    induced skin rashes. *Cancer*. 2008;113:847–853.
39. Duvic M, Nagpal S, Asano AT, Chandraratna RAS. Molecular mechanisms of tazarotene action in pso-
    riasis. *J Am Acad Dermat*. 1997;37(Part 3):S18–S24.
40. Shroot B, Michel S. Pharmacology and chemistry of adapalene. *J Am Acad Dermatol*. 1997;36(suppl):
    S96–S103.
41. Rittie L, Varani J, Kang S, Voorhees JJ, Fisher GJ. Retinoid-induced epidermal hyperplasia is mediated
    by epidermal growth factor receptor activation via specific induction of its ligands, heparin-binding EGF
    and amphiregulin in human skin in vivo. *J Invest Dermatol*. 2006;126:732–739.

42. Bikowski JB. Mechanisms of the comedolytic and anti-inflammatory properties of topical retinoids. *J Drugs Dermatol.* 2005;4:41–47.

43. DeWitt CA, Siroy AE, Stone SP. Acneiform eruptions associated with epidermal growth factor receptor-targeted chemotherapy. *J Am Acad Dermatol.* 2007;56:500–505.

44. Tachihara M, Tokunaga S, Tamura D, Kobayashi K, Ya Funada, Nishimura Y. Successful treatment with adapalene for EGFR-TKI-induced acneiform eruptions. *Jpn J Lung Cancer.* 2014;54:978–982.

45. Vezzoli P, Marzano AV, Onida F, et al. Cetuximab-induced acneiform eruption and the response to isotretinoin. *Acta Derm Venereol.* 2008;88:84–86.

46. Ocvirk J, Rebersek M. Management of cutaneous side effects of cetuximab therapy with vitamin K1 creme. *Radiol Oncol.* 2008;42:215–224.

47. Hirsh V. Managing treatment-related adverse events associated with EGFR tyrosine kinase inhibitors in advanced non-small-cell lung cancer. *Curr Oncol.* 2011;18:126–138.

48. Herbst RS, LoRusso PM, Purdom M, et al. Dermatologic side effects associated with gefitinib therapy: clinical experience and management. *Clin Lung Cancer.* 2003;4:366–369.

49. Balagula Y, Wu S, Xiao S, Feldman DR, Lacouture ME. The risk of hand foot skin reaction to pazopanib, a novel multikinase inhibitor: a systematic review of literature and meta-analysis. *Invest New Drugs.* 2012;30:1773–1781.

50. Hanahan D, Weinberg RA. The hallmarks of cancer. *Cell.* 2000;100(1):57–70.

51. Shibuya M. Vascular endothelial growth factor (VEGF) and its receptor (VEGFR) signaling in angiogenesis: a crucial target for anti- and pro-angiogenic therapies. *Genes Cancer.* 2011;2(12):1097–1105.

52. Simons M, Gordon E, Claesson-Welsh L. Mechanisms and regulation of endothelial VEGF receptor signalling. *Nat Rev Mol Cell Biol.* 2016;17(10):611–625.

53. Belum VR, Wu S, Lacouture ME. Risk of hand-foot skin reaction with the novel multikinase inhibitor regorafenib: a meta-analysis. *Invest New Drugs.* 2013;31:1078–1086.

54. Chu D, Lacouture ME, Fillos T, Wu S. Risk of hand-foot skin reaction with sorafenib: a systematic review and meta-analysis. *Acta Oncol.* 2008;47:176–186.

55. Azad NS, Aragon-Ching JB, Dahut WL, et al. Hand-foot skin reaction increases with cumulative sorafenib dose and with combination anti-vascular endothelial growth factor therapy. *Clin Cancer Res.* 2009;15:1411–1416.

56. Cook KM, Figg WD. Angiogenesis inhibitors: current strategies and future prospects. *CA Cancer J Clin.* 2010;60(4):222–243.

57. Kudo M, Finn RS, Qin S, et al. Lenvatinib versus sorafenib in first-line treatment of patients with unresectable hepatocellular carcinoma: a randomised phase 3 non-inferiority trial. *Lancet.* 2018;391(10126):1163–1173.

58. Choueiri TK, Escudier B, Powles T, et al. Cabozantinib versus everolimus in advanced renal-cell carcinoma. *N Engl J Med.* 2015;373(19):1814–1823.

59. Cortes JE, Kantarjian H, Shah NP, et al. Ponatinib in refractory Philadelphia chromosome-positive leukemias. *N Engl J Med.* 2012;367(22):2075–2088.

60. Hoesly FJ, Baker SG, Gunawardane ND, Cotliar JA. Capecitabine-induced hand-foot syndrome complicated by pseudomonal superinfection resulting in bacterial sepsis and death: case report and review of the literature. *Arch Dermatol.* 2011;147:1418–1423.

61. Degen A, Alter M, Schenck F, et al. The hand-foot-syndrome associated with medical tumor therapy—classification and management. *J Dtsch Dermatol Ges.* 2010;8:652–661.

62. Lipworth AD, Robert C, Zhu AX. Hand-foot syndrome (hand-foot skin reaction, palmar-plantar erythrodysesthesia): focus on sorafenib and sunitinib. *Oncology.* 2009;77:257–271.

63. Sibaud V, Delord JP, Chevreau C. Sorafenib-induced hand-foot skin reaction: a Koebner phenomenon. *Target Oncol.* 2009;4:307–310.

64. Lai SE, Kuzel T, Lacouture ME. Hand-foot and stump syndrome to sorafenib. *J Clin Oncol.* 2007;25:341–343.

65. Boone SL, Jameson G, Von Hoff D, Lacouture ME. Blackberry-induced hand-foot skin reaction to sunitinib. *Invest New Drugs.* 2009;27:389–390.

66. Autier J, Escudier B, Wechsler J, et al. Prospective study of the cutaneous adverse effects of sorafenib, a novel multikinase inhibitor. *Arch Dermatol.* 2008;144:886–892.

67. Jain L, Sissung TM, Danesi R, et al. Hypertension and hand-foot skin reactions related to VEGFR2 genotype and improved clinical outcome following bevacizumab and sorafenib. *J Exp Clin Cancer Res.* 2010;29:95.

68. Otsuka T, Eguchi Y, Kawazoe S, et al. Skin toxicities and survival in advanced hepatocellular carcinoma patients treated with sorafenib. *Hepatol Res.* 2012;2:879–886.

69. Poprach A, Pavlik T, Melichar B, et al. Skin toxicity and efficacy of sunitinib and sorafenib in metastatic renal cell carcinoma: a national registry-based study. *Ann Oncol.* 2012;23:3137–3143.

70. Nakano K, Komatsu K, Kubo T, et al. Hand-foot skin reaction is associated with the clinical outcome in patients with metastatic renal cell carcinoma treated with sorafenib. *Jpn J Clin Oncol.* 2013;43:1023–1029.

71. Lacouture ME, Wu S, Robert C, et al. Evolving strategies for the management of hand-foot skin reaction associated with the multitargeted kinase inhibitors sorafenib and sunitinib. *Oncologist.* 2008;13(9):1001–1011.

72. National Cancer Institute. Cancer Therapy Evaluation Program, Common Terminology Criteria for Adverse Events, Version 3.0. Bethesda, MD: National Cancer Institute; 2006. http://ctep.cancer.gov/protocolDevelopment/electronic_applications/docs/ctcaev3.pdf.

73. National Cancer Institute. Cancer Therapy Evaluation Program, Common Terminology Criteria for Adverse Events, Version 4.0. Bethesda, MD: National Cancer Institute; 2009. http://evs.nci.nih.gov/ftp1/CTCAE/CTCAE_4.03_2010-06-14_QuickReference_8.5x11.pdf.

74. Skin reactions and cancer therapy—guidelines for identifying and managing skin-related side effects during your therapy. West Haven, CT; Emeryville, CA: Bayer Healthcare Pharmaceuticals, Onyx Pharmaceuticals; 2006:1–12.

75. Manchen E, Robert C, Porta C. Management of tyrosine kinase inhibitor-induced hand-foot skin reaction: viewpoints from the medical oncologist, dermatologist, and oncology nurse. *J Support Oncol.* 2011;9:13–23.

76. Anderson R, Jatoi A, Robert C, et al. Search for evidence-based approaches for the prevention and palliation of hand-foot skin reaction (HFSR) caused by the multikinase inhibitors (MKIs). *Oncologist.* 2009;14:291–302.

77. McLellan B, Ciardiello F, Lacouture ME, Segaert S, Van Cutsem E. Regorafenib-associated hand-foot skin reaction: practical advice on diagnosis, prevention, and management. *Ann Oncol.* 2015;26(10):2017–2026.

78. Chren MM, Lasek RJ, Sahay AP, Sands LP. Measurement properties of Skindex-16: a brief quality-of-life measure for patients with skin diseases. *J Cutan Med Surg.* 2001;5:105–110.

79. Lewis V, Finlay AY. 10 years' experience of the Dermatology Life Quality Index (DLQI). *J Investig Dermatol Symp Proc.* 2004;9:169–180.

80. Peuvrel L, Dreno B. Dermatological toxicity associated with targeted therapies in cancer: optimal management. *Am J Clin Dermatol.* 2014;15(5):425–444.

81. Shinohara N, Nonomura N, Eto M, et al. A randomized multicenter phase II trial on the efficacy of a hydrocolloid dressing containing ceramide with a low-friction external surface for hand-foot skin reaction caused by sorafenib in patients with renal cell carcinoma. *Ann Oncol.* 2013;25(2):472–476.

82. De Wit M, Boers-Doets CB, Saettini A, et al. Prevention and management of adverse events related to regorafenib. *Support Care Cancer.* 2014;22(3):837–846.

83. Bozkurt DB, Kara B, Oguz KI, Demiryurek H, Aksungur E. Hand-foot syndrome due to sorafenib in hepatocellular carcinoma treated with vitamin E without dose modification; a preliminary clinical study. *J Buon.* 2011;16(4):759–764.

84. Dietrich EM, Antoniades K. Molecularly targeted drugs for the treatment of cancer: oral complications and pathophysiology. *Hippokratia.* 2012;16(3):196–199.

85. Motzer RJ, Hutson TE, Glen H, et al. Lenvatinib, everolimus, and the combination in patients with metastatic renal cell carcinoma: a randomised, phase 2, open-label, multicentre trial. *Lancet Oncol.* 2015;16:1473–1482.

86. Armstrong AJ, Halabi S, Eisen T, et al. Everolimus versus sunitinib for patients with met-astatic non-clear cell renal cell carcinoma (ASPEN): a multicentre, open-label, randomised phase 2 trial. *Lancet Oncol.* 2016;17:378–388.

87. Choueiri TK, Escudier B, Powles T, et al. Cabozantinib versus everolimus in advanced renal-cell carcinoma. *N Engl J Med.* 2015;373:1814–1823.

88. Martins F, de Oliveira MA, Wang Q, et al. A review of oral toxicity associated with mTOR inhibitor therapy in cancer patients. *Oral Oncol.* 2013;49:293–298.

89. Shameem R, Lacouture M, Wu S. Incidence and risk of high-grade stomatitis with mTOR inhibitors in cancer patients. *Cancer Investig.* 2015;33:70–77.

90. Al-Ansari S, Zecha JA, Barasch A, de Lange J, Rozema FR, Raber-Durlacher JE. Oral mucositis induced by anticancer therapies. *Curr Oral Health Rep.* 2015;2:202–211.

91. Yuan A, Kurtz SL, Barysauskas CM, Pilotte AP, Wagner AJ, Treister NS. Oral adverse events in cancer patients treated with VEGFR-directed multitargeted tyrosine kinase inhibitors. *Oral Oncol.* 2015;51:1026–1033.

92. Boers-Doets CB, Epstein JB, Raber-Durlacher JE, et al. Oral adverse events associated with tyrosine kinase and mammalian target of rapamycin inhibitors in renal cell carcinoma: a structured literature review. *Oncologist.* 2012;17:135–144.

93. United States Department of Health and Human Services, National Institutes of Health, National Cancer Institute (NCI). *Common Terminology Criteria for Adverse Events (CTCAE).* Bethesda, MD: NCI; 2010 Ver. 4.03 http://evs.nci.nih.gov/ftp1/CTCAE/CTCAE_4.03_2010-06-14_ QuickReference_5x7.pdf.

94. Kollmannsberger C, Bjarnason G, Burnett P, et al. Sunitinib in metastatic renal cell carcinoma: recommendations for management of non-cardiovascular toxicities. *Oncologist.* 2011;16:543–553.

95. Widakowich C, de Castro G Jr, de Azambuja E, Dinh P, Awada A. Review: side effects of approved molecular targeted therapies in solid cancers. *Oncologist.* 2007;12:1443–1455.

96. Ferrara N, Davis-Smyth T. The biology of vascular endothelial growth factor. *Endocr Rev.* 1997;18:4–25.

97. Katholnig K, Linke M, Pham H, Hengstschlager M, Weichhart T. Immune responses of macrophages and dendritic cells regulated by mTOR signalling. *Biochem. Soc. Trans.* 2013;41:927–933.

98. Lewkowicz N, Lewkowicz P, Dzitko K, et al. Dysfunction of CD4+ CD25 high T regulatory cells in patients with recurrent aphthous stomatitis. *J Oral Pathol Med.* 2008;37:454–461.

99. Boers-Doets CB, Raber-Durlacher JE, Treister NS, et al. Mammalian target of rapamycin inhibitor-associated stomatitis. *Future Oncol.* 2013;9:1883–1892.

100. Bankvall M, Sjoberg F, Gale G, Wold A, Jontell M, Ostman S. The oral microbiota of patients with recurrent aphthous stomatitis. *J Oral Microbiol.* 2014;6:25739.

101. Hijazi K, Lowe T, Meharg C, Berry SH, Foley J, Hold GL. Mucosal microbiome in patients with recurrent aphthous stomatitis. *J Dent Res.* 2015;94:87S–94S.

102. Slebioda Z, Szponar E, Kowalska A. Recurrent aphthous stomatitis: genetic aspects of etiology. *Postepy Dermatol Alergol.* 2013;30:96–102.

103. Cook KM, Figg WD. Angiogenesis inhibitors: current strategies and future prospects. *CA Cancer J Clin.* 2010;60(4):222–243.

104. Kudo M, Finn RS, Qin S, et al. Lenvatinib versus sorafenib in first-line treatment of patients with unresectable hepatocellular carcinoma: a randomised phase 3 non-inferiority trial. *Lancet.* 2018; 391(10126):1163–1173.

105. Choueiri TK, Escudier B, Powles T, et al. Cabozantinib versus everolimus in advanced renal-cell carcinoma. *N Engl J Med.* 2015;373(19):1814–1823.

106. Cortes JE, Kantarjian H, Shah NP, et al. Ponatinib in refractory Philadelphia chromosome-positive leukemias. *N Engl J Med.* 2012;367(22):2075–2088.

107. Rugo HS, Pritchard KI, Gnant M, et al. Incidence and time course of everolimus-related adverse events in postmenopausal women with hormone receptor-positive advanced breast cancer: insights from BOLERO-2. *Ann Oncol.* 2014;25:808–815.

108. Rugo HS, Hortobagyi GN, Yao J, et al. Meta-analysis of stomatitis in clinical studies of everolimus: incidence and relationship with efficacy. *Ann Oncol.* 2016;27:519–525.

109. Elad S, Raber-Durlacher JE, Brennan MT, et al. Basic oral care for hematology-oncology patients and hematopoietic stem cell transplantation recipients: a position paper from the joint task force of the Multinational Association of Supportive Care in Cancer/International Society of Oral Oncology (MASCC/ISOO) and the European Society for Blood and Marrow Transplantation (EBMT). *Support Care Cancer.* 2015;23:223–236.

110. Lacouture ME, Anadkat MJ, Bensadoun RJ, et al. on behalf of the MASCC Skin Toxicity Study Group. Clinical practice guidelines for the prevention and treatment of EGFR inhibitor–associated dermatologic toxicities. *Support Care Cancer.* 2011;19:1079–1095.

111. Lalla RV, Bowen J, Barasch A, et al. MASCC/ISOO clinical practice guidelines for the management of mucositis secondary to cancer therapy. *Cancer.* 2014;120:1453–1461.

112. McGuire DB, Fulton JS, Park J, et al. Systematic review of basic oral care for the management of oral mucositis in cancer patients. *Support Care Cancer.* 2013;21:3165–3177.

113. Peterson DE, O'Shaughnessy JA, Rugo HS, et al. Oral mucosal injury caused by mammalian target of rapamycin inhibitors: emerging perspectives on pathobiology and impact on clinical practice. *Cancer Med.* 2016;5:1897–1907.

114. Brown CG, Yoder LH. Stomatitis: an overview: protecting the oral cavity during cancer treatment. *Am J Nurs.* 2002;102(suppl 4):20–23.
115. Clark D. How do I manage a patient with aphthous ulcers. *J Can Dent Assoc.* 2013;79:d48.
116. Peterson DE, Boers-Doets CB, Bensadoun RJ, Herrstedt J, Guidelines Committee ESMO. Management of oral and gastrointestinal mucosal injury: ESMO Clinical Practice Guidelines for diagnosis, treatment, and follow-up. *Ann Oncol.* 2015;26:v139–v151.
117. Shameem R, Lacouture M, Wu S. Incidence and risk of high-grade stomatitis with mTOR inhibitors in cancer patients. *Cancer Investig.* 2015;33:70–77.
118. Zecha JA, Raber-Durlacher JE, Nair RG, et al. Low-level laser therapy/photobiomodulation in the management of side effects of chemoradiation therapy in head and neck cancer: part 2: proposed applications and treatment protocols. *Support Care Cancer.* 2016;24:2793–2805.
119. Porta C, Osanto S, Ravaud A, et al. Management of adverse events associated with the use of everolimus in patients with advanced renal cell carcinoma. *Eur J Cancer.* 2011;47:1287–1298.
120. Rugo HS. Dosing and safety implications for oncologists when administering everolimus to patients with hormone receptor-positive breast cancer. *Clin Breast Cancer.* 2016;16:18–22.
121. Belum VR, Marulanda K, Ensslin C, et al. Alopecia in patients treated with molecularly targeted anticancer therapies. *Ann Oncol.* 2015;26:2496–2502.
122. Trueb RM. Chemotherapy-induced alopecia. *Semin Cutan Med Surg.* 2009;28(1):11–14.
123. Rosman S. Cancer and stigma: experience of patients with chemotherapy-induced alopecia. *Patient Educ Couns.* 2004;52(3):333–339.
124. Browall M, Gaston-Johansson F, Danielson E. Postmenopausal women with breast cancer: their experiences of the chemotherapy treatment period. *Cancer Nurs.* 2006;29(1):34–42.
125. Lasheen S, Shohdy KS, Kassem L, Abdel-Rahman O. Fatigue, alopecia and stomatitis among patients with breast cancer receiving cyclin-dependent kinase 4 and 6 inhibitors: a systematic review and meta-analysis. *Expert Rev Anticancer Ther.* 2017;17(9):851–856.
126. Owczarek W, Slowinska M, Lesiak A, et al. The incidence and management of cutaneous adverse events of the epidermal growth factor receptor inhibitors. *Adv Dermatol Allergol.* 2017;34(5):418–428.
127. Robert C, Mateus C, Spatz A, et al. Dermatologic symptoms associated with the multikinase inhibitor sorafenib. *J Am Acad Dermatol.* 2009;60(2):299–305.
128. Osio A, Mateus C, Soria JC, et al. Cutaneous side-effects in patients on long-term treatment with epidermal growth factor receptor inhibitors. *Br J Dermatol.* 2009;161(3):515–521.
129. Hepper DM, Wu P, Anadkat MJ. Scarring alopecia associated with the epidermal growth factor receptor inhibitor erlotinib. *J Am Acad Dermatol.* 2011;64(5):996–998.
130. Hoekzema R, Drillenburg P. Folliculitis decalvans associated with erlotinib. *Clin Exp Dermatol.* 2010;35(8):916–918.
131. Lacouture M. *Dermatologic Principles and Practice in Oncology: Conditions of the Skin, Hair, and Nails in Cancer Patients.* New York: Wiley-Blackwell; 2014.
132. Sobańska K, Szałek E, Grześkowiak E. Cutaneous toxicity of small-molecular EGFR inhibitors. *Farm Współ.* 2013;6:33–40.
133. Jaber SH, Cowen EW, Haworth LR, et al. Skin reactions in a subset of patients with stage IV melanoma treated with anti-cytotoxic T-lymphocyte antigen 4 monoclonal antibody as a single agent. *Arch Dermatol.* 2006;142(2):166–172.
134. Services H. Common Terminology Criteria for Adverse Events v4.0 (CTCAE). http://evs.nci.nih.gov/ftp1/CTCAE/CTCAE_ 4.03_2010-06-14_QuickReference_5x7.pdf.
135. Verma S, Huang Bartlett C, Schnell P, et al. Palbociclib in combination with fulvestrant in women with hormone receptor-positive/HER2-negative advanced metastatic breast cancer: detailed safety analysis from a multicenter, randomized, placebo-controlled, phase III study (PALOMA-3). *Oncologist.* 2016;21(10):1–11.
136. Trüeb RM. Chemotherapy-induced alopecia. *Semin Cutan Med Surg.* 2009;28:11–14.
137. Paus R, Haslam IS, Sharov AA, Botchkarev VA. Pathobiology of chemotherapy-induced hair loss. *Lancet Oncol.* 2013;14(2):e50–e59.
138. Nanney LB, Magid M, Stoscheck CM, King LE Jr. Comparison of epidermal growth factor binding and receptor distribution in normal human epidermis and epidermal appendages. *J Invest Dermatol.* 1984;83(5):385–393.
139. Philpott MP, Kealey T. Effects of EGF on the morphology and patterns of DNA synthesis in isolated human hair follicles. *J Invest Dermatol.* 1994;102(2):186–191.

140. Hansen LA, Alexander N, Hogan ME, et al. Genetically null mice reveal a central role for epidermal growth factor receptor in the differentiation of the hair follicle and normal hair development. *Am J Pathol.* 1997;150(6):1959–1975.

141. Lacouture ME. Mechanisms of cutaneous toxicities to EGFR inhibitors. *Nat Rev Cancer.* 2006;6(10): 803–812.

142. Kawano M, Komi-Kuramochi A, Asada M, et al. Comprehensive analysis of FGF and FGFR expression in skin: FGF18 is highly expressed in hair follicles and capable of inducing anagen from telogen stage hair follicles. *J Invest Dermatol.* 2005;124(5):877–885.

143. Tomita Y, Akiyama M, Shimizu H. PDGF isoforms induce and maintain anagen phase of murine hair follicles. *J Dermatol Sci.* 2006;43(2):105–115.

144. Wang LC, Liu ZY, Gambardella L, et al. Regular articles: conditional disruption of hedgehog signaling pathway defines its critical role in hair development and regeneration. *J Invest Dermatol.* 2000;114(5):901–908.

145. Vijayaraghavan S, Moulder S, Keyomarsi K. et al. Inhibiting CDK in cancer therapy: current evidence and future directions. *Target Oncol.* 2018;13(1):21–38.

146. Duvic M, Lemak NA, Valero V, et al. A randomized trial of minoxidil in chemotherapy-induced alopecia. *J Am Acad Dermatol.* 1996;35:74–78.

147. Rodriguez R, Machiavelli M, Leone B, et al. Minoxidil (Mx) as a prophylaxis of doxorubicine induced alopecia. *Ann Oncol.* 1994;5:769–770.

148. Choi EK, Kim IR, Chang O, et al. Impact of chemotherapy-induced alopecia distress on body image, psychosocial well-being, and depression in breast cancer patients. *Psychooncology.* 2014;23(10):1103–1110.

149. Macdonald JB, Macdonald B, Golitz LE, et al. Cutaneous adverse effects of targeted therapies Part I: Inhibitors of the cellular membrane. *J Am Acad Dermatol.* 2015;72(2):203–218.

150. Melichar B, Nemcova I. Eye complications of cetuximab therapy. *Eur J Cancer Care (Engl).* 2007;16:439–443.

151. Sobańska K, Szałek E, Grześkowiak E. Cutaneous toxicity of small-molecular EGFR inhibitors. *Farm Współ.* 2013;6:33–40.

152. Puzanov I, Amaravadi RK, McArthur GA, et al. Long-term outcome in BRAF(V600E) melanoma patients treated with vemurafenib: patterns of disease progression and clinical management of limited progression. *Eur J Cancer.* 2015;51:1435–1443.

153. Ling P. Incidence and relative risk of cutaneous squamous cell carcinoma with single-agent BRAF inhibitor and dual BRAF/MEK inhibitors in cancer patients: a meta-analysis. *Oncotarget.* 2017;8(47):83280–83291.

154. Wu JH, Cohen DN, Rady PL, Tyring SK. BRAF inhibitor-associated cutaneous squamous cell carcinoma: new mechanistic insight, emerging evidence for viral involvement and perspectives on clinical management. *Br J Dermatol.* 2017;177:914–923.

155. Chapman PB, Hauschild A, Robert C, et al. Improved survival with vemurafenib in melanoma with BRAF V600E mutation. *N Engl J Med.* 2011;364:2507–2516.

156. Flaherty KT, Puzanov I, Kim KB, et al. Inhibition of mutated, activated BRAF in metastatic melanoma. *N Engl J Med.* 2010;363:809–819.

157. Anforth RM, Blumetti TC, Kefford RF, et al. Cutaneous manifestations of dabrafenib (GSK2118436): a selective inhibitor of mutant BRAF in patients with metastatic melanoma. *Br J Dermatol.* 2012;167:1153–1160.

158. Anforth R, Menzies A, Byth K, et al. Factors influencing the development of cutaneous squamous cell carcinoma in patients on BRAF inhibitor therapy. *J Am Acad Dermatol.* 2015;72:809–815.

159. Belum VR, Rosen AC, Jaimes N, et al. Clinico-morphological features of BRAF inhibition-induced proliferative skin lesions in cancer patients. *Cancer.* 2015;121:60–68.

160. Cohen DN, Lumbang WA, Boyd AS, et al. Spindle cell squamous carcinoma during BRAF inhibitor therapy for advanced melanoma: an aggressive secondary neoplasm of undetermined biologic potential. *JAMA Dermatol.* 2014;150:575–577.

161. Ziemer M, Ponitzsch I, Simon JC, et al. Spindle cell squamous cell carcinoma arising from verrucous hyperplasia during BRAF inhibitor therapy for melanoma. *J Dtsch Dermatol Ges.* 2015;13:326–328.

162. Sufficool KE, Hepper DM, Linette GP, et al. Histopathologic characteristics of therapy-associated cutaneous neoplasms with vemurafenib, a selective BRAF kinase inhibitor, used in the treatment of melanoma. *J Cutan Pathol.* 2014;41:568–575.

163. Cohen DN, Lawson SK, Shaver AC, et al. Contribution of beta-HPV infection and UV damage to rapid-onset cutaneous squamous cell carcinoma during BRAF-inhibition therapy. *Clin Cancer Res.* 2015;21:2624–2634.

164. Boussemart L, Routier E, Mateus C, et al. Prospective study of cutaneous side-effects associated with the BRAF inhibitor vemurafenib: a study of 42 patients. *Ann Oncol.* 2013;24:1691–1697.

165. Davies H, Bignell GR, Cox C, et al. Mutations of the BRAF gene in human cancer. *Nature.* 2002; 417(6892):949–954.

166. Xing M. BRAF mutation in papillary thyroid cancer: pathogenic role, molecular bases, and clinical implications. *Endocr Rev.* 2007;28(7):742–762.

167. Wan PT, Garnett MJ, Roe SM, et al. Mechanism of activation of the RAF-ERK signaling pathway by oncogenic mutations of B-RAF. *Cell.* 2004;116(6):855–867.

168. Boussemart L, Malka-Mahieu H, Girault I, et al. eIF4F is a nexus of resistance to anti-BRAF and anti-MEK cancer therapies. *Nature.* 2014;513:105–109. https://doi.org/10.1038/nature13572.

169. Heidorn SJ, Milagre C, Whittaker S, et al. Kinase-dead BRAF and oncogenic RAS cooperate to drive tumor progression through CRAF. *Cell.* 2010;140(2):209–221.

170. Hatzivassiliou G, Song K, Yen I, et al. RAF inhibitors prime wild-type RAF to activate the MAPK pathway and enhance growth. *Nature.* 2010;464(7287):431–435.

171. Poulikakos PI, Zhang C, Bollag G, et al. RAF inhibitors transactivate RAF dimers and ERK signalling in cells with wild-type BRAF. *Nature.* 2010;464(7287):427–430.

172. Robert C, Arnault JP, Mateus C. RAF inhibition and induction of cutaneous squamous cell carcinoma. *Curr Opin Oncol.* 2011;23:177–182.

173. Chapman PB, Hauschild A, Robert C, et al. Improved survival with vemurafenib in melanoma with BRAF V600E mutation. *N Engl J Med.* 2011;364(26):2507–2516.

174. Hauschild A, Grob JJ, Demidov LV, et al. Dabrafenib in BRAF-mutated metastatic melanoma: multicentre, open-label, phase 3 randomised controlled trial. *Lancet.* 2012;380(9839):358–365.

175. Flaherty KT, Infante JR, Daud A, et al. Combined BRAF and MEK inhibition in melanoma with BRAF V600 mutations. *N Engl J Med.* 2012;367(18):1694–1703.

176. Planchard D, Besse B, Groen HJM, et al. Dabrafenib plus trametinib in patients with previously treated BRAF(V600E)-mutant metastatic non-small cell lung cancer: an open-label, multicentre phase 2 trial. *Lancet Oncol.* 2016;17(7):984–993.

177. Subbiah V, Kreitman RJ, Wainberg ZA, et al. Dabrafenib and trametinib treatment in patients with locally advanced or metastatic BRAF V600-mutant anaplastic thyroid cancer. *J Clin Oncol.* 2018;36(1):7–13.

178. Anforth R, Blumetti TC, Clements A, et al. Systemic retinoids for the chemoprevention of cutaneous squamous cell carcinoma and verrucal keratosis in a cohort of patients on BRAF inhibitors. *Br J Dermatol.* 2013;169:1310–1313.

179. George R, Weightman W, Russ GR, et al. Acitretin for chemoprevention of non-melanoma skin cancers in renal transplant recipients. *Australas J Dermatol.* 2002;43:269–273.

180. Lebwohl M, Tannis C, Carrasco D. Acitretin suppression of squamous cell carcinoma: case report and literature review. *J Dermatolog Treat.* 2003;14(suppl. 2):3–6.

181. Chon SY, Sambrano BL, Geddes ER. Vemurafenib-related cutaneous side effects ameliorated by acitretin. *J Drugs Dermatol.* 2014;13:586–588.

182. Fathi R, Kamalpour L, Gammon B, et al. A novel treatment approach for extensive, eruptive, cutaneous squamous cell carcinomas in a patient receiving BRAF inhibitor therapy for metastatic melanoma. *Dermatol Surg.* 2013;39:341–344.

183. Viros A, Hayward R, Martin M, et al. Topical 5-fluorouracil elicits regressions of BRAF inhibitor-induced cutaneous squamous cell carcinoma. *J Invest Dermatol.* 2013;133:274–276.

184. Mays R, Curry J, Kim K, et al. Eruptive squamous cell carcinomas after vemurafenib therapy. *J Cutan Med Surg.* 2013;17:419–422.

185. Wang J, Aldabagh B, Yu J, et al. Role of human papillomavirus in cutaneous squamous cell carcinoma: a meta-analysis. *J Am Acad Dermatol.* 2014;70:621–629.

186. Farzan SF, Waterboer T, Gui J, et al. Cutaneous alpha, beta and gamma human papillomaviruses in relation to squamous cell carcinoma of the skin: a population-based study. *Int J Cancer.* 2013;133:1713–1720.

187. Falchook GS, Rady P, Hymes S, et al. Merkel cell polyomavirus and HPV-17 associated with cutaneous squamous cell carcinoma arising in a patient with melanoma treated with the BRAF inhibitor dabrafenib. *JAMA Dermatol.* 2013;149:322–326.

188. Cohen DN, Lawson SK, Shaver AC, et al. Contribution of beta-HPV infection and UV damage to rapid-onset cutaneous squamous cell carcinoma during BRAF-inhibition therapy. *Clin Cancer Res.* 2015;21:2624–2634.

CHAPTER 16

Cardiovascular Toxicities of Targeted Therapy

Sri Yadlapalli, MD   Ammar Sukari, MD   Misako Nagasaka, MD

Introduction

Cardiotoxicity is one of the worrisome side effects of cancer-directed therapy. Cardiac adverse events can range from mild to severe and vary between classes of targeted agents. Some relevant cardiac adverse events include electrocardiogram (ECG) changes, QT prolongation, hypertension, arrhythmias, pericardial disease, and heart failure. Cardiac toxicities can limit the use of these drugs and warrant their discontinuation. Preexisting comorbidities and cardiac conditions can add to or worsen cardiac toxicity. The Common Terminology Criteria for Adverse Events (CTCAE) provides descriptions and grading for cardiovascular side effects. In this chapter, we will first review the various targeted therapies that are known to cause cardiotoxicities, and then discuss in detail each of the cardiotoxicities and their respective management. Table 16.1 shows the grading of each cardiac toxicity based on the National Cancer Institute (NCI) CTCAE version 5.0.

Targeted Therapies Associated With Cardiotoxicity

- **HER2 targeting antibodies (trastuzumab, pertuzumab, T-DM1):** Trastuzumab and pertuzumab are monoclonal antibodies directed toward the HER2 receptor. They specifically target the erbB2 receptor tyrosine kinase. Trastuzumab is used mainly in HER2-neu-positive breast cancer and in metastatic HER2-neu-positive gastric cancers. These drugs carry a black box warning for cardiomyopathy and heart failure, with an increased risk of heart failure in patients with concomitant use of anthracyclines. T-DM1 (ado-trastuzumab emtansine) is an antibody drug conjugate, which is composed of trastuzumab, a thio linker, and a microtubule inhibitor. This drug had been approved for use in first- or second-line HER2 neu-positive metastatic breast cancer.

MECHANISM OF ACTION

ErbB2/neu is a member of the epidermal growth factor family. Its gene is amplified in many cancer types, and its overexpression is associated with poor prognosis in breast and ovarian cancer. It is overexpressed in 25% to 30% of breast cancer patients.

MECHANISM OF CARDIOTOXICITY

Neuregulins (neu-differentiation factors) and heregulin (ligand with acetyl choline receptor–inducing activity and glial growth factor) along with erbB2 are associated with cardiac myocyte development[1] and have been shown to inhibit the growth of cardiac stem cells and lack capacity for cardiogenic differentiation and vascular formation.[2] Thus interruption of this pathway can lead to cardiac toxicity. Manifestations range from asymptomatic decline in heart function to

TABLE 16.1 ■ **Common Cardiac Adverse Effects as Graded by NCI CTCAE Version 5.0**

CTCAE Term	Grade 1	Grade 2	Grade 3	Grade 4	Grade 5
Heart failure	Asymptomatic with laboratory (e.g., BNP) or cardiac imaging abnormalities	Symptoms with moderate activity or exertion	Symptoms at rest or with minimal activity or exertion; hospitalization; new onset of symptoms	Life-threatening consequences; urgent intervention indicated (e.g., continuous IV therapy or mechanical hemodynamic support)	Death
Left ventricular systolic dysfunction	-	-	Symptomatic due to drop in ejection fraction responsive to intervention	Refractory or poorly controlled heart failure due to drop in ejection fraction; intervention, such as ventricular assist device, intravenous vasopressor support, or heart transplant indicated	Death
Corrected QT interval prolongation on the ECG	Average QTc 450–480 ms	Average QTc 481–500 ms	Average QTc ≥501 ms; >60 ms change from baseline	Torsade de pointes; polymorphic ventricular tachycardia; signs/symptoms of serious arrhythmia	Death
Hypertension	Systolic BP 120–139 mmHg or diastolic BP 80–89 mmHg	Systolic BP 140–159 mmHg or diastolic BP 90–99 mmHg if previously WNL; change in baseline medical intervention indicated; recurrent or persistent (≥24 h); symptomatic increase by >20 mmHg (diastolic) or to >140/90 mmHg; monotherapy indicated or initiated	Systolic BP ≥160 mmHg or diastolic BP ≥100 mmHg; medical intervention indicated; more than one drug or more intensive therapy than previously used indicated	Life-threatening consequences (malignant hypertension, transient or permanent neurologic deficit, hypertensive crisis); urgent intervention indicated	Death

BNP, B-Natriuretic peptide; *BP,* blood pressure; *CTCAE,* Common Terminology Criteria for Adverse Events; *ECG,* electrocardiogram; *ms,* milliseconds; *NCI,* National Cancer Institute; *WNL,* within normal limits.
Adapted from National Institutes of Health, National Cancer Institute. Common Terminology Criteria for Adverse Events (CTCAE), Version 5.0, 2017. https://ctep.cancer.gov/protocoldevelopment/electronic_applications/docs/CTCAE_v5_Quick_Reference_8.5x11.pdf.

symptomatic congestive heart failure. Reported symptoms include tachycardia, palpitations, lower extremity edema, dyspnea on exertion, and clinical heart failure.[3]

- ■ **HER2–targeting tyrosine kinase inhibitors (TKIs) (lapatinib):** Lapatinib is a TKI against EGFR1 and HER2 that results in the inhibition of signaling pathways downstream of HER2. Lapatinib is metabolized in the liver and thus dose adjustments are required in patients with hepatic impairment. Lapatinib has been used in combination with chemotherapy, mostly capecitabine. The most common side effects are diarrhea, rash, and anorexia. Based on a clinical trial comparing lapatinib and capecitabine with capecitabine alone, there were no significant symptomatic cardiac adverse events in the combination treatment arm. Furthermore, no treatment withdrawal or dose reductions due to decreases in left ventricular ejection fraction (LVEF) were reported. There were, however, reports of asymptomatic cardiac events in 4 out of 163 women in the combination treatment arm. One of the four women in the combination arm developed Prinzmetal angina; however, with treatment cessation, her symptoms improved. Due to the decrease in LVEF, the dose was reduced to 1000 mg daily and there was no recurrence of cardiac event noted thereafter.[4]

- Multi-TKIs (sorafenib, sunitinib, pazopanib, axitinib, vandetanib, regorafenib, lenvatinib, cabozantinib)

MECHANISM OF ACTION

An overview of the vascular endothelial growth factor (VEGF) pathway and the mechanism of action of VEGF inhibitors is discussed elsewhere in this book. The specific effects of VEGF inhibition on cardiac tissue are discussed here.

TKIS HAVE ANTITUMOR ACTIVITY IN A VARIETY OF MALIGNANCIES

These TKIs have anti-VEGF activity, but also have activity against growth factor receptors such as EGFR, FGFR, and RET. Their broad coverage is attributed to the similarity of structures at the ATP-binding site region. Because their effects are not limited to VEGF receptors, but also to other growth factor receptors, these drugs are referred to as multitargeted TKIs, or antiangiogenic TKIs. Examples of antiangiogenic TKIs that are in clinical use are sorafenib (inhibits VEGFR2, fms-like tyrosine kinase 3 [FLT3], PDGFR, and fibroblast growth factor receptor [FGFR]-1); sunitinib (inhibits c-kit, VEGFR1-3, PDGFR-alpha, PDGFR-beta, FLT3, CSF-1R, RET); pazopanib (inhibits VEGFR1-3, PDGFR-alpha and -beta, FGFR1 and 3, c-KIT); axitinib (selective VEGFR inhibitor that targets VEGFR1-3); vandetanib (inhibits VEGFR, RET, and EGFR); regorafenib (targets VEGFR1-3 in addition to RET, c-KIT, PDGFR-alpha and -beta, FGFR1 and 2, and other membrane-bound and intracellular kinases); and lenvatinib (targets VEGFRs, RET, and FGFR).

MECHANISM OF CARDIOTOXICITY

VEGF is a protein that upregulates endothelial cell nitric oxides synthase (ecNOS), which upregulates nitric oxide (NO) production, thereby modulating vasodilation, microvascular hyperpermeability, and angiogenesis.[5] VEGF inhibitor-induced hypertension is mediated by suppression of NO production.[6]

TYPES OF CARDIOTOXICITY

In general, the cardiotoxicities associated with anti-VEGF agents are hypertension, thromboembolic disease, left ventricular dysfunction, myocardial ischemia, QT prolongation, and thrombotic angiopathy.[5]

- BCR/ABL and c-KIT inhibitors (imatinib, dasatinib, nilotinib, bosutinib, ponatinib): The mechanism of cardiotoxicity with BCR/ABL and c-KIT targeting drugs is similar to that of multitargeted TKIs.

IMATINIB

Imatinib is known to induce myocyte death by necrosis, autophagy, and apoptosis. The mechanism of imatinib-induced cardiotoxicity was evaluated in animal studies. Dose-related increases in cardiac expression were observed for several genes associated with endoplasmic reticulum stress response, protein folding, and vascular development and remodeling.[7]

DASATINIB

Dasatinib has been approved for the frontline treatment of chronic myeloid leukemia (CML). The most common adverse events associated with dasatinib therapy are cytopenias, particularly neutropenia and thrombocytopenia. Fluid retention, pleural effusion, skin rash, headache, and gastrointestinal disturbances are some other notable side effects. The most common cardiac toxicity associated with dasatinib is fluid retention, especially pleural effusion.

NILOTINIB

Nilotinib has been described to cause QT prolongation and thus must be used with particular caution when combined with other QT-prolonging drugs.

BOSUTINIB

Bosutinib is used in the treatment of CML. It is primarily metabolized in the liver by CYP3A4; thus concurrent use of bosutinib with CYP3A inhibitors and inducers should be avoided whenever possible. P-glycoprotein inhibitors should be avoided, as these can increase the drug concentrations. Most of the cardiotoxicities associated with this drug are reported in the BELA study, a phase III study comparing bosutinib to imatinib in the first-line treatment of CML. Reported cardiac reasons for discontinuation were arrhythmia, pericardial effusion, right bundle branch block, congestive heart failure (CHF), and QT prolongation. Dose reductions due to cardiac toxicities have been reported with bosutinib.[8]

PONATINIB

Ponatinib is also used in the treatment of CML, particularly as a second-line treatment for chronic, accelerated, or blast phase CML, especially in patients who are T315I-positive. Ponatinib is also indicated for Philadelphia-positive acute lymphoblastic leukemia (Ph+ ALL). Ponatinib is associated with multiple cardiotoxicities including hypertension, peripheral vascular disease, arterial ischemia, cerebral ischemia, coronary artery disease, arterial occlusive disease, and mesenteric occlusive disease.
- **VEGF inhibitors (aflibercept, ziv-aflibercept):** Aflibercept is a soluble decoy receptor that binds to all isoforms of VEGF (VEGF-A and -B) and placental growth factor (PIGF). The binding of VEGF with its receptors promotes endothelial proliferation and causes angiogenesis.
- **ALK inhibitors (alectinib, crizotinib, ceritinib, brigatinib):** Anaplastic lymphoma kinase (ALK) is a fusion oncogene that is commonly rearranged in non–small-cell lung cancer (NSCLC). ALK inhibitors, such as alectinib, brigatinib, crizotinib, and ceritinib, are indicated in metastatic NSCLC harboring ALK gene rearrangements.

CRIZOTINIB AND ALECTINIB

Crizotinib was initially developed as a c-MET inhibitor but was later found to have activity in cancers with ALK gene rearrangements and was the first drug to be US Food and Drug Administration (FDA)–approved for use in this setting.[10,11] Crizotinib also inhibits the ROS1 receptor tyrosine kinase. Crizotinib is given at a dose of 250 mg twice daily. However, based on randomized studies, alectinib, which is given 600 mg twice daily, has become a more popular first-line agent when compared with crizotinib.[11] Crizotinib and alectinib have both reported cardiac side effects of bradycardia and QT prolongation.

CERITINIB

The approved dose of ceritinib is 450 mg once daily. The ASCEND-4 trial, an open label phase III study, which led to the approval of first-line ceritinib in ALK-positive metastatic NSCLC, reported no significant cardiac side effects in treated patients except for one patient treated with ceritinib who developed grade 5 myocardial infarction.[9]

BRIGATINIB

Brigatinib is a next generation ALK inhibitor which has also been show to have better efficacy over crizotinib and is approved for in the first line setting. Brigatinib is given as 90 mg daily for 7 days, and if tolerated, the dose is increased to 180 mg daily. The most commonly reported cardiac side effect of brigatinib is hypertension.

- **PARP inhibitors (niraparib, olaparib):** Niraparib is a poly ADP-ribose polymerase (PARP) inhibitor approved for the treatment of ovarian, fallopian, or primary peritoneal cancer. Niraparib blocks both PARP1 and PARP2 enzymes. Niraparib was found to inhibit tumor growth in models with loss of BRCA activity and loss of function mutation of tumor suppressor PTEN proteins.[12] Niraparib is either given at 200 mg daily or 300 mg daily depending on weight and platelet count. Olaparib is used in the treatment of HER2-negative, germline BRCA-mutated (gBRCAm) metastatic breast cancer, advanced ovarian, pancreatic, and prostate cancers. In general, patients should be demonstrated to have homologous recombination deficiency, most commonly in the form of BRCA mutations. The notable exception is in the maintenance treatment of recurrent ovarian cancer. Olaparib is either given at 300 mg tablets twice daily or 400 mg capsules twice daily. Some of the most common side effects of niraparib and olaparib are cytopenias including thrombocytopenia, anemia, and neutropenia. Some cardiac side effects were reported with niraparib and olaparib, the most common of which are hypertension, tachycardia, and palpitations.[13]
- **CDK4/6 inhibitors (ribociclib, palbociclib, abemaciclib):** CDK4/6 inhibitors in combination with endocrine therapy are used in the first-line treatment of many patients with ER/PR-positive, HER2-negative, metastatic breast cancer. The three drugs that are currently approved in this category are ribociclib, palbociclib, and abemaciclib. In the PALOMA-2 trial, which used palbociclib and letrozole, cardiac side effects were not described in detail.[14] However, there were subsequent reports of QT prolongation with this class of drug, and in the mentioned study, patients with baseline QT prolongation were not included.

BRAF INHIBITORS (VEMURAFENIB, DABRAFENIB) VEMURAFENIB

Vemurafenib is an orally available BRAF inhibitor and is approved for the treatment of metastatic melanoma with a BRAF V600E mutation. Vemurafenib is metabolized by CYP3A4, and thus CYP3A4 inducers and inhibitors need to be avoided during treatment, as these can alter drug concentrations.

DABRAFENIB/TRAMETINIB

Dabrafenib is a BRAF inhibitor that is approved for unresectable stage III and stage IV melanoma patients. Dabrafenib was approved after a phase III trial which compared single agent dabrafenib to dacarbazine.[15] Trametinib is a MEK inhibitor given in combination with dabrafenib to improve efficacy. Dabrafenib, when given in combination with trametinib has been associated with cardiotoxicity. Decreased ejection fraction (EF) was noted in a patient who had combination chemotherapy, which improved after cessation of treatment.[16] There are also reports of cases of cardiomyopathy in patients treated with a combination therapy of dabrafenib and trametinib.[16] As there are reports of cardiotoxicity with trametinib, a baseline echocardiogram needs to be obtained, and then periodically while on treatment. If there is a decline in EF of 10% or greater, treatment should be withheld, and cardiac function should be reassessed. If cardiac function improves, the drug can be resumed at a lower dose. Treatment should be discontinued in patients who develop symptomatic heart failure. If the initial decline in the EF is greater than 20%, treatment should be discontinued permanently.

- **EGFR inhibitors (erlotinib, gefitinib, osimertinib)**
  - **Erlotinib:** Rash and diarrhea are the main side effects with this drug. Dyspnea and pneumonitis have been reported, but cardiac side effects are relatively low.[17] Cardiomyopathy causing a decline in EF, which improved with erlotinib cessation, has been reported.[17]
  - **Gefitinib:** Gefitinib-induced cardiotoxicity and cardiac hypertrophy in vivo and in vitro rat models has been described. The mechanism behind these is through cardiac apoptotic cell death and altered oxidative stress pathways.[17] Except for occasional reports of fluid retention, no significant clinical cardiac adverse effects have been reported.
  - **Osimertinib:** Osimertinib is approved as first-line treatment for patients with metastatic NSCLC with sensitizing EGFR mutations. Osimertinib is known to cause QT prolongation. ECGs and electrolytes should be monitored in patients who have a history or predisposition for QT prolongation and in those who are taking medications that are known to cause QT prolongation. Grade 1 or 2 toxicity may require temporary treatment interruption. If clinically significant severe QT prolongation is found, osimertinib should be permanently discontinued (according to the FDA recommendations). Cardiomyopathy has been reported in 1.4% of patients and thus baseline echocardiogram and periodic assessment of LVEF is recommended. In the FLAURA study, which led to the approval of osimertinib in the first-line setting for EGFR-positive metastatic NSCLC, changes in QT interval were reported in a higher percentage of patients in the osimertinib group (10%) compared with the first-generation EGFR-TKI group (5%).[18]

Common Cardiotoxicities Caused by Targeted Therapies

Hypertension

- **Sunitinib:** Sunitinib is a multitargeted TKI used in the treatment of renal cell carcinoma (RCC)[19,20] and gastrointestinal stromal tumor (GIST) in the second-line after imatinib use.[21] The dose of sunitinib varies from 37.5 mg daily to 50 mg daily depending on the indication. The reported incidence of hypertension with sunitinib in various clinical trials ranges from 15.3% to 29.6%.[20,22] Patients receiving sunitinib should be monitored for hypertension and changes in LVEF, especially those with prior cardiac disease.[23]
- **Pazopanib:** Pazopanib is another multitargeted TKI, with a similar side effect profile to sunitinib. In a meta-analysis of phase II and phase III prospective clinical trials using pazopanib, the overall incidence of hypertension was 39.5% for all grades and 6.5% for grades 3 and 4 hypertension.[24] A higher incidence of all-grade hypertension was reported in patients taking axitinib (42%)[25] and pazopanib (36%) compared to sorafenib (29%)[25] and sunitinib (22%).
- **Lenvatinib:** Lenvatinib, a multikinase inhibitor with particular activity against VEGFR kinases, is also reported to have a high incidence of hypertension. Associated risk factors

included a prior history of hypertension, obesity, and age greater than 60 years.[26] Periodic assessments of hypertension are warranted, especially in the initial months of starting treatment, and if required, antihypertensive medications can be prescribed to improve VEGF-TKI medication tolerance. Poorly controlled, prolonged hypertension can lead to cardiomyopathy, decreased LVEF, and CHF.

- **Ramucirumab:** Ramucirumab is a monoclonal antibody targeting against VEGFR2. It is associated with an increased risk of hypertension and arterial thrombotic events.
- **Ziv-aflibercept:** Ziv-aflibercept has been approved for the treatment of metastatic colon cancer in combination with FOLFIRI (5FU, leucovorin, and irinotecan) in patients who have progressed on oxaliplatin-based chemotherapy. It is administered at a dose of 4 mg/kg. Results from the pivotal trial VELOUR, a phase III study of aflibercept and FOLFIRI versus placebo and FOLFIRI for metastatic colorectal cancer as second line-therapy, led to the approval of this drug. Grade 3 hypertension was seen in 19.1% of patients in the aflibercept group compared with only 1.5% of patients in the control group; however, only one patient in the study arm developed grade 4 hypertension. Given this risk, baseline ECG and blood pressure assessment are required. There are no specific guidelines for blood pressure monitoring, and clinical judgement must be exercised.[27] Treatment consists of antihypertensives for grades 1 and 2 hypertension. If a patient develops severe hypertension, temporary discontinuation of the drug is recommended. On some occasions, permanent discontinuation may be necessary.
- **ALK inhibitors:** Patients receiving selective ALK inhibitors have been reported to develop hypertension. Hypertension developed in 21% of patients on brigatinib, 5.9% of whom had grade 3 hypertension.[28] Baseline hypertension screening and periodic blood pressure assessments are recommended, and if elevated, antihypertensive treatment is recommended. It should be noted that ALK inhibitors can cause bradycardia, thus antihypertensives which may cause bradycardia such as beta-blockers should be used carefully.
- **PARP inhibitors:** Some PARP inhibitors, such as niraparib and olaparib, cause hypertension, tachycardia, and palpitations, and thus patients receiving these drugs should be monitored reguarly.[13] The actual proportions of patients who suffer cardiovascular toxicities, however, have not been described in detail. Dose reductions and use of antihypertensive medications may help in uncontrolled hypertension associated with PARP inhibitors.

Congestive Heart Failure

Heart failure is a clinical syndrome in which heart function decreases such that demand is not adequately met. CHF is characterized by symptoms, such as shortness of breath and lower extremity edema, resulting from fluid retention due to inadequate cardiac output. The functional staging of heart failure has been described by the New York Heart Association (NYHA).

- **CHF associated with HER2–targeted therapies (trastuzumab, pertuzumab, ado-trastuzumab emtansine):** The development of CHF in patients who were enrolled in phase II and phase III trials has been retrospectively studied to note the incidence of trastuzumab-related toxicities. In patients who had received concomitant trastuzumab and anthracycline-based chemotherapy, there was an increased risk of cardiac toxicity (27%) compared to patients who had received paclitaxel and trastuzumab (13%). Cardiac toxicity with trastuzumab alone has been reported to be between 3% and 7%. Of the patients who developed cardiomyopathy, 75% were symptomatic.[29]
- Baseline cardiac function should be determined with ECG or multigated acquisition (MUGA) scan (a radionuclide scan used to assess cardiac function) prior to the initiation of HER2–directed therapy. These tests should be repeated every 3 months, or when patients become symptomatic. Periodical assessments of troponin I and pro-BNP levels may aide in the early detection of heart failure.[3] Most patients have improvement in cardiac function

after the cessation of therapy. Treatment can generally be restarted after the return of heart function to baseline. Dose adjustments for cardiotoxicity are determined based on data from clinical trials of adjuvant trastuzumab, such as the NSABP B-31 trial and the NCCTG N9831 trial. Cardiotoxicity is generally neither dose- nor duration-dependent, thus posing a particular problem for clinicians.[30] The risk of cardiotoxicity is thought to be temporary and occurs only when patients are on active treatment. There is no reported evidence of late cardiac adverse effects in patients after completion of treatment.[31]

Cardiac toxicities of T-DM1, the antibody drug conjugate ado-trastuzumab emtansine, were reported in the MARIANNE study. A decrease in EF of less than 50% with more than a 15% decrease in heart function was observed in 0.8% of patients treated with single agent T-DM1 compared to 4.5% of patients treated with trastuzumab plus taxane and 2.5% of patients treated with T-DM1 plus pertuzumab.[32]

CHF ASSOCIATED WITH VEGF INHIBITORS

Sunitinib

An increased incidence of CHF in patients receiving multitargeted TKIs has been reported across various clinical trials for different indications. The studies that led to the approval of sunitinib in RCC observed a concerning incidence of decreased LVEF. In the phase I/II trial, 8 of the 75 patients (11%) who were given continued cycles of sunitinib had a cardiovascular event, with CHF recorded in 6 patients (8%). LVEF reductions of at least 10% occurred in 10 of the 36 patients (28%) treated at the approved sunitinib dose, and 7 patients (19%) had LVEF reductions of 15% or more.[23] In another study, the overall incidence for all-grade and high-grade CHF in patients treated with sunitinib was 4.1% and 1.5%, respectively. The relative risk of all- and high-grade CHF in these patients was reported to be 1.81% and 3.30%, respectively.[33] Although the incidence of CHF was alarming in this setting, CHF and left ventricular dysfunction generally responded well to sunitinib cessation and institution of medical management. Another retrospective study of sunitinib in metastatic RCC and GIST reported that 2.7% of patients who received sunitinib developed heart failure. The mean time of onset was 22 days after the initiation of therapy, and notably, some patients with GIST who received sunitinib did not have a reversal of cardiac dysfunction even after treatment discontinuation.

■ A multicenter analysis of 175 patients who received sunitinib therapy for metastatic RCC showed that 17 patients (9.7%) developed grade 3 hypertension 33 of the 175 (18.9%) patients developed some degree of cardiac abnormality and 12 of the 175 patients developed grade 3 CHF. Based on this analysis, hypertension and coronary artery disease have been considered as independent predictors of cardiac dysfunction.[34]

Bevacizumab

Heart failure associated with bevacizumab has been sporadically reported in several trials.

Pazopanib

Pazopanib has been associated with a decrease in heart function, as noted in the PALETTE trial of pazopanib in sarcoma patients. A decline in heart function was noted in 6.7% of patients compared with 2.4% of placebo-treated patients.[35]

Lenvatinib and regorafenib

Cardiac dysfunction has been reported in patients receiving lenvatinib. In patients receiving regorafenib, biventricular CHF and myocardial ischemia has been reported.

■ In a systematic review and meta-analysis conducted to determine the rates of CHF in patients treated with multitargeted TKIs, a total of 10,647 patients from 16 phase III trials and 5 phase II trials were studied. All-grade CHF occurred in 2.39% of patients treated with VEGFR TKI compared with 0.75% in patients in the non-TKI groups. High-grade CHF occurred in 1.19% of patients receiving VEGFR TKIs compared with 0.65% in patients in the non-TKI groups. The relative risk (RR) of all-grade and high-grade CHF for TKI versus no TKI was 2.69 (*P* < .001; 95% confidence interval [CI]: 1.86–3.87) and 1.65 (*P* = .227, 95% CI: 0.73–3.70), respectively. The RR of relatively specific TKIs (axitinib) was similar to relatively non-specific TKIs (sunitinib, sorafenib, vandetanib, pazopanib).[36] Potentially fatal cardiac failure has been observed in patients treated with axitinib.

- Baseline echocardiogram or MUGA scans should be performed and periodic monitoring of cardiac function should be done thereafter. The FDA recommends permanent cessation of sunitinib in patients who develop severe heart failure. For patients who experience a decrease in EF of between 20% and 50% below baseline values, dose reduction or interruption is recommended.

CHF ASSOCIATED WITH BCR/ABL TARGETING THERAPY

In a study of 103 patients with CML treated with imatinib, there were no significant cardiac side effects. However, there have been subsequent case reports of cardiac toxicity, including a decrease in LVEF, reported with imatinib.[37] Another study of imatinib use in GIST reported a low incidence of cardiac toxicity (0.2%–0.4%).[38] Slight increases in NT-pro BNP levels were noted in some patients, however, these increases were not statistically significant.[39] A study of 90 patients on long-term imatinib for CML (median treatment time of 3.3 years) evaluated EF. In this study, the mean EF was 68 ± 7%; based on this study, imatinib-related cardiotoxicity is considered to be relatively uncommon even when administered long term.[40] Routine cardiac monitoring is not indicated in all patients who are receiving imatinib.[39] There were no differences in cardiac and vascular adverse events between the bosutinib and imatinib groups in the BELA study.[41] The overall incidence of heart failure was 2.9% and grade 3 and 4 toxicity was 0.8%. The discontinuation rates of bosutinib due to cardiac toxicities were higher than in other studies.

CHF ASSOCIATED WITH BRAF INHIBITORS

Cardiomyopathy has been reported with trametinib alone and also with the combination of trametinib and dabrafenib.[16] Baseline echocardiogram should be obtained, and then periodically while patients are on treatment. If there is a decline in EF of 10% or greater, treatment should be withheld, and the patient should be monitored for improvement. If heart function recovers, the drug can be resumed at a lower dose. For patients who develop symptomatic heart failure, treatment should be discontinued permanently. If the initial decline in EF is greater than 20%, treatment should be discontinued, promptly and permanently.

CHF ASSOCIATED WITH EGFR INHIBITORS

Cardiomyopathy has been reported to occur with an incidence of 1.4% of patients treated with osimertinib. These data are based on the FLAURA study, which led to its first-line approval in NSCLC.[18] Baseline echocardiogram and periodic assessment of LVEF is recommended. The treatment of heart failure should be provided per recommendations of the American College of Cardiology/American Heart Association (ACC/AHA).

Thromboembolic Events

- **Arterial thromboembolic events associated with VEGF–targeting agents:** Arterial thromboembolic events (ATE) have been reported in VEGF-TKI drugs, specifically with sorafenib and sunitinib. Based on meta-analyses, the reported incidence is estimated to be around 1.4%.[42] An increased incidence of ATE has also been reported with the use of pazopanib (3%) and lenvatinib (5%). Upon development of ATE, VEGF-TKI should be discontinued promptly and patients should undergo standard treatment for ATE. According to American College of Clinical Pharmacy (ACCP) guidelines, patients at high risk for ATE should receive aspirin for prophylaxis. VEGF-TKIs are not recommended for 6 to 12 months after a serious event such as this.

- An increased incidence of thromboembolic events is associated with bevacizumab, as reported with the use of bevacizumab-containing chemotherapy regimens for advanced colorectal cancer.[43] In a study which reviewed cardiovascular risk factors in 471 patients with bevacizumab in metastatic colorectal cancer, bevacizumab was found to be associated with a slightly increased risk of ATE. Age, previous history of ATE, and vascular risk factors did not seem to increase the risk of ATE in these patients. The effect of aspirinuse in the prevention of ATE in patients on bevacizumab was indeterminate in this particular study.[43] A meta-analyses of over 13,000 patients in 20 randomized trials, which evaluated the relative risk of ATEs had interesting findings. The highest incidence of ATE was seen in patients treated for metastatic colorectal cancer (3.2%, 95% CI: 1.9–5.4), and the lowest was in patients treated for breast cancer (0.7%, 95% CI: 0.1–3.6), a diagnosis that bevacizumab is no longer approved for. Incidence rates of ATE in patients with NSCLC and RCC were 2.5% (95% CI: 1.8–3.7) and 2.3% (95% CI: 1.4–3.7), respectively.[44]

AFLIBERCEPT

In the VELOUR study, an increased risk of arterial thromboembolic events (1.8% vs. 0.5%) and venous thromboembolic events (7.9% vs. 6.3%), was observed in the combination treatment arm of aflibercept and FOLFIRI, compared with placebo and FOLFIRI.[27]

ARTERIAL THROMBOEMBOLIC EVENTS ASSOCIATED WITH PONATINIB

Ponatinib has been evaluated for the treatment of CML in the EPIC study, a phase III randomized trial. The EPIC study was terminated due to the observation of increased ATEs in concurrent trials utilizing ponatinib. Preliminary data from this study suggested an increased risk of ATE with ponatinib as compared with imatinib,[45] although the direct mechanism of these vascular occlusive events is not well understood.

Venous Thromboembolic Events (VTEs)

Meta-analyses of randomized phases II and III trials of sunitinib, sorafenib, pazopanib, vandetanib, and axitinib have studied the incidence of VTE. Based on these meta-analyses, an increased risk of VTEs with these drugs was not detected.[46] Thus these agents are not considered to pose an increased risk of VTEs and can be used safely in patients with a prior history of VTE.[46,47] In general, once a patient develops VTE while taking targeted therapy, the drug can be discontinued temporarily and resumed once adequate anticoagulation is established. The National Comprehensive Cancer Network (NCCN) guidelines do not recommend routine anticoagulation with the use of these drugs. Similar to the TKIs discussed, ramucirumab has not been associated with increased risk of VTE and ATE.[48]

Arrhythmias

- **QT prolongation:** QT prolongation has been described with a variety of targeted therapies. Patients receiving such drugs should undergo baseline ECG monitoring, as well as electrolyte monitoring at regular intervals. Electrolytes, particularly potassium and magnesium levels, should be replenished accordingly. Drug–drug interactions should also be considered to minimize the chance of patients receiving multiple QT prolonging drugs. Although QT prolongation typically does not cause symptoms, it is clinically significant, as it can result in tachyarrhythmias including sustained torsades de pointes.
- **VEGF-TKI:** Sunitinib is known for its dose-dependent QT prolonging effect. When compared with sunitinib, sorafenib has a lesser effect on QT prolongation. Baseline ECG should be obtained in all patients before starting these drugs, and then periodically, although no guidelines specify time intervals. It is also recommended to avoid other concomitant drugs that may prolong the QT interval. Pazopanib and axitinib are not associated with statistically significant risks of QT prolongation. Higher doses of vandetanib are associated with a greater risk of QT prolongation.[49]
- **BCR/ABL targeting TKIs**

NILOTINIB

Nilotinib is known to be associated with QT prolongation at the recommended dose of 800 mg/day. Treatment should be withheld for QTc interval greater than 480 ms. Current recommendations are to resume treatment if QTc interval returns to less than 450 ms. Oftentimes, the dose prior can be resumed. If QT prolongation recurs again, then a dose reduction can be considered. If the QTc remains prolonged even after dose reduction, then permanent discontinuation of treatment is advised.

BOSUTINIB

Bosutinib is also associated with QT prolongation and cardiac arrhythmias. QT prolongation and arrhythmias have been reported (overall 5.7% and grades 3 and 4, 1.5%) in two major studies, which led to the approval of bosutinib.[8] Reported cardiac reasons for discontinuation of bosutinib include cardiac arrhythmias, pericardial effusion, right bundle branch block, CHF, and QT prolongation.[8]

- **ALK inhibitors:** Alectinib is commonly used as a first-line agent for ALK-positive metastatic NSCLC. In the ALEX trial, a phase III trial comparing alectinib versus crizotinib, cardiac disorders like bradycardia were reported in 1% of patients on alectinib compared with 6% of patients on crizotinib.[11] Furthermore, in the J-ALEX study, where crizotinib was compared with alectinib, crizotinib was associated with sinus bradycardia in 6% of patients. Subsequent case reports have also corroborated reports of bradycardia.[50] QT prolongation is also observed with ceritinib.[9] In patients being treated with crizotinib and ceritinib, treatment should be temporarily discontinued if patients develop severe QT prolongation, and the drug should be restarted when the QTc returns to baseline. Recurrent QT prolongation warrants treatment discontinuation.
- **CDK 4/6 inhibitors:** QT prolongation has also been reported in patients treated with CDK 4/6 inhibitors such as ribociclib and abemaciclib. A QTc interval of greater than 480 ms was noted in 3.3% of patients treated with ribociclib at a dose of 600 mg. This side effect is thought to be dose dependent, and thus patients with baseline QT prolongation were excluded from the study. Dose-reduction, interruption, and discontinuation of the drug was required in the study if patients developed QT prolongation.[51] The use of abemaciclib was approved based on the MONARCH-3 trial. This particular drug has the same cardiac side effect profile as the other drugs in this group.

- **BRAF inhibitors:** Vemurafenib is also known to be associated with QT prolongation. Similar to other drugs which cause QT prolongation, this agent should be avoided in patients with baseline prolonged QT interval.
- **EGFR inhibitors:** Osimertinib is also known to cause QT prolongation. Cardiotoxicity, such as changes in QT interval, were reported in a higher percentage of patients in the osimertinib group (29 patients [10%]) than in the first-generation EGFR-TKI group (13 patients [5%]).[18]

Pleural Effusions

- **Bosutinib:** Bosutinib, a BCR/ABL TKI for CML, is known to be associated with pleural effusions. Pleural effusions have been reported in 18.5% of patients on bosutinib, with the majority occurring within 3 months of treatment initiation.[52] Large pleural effusions may require thoracentesis, oxygen supplementation, and diuretics. If severe, dose reduction and treatment interruption should be considered. For grade 3 pleural effusions, treatment should be withheld until the effusion resolves. Another important cardiotoxicity associated with bosutinib is fluid retention, which manifests as peripheral edema.[53]

References

1. Lee KF, Simon H, Chen H, et al. Requirement for neuregulin receptor erbB2 in neural and cardiac development. *Nature*. 1995;378:394–398.
2. Barth AS, Zhang Y, Li T, et al. Functional impairment of human resident cardiac stem cells by the cardiotoxic antineoplastic agent trastuzumab. *Stem Cells Transl Med*. 2012;1:289–297.
3. Keefe DL. Trastuzumab-associated cardiotoxicity. *Cancer*. 2002;95:1592–1600.
4. Geyer CE, Forster J, Lindquist D, et al. Lapatinib plus capecitabine for HER2-positive advanced breast cancer. *N Engl J Med*. 2006;355:2733–2743.
5. Hood JD, Meininger CJ, Ziche M, et al. VEGF upregulates ecNOS message, protein, and NO production in human endothelial cells. *Am J Physiol*. 1998;274:H1054–H1058.
6. Robinson ES, Khankin EV, Choueiri TK, et al. Suppression of the nitric oxide pathway in metastatic renal cell carcinoma patients receiving vascular endothelial growth factor-signaling inhibitors. *Hypertens*. 2010;56:1131–1136.
7. Herman EH, Knapton A, Rosen E, et al. A multifaceted evaluation of imatinib-induced cardiotoxicity in the rat. *Toxicol Pathol*. 2011;39:1091–1106.
8. Cortes JE, Kim DW, Kantarjian HM, et al. Bosutinib versus imatinib in newly diagnosed chronic-phase chronic myeloid leukemia: results from the BELA trial. *J Clin Oncol*. 2012;30:3486–3492.
9. Soria JC, Tan DSW, Chiari R, et al. First-line ceritinib versus platinum-based chemotherapy in advanced ALK-rearranged non-small-cell lung cancer (ASCEND-4): a randomised, open-label, phase 3 study. *Lancet*. 2017;389:917–929.
10. Christensen JG, Zou HY, Arango ME, et al. Cytoreductive antitumor activity of PF-2341066, a novel inhibitor of anaplastic lymphoma kinase and c-Met, in experimental models of anaplastic large-cell lymphoma. *Mol Cancer Ther*. 2007;6:3314–3322.
11. Peters S, Camidge R, Shaw AT, et al. Alectinib versus crizotinib in untreated ALK-positive non-small-cell lung cancer (ALEX). *N Engl J Med*. 2017;377:829–838.
12. Sandhu SK, Schelman WR, Wilding G, et al. The poly(ADP-ribose) polymerase inhibitor niraparib (MK4827) in BRCA mutation carriers and patients with sporadic cancer: a phase 1 dose-escalation trial. *Lancet Oncol*. 2013;14:882–892. http://www.ncbi.nlm.nih.gov/pubmed/23810788.
13. Moore KN, Mirza MR, Matulonis UA. The poly (ADP ribose) polymerase inhibitor niraparib: management of toxicities. *Gynecol Oncol*. 2018;149:214–220.
14. Finn RS, Martin M, Rugo HS, et al. Palbociclib and letrozole in advanced breast cancer. *N Engl J Med*. 2016;375:1925–1936.
15. Long GV, Hauschild A, Santinami M, et al. Adjuvant dabrafenib plus trametinib in stage III *BRAF*-mutated melanoma. *N Engl J Med*. 2017;377:1813–1823.
16. Banks M, Crowell K, Proctor A, et al. Cardiovascular effects of the MEK inhibitor, trametinib: a case report, literature review, and consideration of mechanism. *Cardiovasc Toxicol*. 2017;17:487–493.

17. Shepherd FA, Rodrigues Pereira J, Ciuleanu T, et al. Erlotinib in previously treated non–small-cell lung cancer. *N Engl J Med.* 2005;353:123–132.
18. Soria JC, Ohe Y, Vansteenkiste J, et al. Osimertinib in untreated *EGFR*-mutated advanced non–small-cell lung cancer. *N Engl J Med.* 2018;378:113–125.
19. Motzer RJ, Rini BI, Bukowski RM, et al. Sunitinib in patients with metastatic renal cell carcinoma. *JAMA.* 2006;295:2516.
20. Motzer RJ, Hutson TE, Tomczak P, et al. Sunitinib versus interferon alfa in metastatic renal-cell carcinoma. *N Engl J Med.* 2007;356:115–124.
21. Demetri GD, van Oosterom AT, Garrett CR, et al. Efficacy and safety of sunitinib in patients with advanced gastrointestinal stromal tumour after failure of imatinib: a randomised controlled trial. *Lancet.* 2006;368:1329–1338.
22. Zhu X, Stergiopoulos K, Wu S. Risk of hypertension and renal dysfunction with an angiogenesis inhibitor sunitinib: systematic review and meta-analysis. *Acta Oncol.* 2009;48:9–17.
23. Chu TF, Rupnick MA, Kerkela R, et al. Cardiotoxicity associated with tyrosine kinase inhibitor sunitinib. *Lancet.* 2007;370:2011–2019.
24. Qi WX, Lin F, Sun Y, et al. Incidence and risk of hypertension with pazopanib in patients with cancer: a meta-analysis. *Cancer Chemother Pharmacol.* 2013;71:431–439.
25. Rini BI, Escudier B, Tomczak P, et al. Comparative effectiveness of axitinib versus sorafenib in advanced renal cell carcinoma (AXIS): a randomised phase 3 trial. *Lancet.* 2011;378:1931–1939.
26. Hamnvik OPR, Choueiri TK, Turchin A, et al. Clinical risk factors for the development of hypertension in patients treated with inhibitors of the VEGF signaling pathway. *Cancer.* 2015;121:311–319.
27. Van Cutsem E, Tabernero J, Lakomy R, et al. Addition of aflibercept to fluorouracil, leucovorin, and irinotecan improves survival in a phase III randomized trial in patients with metastatic colorectal cancer previously treated with an oxaliplatin-based regimen. *J Clin Oncol.* 2012;30:3499–3506.
28. Kim DW, Tiseo M, Ahn MJ, et al. Brigatinib in patients with crizotinib-refractory anaplastic lymphoma kinase-positive non-small-cell lung cancer: a randomized, multicenter phase II trial. *J Clin Oncol.* 2017;35:2490–2498.
29. Seidman A, Hudis C, Pierri MK, et al. Cardiac dysfunction in the trastuzumab clinical trials experience. *J Clin Oncol.* 2002;20:1215–1221.
30. Tripathy D, Slamon DJ, Cobleigh M, et al. Safety of treatment of metastatic breast cancer with trastuzumab beyond disease progression. *J Clin Oncol.* 2004;22:1063–1070.
31. Goldhar HA, Yan AT, Ko DT, et al. The temporal risk of heart failure associated with adjuvant trastuzumab in breast cancer patients: a population study. *J Natl Cancer Inst.* 2016;108:djv301.
32. Perez EA, Barrios C, Eiermann W, et al. Trastuzumab emtansine with or without pertuzumab versus trastuzumab plus taxane for human epidermal growth factor receptor 2-positive, advanced breast cancer: primary results from the phase III MARIANNE study. *J Clin Oncol.* 2017;35:141–148.
33. Richards CJ, Je Y, Schutz FAB, et al. Incidence and risk of congestive heart failure in patients with renal and nonrenal cell carcinoma treated with sunitinib. *J Clin Oncol.* 2011;29:3450–3456.
34. Di Lorenzo G, Autorino R, Bruni G, et al. Cardiovascular toxicity following sunitinib therapy in metastatic renal cell carcinoma: a multicenter analysis. *Ann Oncol.* 2009;20:1535–1542.
35. van der Graaf WTA, Blay JY, Chawla SP, et al. Pazopanib for metastatic soft-tissue sarcoma (PALETTE): a randomised, double-blind, placebo-controlled phase 3 trial. *Lancet.* 2012;379:1879–1886.
36. Ghatalia P, Morgan CJ, Je Y, et al. Congestive heart failure with vascular endothelial growth factor receptor tyrosine kinase inhibitors. *Crit Rev Oncol Hematol.* 2015;94:228–237.
37. Ribeiro AL, Marcolino MS, Bittencourt HNS, et al. An evaluation of the cardiotoxicity of imatinib mesylate. *Leuk Res.* 2008;32:1809–1814.
38. Ben Ami E, Demetri GD. A safety evaluation of imatinib mesylate in the treatment of gastrointestinal stromal tumor. *Expert Opin Drug Saf.* 2016;15:571–578.
39. Perik PJ, Rikhof B, de Jong FA, et al. Results of plasma N-terminal pro B-type natriuretic peptide and cardiac troponin monitoring in GIST patients do not support the existence of imatinib-induced cardiotoxicity. *Ann Oncol.* 2008;19:359–361.
40. Marcolino MS, Boersma E, Clementino NCD, et al. The duration of the use of imatinib mesylate is only weakly related to elevated BNP levels in chronic myeloid leukaemia patients. *Hematol Oncol.* 2011;29:124–130.
41. Gambacorti-Passerini C, Cortes JE, Lipton JH, et al. Safety of bosutinib versus imatinib in the phase 3 BELA trial in newly diagnosed chronic phase chronic myeloid leukemia. *Am J Hematol.*

2014 Oct;89(10):947-953. doi: 10.1002/ajh.23788. Epub 2014 Jul 21. PMID: 24944159; PMCID: PMC4305212.

42. Choueiri TK, Schutz FAB, Je Y, et al. Risk of arterial thromboembolic events with sunitinib and sorafenib: a systematic review and meta-analysis of clinical trials. *J Clin Oncol.* 2010;28:2280–2285.

43. Tebbutt NC, Murphy F, Zannino D, et al. Risk of arterial thromboembolic events in patients with advanced colorectal cancer receiving bevacizumab. *Ann Oncol Off J Eur Soc Med Oncol.* 2011;22:1834–1838.

44. Schutz FAB, Je Y, Azzi GR, et al. Bevacizumab increases the risk of arterial ischemia: a large study in cancer patients with a focus on different subgroup outcomes. *Ann Oncol Off J Eur Soc Med Oncol.* 2011;22:1404–1412.

45. Lipton JH, Chuah C, Guerci-Bresler A, et al. EPIC: a phase 3 trial of ponatinib compared with imatinib in patients with newly diagnosed chronic myeloid leukemia in chronic phase (CP-CML). *Blood.* 2014:124.

46. Sonpavde G, Je Y, Schutz F, et al. Venous thromboembolic events with vascular endothelial growth factor receptor tyrosine kinase inhibitors: a systematic review and meta-analysis of randomized clinical trials. *Crit Rev Oncol Hematol.* 2013;87:80–89.

47. Qi WX, Min DL, Shen Z, et al. Risk of venous thromboembolic events associated with VEGFR-TKIs: a systematic review and meta-analysis. *Int J Cancer.* 2013;132:2967–2974.

48. Arnold D, Fuchs CS, Tabernero J, et al. Meta-analysis of individual patient safety data from six randomized, placebo-controlled trials with the antiangiogenic VEGFR2-binding monoclonal antibody ramucirumab. *Ann Oncol Off J Eur Soc Med Oncol.* 2017;28:2932–2942.

49. Ghatalia P, Je Y, Kaymakcalan MD, et al. QTc interval prolongation with vascular endothelial growth factor receptor tyrosine kinase inhibitors. *Br J Cancer.* 2015;112:296–305.

50. Ou SHI, Azada M, Dy J, et al. Asymptomatic profound sinus bradycardia (heart rate ≤45) in non-small cell lung cancer patients treated with crizotinib. *J Thorac Oncol.* 2011;6:2135–2137.

51. Hortobagyi GN, Stemmer SM, Burris HA, et al. Ribociclib as first-line therapy for hr-positive, advanced breast cancer. *N Engl J Med.* 2016;375:1738–1748.

52. Latagliata R, Stagno F, Annunziata M, et al. Frontline dasatinib treatment in a "real-life" cohort of patients older than 65 years with chronic myeloid leukemia. *Neoplasia.* 2016;18:536–540.

53. Khoury HJ, Guilhot F, Hughes TP, et al. Dasatinib treatment for Philadelphia chromosome-positive leukemias. *Cancer.* 2009;115:1381–1394.

CHAPTER 17

Mechanisms of Immune-Related Adverse Events

Pradnya D. Patil, MD ■ Vamsidhar Velcheti, MD

Introduction

■ The origins of immunotherapy can be traced back to the early 1900s when Paul Ehrlich postulated that the host immune system plays a role in the early recognition and elimination of malignant cells.[1] Over the next century, many other researchers built upon this notion. Theories of immunosurveillance[2,3] and cancer immunoediting were conceptualized, to help explain the complex interplay between the immune system and carcinogenesis.[4,5] The theory of immunosurveillance proposed by Macfarlane Burnet and Lewis Thomas states that cellular immunity performs constant surveillance in the human body, and is able to identify and eliminate malignant cells in the early stages of carcinogenesis. This was followed by several experiments in murine models where the incidence of malignancies in athymic mice was studied by researchers. Unfortunately, these showed discordant results and failed to definitively show a relationship between immunosuppression and carcinogenesis.[6–8] Interest in the role of immunity in carcinogenesis waned until the 1990s when new discoveries revived interest in this field.

■ It was during this time that better understanding of the complex interactions between the immune system and malignant cells led to the evolution of the theory of immunoediting. Immunoediting is best described by the three "E's" which represent different stages in the process. The first "E" stands for "Elimination," in which immune cells recognize and eliminate malignant cells. The second "E" represents "Equilibrium," in which the tumor cell variants that escape elimination reach an equilibrium with the immune system. Although the immune system continues to evolve and destroy some of these variants, new variants of tumor cells are constantly being produced resulting in incomplete elimination and an equilibrium between the immune system and the tumor cells. A variety of cytokines and chemokines such as interferon γ, CXCL10, CXCL9, and CXCL11 produced by the tumor cells and the infiltrating immune cells modulate the interactions between the two in the tumor microenvironment. The third "E" stands for "Escape," in which the tumor variants that have evolved to evade recognition by the immune system start to multiply rapidly.[5] This escape is mediated by multiple modalities, such as loss of major histocompatibility complex (MHC) class 1 expression; antigenic mimicry; alteration of the chemokines leading to an increase in immunosuppressant cells, such as regulatory T cells (Tregs) and myeloid-derived suppressor cells (MDSCs); and upregulation of the immune checkpoints leading to T cell exhaustion.

■ Early experiments that attempted to harness host immunity to combat cancer were performed as far back as 1777 when the surgeon to the Duke of Kent tried to create a cancer vaccine by injecting himself with malignant cells. These remained unsuccessful until 1891 when William Coley reported a 10% cure rate in soft-tissue sarcomas by using inactivated streptococci and *Serratia marcescens*.[9] Over the next century recognition of the key role of cytokines led to the successful application of high-dose interleukin (IL)-2 in the treatment of melanoma and renal cell carcinoma. In the last decade, the field of immunotherapy has grown in leaps and bounds with the discovery of immune checkpoint inhibitors. In contrast to high-dose IL-2 which is associated with a number of serious adverse effects, these agents are much better tolerated. They have also shown remarkable efficacy in a wide range of malignancies and are currently approved for use in patients with advanced melanoma, non–small-cell lung cancer, head and neck squamous cell cancer, classic Hodgkin's lymphoma, urothelial carcinoma, renal cell carcinoma, and advanced microsatellite instability (MSI) high/mismatch repair deficient tumors, among others. As immunotherapeutic agents interfere with the physiological pathways that regulate immune homeostasis, a spectrum of untoward side effects that resemble autoimmune diseases have been noted with their use. These adverse events are called immune-related adverse events or irAEs. In this chapter, we will explore the potential pathophysiological mechanisms leading to immune-related adverse events. We will begin by describing the physiological pathways responsible for immune tolerance and then go on to examine how alterations in these pathways can potentially lead to autoimmunity.

Physiological Pathways Involved in the Regulation of Immune Homeostasis

- Both the innate and adaptive immune systems play an important role in generating immune responses in a normal host. Whereas the innate immunity is nonspecific and does not require antigen presentation by the MHC, adaptive immunity is more versatile and leads to the activation and expansion of antigen specific immune cells. Under physiological conditions, adaptive immunity is tightly regulated by costimulatory and inhibitory signals. T cell activation requires two signals—the first one is mediated by engagement of the T cell receptor with an antigenic peptide presented by MHC, and the second is mediated by binding of costimulatory molecules on T cells to ligands on antigen presenting cells. In naïve T cells, the interaction of the costimulatory CD28 with B7-1 and B7-2 (also known as CD80 and CD86, respectively) plays an important role in downstream signaling, which eventually leads to the secretion of proinflammatory cytokines such as IL-12 and interferon-γ, resulting in clonal expansion. The inhibitory signals allow for contraction of the T cell clone upon resolution of the antigenic stimulus.

- The diversity of the T cell receptors (TCR) and B cell receptors (BCR) is a result of the recombination of three separate gene segments—the variable (V), diversity (D), and joining (J) genes—during the differentiation of B cells and T cells in the bone marrow (B cells) and thymus (T cells), respectively. Studies have estimated that between 20% and 50% of TCRs and BCRs generated by this process can have affinity to a self-antigen[10]; however, only a fraction of the general population develops clinical manifestations of autoimmunity. The inhibitory signals or immune checkpoints play an important role in immune tolerance of self-antigens by downregulation of the self-reactive cells. Some of the prominent immune checkpoints include cytotoxic T-lymphocyte–associated protein 4 (CTLA-4), programmed cell death-1 (PD-1), T-cell immunoglobulin and mucin-domain containing-3 (TIM3), and lymphocyte-activation gene 3 (LAG3). Activation of T cells in the lymphoid organs leads to expression of CTLA-4, which is homologous to CD28 but binds to B7-1 and B7-2 with a much higher affinity than CD28, resulting in negative regulation of the T cell response. PD-1 plays an important role in regulation of T cell responses in peripheral tissues. PD-1 binds to its ligands PD-L1 and PD-L2 and leads to apoptosis of antigen-specific T cells and a reduction in the apoptosis of Tregs, therefore dampening the immune response.

Pathophysiology of Immune-Related Adverse Events (irAEs)

- Tumor cells can upregulate immune checkpoint pathways to evade the host immune system. Immune checkpoint inhibitors mediate their antitumor effects by releasing this inhibition and reinvigorating the immune responses to malignant cells. Predictably, this also interferes with the process of immune homeostasis as described previously and can result in immune-mediated adverse effects. The precise pathophysiology of irAEs is unknown; however, emerging evidence suggests that many different aspects of the immune system may play a role. In the following section, we describe the proposed mechanisms for irAEs and the evidence to support each of them.

Shared Antigens, Cross Presentation of Neoantigens and T Cell Epitope Spreading

- **Shared antigens:** Shared antigens amongst cells of various organs and the regulatory proteins that monoclonal antibodies are directed against may be responsible for some of the toxicities seen with immune checkpoint inhibitors. For example, the normal pituitary gland expresses CTLA-4, which may explain the higher incidence of immune-mediated hypophysitis in patients treated with CTLA-4 monoclonal antibodies.[11,12]
- **Epitope spreading:** Tumor-associated antigens that are homologous to native epitopes found on normal cells likely play a role in promoting immune tolerance to malignant cells. Epitope spreading is the process by which the immune response diversifies from targeting a specific epitope to subdominant epitopes in the target protein. Heightened immune responses with immunotherapy can target these shared or homologous antigens on tumor cells and normal tissues, leading to immune-related toxicities. In a report of two cases of fulminant myocarditis following treatment with immune checkpoint blockade, the authors found high expression of muscle specific antigens (desmin and troponin) on tumor cells, further supporting this notion.[13] Likewise, it has been postulated that shared antigens among melanoma cells and melanocytes may explain the higher incidence of vitiligo noted in patients with melanoma treated with immunotherapy.[14]
- **Cross presentation of neoantigens:** One of the mechanisms of action of cancer immunotherapy is by antigen spreading where T cell–mediated destruction of tumor cells leads to the release of additional tumor-associated antigens which can then generate secondary immune responses. Therefore, immunotherapy remodels the immune repertoire of circulating T cells by generation and expansion of new clones. Some of these diversified T cell clonotypes may cross react with antigens on normal tissues and result in autoimmunity.[15] In a retrospective analysis of peripheral blood mononuclear cells PBMCs from patients with metastatic prostate cancer treated with ipilimumab, diversification of the T cell receptor (TCR) repertoire with broad expansion of low frequency clonotypes was associated with the development of irAEs.[16] Specifically, patients who developed irAEs had a significantly greater fraction of new clones that were not present at baseline in comparison with those who did not develop irAEs. In this scenario, it is plausible that the broadening of the clonotypes of T cells rather than priming of T cells with autoantigens is responsible for tissue inflammation and irAEs. Similar findings from a phase II trial of ipilimumab and androgen deprivation therapy in patients with metastatic prostate cancer revealed a correlation between clonal expansion of CD8 T cells and subsequent development of irAEs.[17]

Dysregulation of Other Immune Cells

■ The balance between maintaining immune homeostasis and effective immune responses is tightly regulated by various immune cells and regulatory cytokines. Disruption of this equilibrium by immune checkpoint inhibitors can result in unrestrained immune responses, leading to irAEs. Some of the key modulators of immune responses that appear to play a role in the pathogenesis of irAEs are described below.

1. **Regulatory T cells:** FOXP3 Tregs play a vital role in suppressing autoreactive T cells as well as the regulation of adaptive T cell responses. They are also vital in maintaining mucosal tolerance to commensal bacteria in the gastrointestinal tract. Previous studies have shown that commensal bacteria can induce the formation of adaptive Tregs and IL-10 within the gut, allowing them to persist in the gut without inducing inflammation. In fact, many preclinical models of inflammatory bowel disease highlight the association between depletion of Tregs in the gut and inflammatory bowel disease.[18] Researchers have demonstrated that CTLA-4 is constitutively expressed on the surface of Tregs and of vital importance in the suppressive function. An increase in the ratio of effector T cells to Tregs has been observed after treatment with immunotherapy. Dysregulation of this homeostasis maintained by Tregs is postulated to play a role in some irAEs, particularly colitis. In fact, studies looking at the histopathological findings in patients with inflammatory bowel disease and colitis from immune checkpoint inhibitors have shown a similar number of mucosal Tregs in both populations.[19] However, other studies have reported no difference in the number of mucosal Tregs between patients with and without colitis after treatment with a anti-CTLA-4 antibody.[20]

2. **Eosinophils:** Some patients with dermatological irAEs have been noted to have eosinophilic infiltrates similar to the histopathological findings in a variety of autoimmune skin conditions.[21] In addition, retrospective studies have also shown a relationship between elevated eosinophil counts early in the course of treatment and subsequent development of irAEs.[22,23]

Autoantibodies

■ Although a majority of irAEs are a consequence of T cell–mediated toxicity, some irAEs have been associated with altered humoral responses. A challenge with proving causality of these autoantibodies is that many patients do not have pretherapy antibody titers. Therefore it is difficult to distinguish patients with preexisting antibodies from those who develop new autoantibodies after immunotherapy. Studies have reported thyroid dysfunction associated with antithyroglobulin antibodies after treatment with immune checkpoint inhibitors.[24] Iwama et al. demonstrated that in a murine model after administration of a CTLA-4 monoclonal antibody, pituitary antibodies were detected in those with hypophysitis. These antibodies were directed against the normally expressed CTLA-4 in pituitary cells and led to excessive complement activation and infiltration of the pituitary with lymphocytes.[11] In checkpoint blockade–associated bullous pemphigoid dermatosis, the pathognomonic antibodies to BP180 and BP230 can be detected in the serum.[25] In some patients with diabetes mellitus induced by checkpoint inhibitors, autoantibodies such as anti-glutamic acid decarboxylase have been detected and are thought to be central to the pathogenesis.[26] In certain rheumatological disorders, the presence of preexisting antibodies or development of new antibodies, such as anti-cyclic citrullinated peptide, have been associated with the development of rheumatoid arthritis or other autoimmune phenomenon with therapy.[27]

Cytokines

- Activation of effector T cell function by immune checkpoint inhibitors leads to a surge in proinflammatory cytokines and recruitment of inflammatory cells leading to organ damage. Cytokine release syndrome (CRS) is a potentially life-threatening adverse effect that has been observed with certain antibodies used for the treatment of leukemia and chimeric antigen receptor CAR T-cell therapy. CRS is associated with high circulating levels of many cytokines including IL-6 and interferon-γ.[28] IL-6 appears to be central to the pathogenesis of CRS; therefore blocking this cytokine with tocilizumab (a humanized IL-6R monoclonal antibody) has proven to be an effective management strategy for this syndrome.
- Another downstream effect of immune dysregulation by checkpoint inhibitors is an imbalance between regulatory cytokines. Higher levels of the proinflammatory cytokine IL-17 has been associated with subsequent development of colitis in patients with melanoma treated with ipilimumab.[29] On the other hand, a decrease in the levels of antiinflammatory cytokines such as IL-10 has been observed in patients with irAEs.[30]

Genetic Polymorphisms

- The association between genetic polymorphisms in the PD-1 and CTLA-4 genes and autoimmune conditions is well established.[31] It is plausible that some patients who go on to develop irAEs with immunotherapy have germline genetic polymorphisms in key regulatory genes in immune pathways predisposing them to irAEs. Similarly, high-risk HLA genotypes have been associated with disorders such as type 1 diabetes. There are several reports in the literature of patients with these high-risk genotypes who developed type 1 diabetes with immunotherapy.[26] One group reported that certain germline polymorphisms in the T cell receptor beta variable gene were associated with a higher risk of irAEs. This is likely due to the altered ability of these T cell receptors to interact with HLA, leading to increased autoantigen reactivity.[32] Another group reported that certain single nucleotide polymorphisms in genes that contribute to PD-1-associated T cell responses were associated with adverse effects with nivolumab.[33]

Environmental Modulation of Immune Responses

- There is mounting evidence to suggest that environmental modulation of host immunity, particularly by the gut microbiome, is associated with both the efficacy and toxicity of immune checkpoint inhibitors. Murine models highlight the pivotal role of the gut microbiome in the maturation of the host immune system and regulation of mucosal immunity.[34] It is therefore not surprising that the composition of the host gut microbiome can predispose them to irAEs. Studies have shown that a higher number of commensal bacteria *(Bacteroides)* in the fecal microbiome are associated with a lower incidence of colitis.[35,36] On the other hand, bacteria of the phylum *Firmicutes* have been associated with an increased risk of colitis.[36]

Specific Immunotherapeutic Agents and their Associated Toxicities

- **Cytokines**
  - Cytokines are among the first immunotherapeutic agents to be used in clinical practice. High dose IL-2 was approved for use in patients with melanoma and renal cell carcinoma due to its ability to induce durable responses and cure in a small fraction of patients. Predictably, infusion of high-dose cytokines can lead to a cytokine storm

manifesting as hypotension, cardiac arrhythmias, pulmonary edema, and fever, which can be life threatening. These are direct consequences of the unbridled inflammation induced by the cytokine storm. Some of the novel cytokine superagonists are less likely to result in a cytokine storm.

- **Immune checkpoint inhibitors**
  - The immune checkpoint inhibitors that are currently approved for clinical use target PD-1, PD-L1, or CTLA-4. The profile and incidence of immune-related toxicities observed with PD-1/PD-L1 inhibitors is different from those seen with CTLA-4 inhibitors. Colitis and hypophysitis are reported more commonly with CTLA-4 inhibitors, whereas pneumonitis has been reported more with PD-1 and PD-L1 inhibitors. This is likely a reflection of the role of these proteins in different stages of immune regulation—CTLA-4 regulates the priming phase of T cell activation, whereas PD-1 regulates the effector phase in peripheral tissues. Overall, CTLA-4 inhibitors have been associated with higher incidences of irAEs than have PD-1/PD-L1 inhibitors. Combined PD-1/CTLA-4 inhibition is associated with a higher incidence of irAEs than is either agent alone. The site of primary disease also appears to influence the organ involvement in irAEs. For example, pneumonitis is seen more commonly in patients with non–small-cell lung cancer treated with immunotherapy. This is probably a consequence of organ specific immune response leading to a higher grade of inflammation restricted to that site.
- **Chimeric antigen receptor T (CAR T) cells**
  - CAR T-cell therapy has been approved for patients with refractory acute lymphoblastic leukemia (ALL) and diffuse large B cell lymphoma (DLBCL). A very high incidence of cytokine release syndrome (CRS) is seen with CAR T-cell therapy due to supranormal levels of cytokines such as IL-6. Therapy targeting IL-6 (tocilizumab) has been successful in mitigating symptoms of CRS.
- **Bispecific T cell engagers (BiTEs)**
  - BiTEs are antibodies which link the CD3 molecule expressed on T cells with a specific antigen. In the case of blinatumomab, the target molecule is CD19. Blinatumomab was recently approved for use in Philadelphia chromosome-negative B-ALL and has been associated with CRS and neurological toxicities secondary to immune dysregulation.
- **Oncolytic viruses**
  - irAEs such as glomerulonephritis, pneumonitis, colitis, and vasculitis have been noted with the use of the oncolytic virus talimogene laherparepvec or T-VEC. It is likely that the immunostimulatory properties of this virus mediate these adverse effects.

Conclusion

Immune-mediated toxicities are the expected adverse consequences of the loss of immune tolerance with immunotherapy. As we gain more experience with the clinical use of immunotherapeutic agents, we have also gained more insight into the varied mechanisms of immune-related toxicities. Due to the complex nature of immune modulation by interactions between different entities, both within and outside of the human body, a comprehensive understanding of these immune-mediated toxicities will require in-depth study of each of those entities. A thorough understanding of the mechanisms involved will aide physicians in patient selection for immunotherapy and inform the optimal therapy for immune-mediated toxicities.

References

1. Ehrlich P. Ueber den jetzigen Stand der Karzinomforschung. *Ned Tijdschr Geneeskd*. 1909;5:273–290.
2. Burnet FM. Immunological surveillance in neoplasia. *Transplant Rev*. 1971;7:3–25.
3. Burnet FM. The concept of immunological surveillance. *Prog Exp Tumor Res*. 1970;13:1–27.

4. Dunn GP, Old LJ, Schreiber RD. The three Es of cancer immunoediting. *Annu Rev Immunol.* 2004;22:329–360.
5. Dunn GP, Bruce AT, Ikeda H, et al. Cancer immunoediting: from immunosurveillance to tumor escape. *Nat Immunol.* 2002;3:991–998.
6. Stutman O. Immunodepression and malignancy. *Adv Cancer Res.* 1975;22:261–422.
7. Nishizuka Y, Nakakuki K, Usui M. Enhancing effect of thymectomy on hepatotumorigenesis in Swiss mice following neonatal injection of 20-methylcholanthrene. *Nature.* 1965;205:1236–1238.
8. Burstein NA, Law LW. Neonatal thymectomy and non-viral mammary tumours in mice. *Nature.* 1971;231:450–452.
9. Ichim CV. Revisiting immunosurveillance and immunostimulation: implications for cancer immunotherapy. *J Transl Med.* 2005;3(1):8.
10. Goodnow CC, Sprent J, Fazekas de St Groth B, et al. Cellular and genetic mechanisms of self tolerance and autoimmunity. *Nature.* 2005;435(7042):590–597.
11. Iwama S, De Remigis A, Callahan MK, et al. Pituitary expression of CTLA-4 mediates hypophysitis secondary to administration of CTLA-4 blocking antibody. *Sci Transl Med.* 2014;6:230ra45.
12. Caturegli P, Di Dalmazi G, Lombardi M, et al. Hypophysitis secondary to cytotoxic T-lymphocyte-associated protein 4 blockade: insights into pathogenesis from an autopsy series. *Am J Pathol.* 2016;186:3225–3235.
13. Johnson DB, Balko JM, Compton ML, et al. Fulminant myocarditis with combination immune checkpoint blockade. *N Engl J Med.* 2016;375(18):1749–1755.
14. Larsabal M, Marti A, Jacquemin C, et al. Vitiligo-like lesions occurring in patients receiving anti-programmed cell death-1 therapies are clinically and biologically distinct from vitiligo. *J Am Acad Dermatol.* 2017;76:863–870.
15. Gulley JL, Madan RA, Pachynski R, et al. Role of antigen spread and distinctive characteristics of immunotherapy in cancer treatment. *J Natl Cancer Inst.* 2017;109(4).
16. Oh DY, Cham J, Zhang L, et al. Immune toxicities elicited by CTLA-4 blockade in cancer patients are associated with early diversification of the T-cell repertoire. *Cancer Res.* 2017;77(6):1322–1330.
17. Subudhi SK, Aparicio A, Gao J, et al. Clonal expansion of CD8 T cells in the systemic circulation precedes development of ipilimumab-induced toxicities. *Proc Natl Acad Sci U S A.* 2016;113(42):11919–11924.
18. Yamada A, Arakaki R, Saito M, et al. Role of regulatory T cell in the pathogenesis of inflammatory bowel disease. *World J Gastroenterol.* 2016;22(7):2195–2205.
19. Coutzac C, Adam J, Soularue E, et al. Colon immune-related adverse events: anti-CTLA-4 and anti-PD-1 blockade induce distinct immunopathological entities. *J Crohns Colitis.* 2017;11(10):1238–1246.
20. Lord JD, Hackman RC, Moklebust A, et al. Refractory colitis following anti-CTLA4 antibody therapy: analysis of mucosal FOXP3+ T cells. *Dig Dis Sci.* 2010;55:1396–1405.
21. Jaber SH, Cowen EW, Haworth LR, et al. Skin reactions in a subset of patients with stage IV melanoma treated with anti-cytotoxic T-lymphocyte antigen 4 monoclonal antibody as a single agent. *Arch Dermatol.* 2006;142(2):166–172.
22. Schindler K, Harmankaya K, Kuk D, et al. Correlation of absolute and relative eosinophil counts with immune-related adverse effects in melanoma patients treated with ipilimumab. *J Clin Oncol.* 2014;32 (15 suppl):9096.
23. Diehl A, Yarchoan M, Yang T, et al. Relationship of lymphocyte and eosinophil counts and immune-related adverse events in recipients of programmed death-1 (PD-1) inhibitor therapy: a single-center retrospective analysis. *J Clin Oncol.* 2017;35(15 suppl):e14586.
24. Osorio JC, Ni A, Chaft JE, et al. Antibody-mediated thyroid dysfunction during T-cell checkpoint blockade in patients with non-small-cell lung cancer. *Ann Oncol.* 2017;28:583–589.
25. Naidoo J, Schindler K, Querfeld C, et al. Autoimmune bullous skin disorders with immune checkpoint inhibitors targeting PD-1 and PD-L1. *Cancer Immunol Res.* 2016;4:383–389.
26. Chae YK, Chiec L, Mohindra N, et al. A case of pembrolizumab-induced type-1 diabetes mellitus and discussion of immune checkpoint inhibitor-induced type 1 diabetes. *Cancer Immunol Immunother.* 2017;66(1):25–32.
27. Belkhir R, Burel SL, Dunogeant L, et al. Rheumatoid arthritis and polymyalgia rheumatica occurring after immune checkpoint inhibitor treatment. *Ann Rheum Dis.* 2017;76(10):1747–1750.

28. Lee DW, Gardner R, Porter DL, et al. Current concepts in the diagnosis and management of cytokine release syndrome. *Blood*. 2014;124(2):188–195.
29. Tarhini AA, Zahoor H, Lin Y, et al. Baseline circulating IL-17 predicts toxicity while TGF-β1 and IL-10 are prognostic of relapse in ipilimumab neoadjuvant therapy of melanoma. *J ImmunoTherapy of Cancer*. 2015;3(1):39.
30. Sun J, Schiffman J, Raghunath A, et al. Concurrent decrease in IL-10 with development of immune-related adverse events in a patient treated with anti-CTLA-4 therapy. *Cancer Immun*. 2008;8:9.
31. Patil PD, Burotto M, Velcheti V. Biomarkers for immune-related toxicities of checkpoint inhibitors: current progress and the road ahead. *Expert Rev Mol Diagn*. 2018;18(3):297–305.
32. Looney T, Linch E, Lowman G, et al. Evaluating the link between T cell receptor beta variable gene polymorphism and immune mediated adverse events during checkpoint blockade immunotherapy. *J Clin Oncol*. 2018;36(suppl):e15002.
33. Bins S, Basak E, El Bouazzaoui S, et al. Association between single nucleotide polymorphisms and side effects in nivolumab treated NSCLC patients. *Annals of Oncology*. 2016;27(suppl 8):VIII1.
34. Mazmanian SK, Liu CH, Tzianabos AO, et al. An immunomodulatory molecule of symbiotic bacteria directs maturation of the host immune system. *Cell*. 2005;122(1):107–118.
35. Chaput N, Lepage P, Coutzac C, et al. Baseline gut microbiota predicts clinical response and colitis in metastatic melanoma patients treated with ipilimumab. *Ann Oncol*. 2017;28(6):1368–1379.
36. Dubin K, Callahan MK, Ren B, et al. Intestinal microbiome analyses identify melanoma patients at risk for checkpoint-blockade induced colitis. *Nat Commun*. 2016;7:10391.

CHAPTER 18

Endocrine Toxicities of Immunotherapy

Manu Pandey, MBBS ■ Itivrita Goyal, MBBS ■ Marc S. Ernstoff, MD

Introduction

In the past two decades, the field of cancer immunotherapy evolved from a niche specialty to the frontlines of the fight against cancer. Unlike chemotherapy, immunotherapy unleashes the body's inherent immune system by boosting it and "releasing its breaks." Although we have come far, immunotherapy remains a crude tool, and as collateral damage, we have a new set of toxicities which are labeled as immune-related adverse events (irAEs). Several endocrine irAEs can present with symptoms that overlap with those seen in patients with advanced cancer, some of which can be life-threatening. Diagnosing and managing these conditions requires a collaborative effort between the oncologist, endocrinologist, and primary care physician.

In this chapter, we will discuss the major immunotherapeutic agents which have been approved by the US Food and Drug Administration (FDA). We describe their indications for use, mechanisms of action, endocrine toxicities associated with their use, and management of these toxicities.

Agents and Mechanism of Action

INTERLEUKIN 2 (IL-2)

Interleukin-2 (IL-2) has been used extensively in metastatic melanoma and renal cell carcinoma as monotherapy and in combination with other agents. High-dose IL-2 has a response rate of 25% in patients with renal cell carcinoma and 18% in patients with metastatic melanoma when used as monotherapy.[1,2] IL-2 is associated with significant toxicities and, with the advent of better therapies, its use has largely fallen out of favor.

- **Mechanism of Action**
  - IL-2, after binding to its receptor, causes phosphorylation of Janus tyrosine kinases (JAK) which leads to the activation of signal transducer and activator of transcription (STAT), phosphoinositol-3-kinases (PI3K), and SCH-MAP-RAS pathways which lead to further downstream signaling.[3] IL-2 acts as a double-edged sword in cancer immunotherapy. It regulates both T cell expansion and differentiation into memory and effector cells, natural killer (NK) cell proliferation, and increases cytolytic activity which forms the basis of its antitumor activity. On the other hand, IL-2 also leads to the expansion of regulatory T (Treg) cells, and prolonged exposure to IL-2 leads to activation-induced cell death of T cells, which leads to suppression of antitumor immune responses.[3]
- **Mechanism of Endocrine Toxicity**
  - Thyroid dysfunction is the most common endocrine toxicity with IL-2. Autoimmune destruction is the likely mechanism. An increase in lymphocytic infiltration of the thyroid gland has been seen in patients treated with IL-2.[4,5] An increase in the levels of thyroid autoantibodies (Tab) during treatment with IL-2 has also been reported.[6–8] Whether this leads to thyroid dysfunction is not clear, as a few studies have failed to show the association between increased Tab and hypothyroidism.[9,10]

- **Reported Toxicities**
  - New or worsening of thyroid function is reported in 16% to 47% of patients on IL-2 alone.[6,8,11] In a study of 281 patients treated with IL-2 by Krouse et al., hypothyroidism was more common than hyperthyroidism with about 35% of patients developing hypothyroidism and 7% developing hyperthyroidism. Most patients had subclinical hypothyroidism and only a few required hormone replacement therapy. The median duration of hypothyroidism was around 60 days with an increase in its incidence seen with successive cycles of treatment. No statistical difference in incidence was seen based on age, gender, tumor type, or IL-2 dose.[11] Similar incidences have been reported when IL-2 is used in combination with other agents.[7,9] The use of thyroid dysfunction as a predictive marker for response is controversial, with inconsistent results in several studies.[6,7,9] This has been attributed to the fact that patients who respond to therapy were likely to receive more cycles of IL-2, which would increase their risk of thyroid dysfunction.

    Two cases of acute adrenal insufficiency have been reported: one was due to IL-2 and another due to IL-2/tumor infiltrating lymphocyte combination therapy.[12,13] Cases of new onset insulin dependent diabetes mellitus (DM),[14,15] and changes in levels of β-endorphin, cortisol, and adrenocorticotrophic hormone (ACTH) have been reported.[16] Transient decrease in levels of testosterone, dehydroepiandrosterone, and increase in levels of estradiol have also been reported in men treated with IL-2.[17] These changes suggest a definite endocrine effect caused by IL-2 therapy.

INTERFERON-α (INF-α)

- INF-α2b has been used as an adjuvant treatment in patients with melanoma. It is also approved for use in renal cell cancer, Kaposi sarcoma, and chronic myeloid leukemia but, due to the advent of less toxic and more potent treatments, its use is now restricted to clinical trials.
- **Mechanism of Action**
  - INF-α acts by binding to its receptor on the cell membrane and phosphorylating the intracellular domain along with JAK and tyrosine kinase 2, which are attached to it. This leads to further activation and dimerization of STAT which translocate to the nucleus and leads to the expression of the interferon-regulated genes.[18] INF exerts its anticancer action by (1) inducing apoptosis of tumor cells; (2) inducing activation, proliferation, and cytotoxic activity of dendritic cells, NK cells, CD4+ and CD8+ T cells, and B cells; and (3) decreasing the immunosuppressive action of myeloid-derived suppressor cells and Treg cells.[18]
- **Mechanism of Endocrine Toxicities**
  - Thyroid dysfunction is common with the use of INF-α. Autoimmune thyroiditis (which is mediated by increase in MHC-I expression in thyroid tissue, switching of the immune response to the Th1 pathway, activation of other mediating immune cells, and release of other cytokines) is the likely mechanism, but direct effects of INF-α on thyroid tissue have also been implicated.[19] In-vitro experiments have shown that INF can inhibit thyroid function by a decrease in iodine uptake and secretion of thyroxine.[20]
- **Reported Toxicities**
  - Thyroid dysfunction can present as Hashimoto's thyroiditis, Graves' disease, presence of thyroid antibodies with no clinical disease, and destructive thyroiditis, which presents with biphasic thyroiditis leading to thyrotoxicosis followed by hypothyroidism and resolution.[21] Between 2% and 10% of patients develop hypothyroidism, with a median time of 4 months after beginning therapy, and nearly 60% of these patients will have persistent hypothyroidism.[22] The presence of thyroid autoantibodies is a risk factor for the development of thyroid dysfunction, and prior autoimmune thyroid disorder has been associated with severe hypothyroidism.[23]

- New onset insulin dependent diabetes has also been reported and is associated with high titers of pancreatic autoantibodies with almost all patients requiring insulin even after cessation of treatment.[24] INF-α also causes an increase in the levels of cortisol and adrenocorticotrophic hormone.[25] The effect of INF on sex hormones is unclear. A study in men treated with INF showed a decrease in total and free testosterone and dehydroepiandrosterone-sulphate (DHEAS), and showed a correlation between low testosterone and loss of libido.[26] Another study, however, showed no significant changes,[27] highlighting the need for further investigation.

IMMUNE CHECKPOINT INHIBITORS (ICIS)

In the past decade, ICIs have revolutionized cancer therapeutics. Three classes of ICIs have been approved by the FDA:
- Ipilimumab, an anti-cytotoxic T lymphocyte antigen (CTLA)-4 antibody was the first ICI to be approved for use in melanoma.[28] Tremelimumab is another anti-CTLA-4 which has shown some activity in melanoma, mesothelioma, hepatocellular carcinoma, and colorectal carcinoma but has not received FDA approval for any indication to date.[29]
- Another class of drugs alters the programmed death (PD)-1/programmed death ligand (PDL)-1 pathway. Nivolumab and pembrolizumab are drugs that bind to PD-1. Both are approved for use in melanoma; non–small-cell lung cancer (NSCLC); and head and neck squamous cell, urothelial, and renal cell cancers.[28] Nivolumab is also approved for use in hepatocellular and colorectal carcinomas with high microsatellite instability (MSI) or mismatch repair defects, and pembrolizumab is approved for use in gastric carcinoma and solid tumors with high MSI or mismatch repair defects.[28] Cemiplimab is another PD-1 inhibitor which is approved for advanced squamous cell carcinoma based on it's activity in a phase II trial.[95]
- Atezolizumab (used in NSCLC and urothelial cancer), avelumab (used in Merkel cell carcinoma and urothelial cancer), and durvalumab (used in urothelial carcinoma) bind to PD-L1 and have been approved by the FDA.[28] Recently, PD-L1 agents have also shown benefit with chemotherapy (triple negative breast cancer) and as maintenance therapy (small cell lung cancer, NSCLC and urothelial carcinoma).[96-100]
- **Mechanism of Action of ICIs**
  - CD28 is present on the surface of naïve T cells. It binds to CD80/86 present on the surface of activated antigen presenting cells (APC) providing a costimulatory signal to the interaction between major histocompatibility protein (MHC) and the T cell receptor (TCR). CTLA-4 acts as a competitive antagonist of CD28 expressed on activated T cells and Tregs, and binds to CD80/86 providing an inhibitory signal leading to decrease in T cell activation, proliferation, and IL-2 production.[30] There is some evidence that CTLA-4 might cause trans-endocytosis of CD80/86 leading to its degradation, thereby reducing the number of ligands for CD28.[30] CTLA-4 also enhances the activity of Treg cells leading to more immunosuppression.[31] Blocking of CTLA-4 using monoclonal antibodies (mAbs) was shown to increase T cell activation and proliferation in vitro and decrease tumor growth and tumor rejection in mice models.[31] PD-1, similar to CTLA-4, is also found on the T cell surface, although, unlike CTLA-4, its action is mostly restricted to effector T cells, and peripherally in the tumor microenvironment by binding with its ligands PD-L1 and PD-L2 expressed extensively on tumor cells. This leads to apoptosis and downregulation of T-cell effector functions, which is blocked by antibodies targeting PD-1/PD-L1.[32]
- **Mechanism of Endocrine Toxicity**
  - **Hypophysitis:** Although the exact mechanism has not been defined, autoimmunity is the most popularly theorized mechanism. In a murine model, CTLA-4 was seen in the murine pituitary glands at both RNA and protein levels and administration of anti-CTLA-4 mAb lead to the development of antibodies against pituitary cells, lymphocytic infiltration, and complement deposition in the pituitary: a mechanism similar to type II hypersensitivity

reaction.[33] In the same report, antipituitary antibodies were found in patients who developed hypophysitis after ipiliumumab administration, although not in the other patients without hypophysitis.[33] In an autopsy report of a patient who developed hypophysitis with tremelimumab, high levels of expression of CTLA-4 was seen in the pituitary cells as well as signs of type II and type IV hypersensitivity reactions, ultimately leading to necrosis of the pituitary tissue. None of these changes were seen in patients who did not develop hypophysitis (although one patient had mild lymphocytic infiltration of the pituitary).[34] Although the exact mechanism of hypophysitis with anti-PD-1/PD-L1 is not well described, it does appear to follow the patterns discussed earlier.

- **Thyroid dysfunction:** Genetic susceptibilities linked to HLA phenotypes or polymorphisms in CTLA-4/PD-1 genes have also been associated with the development of Graves' disease and Hashimoto's thyroiditis.[35,36] The current consensus is that thyroid dysfunction is due to autoimmune destruction of the thyroid gland, evidenced by several case series in which patients initially had thyrotoxicosis or subclinical hyperthyroidism before becoming hypothyroid.[37–40] One case study showed that patients at the time of initial thyroid dysfunction had low nuclear uptake or a nonvascular gland on ultrasound, supporting the process of destructive thyroiditis.[40] A recent study described the presence of PD-L1 and PD-L2 on thyroid tissue in patients who developed thyroid dysfunction with nivolumab.[41] It is also possible that the use of PD-1 inhibitors could lead to the loss of peripheral tolerance. Antithyroid antibodies (antithyroglobulin antibodies and antimicrosomal antibodies) may have a role in the pathogenesis of thyroid dysfunction as they are found more commonly in patients who develop thyroid dysfunction but their role in the pathogenesis of ICI induced thyroid dysfunction remains questionable.[39]

- **Other endocrinopathies:** Autoimmune diabetes mellitus is a rare endocrine disorder with ICI therapy, and most cases have been reported with the use of anti-PD-1 or anti-PD-L1 antibodies. Blockade of the PD-1/PD-L1 pathway using anti-PD-1 or anti-PD-L1 antibodies causes destructive insulitis and precipitates DM in nonobese diabetic mice models.[42] It is likely that the PD-1/PD-L1 pathway maintains peripheral tolerance, which is broken down by mAbs (blocking this pathway).

- Primary adrenal insufficiency (PAI) has also been reported with ICI therapy. Polymorphism of the CTLA-4 gene has been associated with the development of this entity.[43,44] Due to its rarity, there are no studies to our knowledge which have thoroughly evaluated its pathogenesis.

- **Reported Toxicities**
- **Hypophysitis**
  - A meta-analysis from 2018 reported that 3.2% of patients developed hypophysitis with ipilimumab.[45] Other studies have reported a higher incidence which is probably due to higher recognition of the condition with more experience with the drug.[46,47] The incidence of hypophysitis is dose-related, with a higher incidence seen with the 10 mg/kg dose versus the 3 mg/kg dose of ipilimumab.[48] The incidence of hypophysitis is more common in men and in elderly patients.[49] The number of cycles received did not differ between patients who developed hypophysitis versus patients who did not.[49] In a study by Faje et al., of 57 patients with ipilimumab-induced hypophysitis, the median time of onset was 2 to 3 months after starting therapy but can occur as early as 4 weeks or have delayed presentation. Most cases involved the anterior pituitary with several hormone axes; thyroid, adrenal, and gonadotrophic deficiencies were commonly reported, whereas growth hormone was usually unaffected. Hyperprolactinemia was rare, whereas low prolactin levels were seen in about 60% of patients. The majority of patients also had radiographic pituitary enlargement at the time of diagnosis, which was transient and resolved in most patients. Thyroid and gonadal axes recovered in about half of the patients, whereas most patients continued to have adrenal axis deficiency. Hypophysitis during treatment with ipilimumab has been associated with improved response to therapy.[50] Interestingly, involvement of the posterior pituitary is exceedingly uncommon, although some cases of diabetes insipidus and syndrome of inappropriate antidiuretic hormone (SIADH) have been reported with ipilimumab.[51,52]

- The incidence of hypophysitis with anti-PD-1 antibody treatment is low- a meta-analysis reported that 0.4% of patients develop hypophysitis with anti-PD-1 antibody.[45] Another article reported the development of hypophysitis to be 0.5% to 0.9% of patients treated with nivolumab with a median time to onset of 5.5 months. With pembrolizumab, the incidence of hypophysitis was reported at 0.8% in patients with melanoma and 0.2% in patients with NSCLC with a time to onset of between 3.3 and 3.7 months.[53] The rate of drug discontinuation due to hypophysitis was less than 1%.[53] The incidence of hypophysitis is greatest with the combination of ICI, with 6.4% developing hypophysitis, whereas anti-PD-L1 antibodies alone cause hypophysitis in less than 0.1% of patients.[45]
- **Thyroid disorders**
  - Barroso et al., in their meta-analysis, reported that 3.8% and 1.7% of patients developed hypothyroidism and hyperthyroidism, respectively, on ipilimumab.[45] No difference in the incidence of hypothyroidism or thyroiditis was noticed between the 3 mg/kg and the 10 mg/kg dose of ipilimumab.[48] The onset of thyroid dysfunction commonly occurred after 2 to 4 infusions.[54] New onset Graves' disease, Graves' ophthalmopathy with normal thyroid stimulating hormone (TSH) levels but elevated thyroid stimulating antibody (TSIAb), and thyroid storm have also been reported.[55-57]
  - Thyroid disorders are more frequently seen with anti-PD-1 therapy compared to ipilimumab. Hypothyroidism is seen in 7.0% and hyperthyroidism is seen in 3.2% of patients.[45] The risk of hyperthyroidism with pembrolizumab is reported to be higher than nivolumab (3.8% vs. 2.3%).[45] New onset hypothyroidism or a transient hyperthyroid state followed by recovery or hypothyroidism have been reported in many studies.[37,38,41] The median time to onset of thyrotoxic phase is 3 to 6 weeks, with resolution in 4 weeks and subsequent hypothyroidism in 6 to 8 weeks.[38]
  - Compared to PD-1 inhibitors, the incidence of thyroid dysfunction with PD-L1 inhibitors is significantly lower: 3.9% of patients developed hypothyroidism, and 0.6% of patients developed hyperthyroidism.[45] The highest incidence of thyroid dysfunction is seen with combination immunotherapy, with 13% and 8% of patients developing hypothyroidism and hyperthyroidism, respectively.[45]
- **Other endocrine disorders**
  - Insulin-dependent DM has been reported with ICIs. The onset is variable with reported times ranging from 1 week to 12 months.[58] Around half of the patients had antibodies against GAD or islet cells. Furthermore, an association with high-risk HLA-genotypes has been shown in some cases.[58] Patients may have variable presentation. Some present with hyperglycemia, whereas others present with diabetic ketoacidosis (DKA). Primary adrenal insufficiency (PAI) is a rare endocrine disorder related to ICI therapy. The incidence with ICI monotherapy is around 0.7%; however, higher incidences were reported with combination therapy.[45] Cases of transient low total testosterone levels without concurrent hypophysitis, suggesting primary gonadal failure, were identified, although most of these patients were receiving high-dose steroids for other irAEs and simultaneous measurement of sex-binding globulins was not done.[59] Autonomous cortisol secretion has been seen in one patient treated with ipilimumab.[59] Hypoparathyroidism leading to symptomatic hypocalcemia has been reported with ipilimumab.[60] Cases of hypercalcemia have also been reported with ipilimumab and nivolumab, although the etiology is unclear.[61]

ONCOLYTIC VIRUSES

- Talimogene laherparepvec (T-VEC) is the first oncolytic virus to receive FDA approval for intralesional use based on a phase III clinical trial which showed significant increase in durable response rate and overall response rate compared to granulocyte macrophage colony stimulating factor (GM-CSF) in melanoma, although without significant change in overall survival.[62] Trials with the combination of T-VEC and ICIs have shown to have clinical benefit and appear to be well tolerated.[63,64]

- **Mechanism of Action**
  - T-VEC is an attenuated herpes simplex virus-1 which can encode for GM-CSF. It is capable of selective replication in tumor cells due to disrupted PRK activity (PKR is a protein which is activated in human cells when infected by a virus and prevents protein translation), and disrupted INF signaling. The replication of viruses in the tumor cell ultimately leads to cell death and release of viruses which can infect neighboring cells. Cell lysis also leads to release of tumor-related antigen and damage-associated protein, which leads to further immune response against the tumor.[65]
- **Reported Endocrine Toxicities**
  - T-VEC is well tolerated. When used as a monotherapy or in combination with ipilimumab, no endocrine toxicities were reported (although when used in combination with ipilimumab only, toxicities with an incidence more than 10% were reported).[62,63] A single case of thyroid dysfunction has been reported with concurrent use of T-VEC, although it was deemed to be not related to T-VEC use.[66]

CHIMERIC ANTIGEN RECEPTOR CAR T-CELL THERAPY

- The FDA has approved CD19 targeting CAR-T cells for use in patients with relapsed/refractory B-cell acute lymphoblastic leukemia (B-ALL) and diffuse large B cell lymphoma (DBCL) who have relapsed after two lines of therapy.[67,68] Several other CAR-T cells targeting various other antigens on hematological and solid malignancies have undergone clinical trials with promising results.[69–71]
- **Mechanism of Action**
  - CAR is an antibody derived single-chain variable fragment which engages the antigen present on the target cell. CAR is attached to a CD3ζ-signaling domain within the T cell via a hinge and transmembrane domain. Further development has led to the addition of costimulatory domains to the CD3ζ-chain signaling domain in second and third generation CAR-T cells.[72]
- **Reported Endocrine Toxicities**
  - Cytokine release syndrome (CRS) and neurological adverse effects are the most common toxicities reported.[73,74] Hyperglycemia was reported as an adverse effect during treatment with CD19 CAR-T cells, although the exact etiology is not known and is may be related to corticosteroids given to treat CRS or neurotoxicity.[73,75] No other endocrine toxicity was reported.

BISPECIFIC T CELL ENGAGER (BiTE)

- Blinatumomab is the first BiTE to be approved by the FDA for use in relapsed/refractory precursor B-ALL in adults and children and has recently gained approval for use in patients with B cell precursor ALL in remission with minimal residual disease.[76] Blinatumomab has shown promising results in phase II trials in patients with relapsed/refractory non-Hodgkin's lymphoma.[77]
- **Mechanism of Action**
  - Blinatumomab consists of two single-chain variable fragments joined together through a linker molecule, with one fragment binding to CD3 on T cells and the other fragment binding to CD19 on B cells.[78] The BiTE brings the T cells and tumor cells into physical proximity, leading to the formation of a transient cytolytic synapse between the two cells. The activated T cell then releases perforins and granzymes which penetrate the tumor cell leading to its apoptosis.[79]

- **Reported Endocrine Toxicities**
  - Neurological adverse events are the most common reported toxicities with BiTE therapy. In a phase II trial, hyperglycemia was reported in about 13% of patients, with about 8% of patients developing grade 3 hyperglycemia.[80] Hyperglycemia is more common in patients over 65 years of age.[81] It is likely related to corticosteroids given to prevent or treat neurotoxicity. No other endocrine toxicity has been reported with blinatumomab.

Pharmacological Management of Toxicities

INTERLEUKIN-2

- Thyroid dysfunction is commonly reported with IL-2 therapy. Krouse et al. based their recommendations on a study of 281 patients treated with IL-2 which proposed that TSH and free T4 (FT4) levels should be measured at regular intervals during treatment with IL-2. In patients who develop moderate and severe hypothyroidism, thyroid hormone replacement should be started, and further IL-2 therapy should be withheld for 2 to 4 weeks. Therapy should be continued for about a year after finishing IL-2 therapy or until thyroid dysfunction resolves. In this study, patients also developed mild and transient hyperthyroidism, which did not require any treatment.[11]

INTERFERON (INF)-α

- Fatigue and depression are common adverse effects of INF therapy and may mimic symptoms of hypothyroidism. Before starting therapy with INF, TSH, and FT4 should be measured. Positive titer of thyroid peroxidase (TPO) Ab prior to treatment is associated with higher risk of developing thyroid dysfunction during treatment with INF.[82] Thyroid function should be checked every 8 to 12 weeks during treatment.[83] Thyroid hormone replacement should be initiated in patients who develop hypothyroidism and should be continued until treatment completion, although in patients who have positive antithyroid antibody titers, lifelong replacement may be required.[83] Patients who develop destructive thyrotoxicosis can be managed with β-blockers, although patients who have uncontrolled symptoms may require withdrawal of INF and recheck of thyroid function in 4 to 6 weeks.[83] Patients with Graves' disease can be managed with antithyroid drugs, although patients with severe disease may need radioiodine ablation. In these cases, INF should be withheld until thyroid function normalizes postablation.[83]

IMMUNE CHECKPOINT INHIBITOR

Thyroid Dysfunction

Hypothyroidism

- A high index of suspicion is necessary as several symptoms of hypothyroidism overlap with those of advanced cancer. Patients present with fatigue, weight gain, hair loss, leg swelling, constipation, and depressed mood. Rarely, patients present with myxedema coma.[84] Biochemical diagnosis requires the presence of high TSH with a low T4 level. In cases of subclinical hypothyroidism, T4 levels will be normal. TSH and FT4 should be obtained at the start of therapy and then every 4 to 6 weeks for the whole duration of treatment.[85] In patients with a biochemical diagnosis of hypothyroidism, thyroid antibodies should also be obtained.[86]
- Treatment is not indicated for patients with grade 1 toxicity and ICI should be continued. Patients should be monitored clinically along with regular monitoring of TSH and FT4 levels.[85,86] Hormone replacement should be initiated for patients with grade 2 toxicity, and ICI may be withheld until replacement produces adequate levels.[85] In patients with no risk factors, a complete replacement dose of 1.6 µg/kg per day can be initiated, whereas elderly

patients or patients with cardiovascular risks should be started on a lower dose of 25–50 μg/day. Levels of TSH should be rechecked in 6 to 8 weeks for adequacy of the replacement, and once stable, the thyroid function can be evaluated annually or with clinical change.[85] Patients with TSH levels persistently greater than 10 mIU/L should be treated similarly, even if asymptomatic, as these patients have higher risk of coronary heart disease (CHD) events, CHD mortality, and total mortality.[85,87]

- Patients with grade 3 or higher toxicity generally need hospitalization for treatment. In these cases, further ICI therapy should be withheld until symptoms resolve. Hormone replacement should be carried out as in grade 2 patients.[85,86] Intravenous levothyroxine should be used in patients who present with myxedema coma.[85] For patients with adrenal insufficiency and hypothyroidism, adrenal hormones should be replaced before thyroid hormone replacement is started[85] as replacement of thyroid hormone in patients with adrenal insufficiency can precipitate an adrenal crisis.[88]

Hyperthyroidism

- Thyrotoxicosis/hyperthyroidism usually presents with symptoms such as palpitations, anxiety, weight loss, diarrhea, and heat intolerance. Cases of thyrotoxic storm as initial presentation have also been reported.[56] Biochemical diagnosis is made by detecting increased T4 or T3 in the setting of a suppressed TSH. Hyperthyroidism can be caused by two different mechanisms: autoimmune destruction of the gland leading to release of thyroxine hormone, and Graves' disease. Thyroid stimulating immunoglobulin or thyroid hormone receptor antibodies, TPO antibodies, and a nuclear iodine uptake scan should be obtained in patients with suspected Graves' disease, because these can help differentiate the clinical syndrome from thyrotoxicosis due to autoimmune thyroiditis.[86] Use of Doppler ultrasound of the thyroid gland is not well defined.

- No intervention is indicated in patients with grade 1 toxicity.[85,86] Assessment of thyroid function should be done every 2 weeks to assess for new hypothyroidism or persistent hyperthyroidism.[85] Grade 2 hyperthyroidism can be managed symptomatically with β-blockers and supportive care.[85,86] Further ICI therapy may be withheld.[85] The role of corticosteroids is controversial as it is not recommended in the American Society of Clinical Oncology (ASCO) and Society for Immunotherapy of Cancer (SITC) guidelines, although European guidelines recommend the use of prednisone 0.5 mg/kg followed by a taper in patients with painful thyroiditis.[85,86,89] ICI therapy should be withheld for grade 3 or higher toxicity and hospitalization is indicated in patients with severe symptoms.[85,86] In addition to treatment indicated for grade 2 toxicity, prednisone 1–2 mg/kg, which is tapered over 1 to 2 weeks, should also be used. Graves' disease should be considered in patients who have persistent hyperthyroidism longer than 4 to 6 weeks.[85,86] Patients with Graves' disease will need antithyroid medications to decrease thyroxine production.[85] Antithyroid medications have no role in autoimmune thyroiditis. Patients who developed ophthalmopathy have been treated successfully with prolonged steroid taper with/without canthotomy.[55,57]

Hypophysitis

- Headache and fatigue are the most common presenting symptoms of hypophysitis,[50,86] but patients can have nausea, vomiting, confusion, anorexia, temperature intolerance and weight loss as well.[50] Patients may present with adrenal crisis as well, a life threatening condition with shock, confusion and electrolyte abnormalities. Symptoms due to mass effect are rare and visual impairment is uncommon as optic structures are rarely involved. In patients in whom hypophysitis is suspected, morning cortisol and ACTH, TSH, and FT4, and electrolytes should be obtained.[85,86] Gonadal hormones, luteinizing hormone (LH) and follicle stimulating hormone (FSH), and MRI of the brain with pituitary cuts can be considered depending on the symptoms of the patients.[85]

- ICI-induced hypophysitis is diagnosed by detecting low ACTH and cortisol, low TSH and FT4, low gonadal hormones, and low FSH/LH. Posterior pituitary involvement may also present with hyponatremia. Radiographic enlargement of the pituitary is seen in the majority of the cases and resolves in almost all cases.[50] Radiographic enlargement of the pituitary on MRI may precede biochemical or clinical onset of disease.[86] A proposed diagnostic criterion includes: ≥1 deficiency of pituitary axis (TSH or ACTH deficiency required) with MRI findings or ≥2 axis deficiency (TSH or ACTH deficiency required) accompanied by headache.[86]

■ Patients with grades 1 and 2 toxicity can be managed with hormone replacement of the deficient axis: hydrocortisone orally 10–20 mg in the morning and 5–10 mg in the early afternoon and levothyroxine based on patient's weight should be started.[85] In patients with deficiency of gonadal hormones, treatment is usually considered in the outpatient setting after consultation with an endocrinologist.[85] Monitoring of thyroid hormone replacement should be evaluated with FT4 levels because TSH levels are inaccurate in patients with central hypothyroidism.[85] In patients presenting with grade 3 toxicity or higher or associated with severe headaches and vision loss, pulse dose therapy with prednisone 1–2 mg/kg, or equivalent, daily tapered over 1 to 2 weeks should be considered, followed by hormone replacement as in grade 1 toxicity.[85] Long-term high-dose steroids (over 3–12 weeks) has not been shown to reduce either residual hormone deficit or time to resolution of symptoms.[90] ICI therapy should be withheld until patients are on a stable dose of replacement hormones.[85]

■ In patients presenting with hypotension, sepsis should always be ruled out. Hormone replacement should be started in critically ill patients who have a high suspicion of hypophysitis even before biochemical diagnosis is made. In patients suspected with adrenal insufficiency, corticosteroids should be started prior to other hormone replacement, especially before thyroid hormone replacement to prevent precipitation of adrenal crisis. The majority of patients will need long-term hormone replacement therapy.[50] Although immunosuppressants like mycophenolate have been frequently used in other irAEs, their use in ICI mediated hypophysitis is not well described.

Primary Adrenal Insufficiency (PAI)

■ PAI, like secondary adrenal insufficiency, presents with nausea, abdominal pain, anorexia, and fatigue and hypotension. Laboratory testing often reveals hyponatremia, hyperkalemia and hypoglycemia. Notably, hyperpigmentation is exclusively seen in PAI compared to patients with secondary adrenal insufficiency, who can have similar presenting complaints.[91] Symptoms of PAI mimic those of disease progression, and requires a high index of suspicion on the clinicians part for diagnosis. In patients with suspicion of PAI, 8:00 a.m. serum cortisol and ACTH levels and serum electrolytes should be obtained. Patients with PAI will have low serum cortisol with high ACTH levels.[85] Plasma renin and aldosterone levels should also be obtained as PAI, unlike secondary insufficiency, will also cause mineralocorticoid deficiency.[91] In patients with an indeterminate result, a cosyntropin test should be obtained.[85] Cortisol level of less than 18 μg/dL at 30 or 60 minutes post-250 μg IV cosyntropin is diagnostic of PAI.[91] Abdominal CT can help to rule out metastasis or hemorrhage as a cause of PAI. Patients should also be evaluated for underlying infection.[85]

■ Further treatment with ICI should be withheld in all cases of PAI until the patient is clinically stable. Expert endocrinology consultation is recommended for patients with suspected PAI.[85] Patients with grade 1 symptoms can be started on a maintenance dose of steroids (prednisone 5–10 mg daily or hydrocortisone 10–20 mg in the morning and 5–10 mg in the afternoon). Fludrocortisone (100 μg/day) will be required in patients with mineralocorticoid deficiency. Patients with grade 2 symptoms will initially need a higher dose of hydrocortisone or equivalent steroid, which can be tapered to maintenance dose as patient's clinical status improve.[85] Patients with higher than grade 3 toxicity should be given

IV hydrocortisone 100 or 4 mg dexamethasone along with adequate fluid resuscitation. Dexamethasone is preferred in cases where the diagnosis is unclear as it does not interfere with cosyntropin stimulation testing.[85] The dose of hydrocortisone should be tapered to maintenance dose as patient's clinical condition improves.[91] Blood cultures and appropriate imaging should be obtained in these patients to rule out sepsis. Further treatment with ICI should be withheld until the patient is on adequate hormone replacement.[85]

Diabetes Mellitus (DM)

- Patients on ICIs can present with worsening of DM or with new onset of insulin-dependent DM. Patients can be asymptomatic or present with symptoms of polyphagia, polydipsia, weight loss, dehydration, and fatigue, or even present in diabetic ketoacidosis (DKA). Blood sugar should be checked at baseline and at regular intervals while patients are on treatment with ICIs.[85,89] Low levels of insulin and C peptide can help differentiate type 1 from type 2 DM.[85,86] In patients with suspected type 1 DM, antiglutamic acid decarboxylase (GAD) 65, anti-insulin and anti-islet cell antibodies can be measured,[85] although antibody negative cases have been reported in the literature.[92]
- Patients with new diagnoses of diabetes should be screened for DM type 1.[85] Patients with grade 1 toxicity can continue with ICI therapy, and oral hypoglycemic medications can be started in patients with DM type 2.[85] In patients with grade 2 toxicity, oral hypoglycemic medications can be up-titrated or patients can be started on insulin if diagnosed with type 1 DM or if the subtype is unclear.[85] Patients with more than grade 3 toxicity will need insulin therapy and an endocrinology consult irrespective of the subtype.[85] In this setting, ICI therapy should be withheld until blood sugars are controlled.[85] Steroids have not shown any benefit in checkpoint induced DM.[93] The role of other immunosupressive agents is not well defined, however, a case of checkpoint induced DM successfully treated with infliximab has been reported.[94]

CAR T-CELL THERAPY AND BITE THERAPY

- Hyperglycemia is frequently seen with both CAR T-cell therapy and with BiTE therapy; however, this is likely due to use of corticosteroids to prevent and treat neurotoxicity and CRS. Patients should be closely monitored with regular blood sugar monitoring, especially if they are diabetic. Insulin-based regimens are preferred due to risk of acute kidney injury, with CRS associated with both therapies. Patients who develop DKA should be managed on established protocols.

Non-Pharmacological Management

- Medical alert bracelets should be provided to patients with primary and secondary adrenal insufficiency.[85] Patients should be made aware of the need to increase steroid dosage with concurrent illness. Similarly, doses should also be increased prior to any major surgery, in consultation with an endocrinologist.[85] Patients with thyroid dysfunction and diabetes are at a higher risk of CHD, and risk factor for CHD should be optimized.

References

1. McDermott DF, Cheng SC, Signoretti S, et al. The high-dose aldesleukin "select" trial: a trial to prospectively validate predictive models of response to treatment in patients with metastatic renal cell carcinoma. *Clin Cancer Res.* 2015;21(3):561–568.
2. Davar D, Ding F, Saul M, et al. High-dose interleukin-2 (HD IL-2) for advanced melanoma: a single center experience from the University of Pittsburgh Cancer Institute. *J Immunother Cancer.* 2017;5(1):74.
3. Sim GC, Radvanyi L. The IL-2 cytokine family in cancer immunotherapy. *Cytokine Growth Factor Rev.* 2014;25(4):377–390.

4. Kragel AH, Travis WD, Feinberg L, et al. Pathologic findings associated with interleukin-2-based immunotherapy for cancer: a postmortem study of 19 patients. *Hum Pathol.* 1990;21(5):493–502.
5. Pichert G, Jost L, Zöbeli L, Odermatt B, Pedia G, Stahel R. Thyroiditis after treatment with interleukin-2 and interferon α-2a. *Br J Cancer.* 1990;62(1):100.
6. Weijl N, Van der Harst D, Brand A, et al. Hypothyroidism during immunotherapy with interleukin-2 is associated with antithyroid antibodies and response to treatment. *J Clin Oncol.* 1993;11(7):1376–1383.
7. Atkins MB, Mier JW, Parkinson DR, Gould JA, Berkman EM, Kaplan MM. Hypothyroidism after treatment with interleukin-2 and lymphokine-activated killer cells. *N Engl J Med.* 1988;318(24):1557–1563.
8. Vialettes B, Guillerand MA, Viens P, et al. Incidence rate and risk factors for thyroid dysfunction during recombinant interleukin-2 therapy in advanced malignancies. *Acta Endocrinol (Copenh).* 1993;129(1):31–38.
9. Schwartzentruber DJ, White DE, Zweig MH, Weintraub BD, Rosenberg SA. Thyroid dysfunction associated with immunotherapy for patients with cancer. *Cancer.* 1991;68(11):2384–2390.
10. Vassilopoulou-Sellin R, Sella A, Dexeus FH, Theriault RL, Pololoff DA. Acute thyroid dysfunction (thyroiditis) after therapy with interleukin-2. *Horm Metab Res.* 1992;24(9):434–438.
11. Krouse RS, Royal RE, Heywood G, et al. Thyroid dysfunction in 281 patients with metastatic melanoma or renal carcinoma treated with interleukin-2 alone. *J Immuno Emphasis Tumor Immunol.* 1995;18(4):272–278.
12. Wahle JS, Hanson JP, Shaker JL, Findling JW. Autoimmune Addison's disease after treatment with interleukin-2 and tumor-infiltrating lymphocytes. *Endocr Pract.* 1995;1(1):14–17.
13. Van der Molen LA, Smith JW 2nd, Longo DL, Steis RG, Kremers P, Sznol M. Adrenal insufficiency and interleukin-2 therapy. *Ann Intern Med.* 1989;111(2):185.
14. Fraenkel PG, Rutkove SB, Matheson JK, et al. Induction of myasthenia gravis, myositis, and insulin-dependent diabetes mellitus by high-dose interleukin-2 in a patient with renal cell cancer. *J Immunother.* 2002;25(4):373–378.
15. Soni N, Meropol NJ, Porter M, Caligiuri MA. Diabetes mellitus induced by low-dose interleukin-2. *Cancer Immunol Immunother.* 1996;43(1):59–62.
16. Denicoff KD, Durkin TM, Lotze MT, et al. The neuroendocrine effects of interleukin-2 treatment. *J Clin Endocrinol Metab.* 1989;69(2):402–410.
17. Meikle AW, Cardoso de Sousa JC, Ward JH, Woodward M, Samlowski WE. Reduction of testosterone synthesis after high dose interleukin-2 therapy of metastatic cancer. *J Clin Endocrinol Metab.* 1991;73(5):931–935.
18. Parker BS, Rautela J, Hertzog PJ. Antitumour actions of interferons: implications for cancer therapy. *Nat Rev Cancer.* 2016;16(3):131–144.
19. Tomer Y, Blackard JT, Akeno N. Interferon alpha treatment and thyroid dysfunction. *Endocrinol Metab Clin North Am.* 2007;36(4):1051–1066; x–xi.
20. Yamazaki K, Kanaji Y, Shizume K, et al. Reversible inhibition by interferons alpha and beta of 125I incorporation and thyroid hormone release by human thyroid follicles in vitro. *J Clin Endocrinol Metab.* 1993;77(5):1439–1441.
21. Mandac JC, Chaudhry S, Sherman KE, Tomer Y. The clinical and physiological spectrum of interferon-alpha induced thyroiditis: toward a new classification. *Hepatology.* 2006;43(4):661–672.
22. Hamnvik OP, Larsen PR, Marqusee E. Thyroid dysfunction from antineoplastic agents. *J Natl Cancer Inst.* 2011;103(21):1572–1587.
23. Vial T, Choquet-Kastylevsky G, Liautard C, Descotes J. Endocrine and neurological adverse effects of the therapeutic interferons. *Toxicology.* 2000;142(3):161–172.
24. Zornitzki T, Malnick S, Lysyy L, Knobler H. Interferon therapy in hepatitis C leading to chronic type 1 diabetes. *World J Gastroenterol.* 2015;21(1):233–239.
25. Muller H, Hammes E, Hiemke C, Hess G. Interferon-alpha-2-induced stimulation of ACTH and cortisol secretion in man. *Neuroendocrinology.* 1991;54(5):499–503.
26. Kraus MR, Schafer A, Bentink T, et al. Sexual dysfunction in males with chronic hepatitis C and antiviral therapy: interferon-induced functional androgen deficiency or depression? *J Endocrinol.* 2005;185(2):345–352.
27. Piazza M, Tosone G, Borgia G, et al. Long-term interferon-alpha therapy does not affect sex hormones in males with chronic hepatitis C. *J Interferon Cytokine Res.* 1997;17(9):525–529.
28. Postow MA, Sidlow R, Hellmann MD. Immune-related adverse events associated with immune checkpoint blockade. *N Engl J Med.* 2018;378(2):158–168.

29. Zhao Y, Yang W, Huang Y, Cui R, Li X, Li B. Evolving roles for targeting CTLA-4 in cancer immuno-therapy. *Cell Physiol Biochem*. 2018;47(2):721–734.
30. Gardner D, Jeffery LE, Sansom DM. Understanding the CD28/CTLA-4 (CD152) pathway and its implications for costimulatory blockade. *Am J Transplant*. 2014;14(9):1985–1991.
31. Mocellin S, Nitti D. CTLA-4 blockade and the renaissance of cancer immunotherapy. *Biochim Biophys Acta*. 2013;1836(2):187–196.
32. Ott PA, Hodi FS, Robert C. CTLA-4 and PD-1/PD-L1 blockade: new immunotherapeutic modalities with durable clinical benefit in melanoma patients. *Clin Cancer Res*. 2013;19(19):5300–5309.
33. Iwama S, De Remigis A, Callahan MK, Slovin SF, Wolchok JD, Caturegli P. Pituitary expression of CTLA-4 mediates hypophysitis secondary to administration of CTLA-4 blocking antibody. *Sci Transl Med*. 2014;6(230):230ra45.
34. Caturegli P, Di Dalmazi G, Lombardi M, et al. Hypophysitis secondary to cytotoxic T-lympho-cyte-associated protein 4 blockade: insights into pathogenesis from an autopsy series. *Am J Pathol*. 2016;186(12):3225–3235.
35. Kouki T, Sawai Y, Gardine CA, Fisfalen ME, Alegre ML, DeGroot LJ. CTLA-4 gene polymorphism at position 49 in exon 1 reduces the inhibitory function of CTLA-4 and contributes to the pathogenesis of Graves' disease. *J Immunol*. 2000;165(11):6606–6611.
36. Kotsa K, Watson PF, Weetman AP. A CTLA-4 gene polymorphism is associated with both Graves disease and autoimmune hypothyroidism. *Clin Endocrinol (Oxf)*. 1997;46(5):551–554.
37. Morganstein DL, Lai Z, Spain L, et al. Thyroid abnormalities following the use of cytotoxic T-lympho-cyte antigen-4 and programmed death receptor protein-1 inhibitors in the treatment of melanoma. *Clin Endocrinol (Oxf)*. 2017;86(4):614–620.
38. Orlov S, Salari F, Kashat L, Walfish PG. Induction of painless thyroiditis in patients receiving pro-grammed death 1 receptor immunotherapy for metastatic malignancies. *J Clin Endocrinol Metab*. 2015;100(5):1738–1741.
39. Osorio JC, Ni A, Chaft JE, et al. Antibody-mediated thyroid dysfunction during T-cell checkpoint blockade in patients with non-small-cell lung cancer. *Ann Oncol*. 2017;28(3):583–589.
40. Alhusseini M, Samantray J. Hypothyroidism in cancer patients on immune checkpoint inhibitors with anti-PD1 agents: insights on underlying mechanisms. *Exp Clin Endocrinol Diabetes*. 2017;125(4):267–269.
41. Yamauchi I, Sakane Y, Fukuda Y, et al. Clinical features of nivolumab-induced thyroiditis: a case series study. *Thyroid*. 2017;27(7):894–901.
42. Ansari MJ, Salama AD, Chitnis T, et al. The programmed death-1 (PD-1) pathway regulates autoim-mune diabetes in nonobese diabetic (NOD) mice. *J Exp Med*. 2003;198(1):63–69.
43. Brozzetti A, Marzotti S, Tortoioli C, et al. Cytotoxic T lymphocyte antigen-4 Ala17 polymorphism is a genetic marker of autoimmune adrenal insufficiency: Italian association study and meta-analysis of European studies. *Eur J Endocrinol*. 2010;162(2):361–369.
44. Falorni A, Brozzetti A, Perniola R. From genetic predisposition to molecular mechanisms of autoim-mune primary adrenal insufficiency. *Front Horm Res*. 2016;46:115–132.
45. Barroso-Sousa R, Barry WT, Garrido-Castro AC, et al. Incidence of endocrine dysfunction following the use of different immune checkpoint inhibitor regimens: a systematic review and meta-analysis. *JAMA Oncol*. 2018;4(2):173–182.
46. Weber J, Mandala M, Del Vecchio M, et al. Adjuvant nivolumab versus ipilimumab in resected stage III or IV melanoma. *N Engl J Med*. 2017;377(19):1824–1835.
47. Eggermont AM, Chiarion-Sileni V, Grob JJ, et al. Adjuvant ipilimumab versus placebo after complete resection of high-risk stage III melanoma (EORTC 18071): a randomised, double-blind, phase 3 trial. *Lancet Oncol*. 2015;16(5):522–530.
48. Ascierto PA, Del Vecchio M, Robert C, et al. Ipilimumab 10 mg/kg versus ipilimumab 3 mg/kg in pa-tients with unresectable or metastatic melanoma: a randomised, double-blind, multicentre, phase 3 trial. *Lancet Oncol*. 2017;18(5):611–622.
49. Faje AT, Sullivan R, Lawrence D, et al. Ipilimumab-induced hypophysitis: a detailed longitudinal analysis in a large cohort of patients with metastatic melanoma. *J Clin Endocrinol Metab*. 2014;99(11):4078–4085.
50. Faje A. Immunotherapy and hypophysitis: clinical presentation, treatment, and biologic insights. *Pitu-itary*. 2016;19(1):82–92.
51. Nallapaneni NN, Mourya R, Bhatt VR, Malhotra S, Ganti AK, Tendulkar KK. Ipilimumab-induced hypophysitis and uveitis in a patient with metastatic melanoma and a history of ipilimumab-induced skin rash. *J Natl Compr Canc Netw*. 2014;12(8):1077–1081.

52. Barnard ZR, Walcott BP, Kahle KT, Nahed BV, Coumans JV. Hyponatremia associated with ipilimum-ab-induced hypophysitis. *Med Oncol.* 2012;29(1):374–377.
53. Torino F, Corsello SM, Salvatori R. Endocrinological side-effects of immune checkpoint inhibitors. *Curr Opin Oncol.* 2016;28(4):278–287.
54. Torino F, Barnabei A, Paragliola R, Baldelli R, Appetecchia M, Corsello SM. Thyroid dysfunction as an unintended side effect of anticancer drugs. *Thyroid.* 2013;23(11):1345–1366.
55. Borodic G, Hinkle DM, Cia Y. Drug-induced Graves disease from CTLA-4 receptor suppression. *Ophthal Plast Reconstr Surg.* 2011;27(4):e87–e88.
56. McMillen B, Dhillon MS, Yong-Yow S. A rare case of thyroid storm. *BMJ Case Rep.* 2016;2016. doi:10.1136/bcr-2016-214603.
57. Min L, Vaidya A, Becker C. Thyroid autoimmunity and ophthalmopathy related to melanoma biological therapy. *Eur J Endocrinol.* 2011;164(2):303–307.
58. Chae YK, Chiec L, Mohindra N, Gentzler R, Patel J, Giles F. A case of pembrolizumab-induced type-1 diabetes mellitus and discussion of immune checkpoint inhibitor-induced type 1 diabetes. *Cancer Immunol Immunother.* 2017;66(1):25–32.
59. Ryder M, Callahan M, Postow MA, Wolchok J, Fagin JA. Endocrine-related adverse events following ipilimumab in patients with advanced melanoma: a comprehensive retrospective review from a single institution. *Endocr Relat Cancer.* 2014;21(2):371–381.
60. Win MA, Thein KZ, Qdaisat A, Yeung SJ. Acute symptomatic hypocalcemia from immune checkpoint therapy-induced hypoparathyroidism. *Am J Emerg Med.* 2017;35(7):1039.e5–1039.e7.
61. Mills TA, Orloff M, Domingo-Vidal M, et al. Parathyroid hormone-related peptide-linked hypercalcemia in a melanoma patient treated with ipilimumab: hormone source and clinical and metabolic correlates. *Semin Oncol.* 2015;42(6):909–914.
62. Andtbacka RH, Kaufman HL, Collichio F, et al. Talimogene laherparepvec improves durable response rate in patients with advanced melanoma. *J Clin Oncol.* 2015;33(25):2780–2788.
63. Puzanov I, Milhem MM, Minor D, et al. Talimogene laherparepvec in combination with ipilimumab in previously untreated, unresectable stage IIIB-IV melanoma. *J Clin Oncol.* 2016;34(22):2619–2626.
64. Long GV, Dummer R, Ribas A, et al. Efficacy analysis of MASTERKEY-265 phase 1b study of talimogene laherparepvec (T-VEC) and pembrolizumab (pembro) for unresectable stage IIIB-IV melanoma. *Am Soc Clin Oncol.* 2016;34(15 suppl):9568.
65. Kohlhapp FJ, Kaufman HL. Molecular pathways: mechanism of action for talimogene laherparepvec, a new oncolytic virus immunotherapy. *Clin Cancer Res.* 2016;22(5):1048–1054.
66. Chalan P, Di Dalmazi G, Pani F, De Remigis A, Caturegli P. Thyroid dysfunctions secondary to cancer immunotherapy. *J Endocrinol Invest.* 2018;41(6):625–638.
67. FDA approves second CAR T-cell therapy. *Cancer Discov.* 2018;8(1):5–6.
68. Mullard A. FDA approves first CAR T therapy. *Nat Rev Drug Discov.* 2017;16(10):669.
69. Ramos CA, Ballard B, Zhang H, et al. Clinical and immunological responses after CD30-specific chimeric antigen receptor-redirected lymphocytes. *J Clin Invest.* 2017;127(9):3462–3471.
70. Ahmed N, Brawley V, Hegde M, et al. HER2-specific chimeric antigen receptor-modified virus-specific T cells for progressive glioblastoma: a phase 1 dose-escalation trial. *JAMA Oncol.* 2017;3(8):1094–1101.
71. Wang Y, Chen M, Wu Z, et al. CD133-directed CAR T cells for advanced metastasis malignancies: a phase I trial. *Oncoimmunology.* 2018;7(7):e1440169.
72. Maus MV, Grupp SA, Porter DL, June CH. Antibody-modified T cells: CARs take the front seat for hematologic malignancies. *Blood.* 2014;123(17):2625–2635.
73. Schuster SJ, Svoboda J, Chong EA, et al. Chimeric antigen receptor T cells in refractory B-cell lymphomas. *N Engl J Med.* 2017;377(26):2545–2554.
74. Park JH, Riviere I, Gonen M, et al. Long-term follow-up of CD19 CAR therapy in acute lymphoblastic leukemia. *N Engl J Med.* 2018;378(5):449–459.
75. Maude SL, Laetsch TW, Buechner J, et al. Tisagenlecleucel in children and young adults with B-cell lymphoblastic leukemia. *N Engl J Med.* 2018;378(5):439–448.
76. Blinatumomab approval expanded based on MRD. *Cancer Discov.* 2018;8(6):OF3.
77. Viardot A, Goebeler ME, Hess G, et al. Phase 2 study of the bispecific T-cell engager (BiTE) antibody blinatumomab in relapsed/refractory diffuse large B-cell lymphoma. *Blood.* 2016;127(11):1410–1416.
78. Brinkmann U, Kontermann RE. The making of bispecific antibodies. *MAbs.* 2017;9(2):182–212.
79. Nagorsen D, Baeuerle PA. Immunomodulatory therapy of cancer with T cell-engaging BiTE antibody blinatumomab. *Exp Cell Res.* 2011;317(9):1255–1260.

80. Topp MS, Gokbuget N, Stein AS, et al. Safety and activity of blinatumomab for adult patients with relapsed or refractory B-precursor acute lymphoblastic leukaemia: a multicentre, single-arm, phase 2 study. *Lancet Oncol.* 2015;16(1):57–66.

81. Kantarjian HM, Stein AS, Bargou RC, et al. Blinatumomab treatment of older adults with relapsed/refractory B-precursor acute lymphoblastic leukemia: results from 2 phase 2 studies. *Cancer.* 2016;122(14):2178–2185.

82. Monzani F, Caraccio N, Dardano A, Ferrannini E. Thyroid autoimmunity and dysfunction associated with type I interferon therapy. *Clin Exp Med.* 2004;3(4):199–210.

83. Carella C, Mazziotti G, Amato G, Braverman LE, Roti E. Clinical review 169: Interferon-alpha-related thyroid disease: pathophysiological, epidemiological, and clinical aspects. *J Clin Endocrinol Metab.* 2004;89(8):3656–3661.

84. Khan U, Rizvi H, Sano D, Chiu J, Hadid T. Nivolumab induced myxedema crisis. *J Immunother Cancer.* 2017;5:13.

85. Brahmer JR, Lacchetti C, Schneider BJ, et al. Management of immune-related adverse events in patients treated with immune checkpoint inhibitor therapy: American Society of Clinical Oncology Clinical Practice Guideline. *J Clin Oncol.* 2018;36(17):1714–1768.

86. Puzanov I, Diab A, Abdallah K, et al. Managing toxicities associated with immune checkpoint inhibitors: consensus recommendations from the Society for Immunotherapy of Cancer (SITC) Toxicity Management Working Group. *J Immunother Cancer.* 2017;5(1):95.

87. Rodondi N, den Elzen WP, Bauer DC, et al. Subclinical hypothyroidism and the risk of coronary heart disease and mortality. *JAMA.* 2010;304(12):1365–1374.

88. Wang G, Cai C, Wu B. Thyroid hormones precipitate subclinical hypopituitarism resulted in adrenal crisis. *J Am Geriatr Soc.* 2010;58(12):2441–2442.

89. Haanen J, Carbonnel F, Robert C, et al. Management of toxicities from immunotherapy: ESMO Clinical Practice Guidelines for diagnosis, treatment and follow-up. *Ann Oncol.* 2017;28(suppl 4):iv119–iv142.

90. Min L, Hodi FS, Giobbie-Hurder A, et al. Systemic high-dose corticosteroid treatment does not improve the outcome of ipilimumab-related hypophysitis: a retrospective cohort study. *Clin Cancer Res.* 2015;21(4):749–755.

91. Bornstein SR, Allolio B, Arlt W, et al. Diagnosis and treatment of primary adrenal insufficiency: an endocrine society clinical practice guideline. *J Clin Endocrinol Metab.* 2016;101(2):364–389.

92. Hughes J, Vudattu N, Sznol M, et al. Precipitation of autoimmune diabetes with anti-PD-1 immunotherapy. *Diabetes Care.* 2015;38(4):e55–e57.

93. Aleksova J, Lau PK., Soldatos G, McArthur G. Glucocorticoids did not reverse type 1 diabetes mellitus secondary to pembrolizumab in a patient with metastatic melanoma. *Case Reports.* 2016;bcr2016217454.

94. Trinh B, Donath MY, Läubli H. Successful treatment of immune checkpoint inhibitor–induced diabetes with infliximab. *Diabetes care.* 2019;42(9):e153–e154.

95. Migden MR, Rischin D, Schmults CD, Guminski A, Hauschild A, Lewis KD, Rabinowits G. PD-1 blockade with cemiplimab in advanced cutaneous squamous-cell carcinoma. *New Eng J Med.* 2018;379(4):341–351.

96. Schmid P, Adams S, Rugo HS, Schneeweiss A, Barrios CH, Iwata H, Henschel V. Atezolizumab and nab-paclitaxel in advanced triple-negative breast cancer. *New Eng J Med.* 2018;379(22):2108–2121.

97. Horn L, Mansfield AS, Szczęsna A, Havel L, Krzakowski M, Hochmair MJ, Reck M. First-line atezolizumab plus chemotherapy in extensive-stage small-cell lung cancer. *New Eng J Med.* 2018;379(23):2220–2229.

98. Paz-Ares L, Dvorkin M, Chen Y, Reinmuth N, Hotta K, Trukhin D, Voitko O. Durvalumab plus platinum–etoposide versus platinum–etoposide in first-line treatment of extensive-stage small-cell lung cancer (CASPIAN): a randomised, controlled, open-label, phase 3 trial. *The Lancet.* 2019;394(10212):1929–1939.

99. Faivre-Finn C, Vicente D, Kurata T, Planchard D, Paz-Ares L, Vansteenkiste JF, Naidoo J. LBA49 Durvalumab after chemoradiotherapy in stage III NSCLC: 4-year survival update from the phase III PACIFIC trial. *Annals of Oncology.* 2020;31:S1178–S1179.

100. Powles T, Park SH, Voog E, Caserta C, Valderrama BP, Gurney H, Loriot Y. Avelumab maintenance therapy for advanced or metastatic urothelial carcinoma. *New Eng J Med.* 2020;383(13):1218–1230.

Gastrointestinal Toxicities of Immunotherapy

Shipra Gandhi, MD   Aman Gupta, MD   Marc S. Ernstoff, MD

Introduction

Novel agents have revolutionized the treatment of cancer, resulting in many benefits for patients. These same agents, however, have been associated with new toxicity profiles compared with traditional chemotherapy. Most of these adverse events have been classified as mild or moderate, but unfortunately, severe and life-threatening complications also occur. This section will focus specifically on immunotherapy and subsequent gastrointestinal toxicity. The various approaches that will be discussed in this section include immune checkpoint inhibitors (ICIs), bispecific antibodies (BABs), chimeric antigen receptor (CAR) T cells, interleukin-2 (IL-2) and interferon-α (IFN-α), which attack cancer cells by activating the immune effector cells and disrupting immune tolerance. Immune therapies can be associated with durable responses; however, they are also associated with multiple toxicities as the activated immune system also attacks normal body cells along with the tumor tissue, resulting in several toxicities. The gastrointestinal system is significantly impacted, resulting in nausea, vomiting, anorexia, diarrhea, colitis, and hepatitis. There have been reports of acute pancreatitis due to ICIs, but clinical pancreatitis is rare and may be considered anecdotal at this time.

Description

IMMUNE CHECKPOINT INHIBITORS

Currently, there are several ICIs that are approved by the US Food and Drug Administration (FDA). Ipilimumab, an anti-cytotoxic T-lymphocyte–associated protein 4 (anti-CTLA-4) antibody, was the first ICI approved to be used in metastatic melanoma. Nivolumab and pembrolizumab, which target programmed cell death protein-1 (PD-1) have been approved for use in melanoma, metastatic non–small-cell lung cancer (NSCLC), head and neck squamous cell cancer, urothelial carcinoma, gastric adenocarcinoma, and mismatch repair deficient solid tumors, as well as for classic Hodgkin's lymphoma. Nivolumab is also approved for use in hepatocellular carcinoma and in patients with renal cell carcinoma. The combination of nivolumab and ipilimumab has been approved by the FDA for treatment of metastatic melanoma, renal cell carcinoma, and non-small cell lung cancer. Recently, programmed cell death protein-ligand 1 (PD-L1) antibodies have been approved, namely, atezolizumab (urothelial cancer, triple negative breast cancer and NSCLC) durvalumab (urothelial cancer) and avelumab (Merkel cell carcinoma and urothelial cancer) which also block the PD-1 pathway. This field is rapidly evolving, as new agents and combinations continue to be discovered and tested.[1]

BISPECIFIC ENGAGER OF T-CELL ACTIVITY

Blinatumomab is a novel agent for the treatment of B-precursor acute lymphoblastic leukemia (ALL) that has demonstrated encouraging response rates in the setting of minimal residual disease (MRD)-positive (80% complete remission) and relapsed/refractory (R/R) patients. Blinatumomab is a monoclonal antibody which functions as a bispecific T cell engager, or BiTE, that is directed against CD19 on B cells and against CD3 on T cells. It is approved by the FDA for the treatment of R/R, Philadelphia (Ph)-negative and positive B-precursor ALL in adults and children. Due to the above success, the incorporation of blinatumomab in ALL patients in combination with chemotherapy, targeted therapies, or other immunotherapeutic approaches is currently being actively investigated.[2]

CHIMERIC ANTIGEN RECEPTOR T CELLS

In this emerging treatment modality, T cells are isolated from a patient, genetically engineered to express a CAR, and reintroduced into the patient. CAR T cells have demonstrated efficacy primarily in the treatment of relapsed or refractory ALL, chronic lymphocytic leukemia (CLL), and non-Hodgkin's lymphoma.[3] In August 2017, the FDA approved the first anti-CD19 CAR T cell product, tisagenlecleucel, for the treatment of pediatric and young adult patients with relapsed and/or refractory B-cell precursor ALL.[4] In October 2017, the FDA approved axicabtagene ciloleucel for the treatment of relapsed/refractory diffuse large B-cell lymphoma (DLBCL).[5]

INTERLEUKIN-2

High-dose IL-2 was the first immunotherapy approved for treatment of metastatic melanoma based on durable responses observed, but recently its use has fallen out of favor due to significant toxicities. IL-2 is also approved for the treatment of renal cell carcinoma.[6]

INTERFERON-α

Patients with resected stage II or III melanoma are at high risk of recurrence. Adjuvant IFN-α has been used in the past to decrease the risk of recurrence of melanoma.[7]

Agents and Mechanism of Action

IMMUNE CHECKPOINT INHIBITORS

Checkpoint inhibitors work by the mechanism of "inhibition of inhibition" and thereafter stimulating the immune system by attenuating tolerance and can result in overwhelming inflammation, tissue damage, and autoimmunity. Checkpoint inhibitors work by inhibition of CTLA-4, PD-1 or PD-2; their ligands that normally limit immune reactions in order to avoid tissue damage, allow tolerance. Ipilimumab inhibits CTLA-4, an inhibitory receptor that is constitutively expressed on CD25(+) CD4(+) T-regulatory cells. CTLA-4 is upregulated on activated T cells and transmits an inhibitory signal to downregulate the immune response, thus acting as an immune checkpoint.[8] As ipilimumab inhibits this signaling, it depletes T-regulatory cells and impairs their function in the blood or tumor microenvironment, thus maintaining T-effector cell activation, and increasing antitumor immunity.[9] PD-1 is an immune checkpoint expressed on the surface of activated T cells. PD-L1 is selectively expressed on many tumors and on cells within the tumor microenvironment in response to inflammatory stimuli, such as interferon-γ.[10] Signaling through the PD-1 pathway results in inhibition of cytokine production and apoptosis of PD-1+ tumor-infiltrating T cells.[11] Along with the activation of the effector T lymphocytes, the ICI leads to the depletion of the regulatory T cells.[10] Depletion of the regulatory T cells removes one of the most important antiinflammatory mechanisms of the immune system because these cells are responsible for the production of inhibitory cytokines, including, transforming growth factor-β, IL-10, and IL-35.[12]

By inhibition of this tolerance mechanism, ICIs stimulate cytotoxic T lymphocytes to kill tumor cells, and, as an off-target effect, also result in immune system activation and reactivity against the body's own organs and tissues. They are known as immune related adverse events (irAEs) and are reported in about 85% of patients after treatment with ipilimumab[13] and up to 70% of patients after blockade of the PD-1 axis.[14] The frequency of severe, life-threatening or even fatal (grade ≥3) events is higher after ipilimumab (10%–40%) compared to nivolumab or pembrolizumab (<5%).[14,15] Combination of ICIs results in an increase in the incidence of severe toxicity.[16] The various gastrointestinal (GI) manifestations of ICIs include nausea, vomiting, diarrhea, colitis, and hepatitis.

GI Manifestations With Immune Checkpoint Inhibitors

Anti-CTLA-4. Gastrointestinal tract irAEs following anti-CTLA-4 inhibitors can range from mild diarrhea to severe colitis, or even death.[17] The most common presentation is diarrhea (27%),[18] followed by colitis. Severe enterocolitis unresponsive to immunosuppressive therapy that may even require a subtotal colectomy, as well as perforation or intractable diarrhea, has been reported in the early trials. These are now rare as the condition is recognized and treated aggressively.[19] The median time of onset of ipilimumab-associated colitis is about 34 days.[12] Some reports, however, note a correlation between adverse events and tumor regression, suggesting that toxicity may serve as evidence of immune activation.[12]

Anti-PD-1. The number of adverse events with anti-PD-1 therapies has been reported to be less than with anti-CTLA-4.[20] Nivolumab treatment resulted in diarrhea and colitis in 17% of melanoma patients, with grade 3 toxicities in only 1.2% of patients. Pembrolizumab resulted in colitis in 2.8% of patients, and here a positive correlation was noted between the dosage and the adverse events. The median time of onset of irAE was longer for pembrolizumab (18 weeks) than for nivolumab (6 weeks).[20]

Combination Anti-CTLA-4 and Anti-PD-1 Therapy. The frequency of colitis reported in the literature ranges from 8% to 27%, but the incidence of diarrhea is around 54% in patients treated with anti-CTLA-4 and anti-PD-1 combination therapy.[21] In a meta-analysis of patients treated with ICIs, the relative risk (RR) of all-grade diarrhea and colitis was 1.64 (95% confidence interval [CI], 1.19 to 2.26; P = .002) and 10.35 (95% CI, 5.78 to 18.53; P < .001), the RR of high-grade diarrhea and colitis was reported to be 4.46 (95% CI, 1.46 to 13.57; P = .008) and 15.81 (95% CI, 6.34 to 39.42; P < .001), respectively. RR of upper-GI symptoms (e.g., vomiting) was not significant.[22] Frequency of intestinal perforation has been described at approximately 1%.[23] Compared with lower GI toxicities, the incidence of upper GI toxicities, namely, dysphagia, nausea/vomiting, and epigastric pain, is much less common.

Hepatitis Associated With Immune Checkpoint Inhibitors

Hepatitis is a less frequent complication of ICI therapy. It is characterized by elevated alanine aminotransferase (ALT) or aspartate aminotransferase (AST), with or without increased bilirubin. The median onset of transaminase elevation is approximately 6 to 14 weeks after starting ICIs.[24] Hepatitis is generally picked up on routine laboratory evaluation, but some patients may also present with fever or abdominal discomfort. Any-grade hepatic toxicities with ipilimumab 3 mg/kg monotherapy is less than 4% and this increases to up to 15% when ipilimumab is dosed at 10 mg/kg.[18,25] The incidence of hepatitis is about 5% in patients treated with anti-PD-1 inhibitors only, but this increases to about 25% to 30% grade 3-15% in patients on combination ipilimumab and nivolumab.[24]

Pancreatitis Associated With Immune Checkpoint Inhibitors

Reports of acute pancreatitis with ICIs are rare,[26] whereas asymptomatic elevation of lipase and amylase are more common. Of note is the rare complication of autoimmune endocrine dysfunction of the pancreas with acute onset of type 1 diabetes.

Celiac Disease Associated With Immune Checkpoint Inhibitors

Rare irAE such as celiac disease have also been observed with ICI treatment presenting with nausea, vomiting, diarrhea or abdominal pain. Histological features include intraepithelial lymphocytosis, lymphoplasmacytic inflammation of the lamina propria, villous atrophy and crypt hyperplasia on small bowel biopsy. A gluten-free diet is a reasonable strategy for these patients (either alone or in combination with immunosuppression).[27]

Mechanism of Immune Checkpoint Inhibitor–Mediated GI and Hepatic Manifestations

Biomarkers Predictive of GI irAE. A study with 162 advanced melanoma patients with pretreatment blood samples for biomarkers showed higher baseline levels of immune-related genes (CD3E, IL2RG, CD4, CD37, IL-32, and RAC-2), cell-cycle associated genes (SPATAN1, BANF1, BAT1, PCGF1, FP36L2, and WDR1) and genes involved in vesicle trafficking (PICALM, SNAP23, and VAMP3) in patients who developed GI irAEs compared to those who did not. Biomarkers were also studied 3 weeks after treatment with ICIs; CD177, a unique neutrophil surface marker that plays an essential role in neutrophil activation and also mediates migration, was noted to be elevated. Carcino-embryonic antigen-related cell adhesion molecule (CEACAM), an adherence mediator important in neutrophil migration, was also found to be significantly increased in the GI irAE group.[28] Another inflammatory cytokine, IL-17, has also been proposed as a predictor of irAEs, and has been correlated with the development of grade 3 GI toxicities.[29]

Role of the Gut Microbiome. The gut microbiome has been implicated in the response to ICI therapy. This holds significant promise as fecal transplants in addition to ICI therapy may play a role in enhancing therapy. Fecal abundance of *Bacteroides fragilis* negatively correlated with tumor size following CTLA-4 blockade. Interestingly, as the *B. fragilis* polysaccharide capsule is known to induce IL-12–dependent TH1 immune responses, these immunogenic bacteria show potential to act as "anticancer probiotics."[30]

The gut microbiota plays an important role in maintaining mucosal tolerance by promoting T-regulatory cell expansion or by stimulating anti-inflammatory cytokines. The intestinal microbial composition was sampled in a prospective study from 34 melanoma patients prior to CTLA-4 blockade. Although the patients all shared a similar proportion of *Firmicutes*, the *Bacteroidaceae* family was underrepresented in patients who later developed immune-mediated colitis. *Bacteroidetes* exert anti-inflammatory effects through various pathways. The combination of (1) polyamine transport system and (2) the biosynthesis of vitamins riboflavin (B2), pantothenate (B5), and thiamine (B1) resulted in 70% sensitivity and 83% specificity for predicting patients at risk of developing colitis.[31] Thus, the microbiome may play a role in developing immune-related colitis. Further supporting this hypothesis is the observation that intestinal reconstitution of germ-free mice with the combination of *B. fragilis* and *Burkholderia cepacia* reduced histopathological signs of colitis.[30]

Histological Presentation

Diarrhea and Colitis

- **Anti-CTLA-4:** Colitis seen after anti-CTLA-4 inhibitors is characterized by the presence of neutrophilic inflammation with increased intraepithelial lymphocytes, crypt epithelial cell apoptosis, and few or no features of chronicity.[32]
- **Anti-PD-1:** Two patterns of colitis are seen following the use of anti-PD-1: active colitis (active inflammation, neutrophilic crypt micro-abscesses, increased crypt epithelial cell apoptosis, and presence of crypt atrophy/dropout) or lymphocytic colitis (increased intraepithelial lymphocytes in surface epithelium, surface epithelial injury, and expansion of the lamina propria). Similar histological changes can also be observed outside of the colon in the duodenum, stomach, and/or small bowel.[33] Features of inflammatory bowel disease (IBD)-type chronicity are seen in patients with recurrent anti-PD-1 colitis, which may develop many months after stopping anti-PD-1 therapy.[34]

Nausea/Vomiting/Epigastric Pain. Patchy chronic duodenitis or chronic gastritis with rare granulomas can be seen.[32] These findings suggest the possibility of immune mechanisms which are directed towards region-specific epitopes.

Hepatitis. Liver biopsies of patients on ICIs, reveal a pan-lobular active hepatitis with a predominant CD8-positive inflammatory infiltrate, and hence, the pathological presentation mimics autoimmune hepatitis, and suggests underlying injury to hepatocytes.[35] The cytotoxic T cell infiltrate can also result in injury to the bile ducts, manifesting as mild portal mononuclear infiltrate around the proliferated bile ductules.[36]

BISPECIFIC ENGAGER OF T CELL ACTIVITY/BLINATUMOMAB

Blinatumomab is a bispecific antibody that belongs to a class of agents, which work as engagers of T cell activity via binding to CD19 and CD3. The drug is approved for relapsed or refractory B-precursor ALL. It is administered as a 4-week continuous infusion. Blinatumomab infusion is associated with cytokine release syndrome (CRS), which is a potentially life-threatening systemic inflammatory reaction observed after infusion of agents targeting different immune effectors and also with hemophagocytic lymphohistiocytosis/macrophage activation syndrome (HLH/MAS). The frequency of grade 3 or higher CRS ranged from 2% to 6% in clinical trials in adult patients with relapsed/refractory ALL,[37] and was 6% in a trial conducted in children.[38] Fortunately, CRS is fatal in a very small number of patients. The syndrome manifests with symptoms of fever, chills, hypotension, and tachycardia during or immediately after drug administration.

GI, Hepatic, and Pancreatic Manifestations of Blinatumomab

Blinatumomab can present with a broad spectrum of constitutional and organ-related disorders, and numerous blood test abnormalities. Patients present with nausea, vomiting, diarrhea, and hepatotoxicity (grade ≥3 increased ALT and AST in 9%–16% cases).[37,39]
- Cases of pancreatitis have been reported during blinatumomab treatment; this has been observed mostly during clinical trials. It is important for physicians to be alert, and monitor amylase and lipase if clinically indicated.[40]
- HLH/MAS has also been observed in patients receiving blinatumomab infusion.[41]

Mechanism of Blinatumomab-Mediated GI and Hepatic Toxicities

The two blinatumomab-mediated mechanisms for hepatotoxicity are CRS and HLH/MAS.
- CRS is characterized by an increase in inflammatory cytokine release after the activation and cytotoxic damage of monocytes, macrophages, and different lymphocyte populations. This is associated with extensively high levels of IL-6, which plays a central role in the pathophysiology of these toxicities.[42] Other effects that could be mediated by the release of cytokines include nausea/vomiting and increased AST/ALT levels. The increase in cytokine levels coincides with the early peak in the adverse events' incidence and the development of severe peripheral B lymphocytopenia within days of blinatumomab initiation.
- HLH is a rare condition characterized by inappropriate immune activation and cytokine release that typically presents with fever and splenomegaly in association with hyperferritinemia, coagulopathy, hypertriglyceridemia, and cytopenias.

ADOPTIVE CELLULAR THERAPY (CAR T CELL AND T CELL RECEPTOR GENE THERAPIES)

Cellular immunotherapy consists of autologous or allogenic T cells which have been genetically engineered to express CARs or T cell receptors (TCRs) to redirect cytotoxicity specifically towards cancer cells. These therapies are currently emerging as a promising modality for a broad range of cancers. In August 2017, the FDA approved the first anti-CD19 CAR T cell product, tisagenlecleucel, for the treatment of pediatric and young adult patients with relapsed and/or refractory B-cell precursor ALL. Currently, novel targets such as CD20, NY-ESO-1, and B-cell maturation antigens, are being explored with CAR-based and TCR-redirected cell therapies in preclinical studies and early phase clinical trials, in hematological and non-hematological malignancies.[43] The release of the multitude of chemokines and cytokines results in CRS with diverse manifestations including different organ systems, such as cardiovascular, respiratory, integumentary, GI, hepatic, renal, hematological, and nervous system, and manifests as high fever, hypotension, hypoxia, and/or multiorgan toxicity.[44] There is a high risk of development of CRS in patients with bulky disease.

GI and Hepatic Manifestations With CAR T-Cell Therapy

- The GI and hepatic manifestations of CRS include nausea, vomiting, diarrhea (GI), and increased AST, ALT, or bilirubin levels (hepatic), which are reversible with CRS resolution. In a phase I clinical trial of axicabtagene ciloleucel CAR T-cell therapy in refractory large B-cell lymphoma by Neelapu et al., the incidence of any grade nausea was 58%, any grade anorexia and grade 3 or higher anorexia was 50% and 2%, respectively; any grade diarrhea and grade 3 or higher diarrhea was 43% and 4%, respectively; and any grade vomiting and grade 3 or higher vomiting was 34% and 1%, respectively.[5] Phase I results of the ZUMA-1 study showed that 1/7 patients (14%) developed grade 3 or higher ascites and one in seven patients (14%) developed grade 3 AST elevation.[45] There are studies which have shown that high serum levels of IL-6, soluble gp 130, IFN-γ, IL-15, IL-8, and/or IL-10, either 1 day before or 1 day after CAR T cell infusion, are associated with the subsequent development of CRS, but prospective validation is required for the above tests.[46] The onset of symptoms of CRS toxicity is usually seen within the first week after treatment with CAR T cells and typically peaks within 1 to 2 weeks of cell administration.

Mechanism of CAR T Cell–Mediated GI and Hepatic Toxicities

The three mechanisms responsible for GI and hepatic toxicity with cellular immunotherapy (CAR T cells, TCR-gene therapies) are CRS (most common acute toxicity of CAR T cells), off-target effects, and HLH/MAS.

- **CRS:** The most common toxicity associated with the use of cellular immunotherapy is mediated by the activation of T cells or engagement of their T cell receptors or CARs with antigens which are expressed by the tumor cells. Thus, the activated T cells release cytokines and chemokines, namely IL-2, soluble IL-2Rα, IFN-γ, IL-6, soluble IL-6R, and GM-CSF, and result in hypotension and capillary leak syndrome.[45]
- **Off-target effects:** CAR T cells can also potentially damage normal tissues by targeting a tumor-associated antigen that is also expressed on those tissues.[47] Examples of this mechanism of action have been reported in the literature. In one study, 3 patients with metastatic renal cell carcinoma who were treated with CAR T cells targeting carboxy-anhydrase-IX experienced grade 3 to 4 increases in ALT, AST, or total bilirubin.[48] Liver biopsies of these affected patients demonstrated cholangitis with T cell infiltration surrounding the bile ducts. Surprisingly, bile duct epithelial cells were found to express carboxy-anhydrase-IX.[48]
- **HLH/MAS:** There have also been reports of fulminant HLH/MAS with CAR T-cell therapy. HLH/MAS is marked by severe immune activation, lymphohistiocytic tissue infiltration, and immune-mediated multiorgan failure. A diagnosis of CAR T cell–related HLH/MAS can be made if a patient has a peak ferritin >10,000 ng/mL during the CRS phase (typically observed within the first 5 days after cell infusion) and has developed any two of the following: grade 3 or higher organ toxicities involving the liver, kidney, or lung, or hemophagocytosis in the bone marrow or other organs. HLH/MAS belongs to a spectrum of systemic hyperinflammatory disorders, and thus it is not surprising that these syndromes can occur with cellular therapies. Fulminant refractory HLH/MAS is observed in 1% of patients treated with CAR T-cell therapy.

INTERLEUKIN-2

Interleukin-2 (IL-2) is a cytokine, or biologic response modifier, produced by activated natural killer (NK) cells which promotes clonal T cell expansion during an immune response. It also helps develop and mature T regulatory cells, promotes NK cell activity, and mediates immune tolerance by activation-induced cell death. It mainly binds to IL-2 receptors of either high-affinity containing α(CD25)-, β(CD122)- and γ(CD132)-chains or low-affinity receptors that contain only α- and β-chains. IL-2 induces proliferation and differentiation of both CD4+ and CD8+ cells to effector cells or memory cells. IL-2 elicits a combination of immune responses, including both activation of innate immune effectors including NK cells and macrophages, and specific immune responses mediated by T effector and memory cells for long-term control of tumor recurrence. Subsequent release of various cytokines, including other interleukins, interferons, and colony stimulating factors, is also believed to be important in induction of tumor regression.

GI and Hepatic Manifestations of High-Dose IL-2

Nausea and vomiting are very common adverse events related to IL-2. These symptoms are likely related to the emetogenic potential of IL-2 and the use of nonsteroidal anti-inflammatory drugs as premedication. Anorexia is also very common during IL-2 therapy and may be secondary to systemic inflammation. When IL-2 is associated with diarrhea, it is usually secretory in nature. Hepatic enzyme and function abnormalities are commonly noticed during IL-2 treatment. This can range from asymptomatic laboratory elevations to symptomatic signs of hepatitis. This tends to accumulate in severity as cumulative dose increases. In the PROCLAIM registry, fewer than 5% of patients had hepatitis that required intervention (i.e., holding IL-2).[49] Patients can present with several laboratory abnormalities including low albumin, mild coagulopathy, hyperbilirubinemia, and hepatic enzyme elevation. Clinically, IL-2–related hepatitis can present with jaundice, right upper quadrant abdominal pain, anorexia, nausea, vomiting, and mild abdominal tenderness.

Mechanism of IL-2 Mediated GI and Hepatic Toxicities

In general, toxicities of IL-2 are directly related to the systemic effects of IL-2 and also subsequent cytokines released by T cell activation.

INTERFERON-α

IFN-α induces the transcription of several genes via the JAK-STAT pathway and other signaling pathways.[50] The antitumor mechanism of IFN-α is the cumulative result of cytostatic, anti-angiogenic, and immune-modulatory activities. The immune-modulatory effects of IFN-α include induction of cytokines, upregulation of major histocompatibility antigen expression, enhancement of phagocytic activity of NK cells and macrophages, and augmentation of T cell cytotoxicity against tumor cells.[7]

GI and Hepatic Manifestations With IFN-α

IFN-α2b is the most widely recognized adjuvant IFN-α therapy for patients with resected melanoma who are at high risk for relapse. However, the regimen is associated with significant toxicity. IFN-α is associated with all-grade nausea (66%), vomiting (66%), anorexia (69%), and transaminitis (63%). Grade 3/4 adverse events observed are nausea (9%), vomiting (6%), and transaminitis (14%–29%).[51] Hepatotoxicity occurs soon after initiation of treatment but can occur anytime during treatment. Other causes of elevated liver function tests, such as alcohol, hepatitis B, and hepatitis C, should be considered in this group of patients. Hepatotoxicity, generally manifested as transaminitis, is a common but serious adverse event; as an example, two patients died of liver failure in the E1684 trial.[52]

Mechanism of IFN-α Mediated GI and Hepatic Toxicities

Nausea and Vomiting. Increased activity of IFN-α, IL-1 and other proinflammatory cytokines are implicated in the pathophysiology of nausea and vomiting. These cytokines act on the mono-amine transmitters, especially serotonin. The enterochromaffin cells in the GI mucosa become activated in response to the cytokines to increase the production of 5-HT3.[53]

Anorexia. Cytokines such as IFN-α, IL-1, and TNF-α are implicated in anorexia through their impact systemically as well as within the central nervous system.[53]

Acute Pancreatitis. Hypertriglyceridemia over 1000 mg/dL is associated with acute pancreatitis, and has been anecdotally reported in patients treated with IFN-α.[54] IFN-α decreases the clearance of lipoproteins rich in triglycerides and hence induces hepatic lipogenesis, resulting in hypertriglyceridemia.

Hepatotoxicity. IFN-α acts on the CYP450 enzyme system and suppresses the activation of certain isoenzymes. This plays an important role in the potential for drug interactions as 90% of drug metabolism occurs through the CYP 450 system.[53]

Pharmacologic Approaches for Management and Treatment

IMMUNE CHECKPOINT INHIBITORS

Approach to a Patient With Diarrhea and/or Colitis

The most common clinical presentation of immune-related GI toxicities vary from very frequent loose stools to colitis symptoms (mucus in the stools, abdominal pain, fever, rectal bleeding).[21] The symptom onset is in the range of 5 to 10 weeks after initiation of ICIs, but it can occur even months after discontinuation of ICIs.[21]

Diagnostic Evaluation. The distinction between ICI-associated diarrhea and colitis is a subtle yet important one. Clinicians should be vigilant as to the presence of abdominal pain, rectal bleeding, mucus in the stool, or fever, as these findings may signal colitis, a potentially life-threatening complication of ICIs. Furthermore, cases of intestinal perforation have been described and thus urgent assessment and management is recommended in suspicious cases.[24,55] ICI-associated colitis can be distributed uniformly or can be localized to certain areas, more commonly the proximal colon.[23,56] Diarrhea and/or colitis has been observed months after discontinuation of immunotherapy and can mimic IBD,[57] and thus careful history taking is important in establishing this diagnosis.

Differential Diagnosis of Colitis. Active colitis with an apoptotic pattern on biopsy should include other causes of colitis with prominent apoptosis, such as:
1. Infections (cytomegalovirus [CMV])
2. Acute graft versus host disease (GVHD)[58]
3. Autoimmune enteropathy[59]
4. Medications: There are many medications associated with colitis, most of which are immu-nosuppressants. Patients receiving ICIs are unlikely to be receiving these immunosuppressive medications; however, this bears mention, as some chemotherapeutic agents fall within this category. Colitis secondary to mycophenolate mofetil (MMF)[60] may be apoptosis-predominant and show apoptotic microabscesses. 5-Fluorouracil (5-FU) and anti-TNF antibody have also been reported to substantially cause crypt apoptosis.[61] Methotrexate (MTX) and capecitabine can cause crypt apoptosis, dilated damaged crypts, and architectural distortion.[61] The PI3 kinase inhibitor, idelalisib, can cause acute inflammation, increased intraepithelial lymphocytes, and prominent apoptosis.[62]

5. Idiopathic inflammatory disease: Chronic idiopathic inflammatory bowel disease has been classified into Crohn's disease (CD) and ulcerative colitis (UC). The histological features of CD include granulomas, focal crypt distortion, and ileal involvement. On the other hand, biopsies of patients with UC show type II NK cells that produce significant quantities of IL-13. Also observed in UC are diffuse chronic inflammation, diffuse crypt atrophy, mucin depletion, and absence of ileal inflammation.[63]

Diagnostic Workup for Grades 2, 3, and 4 Colitis.[1] When a patient presents with acute diarrhea, it is important to rule out infectious and inflammatory causes of diarrhea, and hence, should obtain the workup detailed below:

1. Complete blood count (CBC) and comprehensive metabolic panel (CMP), thyroid stimulating hormone (TSH), erythrocyte sedimentation rate (ESR), C-reactive protein (CRP)
2. Stool culture to evaluate for bacterial infectious etiology
3. *Clostridium difficile* testing to evaluate for *C. difficile* colitis
4. CMV DNA polymerase chain reaction (PCR) to evaluate for CMV colitis
5. Stool ova and parasites to evaluate for parasitic infections
6. Inflammatory markers (fecal leukocytes/lactoferrin, fecal calprotectin) and fecal occult blood test (FOBT) to evaluate for inflammatory etiology
7. Screening laboratory work (HIV, viral hepatitis testing, and blood QuantiFERON for TB) in the event that patients will need to be given infliximab (infliximab can cause reactivation of viral hepatitis and TB, and can increase the risk of opportunistic infections in patients with HIV)
8. Computed tomography (CT) scan of the abdomen and pelvis to evaluate for extent of colitis and concomitant inflammation and/or infection
9. GI endoscopy with biopsy (colonoscopy): The presence of ulcerations in the colon predicts a corticosteroid-refractory disease, and thus these patients may require early infliximab. For grade 2 or higher diarrhea, once infectious etiology has been ruled out, systemic immunosuppression should be initiated promptly. Colitis can be associated with a normal mucosa; however, colonoscopy may be helpful as it may identify certain inflammatory features, such as CMV infection on immunohistochemical staining.

    Colitis secondary to anti-CTLA-4 can manifest in two ways: diffuse colitis characterized by mesenteric vessel engorgement and segmental colitis with moderate wall thickening and pericolonic fat stranding (seen on CT).[64] The most accurate means of evaluating the extent and the severity of the colitis is via colonoscopy because recent data has shown that the presence of ulceration on endoscopy predicts for steroid-refractory disease.[65] Colonoscopic examination is recommended for persistent grade 2 or higher diarrhea because of the risks associated with endoscopic procedures.[20] Endoscopic examination often shows inflammatory changes in a continuous pattern throughout the gastrointestinal tract, such as exudates, granularity, loss of vascularity, and ulcerations.[56] Although colonoscopy is considered the gold standard exploratory technique, rectosigmoidoscopy also appears to be a feasible option. Whereas on one hand, colonoscopy requires an efficient bowel preparation and general sedation in the vast majority of patients, a rectosigmoidoscopy can be performed without sedation with a simple enema preparation and can lead to a rapid diagnosis. Even in the absence of morphological abnormalities, biopsies should be taken to evaluate for colitis.[19]

10. Patients not responding to immunosuppressive agents may need repeat endoscopy. This is particularly important in patients with grades 3 and 4 toxicity. Repeating endoscopy for disease monitoring should be offered when it is clinically indicated or when the plan is to resume therapy.

Restarting Checkpoint Inhibitors

- Grades 2 or 3: If patients improve from their irAE after adequate treatment, they can be rechallenged with anti-PD-1 therapy as only a small proportion of patients with ICI-related colitis experience recurrences with anti-PD-1 resumption alone.[66]
- Grade 4 diarrhea/colitis: ICI therapy should be permanently discontinued.

Approach to a Patient With Nausea/Vomiting/Epigastric Pain

The approach to these patients is similar to that of patients with colitis. Initial treatment is corticosteroids followed by TNF-α blockers for refractory cases. Notably, the evidence for this approach is based on case studies.[65]

Expert Consultation

When patients present with diarrhea/colitis and previous immunotherapy exposure is considered a possible etiology, the patient should be referred to a gastroenterologist experienced with immunotherapy-related colitis and an endoscopy with biopsy should be performed. In some cases, colitis can progress to chronic IBD long term.[12] These patients should continue to follow up with a gastroenterologist long-term.

Table 19.1 describes the management of ICI-mediated grade 2 to 4 diarrhea based on the Society for Immunotherapy of Cancer (SITC) Toxicity Management Working Group[67] and the American Society of Clinical Oncology (ASCO) Clinical Practice Guidelines.[1]

Preventive Treatment

Currently, no preventive treatment has shown sufficient efficacy. In a double-blind phase II study by Weber et al., comparing the tolerability and efficacy of ipilimumab with or without prophylactic budesonide in patients with unresectable stage III or IV melanoma, the rate of grade 2 or higher diarrhea was no different between the group receiving budesonide compared with the group receiving placebo.[25]

Concomitant *Clostridium difficile* Colitis

Clostridium difficile colitis can coexist with immune-mediated colitis; therefore, potential *C. difficile* infection should be assessed by *C. difficile* toxin polymerase chain reaction (PCR) in the stool and be treated (metronidazole or oral vancomycin). Concomitant treatment with both antibiotics and steroids for patients on checkpoint inhibitors is not uncommon.

Patient Education

Because there is a 10% to 30% incidence of GI side effects associated with the use of ICIs, it is very important to educate patients about the signs and symptoms to expect with treatment as this can decrease diagnostic delay.[68]

ICI Use in Patients With Autoimmune Disease

Patients with autoimmune diseases were generally excluded from clinical trials with ICIs and, hence, minimal data about the safety and efficacy of CTLA-4 and PD-1 inhibitors in this group is available. Retrospective studies have shown exacerbation of preexisting disease after treatment with ICIs.[69] Some have even raised the possibility of prophylactic colectomy prior to ipilimumab therapy in patients with underlying IBD when no other treatment options exist.[70] From the very limited data that is available, ICIs have been administered to patients with underlying autoimmune diseases, but careful monitoring is essential.[69] Further study is necessary to determine the safety of ICIs in patients with underlying autoimmune disorders.

Approach to a Patient With Hepatitis

Baseline Workup. Prior to initiating ICI therapy, baseline testing, including viral hepatitis serologies, transaminase levels (AST, ALT), and bilirubin, should be performed. The various viral serologies, which should be ordered prior to initiating ICIs, include: Hepatitis-B virus (HBV) surface antigen (HbsAg), Hepatitis-B core antibody (HBcAb), and Hepatitis C virus (HCV) antibody. A positive HBsAg or HBcAb serology should prompt evaluation of HBV DNA and a positive HCV antibody should be followed by HCV RNA levels. It is important for clinicians to obtain a hepatology

TABLE 19.1 ■ Management of Immune Checkpoint Inhibitor-Mediated Grades 2–4 Diarrhea[a]

Grade	CTCAE Description	Management
2	Increase of 4 to 6 stools per day over baseline, mild increase in ostomy output compared with baseline	- Withhold ICI until symptoms recover to grade 1 or less. Can consider to permanently discontinue anti-CTLA-4 agents and may restart PD-1, PD-L1 agents if patient recovers to grade 1 or less. - Immunosuppressive maintenance therapy (<10 mg prednisone equivalent dose) - Imodium if infection ruled out. - Gastroenterology consult for grade 2 or higher. - Prednisone or equivalent 1–2 mg/kg/day if infection ruled out. - When symptoms improve to grade 1 or less, taper corticosteroids over 4–6 weeks before resuming treatment. - EGD/colonoscopy for cases grade 2 or higher, to determine when to start early infliximab and for safety of resuming PD-1/PD-L1 therapy. - Stool lactoferrin or calprotectin to differentiate functional versus inflammatory diarrhea. - Repeat colonoscopy is optional and may be offered for cases grade 2 or higher for disease activity monitoring.
3	Increase of 7 or more stools per day over baseline, incontinence, hospitalization indicated, severe increase in ostomy output compared with baseline, limiting self-care ADL	- Hospitalization or outpatient facility treatment of dehydrated. - Permanently discontinue CTLA-4 agents and may restart PD-1, PD-L1 agents if patients recover to grade 1 or less. - Corticosteroids (1–2 mg/kg/day) prednisone or equivalent. - If symptoms persist ≥3–5 days or recur after improvement, IV corticosteroids or noncorticosteroid (infliximab). - Colonoscopy may be offered if patients have been immunosuppressed or at risk of opportunistic infections (CMV colitis) or on anti-TNF agents, or steroid refractory.
4	Life-threatening consequences, urgent intervention indicated	- Admit patients if clinically indicated. If outpatient, closely monitor. - Permanently discontinue ICI. - IV steroids, until symptoms improve to grade 1, taper over 4–6 weeks. - Early infliximab 5–10 mg/kg if symptoms refractory to steroids within 2–3 days. - If symptoms refractory to infliximab, and/or contraindicated to TNF-α blocker, vedolizumab (anti-integrin α4β7 antibody) can be used on an individual basis. - GI endoscopy if symptoms refractory despite treatment.

[a]Based on Society for Immunotherapy of Cancer (SITC) Toxicity Management Working Group and ASCO Clinical Practice Guidelines.

ADL, Activities of daily living; ASCO, American Society of Clinical Oncology; CMV, cytomegalovirus; CTCAE, common terminology criteria for adverse events; CTLA-4, cytotoxic T-lymphocyte–associated protein 4; EGD, esophagogastroduodenoscopy; GI, gastrointestinal; ICI, immune checkpoint inhibitor; PD-1, programmed cell death protein-1; PD-L1, programmed cell death protein-ligand 1.

consultation for patients with positive viral serology, in order to consider treatment for viral hepatitis, either prior to starting ICIs or while concurrently on ICIs. Factors which dictate initiating treatment for viral hepatitis include viral load, liver enzymes, and underlying liver conditions. Other causes which can lead to liver enzyme elevations such as alcohol use, viral infection, thromboembolic and outflow obstructive etiology, other medications, and cancer progression, must be ruled out.

Monitoring on Immune Checkpoint Inhibitors. While a patient is on ICIs, being cognizant of the potential hepatotoxicity of the regimen is important, but at the same time, it is important to rule out other factors that could also lead to elevation of the liver enzymes. These include concurrent or prior treatments, underlying malignancy, infection, or inflammation. Isolated increases in ALT in patients with known HBV or HCV infection could be due to activation of the immune system, hence leading to an increased immune response to HBV and HCV and a subsequent decrease in the viral load.

- Liver function tests should be repeated prior to every dose of the ICI. If an elevation in liver enzymes of more than twice the upper limit is noted, it should immediately prompt workup for other causes of liver injury. The various questions that should be asked include current medications/alternative therapy/herbal medications and any suspicious hepatotoxic drugs that the patient could be taking. Additional testing should include ANA, anti-smooth muscle antibody (SMA), antineutrophil cytoplasmic antibodies, Epstein Barr Virus (EBV) IgM, and CMV PCR on a case-by-case basis for investigating liver dysfunction.[71] In patients with elevated ALP alone, γ-glutamyl transferase (GGT) should be tested.

Imaging. Imaging findings can vary in hepatitis. In mild cases, findings on abdominal CT may look normal. In more severe cases, patients can present with hepatomegaly, edema, enlarged periportal lymph nodes, and attenuated liver parenchyma on CT and magnetic resonance imaging (MRI). Ultrasound findings can also show prominent periportal echogenicity and gallbladder wall edema. Anatomical etiology, such as progression of hepatic metastases, should be considered in these patients and thus prompt ultrasound or CT scan imaging is indicated. Furthermore, hyperprogressive disease is also possible. Hyperprogressive disease is characterized by its accelerated progression in a slowly progressive disease in up to 9% patients on initiating ICIs (anti-PD-1/PD-L1 therapy).[72]

Liver Biopsy. Liver biopsy should be considered in patients with negative viral hepatitis serologies who continue to have persistent grade 2 hepatotoxicity despite 3 to 4 days of adequate steroid therapy, and in patients who present with grade 3 and 4 toxicity. Liver biopsy, if performed, can demonstrate hepatocyte injury (acute hepatitis pattern) with sinusoidal infiltrates, central hepatic vein damage and endothelial inflammation similar to autoimmune hepatitis, or predominant bile duct injury (biliary pattern with portal inflammation).[35,36] Rarely, fibrin ring granulomas have also been reported.[73] However, as evident, there is significant overlap between features of autoimmune hepatitis and ICI-related liver injury.

Pharmacological Management of ICI-Associated Hepatitis. Table 19.2 shows the pharmacological management of ICI-mediated grade 2 to 4 hepatitis based on the SITC Toxicity Management Working Group[67] and ASCO Clinical Practice Guidelines.[1] Notably, *Pneumocystis carinii* prophylaxis should be provided to patients who receive prednisone equivalent of 20 mg or more for longer than 4 weeks.[74]

Inpatient Admission. Patients who present with rising AST/ALT despite treatment with prednisone, or patients who experience liver enzyme increase of more than 10 times the upper limit of normal (ULN) (with or without bilirubin elevation >5 times the ULN), should be admitted for management in the inpatient setting. IV methylprednisolone should be started at 4 mg/kg/day emergently, hepatology consult should be obtained, and liver biopsy should be strongly considered. Liver function tests (LFTs) should be monitored daily until the AST/ALT is less than 8 times the ULN. If LFTs do not respond to IV steroids after 2 days, MMF should be added. Patients with refractory hepatitis that does not respond to steroids and MMF usually respond to antithymocyte globulin (ATG) therapy.[75] Infliximab, which is usually effective in severe autoimmune adverse reactions, should be avoided in autoimmune hepatitis as it can by itself be hepatotoxic.

Restarting Checkpoint Inhibitors. The decision to resume checkpoint inhibitors after an episode of checkpoint-inhibitor–related toxicity should be based on the degree of hepatocyte damage and the duration of toxicity. Checkpoint inhibitors should not be restarted if: (1) peak AST/ALT

TABLE 19.2 ■ **Pharmacological Management of Immune Checkpoint Inhibitor-Mediated Grades 2–4 Hepatitis[a]**

Grade	CTCAE Description	Management
2	Asymptomatic (AST, ALT > 3–≤5 × ULN; and/or total bilirubin >1.5–≤3 × ULN)	- Withhold ICI treatment temporarily and resume if recover to grade 1 or less on prednisone ≤10 mg/day. - Steroids 0.5–1 mg/kg/day if abnormal elevation persists with significant clinical symptoms in 3–5 days. - Laboratory monitoring every 3 days. - May resume ICI treatment followed by taper when symptoms improve to grade 1 or less on steroids ≤10 mg/day. - Stop any known hepatotoxic drugs.
3	Symptomatic liver dysfunction, fibrosis by biopsy, compensated cirrhosis, reactivation of chronic hepatitis (AST, ALT 5–20 × ULN; and/or total bilirubin 3–10 × ULN)	- May offer inpatient monitoring for patients with AST/ALT ≥8 times ULN and/or elevated bilirubin ≥3 times ULN. - Permanently discontinue treatment with ICI. - Corticosteroid 1–2 mg/kg initial dose. Taper over 4–6 weeks. - If steroid refractory or no improvement after 3 days, may give mycophenolate mofetil or azathioprine (test for thiopurine methyltransferase deficiency). - Laboratory monitoring every 1–2 days. - Can use non-TNF-α agents as systemic immunosuppressants. - If no improvement, referral to hepatologist for pathologic evaluation of hepatitis.
4	Decompensated liver function (ascites, coagulopathy, encephalopathy, coma; AST/ALT >20 × ULN and/or total bilirubin >10 × ULN)	- May offer inpatient monitoring. Monitor labs daily. - Permanently discontinue treatment with ICI. - 2 mg/kg/day methylprednisolone equivalent. Steroid taper over 4–6 weeks when symptoms improve to grade 1 or less, re-escalate if needed. Optimal duration unclear. - If corticosteroid refractory or no improvement after 3 days, may offer mycophenolate mofetil. TNF-α blocker infliximab is not recommended due to concern of liver toxicity, despite lack of evidence. - Refer to hepatology if no improvement achieved with steroids. - Consider transfer to tertiary hospital if needed.

[a]Based on the Society for Immunotherapy of Cancer (SITC) Toxicity Management Working Group and ASCO Clinical Practice Guidelines.

ALT, Alanine aminotransferase; *ASCO*, American Society of Clinical Oncology; *AST*, aspartate aminotransferase; *CTCAE*, common terminology criteria for adverse events; *ICI*, immune checkpoint inhibitor; *ULN*, upper limit of normal.

elevation is more than 5 times ULN; (2) levels of AST/ALT do not improve to grade 1 levels (or baseline levels); and (3) patients show signs of liver decompensation, such as an increasing INR.[71]

Approach to a Patient With Colitis and Hepatitis

Patients with both hepatitis and colitis are rare. Management should include permanently discontinuing the ICI and offering other immunosuppressant medications.

Approach to a Patient With Pancreatitis

Routine monitoring of amylase/lipase in asymptomatic patients is not recommended unless pancreatitis is clinically suspected. In the absence of symptoms, steroid treatment is not indicated for modest elevations in serum amylase and lipase.[76]

BISPECIFIC ANTIBODIES AND CAR T-CELL THERAPY

Prophylaxis Prior to Blinatumomab Infusion

There is a high incidence of CRS associated with blinatumomab infusion, and thus, patients with high tumor burdens, such as blast infiltration of the bone marrow of more than 50%, 15,000 blasts/μL or higher in the peripheral blood, or other signs of increased leukemia load, such as high lactate dehydrogenase (LDH), should be pretreated with dexamethasone for up to 5 days in order to reduce tumor load.[77] In all patients, premedication with dexamethasone 20 mg for adult patients, or 5 mg/m^2 for pediatric patients up to a maximum dose of 20 mg should be given 1 hour before treatment to decrease the risk of CRS. Because of the possibility of adverse events with blinatumomab during the early phase of therapy, it is recommended that patients be hospitalized for the beginning of each cycle, and at each time the dose is increased.[77]

CRS Management

CRS secondary to the use of bispecific antibodies or CAR T cells presents with multiple organ abnormalities, including transaminitis. The treatment for both etiologies remains the same and is generally administration of the monoclonal antibody against IL-6, tocilizumab. Tocilizumab represents a therapeutic option to neutralize a key mediator of the inflammatory syndrome and to interrupt progression of the inflammatory process. However, since tocilizumab is costly and is associated with multiple serious adverse events, including infections, reactivation of viruses and tuberculosis, and hepatotoxicity, treatment with tocilizumab should be limited to critically ill patients. Notably based on the National Cancer Institute (NCI) recommendations for the use of tocilizumab, hepatotoxicity is not an indication for its use.[44]

CRS Due to CAR T-Cell Therapy. For patients who present with CRS grade 2 (grade 2 colitis, diarrhea, or transaminitis), CRS grade 3 (grade 3 colitis, diarrhea, or grade 3 or 4 transaminitis), or CRS grade 4 (grade 4 colitis or diarrhea): supportive care and tocilizumab is recommended. Repeat dosing of tocilizumab is recommended if clinical improvement does not occur within 24 to 48 hours. Alternative options include administration of a second immunosuppressive agent, such as corticosteroids.[42]

CRS Due to Bispecific Antibodies[78]
- **Grade 3 CRS (grade 3 diarrhea, grade 3 colitis or grade 3/4 transaminitis):** In adult patients with grade 3 CRS, blinatumomab should be withheld until complete resolution of CRS; it can then be reinitiated at 9 μg/day and dose-escalated to 28 μg/day after 7 days. Grade 3 CRS can also be treated with corticosteroids and tocilizumab (experience limited) as clinically appropriate.
- **Grade 4 CRS (grade 4 diarrhea/colitis):** Grade 4 CRS warrants permanent discontinuation of blinatumomab. Again, these patients should be treated with corticosteroids and tocilizumab (experience limited).

Management of HLH/MAS. Rare manifestations of CRS such as secondary HLH/MAS, have been described with blinatumomab and with CAR T-cell therapies, and may require cytokine-directed therapies.[41] Patients on CAR T-cell therapy who have suspected HLH/MAS should be managed with anti-IL-6 therapy and with corticosteroids for grade 3 or higher toxicities as per CRS recommendations. Cytokine-directed therapy has been successful in patients who have developed HLH/MAS after receiving blinatumomab. This treatment resulted in resolution of multisystem organ failure without reversing anti-leukemic activity.[41] Strategies developed with CAR T-cell therapy have also been used successfully in patients with progressive blinatumomab-related CRS, though experience is limited. Tocilizumab (8 mg/kg IV, 1-time dose) is currently the agent of choice for patients ≥30 kg, but, its exact role remains unclear.[79] The role of tocilizumab with CAR T cells cannot be directly extrapolated to blinatumomab, due to the long and short durations of IL-6 elevation, respectively, between the two therapeutic modalities.[3,80] In cases of HLH/MAS where no improvement is observed after 48 hours, additional therapy with etoposide 75–100 mg/m^2 should be considered.[81] Etoposide can be used in patients with liver and kidney dysfunction. Although etoposide is used in patients with familial and malignancy-associated HLH, evidence to use the same in HLH induced by CAR T-cells therapy is currently lacking and needs to be investigated further.

■ The goal of therapy in HLH is suppression of overactive CD8+ T cells and macrophages that are responsible for this immunological syndrome. In the future, agents targeting IFN-γ may be useful as this is the primary mediator of HLH. For example, a humanized anti-IFN-γ mAb, empalumab, produced responses in 63% children with refractory primary HLH, with good tolerability.[82]

INTERLEUKIN-2

Nausea and Vomiting

Antiemetics are recommended both prophylactically and as needed for breakthrough nausea and vomiting in patients receiving IL-2. Some patients may need more intensive antinausea medications. Preferred drugs are ondansetron and granisetron, but prochlorperazine can be added if necessary.

Mucositis

Mucositis associated with IL-2 is treated similar to chemotherapy-associated mucositis, and is generally self-limiting and treated with nonalcohol–containing mouthwashes.

Diarrhea

In severe cases, some centers postpone IL-2 dosing until diarrhea resolves, whereas others withhold IL-2 for diarrhea greater than 1000 mL/12 hours and stop IL-2 for diarrhea greater than 2000 mL/12 hours. Antidiarrheals, like Imodium and Lomotil, can also be used. *Clostridium difficile* should also be considered. A single dose of vancomycin can also be given to decrease the impact of diarrhea.[83]

INTERFERON-α

Nausea and Vomiting

Nausea and vomiting associated with IFN-α typically occurs 1 to 2 hours post-dose and is manageable with standard antiemetics; acetaminophen and/or nonsteroidal anti-inflammatory agents can be added for associated abdominal discomfort.[53]

Anorexia

Anorexia associated with IFN-α is typically managed the same way as with any other treatment. First, the underlying cause should be treated. If nausea is the predominant problem, antiemetics can be used. If gastrointestinal dysmotility is present, a prokinetic agent such as metoclopramide can be used. Pain and depression should be assessed and treated appropriately. If the underlying cause cannot be addressed, then a concerted effort must be made to maximize nutritional intake whenever possible.[53]

Nonpharmacological Approaches for Management and Treatment

IMMUNE CHECKPOINT INHIBITORS

Diarrhea

Patients presenting with fewer than six stools per day over baseline (grade 1 or 2 diarrhea based on NCI CTC v4), can be managed in the outpatient setting. No specific diagnostic workup is recommended for grade 1 adverse events. Treatment continuation is possible in the case of grade I diarrhea (<4 stools/day over baseline) with close medical supervision. However, it is important

TABLE 19.3 ■ Nonpharmacological Management of Grade 1 Diarrhea and Grade 1 Hepatitis[a]

Grade	CTCAE Description	Management
1	Asymptomatic; clinical or diagnostic observations only; intervention not indicated (Grade 1 diarrhea frequency ≤4/day)	Close follow up within 24–48 h for changes or progression • Continue ICI • If symptoms persist, start routine stool and blood tests • Bland diet advisable during period of acute diarrhea • Antidiarrheal medication is optional but not highly recommended when infectious workup is negative.

[a]Based on the SITC Toxicity Management Working Group and ASCO Clinical Practice Guidelines.

ASCO, American Society of Clinical Oncology; *CTCAE*, common terminology criteria for adverse events; *ICI*, immune checkpoint inhibitor; *SITC*, Society for Immunotherapy of Cancer.

to note that in the case of persistent or worsening of symptoms, ICI treatment should be withheld. Treatment may be considered upon resolution to grade 0 to 1 symptoms. Patients should be monitored for dehydration and dietary changes should be recommended. For prolonged grade 1 cases, gastroenterology consult should be obtained. Further testing to evaluate for infectious etiology should be performed.

Hepatitis

Patients should be monitored for abnormal liver blood tests: AST, ALT, and bilirubin levels prior to each infusion and weekly if there are grade 1 LFT elevations. ICIs can generally be continued in grade 1 liver dysfunction, but with close monitoring.
  ■ Tables 19.3 and 19.4 show the nonpharmacological management of grade 1 diarrhea and grade 1 hepatitis based on the SITC Toxicity Management Working Group[67] and ASCO Clinical Practice Guidelines.[1]

BISPECIFIC ANTIBODIES AND CAR T-CELL THERAPY

Both bispecific antibodies and CAR T-cells therapy may result in elevation in LFTs as part of CRS and HLH/MAS. However, it has been observed that these liver abnormalities can occur at any time during the course of the treatment and, hence, need intermittent monitoring and drug interruption if AST or ALT levels exceed 5 times the ULN or total bilirubin exceeds 3 times the ULN.[77] Liver enzymes generally transiently increase during the first treatment week, without any

TABLE 19.4 ■ Nonpharmacologic Management of Grade 1 Diarrhea and Grade 1 Hepatitis[a]

Grade	CTCAE Description	Management
1	Asymptomatic (AST, ALT > ULN– 3 × ULN; and/or total bilirubin > ULN–1.5 × ULN)	Continue ICI with close monitoring. Consider alternate etiologies. Monitor labs once or twice weekly. Manage with supportive care for symptom control.

[a]Based on the SITC Toxicity Management Working Group and ASCO Clinical Practice Guidelines.

ALT, Alanine aminotransferase; *ASCO*, American Society of Clinical Oncology; *AST*, aspartate aminotransferase; *CTCAE*, common terminology criteria for adverse events; *ICI*, immune checkpoint inhibitor; *SITC*, Society for Immunotherapy of Cancer; *ULN*, upper limit of normal.

clinical symptoms, and reverse to baseline levels within several weeks, and do not usually require any infusion interruptions.[85]

It is recommended that patients be hospitalized for about 1 week after CAR T cell infusion. They should have assessment of vital signs regularly and complete metabolic profile evaluation daily. It may be imperative to perform a chemistry panel more than once daily, especially in patients with high risk of CRS, such as patients with high tumor burden, who are at risk of having tumor cell lysis. It is important to monitor their daily fluid balance and body weight, and maintenance intravenous hydration is recommended for all patients who are at risk of developing CRS. These patients should have central venous access even before infusion of CAR T cells is begun in order to prepare for the medication administration needed to manage toxicities.

INTERLEUKIN-2

Anorexia

Anorexia generally resolves within 24 hours of stopping IL-2. Given the short duration of anorexia, it is acceptable for patients not to eat during treatment.

Hepatotoxicity

Hepatotoxicity usually resolves with cessation of IL-2 treatment. Hepatic enzymes should be monitored daily during treatment. Consensus recommendations suggest discontinuing IL-2 for bilirubin higher than 7 mg/dL or for severe, unrelenting abdominal pain.[83]

INTERFERON-α

Hepatotoxicity

LFTs should be assessed at baseline and monitored regularly. Abnormal LFTs require more frequent monitoring. Grade 3+ transaminitis (ALT or AST >5 × ULN) requires withholding IFN-α treatment. Resumption of IFN-α2b at a reduced dose should only be considered upon resolution to grade 1 transaminitis or less.[53]

Pancreatitis

Serum triglyceride levels rapidly decline after discontinuation of IFN-α therapy and return to normal levels within a few weeks.[54] Dietary modifications and gemfibrozil therapy may also be helpful in this case.

References

1. Brahmer JR, Lacchetti C, Schneider BJ, et al. Management of immune-related adverse events in patients treated with immune checkpoint inhibitor therapy: American Society of Clinical Oncology Clinical Practice Guideline. *J Clin Oncol.* 2018;36(17):1714–1768.
2. Przepiorka D, Ko CW, Deisseroth A, et al. FDA approval: blinatumomab. *Clin Cancer Res.* 2015; 21(18):4035–4039.
3. Grupp SA, Kalos M, Barrett D, et al. Chimeric antigen receptor-modified T cells for acute lymphoid leukemia. *N Engl J Med.* 2013;368(16):1509–1518.
4. Liu Y, Chen X, Han W, et al. Tisagenlecleucel, an approved anti-CD19 chimeric antigen receptor T-cell therapy for the treatment of leukemia. *Drugs Today (Barc).* 2017;53(11):597–608.
5. Neelapu SS, Locke FL, Bartlett NL, et al. Axicabtagene ciloleucel CAR T-cell therapy in refractory large B-cell lymphoma. *N Engl J Med.* 2017;377(26):2531–2544.
6. Atkins MB, Lotze MT, Dutcher JP, et al. High-dose recombinant interleukin 2 therapy for patients with metastatic melanoma: analysis of 270 patients treated between 1985 and 1993. *J Clin Oncol.* 1999; 17(7):2105–2116.

7. Jonasch E, Haluska FG. Interferon in oncological practice: review of interferon biology, clinical applications, and toxicities. *Oncologist.* 2001;6(1):34–55.
8. Chambers CA, Kuhns MS, Egen JG, et al. CTLA-4-mediated inhibition in regulation of T cell responses: mechanisms and manipulation in tumor immunotherapy. *Annu Rev Immunol.* 2001;19:565–594.
9. Simpson TR, Li F, Montalvo-Ortiz W, et al. Fc-dependent depletion of tumor-infiltrating regulatory T cells co-defines the efficacy of anti-CTLA-4 therapy against melanoma. *J Exp Med.* 2013;210(9):1695–1710.
10. Pardoll DM. The blockade of immune checkpoints in cancer immunotherapy. *Nat Rev Cancer.* 2012;12(4):252–264.
11. Brahmer JR, Tykodi SS, Chow LQ, et al. Safety and activity of anti-PD-L1 antibody in patients with advanced cancer. *N Engl J Med.* 2012;366(26):2455–2465.
12. Marthey L, Mateus C, Mussini C, et al. Cancer immunotherapy with anti-CTLA-4 monoclonal antibodies induces an inflammatory bowel disease. *J Crohns Colitis.* 2016;10(4):395–401.
13. Horvat TZ, Adel NG, Dang TO, et al. Immune-related adverse events, need for systemic immunosuppression, and effects on survival and time to treatment failure in patients with melanoma treated with ipilimumab at Memorial Sloan Kettering Cancer Center. *J Clin Oncol.* 2015;33(28):3193–3198.
14. Michot JM, Bigenwald C, Champiat S, et al. Immune-related adverse events with immune checkpoint blockade: a comprehensive review. *Eur J Cancer.* 2016;54:139–148.
15. Weber JS, Antonia SJ, Topalian SL, et al. Safety profile of nivolumab (NIVO) in patients (pts) with advanced melanoma (MEL): a pooled analysis. *J Clin Oncol.* 2015;33(15).
16. Larkin J, Chiarion-Sileni V, Gonzalez R, et al. Combined nivolumab and ipilimumab or monotherapy in untreated melanoma. *N Engl J Med.* 2015;373(1):23–34.
17. Gonzalez-Cao M, Boada A, Teixidó C, et al. Fatal gastrointestinal toxicity with ipilimumab after BRAF/MEK inhibitor combination in a melanoma patient achieving pathological complete response. *Oncotarget.* 2016;7(35):56619–56627.
18. Hodi FS, Hodi FS, O'Day SJ, et al. Improved survival with ipilimumab in patients with metastatic melanoma. *N Engl J Med.* 2010;363(8):711–723.
19. Beck KE, Blansfield JA, Tran KQ, et al. Enterocolitis in patients with cancer after antibody blockade of cytotoxic T-lymphocyte-associated antigen 4. *J Clin Oncol.* 2006;24(15):2283–2289.
20. Eigentler TK, Hassel JC, Berking C, et al. Diagnosis, monitoring and management of immune-related adverse drug reactions of anti-PD-1 antibody therapy. *Cancer Treat Rev.* 2016;45:7–18.
21. Kumar V, Chaudhary N, Garg M, et al. Current diagnosis and management of immune related adverse events (irAEs) induced by immune checkpoint inhibitor therapy. *Front Pharmacol.* 2017;8:49.
22. Abdel-Rahman O, El Halawani H, Fouad M. Risk of gastrointestinal complications in cancer patients treated with immune checkpoint inhibitors: a meta-analysis. *Immunotherapy.* 2015;7(11):1213–1227.
23. Gupta A, De Felice KM, Loftus EV Jr, et al. Systematic review: colitis associated with anti-CTLA-4 therapy. *Aliment Pharmacol Ther.* 2015;42(4):406–417.
24. Spain L, Diem S, Larkin J. Management of toxicities of immune checkpoint inhibitors. *Cancer Treat Rev.* 2016;44:51–60.
25. Weber J, Thompson JA, Hamid O, et al. A randomized, double-blind, placebo-controlled, phase II study comparing the tolerability and efficacy of ipilimumab administered with or without prophylactic budesonide in patients with unresectable stage III or IV melanoma. *Clin Cancer Res.* 2009;15(17):5591–5598.
26. Oble DA, Mino-Kenudson M, Goldsmith J, et al. Alpha-CTLA-4 mAb-associated panenteritis: a histologic and immunohistochemical analysis. *Am J Surg Pathol.* 2008;32(8):1130–1137.
27. Badran YR, Shih A, Leet D, et al. Immune checkpoint inhibitor-associated celiac disease [published correction appears in J Immunother Cancer. 2020 Jul;8(2):]. *J Immunother Cancer.* 2020;8(1):e000958. doi:10.1136/jitc-2020-000958
28. Shahabi V, Berman D, Chasalow SD, et al. Gene expression profiling of whole blood in ipilimumab-treated patients for identification of potential biomarkers of immune-related gastrointestinal adverse events. *J Transl Med.* 2013;11:75.
29. Tarhini AA, Zahoor H, Lin Y, et al. Baseline circulating IL-17 predicts toxicity while TGF-beta1 and IL-10 are prognostic of relapse in ipilimumab neoadjuvant therapy of melanoma. *J Immunother Cancer.* 2015;3:39.
30. Vetizou M, Pitt JM, Daillère R, et al. Anticancer immunotherapy by CTLA-4 blockade relies on the gut microbiota. *Science.* 2015;350(6264):1079–1084.

31. Dubin K, Callahan MK, Ren B, et al. Intestinal microbiome analyses identify melanoma patients at risk for checkpoint-blockade-induced colitis. *Nat Commun.* 2016;7:10391.
32. Verschuren EC, van den Eertwegh AJ, Wonders J, et al. Clinical, endoscopic, and histologic characteristics of ipilimumab-associated colitis. *Clin Gastroenterol Hepatol.* 2016;14(6):836–842.
33. Gonzalez RS, Salaria SN, Bohannon CD, et al. PD-1 inhibitor gastroenterocolitis: case series and appraisal of 'immunomodulatory gastroenterocolitis'. *Histopathology.* 2017;70(4):558–567.
34. Venditti O, De Lisi D, Caricato M, et al. Ipilimumab and immune-mediated adverse events: a case report of anti-CTLA4 induced ileitis. *BMC Cancer.* 2015;15:87.
35. Johncilla M, Misdraji J, Pratt DS, et al. Ipilimumab-associated hepatitis: clinicopathologic characterization in a series of 11 cases. *Am J Surg Pathol.* 2015;39(8):1075–1084.
36. Kim KW, Ramaiya NH, Krajewski KM, et al. Ipilimumab associated hepatitis: imaging and clinicopathologic findings. *Invest New Drugs.* 2013;31(4):1071–1077.
37. Kantarjian H, Stein A, Gökbuget N, et al. Blinatumomab versus chemotherapy for advanced acute lymphoblastic leukemia. *N Engl J Med.* 2017;376(9):836–847.
38. von Stackelberg A, Locatelli F, Zugmaier G, et al. Phase I/phase II study of blinatumomab in pediatric patients with relapsed/refractory acute lymphoblastic leukemia. *J Clin Oncol.* 2016;34(36):4381–4389.
39. Kantarjian HM, Stein AS, Bargou RC, et al. Blinatumomab treatment of older adults with relapsed/refractory B-precursor acute lymphoblastic leukemia: results from 2 phase 2 studies. *Cancer.* 2016;122(14):2178–2185.
40. Blinatumomab product sheet. https://www.Arzneimittelsicherheit/RHB/20161025.pdf.
41. Teachey DT, Rheingold SR, Maude SL, et al. Cytokine release syndrome after blinatumomab treatment related to abnormal macrophage activation and ameliorated with cytokine-directed therapy. *Blood.* 2013;121(26):5154–5157.
42. Lee DW, Gardner R, Porter DL, et al. Current concepts in the diagnosis and management of cytokine release syndrome. *Blood.* 2014;124(2):188–195.
43. Rosenberg SA, Restifo NP. Adoptive cell transfer as personalized immunotherapy for human cancer. *Science.* 2015;348(6230):62–68.
44. Brudno JN, Kochenderfer JN. Toxicities of chimeric antigen receptor T cells: recognition and management. *Blood.* 2016;127(26):3321–3330.
45. Locke FL, Neelapu SS, Bartlett NL, et al. Phase 1 results of ZUMA-1: a multicenter study of KTE-C19 anti-CD19 CAR T cell therapy in refractory aggressive lymphoma. *Mol Ther.* 2017;25(1):285–295.
46. Teachey DT, Lacey SF, Shaw PA, et al. Identification of predictive biomarkers for cytokine release syndrome after chimeric antigen receptor T-cell therapy for acute lymphoblastic leukemia. *Cancer Discov.* 2016;6(6):664–679.
47. Morgan RA, Yang JC, Kitano M, et al. Case report of a serious adverse event following the administration of T cells transduced with a chimeric antigen receptor recognizing ERBB2. *Mol Ther.* 2010;18(4):843–851.
48. Lamers CH, Sleijfer S, Vulto AG, et al. Treatment of metastatic renal cell carcinoma with autologous T-lymphocytes genetically retargeted against carbonic anhydrase IX: first clinical experience. *J Clin Oncol.* 2006;24(13):e20–e22.
49. Curti B, Daniels GA, McDermott DF, et al. Improved survival and tumor control with interleukin-2 is associated with the development of immune-related adverse events: data from the PROCLAIM^SM registry. *J Immunother Cancer.* 2017;5(1):102.
50. Fish EN, Platanias LC. Interferon receptor signaling in malignancy: a network of cellular pathways defining biological outcomes. *Mol Cancer Res.* 2014;12(12):1691–1703.
51. Kirkwood JM, Ibrahim JG, Sondak VK, et al. High- and low-dose interferon alfa-2b in high-risk melanoma: first analysis of intergroup trial E1690/S9111/C9190. *J Clin Oncol.* 2000;18(12):2444–2458.
52. Kirkwood JM, Strawderman MH, Ernstoff MS, et al. Interferon alfa-2b adjuvant therapy of high-risk resected cutaneous melanoma: the Eastern Cooperative Oncology Group Trial EST 1684. *J Clin Oncol.* 1996;14(1):7–17.
53. Kirkwood JM, Bender C, Agarwala S, et al. Mechanisms and management of toxicities associated with high-dose interferon alfa-2b therapy. *J Clin Oncol.* 2002;20(17):3703–3718.
54. Eland IA, Rasch MC, Sturkenboom MJ, et al. Acute pancreatitis attributed to the use of interferon alfa-2b. *Gastroenterology.* 2000;119(1):230–233.

55. Kwon ED, Drake CG, Scher HI, et al. Ipilimumab versus placebo after radiotherapy in patients with metastatic castration-resistant prostate cancer that had progressed after docetaxel chemotherapy (CA184-043): a multicentre, randomised, double-blind, phase 3 trial. *Lancet Oncol.* 2014;15(7):700–712.

56. Berman D, Parker SM, Siegel J, et al. Blockade of cytotoxic T-lymphocyte antigen-4 by ipilimumab results in dysregulation of gastrointestinal immunity in patients with advanced melanoma. *Cancer Immun.* 2010;10:11.

57. Cramer P, Bresalier RS. Gastrointestinal and hepatic complications of immune checkpoint inhibitors. *Curr Gastroenterol Rep.* 2017;19(1):3.

58. Kreisel W, Dahlberg M, Bertz H, et al. Endoscopic diagnosis of acute intestinal GVHD following allogeneic hematopoietic SCT: a retrospective analysis in 175 patients. *Bone Marrow Transplant.* 2012;47(3):430–438.

59. Masia R, Peyton S, Lauwers GY, et al. Gastrointestinal biopsy findings of autoimmune enteropathy: a review of 25 cases. *Am J Surg Pathol.* 2014;38(10):1319–1329.

60. Lee S, de Boer WB, Subramaniam K, et al. Pointers and pitfalls of mycophenolate-associated colitis. *J Clin Pathol.* 2013;66(1):8–11.

61. Soldini D, Gaspert A, Montani M, et al. Apoptotic enteropathy caused by antimetabolites and TNF-alpha antagonists. *J Clin Pathol.* 2014;67(7):582–586.

62. Louie CY, DiMaio MA, Matsukuma KE, et al. Idelalisib-associated enterocolitis: clinicopathologic features and distinction from other enterocolitides. *Am J Surg Pathol.* 2015;39(12):1653–1660.

63. Feakins RM. Ulcerative colitis or Crohn's disease? Pitfalls and problems. *Histopathology.* 2014;64(3):317–335.

64. Kim KW, Ramaiya NH, Krajewski KM, et al. Ipilimumab-associated colitis: CT findings. *AJR Am J Roentgenol.* 2013;200(5):W468–W474.

65. Jain A, Lipson EJ, Sharfman WH, et al. Colonic ulcerations may predict steroid-refractory course in patients with ipilimumab-mediated enterocolitis. *World J Gastroenterol.* 2017;23(11):2023–2028.

66. Pollack MH, Betof A, Dearden H, et al. Safety of resuming anti-PD-1 in patients with immune-related adverse events (irAEs) during combined anti-CTLA-4 and anti-PD1 in metastatic melanoma. *Ann Oncol.* 2018;29(1):250–255.

67. Puzanov I, Diab A, Abdallah K, et al. Managing toxicities associated with immune checkpoint inhibitors: consensus recommendations from the Society for Immunotherapy of Cancer (SITC) Toxicity Management Working Group. *J Immunother Cancer.* 2017;5(1):95.

68. Champiat S, Lambotte O, Barreau E, et al. Management of immune checkpoint blockade dysimmune toxicities: a collaborative position paper. *Ann Oncol.* 2016;27(4):559–574.

69. Johnson DB, Sullivan RJ, Ott PA, et al. Ipilimumab therapy in patients with advanced melanoma and preexisting autoimmune disorders. *JAMA Oncol.* 2016;2(2):234–240.

70. Bostwick AD, Salama AK, Hanks BA. Rapid complete response of metastatic melanoma in a patient undergoing ipilimumab immunotherapy in the setting of active ulcerative colitis. *J Immunother Cancer.* 2015;3:19.

71. Sanjeevaiah A, Kerr T, Beg MS. Approach and management of checkpoint inhibitor-related immune hepatitis. *J Gastrointest Oncol.* 2018;9(1):220–224.

72. Champiat S, Dercle L, Ammari S, et al. Hyperprogressive disease is a new pattern of progression in cancer patients treated by anti-PD-1/PD-L1. *Clin Cancer Res.* 2017;23(8):1920–1928.

73. Everett J, Srivastava A, Misdraji J. Fibrin ring granulomas in checkpoint inhibitor-induced hepatitis. *Am J Surg Pathol.* 2017;41(1):134–137.

74. National Comprehensive Cancer Network Guidelines. https://www.nccn.org/professionals/physician_gls/f_guidelines.aspx.

75. Chmiel KD, Suan D, Liddle C, et al. Resolution of severe ipilimumab-induced hepatitis after antithymocyte globulin therapy. *J Clin Oncol.* 2011;29(9):e237–e240.

76. Postow M, Wolchok J. Toxicities associated with checkpoint inhibitor immunotherapy. UpToDate, Waltham, MA 2016 (Accessed on December 15, 2015).

77. Topp MS, Gökbuget N, Stein AS, et al. Safety and activity of blinatumomab for adult patients with relapsed or refractory B-precursor acute lymphoblastic leukaemia: a multicentre, single-arm, phase 2 study. *Lancet Oncol.* 2015;16(1):57–66.

78. Ribera JM. Efficacy and safety of bispecific T-cell engager blinatumomab and the potential to improve leukemia-free survival in B-cell acute lymphoblastic leukemia. *Expert Rev Hematol.* 2017;10(12):1057–1067.

79. Brandl C, Haas C, d'Argouges S, et al. The effect of dexamethasone on polyclonal T cell activation and redirected target cell lysis as induced by a CD19/CD3-bispecific single-chain antibody construct. *Cancer Immunol Immunother.* 2007;56(10):1551–1563.
80. Hijazi Y, Klinger M, Schub A, et al. Blinatumomab exposure and pharmacodynamic response in patients with non-Hodgkin lymphoma (NHL). *J Clin Oncol.* 2013;31(15).
81. Jordan MB, Allen CE, Weitzman S, et al. How I treat hemophagocytic lymphohistiocytosis. *Blood.* 2011; 118(15):4041–4052.
82. Locatelli F, Jordan MB, Allen C, et al. Empalumab in children with primary hemophagocytic lympho-histiocytosis. *N Engl J Med.* 2020;382:1811-1822.
83. Marabondo S, Kaufman HL. High-dose interleukin-2 (IL-2) for the treatment of melanoma: safety considerations and future directions. *Expert Opin Drug Saf.* 2017;16(12):1347–1357.
85. Huguet F, Tavitian S. Emerging biological therapies to treat acute lymphoblastic leukemia. *Expert Opin Emerg Drugs.* 2017;22(1):107–121.

CHAPTER 20

Neurological Toxicities of Immunotherapy

Manu R. Pandey, MBBS ■ Marc S. Ernstoff, MD

Introduction

Cancer immunotherapy has a rich history. In the late 19th century, William Coley treated sarcoma patients with intratumoral bacteria and bacterial products and demonstrated tumor shrinkage. Over the years, we have added significantly to the "immunological armament" against cancer. In the past two decades, there has been an explosion of immunotherapies which have brought this field to the forefront of oncology. These new agents activate the immune system against cancers but, in the process, create a new set of toxicities including adverse events in both the central and the peripheral nervous systems. In this chapter, we will discuss the major immunological agents, their mechanisms of action, mechanisms of action as pertaining to their neurological toxicities, and major reported neurotoxicities. We will further describe the management of these toxicities.

Agents

INTERLEUKIN

- Interleukin 2 (IL-2) has been extensively studied in metastatic melanoma and renal cell carcinoma (RCC). High dose IL-2 (HDIL-2) has been used as monotherapy for metastatic melanoma (MM) and metastatic renal cell carcinoma (mRCC) with objective response rates of 14% to 18% for mRCC and 15% to 16% for MM with few patients showing durable responses of over 10 years.[1-3]
- **Mechanism of Action**
  - IL-2 binds to its receptors, expressed on regulatory T cells (Tregs), activated CD8+, CD4+, CD56 high, dendritic cells, and endothelial cells, which leads to signaling via the Janus family tyrosine kinase (JAK). This further activates downstream signaling, causing T and NK cell expansion, T cell effector differentiation, and expansion of CD8+ memory T cells; the increased cytolytic activity of the T and NK cells is responsible for its antitumor effect.[4] Interestingly IL-2 also causes expansion of immunosuppressive Tregs.[4]
- **Mechanism of Neurotoxicity**
  - Several mechanisms have been proposed for IL-2 medicated neurotoxicity. IL-2 has shown to have effects on neuronal cells, major neurotransmitters, and electrical activity.[5] IL-2 can also lead to increase in the total water content of the brain, likely due to an increase in tumor vascular permeability or due to an overall increase in the total body water content.[6]
- **Reported Neurotoxicity**
  - Patients on IL-2 can develop delirium, lethargy, fatigue, insomnia, memory loss, dizziness, cognitive decline, and restlessness. In a large study with HDIL-2, multiple events of all-grade neurological toxicity were reported, including coma, somnolence, and dizziness, whereas another study reported grades 3 and 4 neurological toxicity or seizure in about 35% of patients.[7,8] Mood symptoms are also frequently seen with IL-2. Two studies found

a significant increase in depression scores during IL-2 therapy.[9,10] In one study, patients developed new-onset neurological deficits which were associated with lesions in the white and grey matter. These lesions resolved and the neurological status improved in the majority of the patients once IL-2 therapy was withdrawn.[11] Peripheral nerve entrapment due to fluid retention can be seen.[12] Cases of brachial plexopathy have also been reported.[13]

INTERFERON

- Interferon (INF)-α2b has been extensively used as an adjuvant therapy in patients with melanoma. It was also approved for use in RCC, chronic myelogenous leukemia, Kaposi's sarcoma, and follicular lymphoma. With the advent of better drugs, however, it is no longer commonly used.
- **Mechanism of Action**
  - INF-α works intrinsically on the tumor by decreasing tumor proliferation, inducing apoptosis, and extrinsically by increasing the proliferation and cytotoxicity of T and NK cells, decreasing proliferation of Treg cells, and decreasing the immunosuppressive activity of Treg and myeloid-derived suppressor cells, increasing major histocompatibility complex-1 (MHC-1) and tumor antigen presentation, increasing activation and signaling of dendritic cells, and inducing release of other cytokines.[14]
- **Mechanism of Neurotoxicity**
  - INF-α acts directly on neurons, leading to a decrease in the length and branching of the dendritic processes via the breakdown of MAP-2 (a cytoskeletal protein), decreasing signal transmission, and through the release of other cytokines.[15] Indirectly, INF-α causes a decrease in levels of dopamine and serotonin and has effects on the hypothalamic-pituitary-adrenal axis.[16]
- **Reported Neurotoxicities**
  - Psychiatric symptoms are commonly reported with use of INF-α. Utilization of mental health care facilities was found to be more common among patients receiving adjuvant INF-α for melanoma compared with controls, with a higher risk of treatment discontinuation in patients who develop mental health problems.[17] Depressive symptoms have been reported in between 8% and 48% of patients receiving INF-α.[16] Risk factors for depression with INF-α therapy including higher dose and longer duration of treatment, history of psychiatric illness, ongoing psychiatric treatment, and lack of social support.[18] In a clinical trial of patients with melanoma treated with INF, depression, anxiety, and action tremors were more common compared to controls.[19] Other neuropsychiatric symptoms seen with the use of INF-α include mania, suicidal ideation, acute psychosis, difficulty concentrating, impaired memory, and insomnia.[16] New onset seizures have been reported in about 1% of patients treated with INF-α.[20] Development of Parkinson's disease has also been seen with the use of INF-α.[21]

IMMUNE CHECKPOINT INHIBITORS

- In recent years, immune checkpoint inhibitors (ICIs) have revolutionized the treatment of cancer and have shown efficacy in multiple tumors. The US Food and Drug Administration (FDA) has approved multiple ICIs for various indications. Ipilimumab, a fully humanized immunoglobulin (Ig) G1 monoclonal antibody (mAb) that binds to cytotoxic T cell lymphocyte antigen-4 (CTLA-4),[22] was the first anti-CTLA-4 antibody to be approved for use in melanoma.[23] Tremelimumab is a human IgG2 mAb that also binds CTLA-4.[24] It has been studied in malignant mesothelioma, although a recent phase 2 trial did not show any difference in overall survival when compared with placebo.[25]
- Anti–programmed death-1 (PD-1) antibodies are another group of ICIs. Nivolumab and pembrolizumab are both fully humanized IgG4 antibodies that bind PD-1.[26] They have been

FDA–approved for used in melanoma, non–small-cell lung cancer (NSCLC), urothelial carcinoma, head and neck squamous cell cancer, and classic Hodgkin's lymphoma. Apart from the above indications, pembrolizumab is approved for used in gastric cancer and solid tumors with high microsatellite instability (MSI) and mismatch repair deficiency, whereas nivolumab is approved for use in RCC, colorectal cancer with high MSI, and hepatocellular carcinoma.[23] Cemipilimab, in another anti-PD-1 antibody which has shown activity in patient with advanced cutaneous squamous cell carcinoma, and has been approved for use by the FDA.[160]

- Anti–program death ligand-1 (PD-L1) antibodies also block the PD-1 pathway. Three drugs from this group have been FDA–approved for use. Atezolizumab has been approved for use in NSCLC and urothelial cancer, avelumab has been approved for use in Merkel cell carcinoma and urothelial carcinoma, and durvalumab has been approved for use in urothelial cancer.[23] Anti-PDL1 agents have also shown survival benefit as maintenance therapy in SCLC (atezolizumab and durvalumab), NSCLC (durvalumab) and urothelial carcinoma (avelumab).[161-164]

- **Mechanism of Action**
  - CTLA-4 present on the T cell surface competes with CD28 to bind with B7 on antigen presenting cells (APCs).[27] Binding of CD28 leads to T cell proliferation by the production of IL-2 and anti-apoptotic factor, an action that is blocked by CTLA-4.[27] Not only does it block CD28, but CTLA-4 also increases inhibitory signaling through tryptophan catabolism.[27] Binding of CTLA-4 leads to downstream signaling inhibition of both CD4+ and CD8+ T cells and enhancement of Treg cells.[27] Blockade of CTLA-4 in vivo has been shown not only to increase T cell activation and proliferation but also cause reduction in tumor growth in several animal models.[27]

    PD-1 is a transmembrane receptor which is expressed on mature T and B cells, thymocytes, and macrophages, whereas its ligands, PD-L1 and PD-L2, are expressed on several tissues and tumor cells. Binding of PD-1 with its ligand leads to decrease in T cell proliferation as well as tumor lysis.[28] Blockade of the PD-1/PD-L1 pathway has shown to decrease tumorigenesis, increase proliferation and cytokine production by T helper cells and memory cells, increase cytolytic activity of T effector cells, and increase proliferation of memory cells, as well as other antitumor effects.[29]

- **Mechanism of Neurotoxicity**
  - Various mechanisms have been proposed to explain the neurological adverse effects seen with ICIs. Perivascular lymphocytic infiltration by both CD4+ and CD8+ T cells observed in this situation supports a T cell-mediacted mechanism.[30] On the other hand, development of new-onset myasthenia gravis (MG), the presence of anti-NMDA and anti-HU antibodies in patients with acute encephalitis, and the presence of anti-exosome antibodies in patients with myositis points towards a mechanism of ICI which involves the production of these pathogenic antibodies.[31-35]

- **Reported Neurotoxicities**
  - The incidence of any grade adverse effects was 3.8% with anti-CTLA-4 antibodies, 6.1% for anti-PD-1 antibodies, and 12% with the combination of anti-CTLA-4 with anti-PD-1 antibodies.[30] The incidence of grades 3 to 4 adverse effects is less than 1% with all agents, including anti-PD-L1 antibodies.[30,36] Neurological adverse effects are seen more commonly in men, with a median time of onset 6 weeks after starting therapy, with recovery seen in most patients after a 4-week interruption of treatment.[30] No difference was seen in the incidence of neurological adverse effects when a higher dose of ipilimumab was used.[30,36] A higher incidence was reported with higher doses of nivolumab, whereas the opposite was seen with pembrolizumab[30,36]

    The most common neurological adverse events are grades 1 to 2 and are nonspecific, such as headache, dysgeusia, sensory impairment, or dizziness.[30] Hypophysitis, which can present with headaches, has also been reported; a higher incidence is seen with the use of anti-CTLA-4 antibodies compared with the anti-PD-1 antibodies.[37] Other central nervous system (CNS) toxicities include encephalitis and aseptic meningitis, which occur in about 0.1% to 0.2% of cases.[36] Cases of cerebral edema, multiple sclerosis, transverse myelitis, posterior reversible encephalopathy (PRES), and CNS vasculitis have also been seen with the use of ICIs.[38–44] De novo MG, worsening of MG, Guillain-Barre syndrome (GBS)/chronic demyelinating polyneuropathy, radiculopathy, and myositis have also been reported.[31,45–47]

CHIMERIC ANTIGEN RECEPTOR T-CELL THERAPY

■ Novartis's CTL019 (tisagenlecleucel) and Kite's KTE-C19 (axicabtagene ciloleucel) have been approved by the FDA for use in relapsed/refractory B-cell acute lymphoblastic leukemia (B-ALL) and large B cell lymphoma (BCL) patients who have relapsed after two lines of therapy, respectively.[48,49] Several trials have also looked at the use of chimeric antigen receptor (CAR) T cells in solid tumors with disappointing results due to differing antigen densities on the tumor, presence of tumor antigens on normal tissues leading to cross reactivity, and the immunosuppressive tumor microenvironment.[50]

■ **Mechanism of Action**
  ■ CAR T cells are genetically modified T cells that express an antibody-derived single-chain variable region, which attaches to the tumor antigen, and is linked to an intracellular T cell signaling domain (along with other costimulatory molecules in second and third generation CAR T cells) leading to T cell activation.[51]

■ **Mechanism of Neurotoxicity**
  ■ Neurological toxicity and cytokine release syndrome (CRS) are the most common toxicities with use of CAR T-cell therapy.[52] The major mechanism that has been proposed for neurotoxicity is through activation of endothelial cells and disruption of the blood-brain barrier (BBB). Gust et al. showed a correlation of neurotoxicity with endothelial cell activation, supporting this theory. Increase in angiopoietin (ANG) 2, an enzyme which is released from activated endothelial cells, increased ANG2:ANG1 ratio (ANG1 helps maintain endothelial cell quiescence), and increased von Willebrand factor (which, like ANG2, is stored in endothelial cells and is released upon activation) were found in patients with grade 4 or 5 neurotoxicity.[53] In an animal model, use of CD20 CAR T cell was associated with an increase in multiple proinflammatory cytokines and T cell accumulation in the cerebrospinal fluid (CSF).[54] Similar results have also been seen in humans treated with CD19 CAR T cells, with an increase in proteins and cells in CSF.[53] Gust et al. also showed an increase in the IL-6, INF and tumor necrosis factor (TNF)-α in the CSF. These cytokines have been implicated in the activation of endothelial cells and increase in the BBB permeability.[53] Although CAR T cells may cross-react with normal tissues, to date, CD19 expression has not been described in the nervous system, thus suggesting that CD19 CAR T cells do not cause toxicity by this mechanism. Recent evidence also implicates granulocyte macrophage–colony stimulating factor (GM-CSF), in the development of neurotoxicity and CRS.[55] Lenzilumab, an anti–GM-CSF mAb, not only abrogated neurotoxicity but also improved the antitumor effect of CAR T cells.[55]

■ **Reported Neurotoxicity**
  ■ In published studies and clinical trials, any grade neurological toxicity has been reported in 28% to 64% of patients, with development of grade 3 or higher toxicity seen in 11% to 28% and a median onset of 4 to 5 days.[53,56–60] In a study of 133 patients treated with CD19 CAR T-cell therapy, delirium and headache were the two most commonly reported neurological symptoms.[53] Language disturbances, decreased level of consciousness, memory impairment, ataxia and movement abnormality, seizures, and intracranial hemorrhage were some of the other neurological disorders reported.[53,56,57] Complete resolution of neurotoxicity is seen in most patients.[53] Factors associated with the development of neurological toxicity included

young age, B-ALL, high disease burden, higher dose, and peak expansion value of CAR T cells, and preexisting neurological disease.[53,61] Development of grade 4 or higher CRS was linked to the development of grade 3 or higher neurotoxicity in several studies.[58–60] Other factors associated with grade 4 or higher neurotoxicity included pre-lymphodepletion higher ANG2:ANG1 ratio, a higher peak of ferritin c-reactive protein (CRP) and other cytokines.[53] Usually there are no changes in the magnetic resonance image (MRI) or computed tomography (CT) scans observed in these patients.[53,57,62] Anatomical changes seen on MRI are a poor prognostic marker as seen in the study by Gust et al., where 4 out of the 7 patients who developed MRI changes died.[53] On electroencephalogram (EEG), generalized slowing is the most common finding.[53,63]

ONCOLYTIC VIRUSES

- Intralesional talimogene laherparepavec (T-VEC) is the first oncolytic virus to be FDA–approved for use as local treatment of unresectable cutaneous, subcutaneous, and nodal lesions in patients with melanoma recurrence after surgery. This approval was based on a phase III trial which showed a greater than 50% decrease in 64% of the injected lesions and in uninjected lesions (34% nonvisceral and 15% visceral), and improvement in durable response rates compared with GM-CSF, although no difference was seen in the overall survival.[64,65] T-VEC has also been studied in combination with ICIs and has shown promising results in early phase trials.[66,67]
- **Mechanism of Action**
- T-VEC is an attenuated herpes simplex virus-1 encoding for GM-CSF.[68] Tumor cells have disrupted activity of PKR which blocks protein translation in healthy cells.[68] Type 1 INF signaling, which controls multiple transcription factors and cytokines which prevent viral replication, and is also disrupted in tumor cells.[68] In the absence of PKR and INF signaling, the virus undergoes unchecked replication, ultimately leading to cell lysis and subsequent infection of more tumor cells.[68] The release of tumor antigen and release of GM-CSF in the tumor microenvironment augments the action of the vaccine.[68]
- **Mechanism of Neurotoxicity**
- The mechanism of neurotoxicity associated with oncolytic viruses is not known.
- **Reported Neurotoxicities**
- In a phase III trial, fatigue was the most common toxicity and was reported in about 50% of patients. Most of these were low grade with grade 3 or higher toxicity reported in only 2% of patients. Any grade headache was reported in about 19% of patients with 0.7% reporting grade 3 or higher. Other common toxicities include influenza-like illness, injection site pain, chills, nausea, vomiting, nausea, and pyrexia.[65]

BISPECIFIC T CELL ENGAGERS

- Bispecific T cell engagers (BiTEs) are a form of immunological agents called bispecific antibodies which have two unique antigen binding sites.[69] Blinatumomab was the first BiTE to be FDA–approved and is currently approved for relapsed/refractory precursor B cell ALL in adult and children.[70] It has also recently gained approval for use in B cell precursor ALL in remission with positive minimal residual disease.[71] Studies have also shown promising results with blinatumomab in relapsed/refractory non-Hodgkin's lymphoma (NHL).[72,73] There are ongoing early phase trials of BiTE cells in acute myelogenous leukemia (AML) and other solid tumors including gastrointestinal adenocarcinoma and prostate cancer.[74]

- **Mechanism of Action**
  - BiTEs consist of two single-chain variable fragments which are joined together by a linker molecule, one of which binds to T cells, whereas the other binds to a tumor antigen.[69] The simultaneous binding of BiTE cells to T cells and tumor antigens causes T-cell activation and release of cytokines, including γ-interferon, TNF-α, IL-6, and IL-2.[75] BiTE cells also lead to the formation of a cytolytic synapse through which transfer to perforin and granzyme takes place from activated T cells to target tumor cells, leading to apoptosis of the tumor cell.[76]
- **Mechanism of Neurotoxicity**
  - Blinatumomab causes a transient increase in cytokines including IL-6, TNF-α, and INF-γ, generally with the first cycle of treatment. This increase in cytokines, however, is not reproduced with later cycles.[77] These cytokines have been shown to increase endothelial cell activation and BBB permeability.[53] Interestingly, neurological toxicity is most often reported after the first cycle of blinatumomab.[73,78] A study also showed an increase in T cell adhesion to the endothelium with blinatumomab infusion, leading to the redistribution of T cells into neural tissues.[79] Although there is no direct evidence of the mechanism of neurological toxicity from blinatumomab, it appears to be due to the release of cytokines from activated T cells.
- **Reported Neurotoxicities**
  - Any grade neurological adverse events developed in 47% to 71% of patients.[80,81] Severe toxicity developed in about 7% to 22% of patients.[78,80–82] Headache, dizziness, and tremors are the most common neurological toxicities reported, with other adverse effects reported including encephalopathy, seizures, convulsions, apraxia, memory impairment, aphasia, hemiparesis, and cerebral hemorrhage.[78,81–84] Neurological adverse effects are more common in patients aged 65 years or older, although overall adverse effects remain unchanged in this group.[83] The incidence of neurological adverse effects is directly proportional to the dose of blinatumomab administered, as seen in a phase 1 study in NHL where 3 out of 4 patients developed dose-limiting toxicity when treated at the highest dose level.[73] In most patients, neurological adverse events abated after interruption of the drug.[72,73,78,81]

OTHER MONOCLONAL ANTIBODYS

Antibody-Drug Conjugates

- Antibody-drug conjugates (ADCs) are a group of immunological agents where a cytotoxic agent is bound to a mAb targeting a tumor specific antigen. The ADC is internalized by the tumor cell leading to release of the cytotoxic agent and subsequent tumor death.[85] The first drug of this class to be FDA–approved was gemtuzumab ozogamicin (GO), a CD33 binding ADC initially used in patients with AML, but it was later withdrawn from the market due to lack of survival benefit when added to standard therapy, and increased rate of non-hematological grade 4 and fatal toxicity during induction.[86] Although a recent phase III study which used a lower dose of the drug led to its re-approval in the US along with combination chemotherapy or monotherapy.[87] Brentuximab vedotin, another ADC, is approved for use in Hodgkin's lymphoma, CD30-positive mycosis fungoides, and in systemic and cutaneous large B cell lymphoma in patients who have failed prior systemic chemotherapy.[88] Ado-trastuzumab emtansine is FDA–approved for human epidermal growth factor-2 (HER2)–positive metastatic breast cancer in patients who have received trastuzumab with or without a taxane.[89]
  - **Mechanism of Action.** Brentuximab vedotin (BV) is an anti-CD30 targeting antibody conjugated with monomethyl auristatin-E (MMAE).[90] Upon binding to CD30, the molecule is endocytosed, then cleaved in lysosomes, leading to release of MMAE, a tubulin inhibitor which prevents polymerization of microtubulin, subsequently causing arrest of cell division and growth.[89]

Ado-trastuzumab emtansine (T-DM1) is a HER2-targeting antibody conjugated with a derivative of maytansine (DM-1), which upon internalization, is broken down to release DM-1, a potent tubulin inhibitor, causing inhibition of microtubule assembly leading to cell death.[91] T-DM1 still retains the action of trastuzumab by blocking the HER2 downstream signaling. It inhibits shedding of the extracellular HER2 domain and promotes antibody-dependent cellular cytotoxicity (ADCC).[91]

Gemtuzumab ozogamicin (GO) is a CD33 binding ADC linked to N acetyl-calicheamicin, which, once internalized by myeloid blast cells, releases calicheamicin, a cytotoxic agent that damages DNA by introducing breaks in its structure.[87]

- **Mechanism of Neurotoxicity.** MMAE, like other tubulin inhibitors, predisposes patients to peripheral neuropathy by disrupting axonal transport in the neuron.[92] Neurons do not express CD30 on their surface[93]; however, toxicity is likely due to the bystander effect in the surrounding tissue caused by the diffusion of the drug from the tumor cells.[90] T-DM1 likely causes neurotoxicity through a similar mechanism.

- **Reported Neurotoxicity.** Peripheral neuropathy (PN) is one of the most common toxicities of ADCs and has been reported in 42% to 67% of patients with about 8% to 12% of patients developing grade 3 or higher toxicities. This often leads to treatment discontinuation, treatment delay, and dose reduction in a significant number of patients.[94–96] Both motor and sensory nerves can be involved, although sensory neuropathy is more common.[94,97] Complete resolution has been seen in about 50% of patients, with time to resolution varying from 13 to 41 weeks.[94,96] PN can be managed in most cases with dose delays and dose reductions. Cases of progressive multifocal leukoencephalopathy (PML) have also been described with brentuximab vedotin (BV).[98,99] Peripheral neuropathy has been reported with T-DM1, although at significantly lower rates when compared with BV.[100,101] GO, owing to its action of mechanism which is different from the other ADCs, is well tolerated neurologically and no neurological adverse effects were reported in a phase III trial.[102]

CD20–Directed Antibodies

- Rituximab, a chimeric antibody made up of murine variable regions which bind to CD20 and a human Fc region, was the first anti-CD20 mAb to be approved.[103] It is approved for use in several hematological malignancies as well as some autoimmune disorders. Its action is based on antibody-dependent cell-mediated cytoxicity (ADCC), complement-dependent cytotoxicity (CDC), complement-dependent phagocytosis, and direct apoptosis.[103] Ofatumumab and obintuzumab are other CD20-directed antibodies with similar action to that of rituximab.[104,105] Ibritumomab tiuxetan contains a CD20-targeting mAb bound to tiuxetan, a chelator, which is further bound to 90Y, a radioactive isotope, which releases high energy beta particles, and causes cytotoxicity by an antibody- and complement-dependent manner as well as directly through beta emmision.[106]

- **Reported Toxicities.** Neurological adverse effects are uncommon with rituximab, although headache was reported in 16% of patients in one clinical trial.[107] Several cases of PML have been reported with use of rituximab.[108] Other mAbs are also generally well tolerated.

CD52–Directed Antibodies

- Alemtuzumab is a mAb which binds to CD52, a CD marker expressed on both T and B cells.[109] Alemtuzumab has been approved for use as monotherapy in chronic lymphocytic leukemia and has shown activity in patients with certain T cell lymphomas and leukemias. Alemtuzumab has also shown activity in the prevention of graft versus host disease (GVHD) after stem cell transplantation.[109]

- **Reported Toxicity.** Neurological complications are uncommon with alemtuzumab, although a study did report an increase in peripheral neuropathy and myelitis in patients who received alemtuzumab-based reduced-intensity allogeneic transplants.[110] A case of PML has also been reported with alemtuzumab.[111]

CD38–Directed Antibodies and Signal Lymphocytic Activation Molecule-7–Directed Antibodies

- Daratumumab is a mAB directed against CD38 and has been approved for use in multiple myeloma patients who have progressed through one line of therapy.[112] Like other mAbs, daratumumab also causes ADCC and complement-dependent cytotoxicity (CDC) leading to the lysis of normal and malignant plasma cells.[113]

    Elotuzumab is a signal lymphocytic activation molecule (SLAM)-7–directed antibody that has been approved for use in combination with dexamethasone and lenalidomide in patients with multiple myeloma who have received one to three prior therapies.[114,115] Elotuzumab is a humanized mAb that binds to SLAM7 and induces ADCC and natural killer (NK) cell–dependent direct cytotoxicity.[116]

- **Reported Toxicities.** When used as monotherapy, neurological adverse effects due to daratumumab were rare, with one phase II trial reporting headache and dizziness in 3% and 6% of patients, respectively.[117,118] Peripheral neuropathy, headache, insomnia, and dizziness have been reported with the combination of elotuzumab with dexamethasone and lenalidomide, although nearly all of these were grade 2 or lower.[119]

Epidermal Growth Factor Receptor–Directed Antibodies

Epidermal growth factor receptor (EFGR) is mutated and/or overexpressed in a number of malignancies and has become a well-exploited target. EGFRs belong to the group of transforming growth factor receptors. Their activation lead to downstream signaling via tyrosine kinases which, in turn, lead to an increase in proliferation, and a decrease in apoptosis.[120] Cetuximab, a chimeric mAb directed against EGFR, not only blocks this downstream signaling but can also cause cell cycle arrest in the G1 phase, decrease angiogenesis, decrease tumor invasion and metastasis, induce apoptosis in tumor cells, and thus can potentiate the action of chemotherapy and radiotherapy.[121] Cetuximab is approved for use in patients with wild-type KRAS metastatic colorectal carcinoma along with irinotecan or as monotherapy, and in head and neck cancers with radiation, in combination with platinum-based chemotherapy or as monotherapy.[122] Panitumumab is a fully humanized antibody against EGFR with a mechanism of action similar to that of cetuximab; in addition, it also causes ADCC and autophagy.[123] Panitumumab is approved for use as monotherapy in wild-type KRAS metastatic colon cancer which does not respond to chemotherapy.[124]

- **Reported Neurological Toxicity.** When used as monotherapy, headache is the most common neurological adverse effect reported; other neurological adverse effects are uncommon.[125,126] Cases of aseptic meningitis have been reported with cetuximab with recovery after symptomatic treatment.[127] Although dermatological toxicities were common, neurological toxicities were not reported in studies with panitumumab as monotherapy.[128,129]

Human Epidermal Growth Factor 2–Directed Antibodies

- HER2 is a group of tyrosine kinases, which promote cell growth and proliferation, prevent apoptosis, and are overexpressed in 20% to 30% of patients with invasive breast cancer.[130] Trastuzumab is a humanized IgG1 monoclonal antibody which binds to HER2 and not only prevents downstream signaling but also results in ADCC, prevents angiogenesis, and has been approved for use in HER2 positive breast cancer both in the metastatic and adjuvant settings.[130] Pertuzumab is another HER2-directed mAb and has shown improvement in overall survival when used in combination with trastuzumab and docetaxel in patients with HER2+ metastatic breast cancer.[131]

Reported Neurological Toxicity. Cardiac toxicity and neutropenia/neutropenic fever are common toxicities reported with HER2-directed therapy. Severe neurological toxicities are uncommon, although fatal cases of cerebrovascular accident (CVA) and hemorrhage have been noted in clinical trials.[132] When used as monotherapy in a phase II trial in patients with ovarian cancer, 14 out of 41 patients developed neurotoxicity, although only one patient developed grade 3 or higher toxicity.[133] Like trastuzumab, the combination of pertuzumab with docetaxel and trastuzumab did not have significant neurotoxicity except headache, which was seen in about 17% of the patients in the combination group compared with 12% of the patients in the control group.[131]

Clinical Approach and Pharmacological Management of Toxicity

INTERLEUKIN-2

- Neuropsychiatric symptoms are commonly seen with IL-2. Although some guidelines recommend the use of benzodiazepines for insomnia/irritability, the risk of delirium must be considered prior to administration. Given this, other medications that are known to worsen delirium should be stopped. Antipsychotic medications can be considered in select cases. Progressive changes in personality, hallucinations, hostility, disorientation, and confusion are indications to stop treatment.[134]
- In patients with depressive symptoms, escitalopram can be used, as it has shown to decrease depressive symptoms compared with placebo.[10]
- Conservative management of peripheral neuropathy with pain medications and dose reduction of IL-2 is usually sufficient as many of these symptoms are self-limiting.

INTERFERON-α

- Hypothyroidism is commonly seen with INF use. It can mimic symptoms of depression and should be considered when evaluating patients with neurotoxicity.
- Patients with a history of, or who are currently suffering from, psychiatric disorders should be co-managed with the help of a psychiatrist.[18] Pretreatment of patients with paroxetine has shown to decrease the incidence of depression and anxiety in patients treated with INF and can be used prophylactically in patients with high risk of depression.[18,135] In patients with new-onset depression, use of drugs that affect both the serotonin and dopaminergic/noradrenergic pathways, including serotonin norepinephrine reuptake inhibitors (SNRIs), psychostimulants like modafinil and methylphenidate, and bupropion, may be more beneficial than selective serotonin reuptake inhibitors (SSRIs), as they can also improve fatigue and other neurovegetative symptoms, such as anorexia and pain, which are commonly seen in patients receiving INF.[18]
- Development of mania is an indication to stop INF. However, gabapentin has been successfully used in patients who develop mania and bipolar disorder with INF treatment.[136]

IMMUNE CHECKPOINT INHIBITORS

CNS Involvement

- **Meningitis/Encephalitis.** Patients with meningitis present with headache, nausea and vomiting, photophobia, and neck stiffness. Encephalitis can present with similar symptoms; in addition, patients may have altered mental status (AMS) or focal neurological deficits. Several pathologies including the metastatic spread of the tumor to CNS/leptomeninges, CVA, infection, autoimmune diseases, and metabolic derangement may present with similar features and should be considered in the differential. In patients presenting with headache with visual disturbances, fatigue, or hypotension, hypophysitis should be considered as a potential etiology.
- Testing, including metabolic panel, imaging (usually MRI), and CSF analysis will help in differentiating the underlying cause. In patients presenting with AMS or focal deficits, increased intracranial pressure should be ruled out before attempting a lumbar puncture.

Serum cortisol and serum adrenocorticotropic hormone (ACTH) levels should be obtained in patients to evaluate for adrenal insufficiency.[137] Other recommended workup includes erythrocyte sedimentation rate (ESR), CRP, antineutrophil cytoplasmic antibodies (ANCA), thyroid panel, and peripheral smear to evaluate for thrombotic thrombocytopenic purpura (TTP), and inflammatory or autoimmune conditions. Electroencephalogram should be obtained in patients with AMS and neurology consultation should be obtained.[137]

- Patients who present with symptoms of meningitis should receive appropriate antibiotic coverage until infectious causes are ruled out. Once infectious etiology has been ruled out, steroids (prednisone 0.5–1 mg/kg or methylprednisolone 1–2 mg/kg for severe disease) are recommended, and further ICIs should be withheld.[137,138] The management of patients who present with encephalitis is similar, although in patients with progressive symptoms or presence of oligoclonal bands in CSF, pulse dose steroids (methylprednisolone 1 g/day for 3–5 days) and intravenous immunoglobulin (IVIG) 2 g/kg over 5 days may be considered.[137] A slow taper of steroids over several weeks has been used in most reported cases of ICI-associated encephalitis.[32,33,41,139] Patients with autoimmune encephalopathy showing no improvement with steroids can be considered for plasmapheresis or rituximab therapy.[137] A case of steroid- and IVIG-resistant NMDAR-positive encephalitis successfully treated with rituximab has been reported.[140]

- **Transverse Myelitis.** Patients with transverse myelitis (TM) usually present with acute or subacute symptoms. A rapid onset over a few hours or a prolonged progressive deficit over weeks is uncharacteristic of TM, and such patients should be considered for alternative diagnoses.[141] TM can involve the entire spinal cord, leading to complete plegia, as well as sensory and autonomic deficits.[141]

- MRI of the spine is required for diagnosis. MRI of the brain, serum B12 levels, HIV testing, syphilis serology, TSH, anti-Ro and La antibodies, anti-aquaporin 4-IgG, and CSF analysis, including oligoclonal bands and onconeural antibodies, should also be obtained in patients with suspected TM.[137,138] Patients with the involvement of spinal cord of more than three vertebral segments should have an extensive autoimmune workup.[141] Other etiologies of TM include infections, metabolic abnormalities, and autoimmune disorders, all of which should be ruled out depending on the clinical scenario.[141] Interestingly, many malignancies, including lung and ovarian cancer, can also cause paraneoplastic TM and are associated with specific antibodies.[141]

- In patients who develop TM, ICIs should be permanently discontinued and patients should be started on high-dose steroids (methylprednisolone 2 mg/kg); pulse dose steroids (1 g/day for 3–5 days) and IVIG (2 g/kg over 5 days) should be considered in these patients.[137] Plasmapheresis has also been recommended in patients not responsive to steroids.[138]

PNS Involvement

- **Myasthenia Gravis.** Patients with MG classically present with diplopia which gets worse during the day. Other symptoms include ptosis, bulbar muscle weakness leading to dysarthria, dysphagia, and respiratory muscle involvement occurs in severe cases. The Miller-Fischer variant of GBS presents with ophthalmoplegia, ataxia, and absent reflexes, and can often be mistaken for MG.[142]

- Neurology consultation should be obtained in patients with suspected MG.[137,138] Diagnosis is made based on clinical symptoms and a positive anticholinesterase antibody (AChR). Historically, 80% of patients with a diagnosis of classic MG will have AChR antibody.[143] Interestingly, a case series reported about 40% of patients without AChR antibodies who developed MG during treatment with ICIs.[31] Anti–muscle-specific kinase (MuSK) and lipoprotein-related antibody 4 should be tested in patients with negative AchR.[137] Several patients also have elevated levels of creatinine kinases (CK), unlike non–ICI-mediated MG, which is related to concomitant myositis along with MG.[31] Creatinine phosphokinase, aldolase, ESR, and CRP can be used to help rule out concomitant myositis.[137] Other recommended workup includes MRI brain and/or spine; electrodiagnostic (EDX) studies can be used to help rule out peripheral neuropathy or concomitant myositis.[137] Cardiac involvement can be seen with MG and is often overlooked. In a study of 58 patients with MG and no underlying cardiac abnormalities nearly 60% of patients had new electrocardiogram (ECG) changes and 5 patients had a reduction in their ejection fraction.[144] Creatinine phosphokinase and troponin T should also be obtained in patients with MG and if elevated, further workup with ECG and echocardiogram should be done.[137]

- Treatment usually entails pyridostigmine and corticosteroids with cessation of further treatment with ICI.[137,138] Patients presenting with grade 2 toxicity should be treated with prednisone (1–1.5 mg/kg) and pyridostigmine starting at 30 mg three times a day, gradually increasing to a maximum 120 mg 4 times a day based on improvement of symptoms.[137] Patients with grade 3–4 disease should be monitored in the ICU, and apart from the above, IVIG 2 g/day or plasmapheresis should be considered along with permanent discontinuation of ICI.[137] Use of other immunosuppressants like azathioprine has been reported.[145] Immunosuppressants have a role in this entity, but the risk of disease progression and toxicity should be weighed with the benefit of the medication.[138] Some medications can worsen MG and should be avoided.[137]

- **Guillain-Barre Syndrome.** GBS classically presents as an ascending muscle weakness with absent reflexes, which progresses over hours to days. Dysautonomia including cardiac arrhythmias can also occur. Respiratory muscles can also be involved in severe cases and cranial nerve involvement can also be seen. Sensory symptoms like back pain, paresthesias, and meningismus may precede motor symptoms in one-third of cases.[142] Five different variants on GBS exist, all of which have varied clinical presentations.[142]

- Diagnostic workup for GBS requires MRI of the spine, EDX, CSF analysis, serum antiganglioside antibody testing, and pulmonary function testing.[137] Classic GBS shows an albuminocytological gap without pleocytosis in the CSF.[142] Interestingly, there have been reports of GBS and chronic inflammatory demyelinating neuropathy associated with ICIs with pleocytosis in the CSF, unlike classic GBS.[45] In the same study, the patient with an axonal pattern on EDX, again unlike classic GBS, was seen.[45]

- Neurology consultation should be obtained in all patients with suspected GBS. ICIs should be discontinued immediately. IVIG (2 g/kg over 5 days) and plasmapheresis are the main treatment modalities used.[137] Treatment with steroids is generally not useful in classic GBS,[45] but can be used in patients with ICI-mediated GBS. Methylprednisolone (2–4 mg/kg) followed by a taper for patients with grade 2 GBS, and pulse dose steroids (1 g/day for 5 days) for patients with grade 3–4 GBS, can be considered along with the other previously mentioned therapies.[137] Neuropathic pain in this group of patients can be treated with gabapentin or carbamazepine.[142]

- **Other Toxicities.** Several cases of peripheral nerve involvement have been reported with use of ICIs. This peripheral nerve involvement can have varied presentation including sensory neuropathy, motor neuropathy, and polyradiculitis.[146,147] Enteric neuropathy presenting as constipation has also been reported in the literature.[148] Workup of peripheral neuropathy should include EDX as well as evaluation for other potential diagnoses.[137]

- Whereas patients with grade 1 peripheral neuropathy can be managed conservatively, patients with grade 2 toxicity should be treated with corticosteroids (prednisone 0.5–1 mg/kg), and patients with grades 3 and 4 toxicity should be managed as mentioned under the GBS section.[137] Patients with autonomic neuropathy can be managed similarly, although grades 3 and 4 toxicity generally require pulse dose steroids followed by a taper.[137]

CHIMERIC ANTIGEN RECEPTOR T-CELL THERAPY

- Neelapu et al. have proposed a grading system for CNS toxicity which can be used to guide management of patients receiving CAR T-cell therapy, referred to as CARTOX. CARTOX is a 10-point neurological assessment that is done three times a day. Points are assigned for orientation, naming, ability to follow commands, writing, and attention; a score of 10 denotes no impairment, but a lower score denotes grade 2 through 4 immune effector cell–associated neurotoxicity syndrome (ICANS).[63] All patients should have a baseline neurological examination prior to initiation of treatment and should undergo regular CARTOX evaluation. Prophylactic use of levetiracetam 750 mg every 12 hours for 1 month after starting therapy, regular clinical examination, and daily grading of neurotoxicity is recommended.[63] Patients with suspected neurotoxicity should undergo neurology consultation, evaluation for papilledema, EEG, and MRI/CT of the brain, and should be treated with antipyretics, antipsychotics, and ventilator support as required.[63] Of note, use of GM-CSF should be avoided in these patients as it has been implicated in the development of CRS and neurotoxicity.[55] A clinical trial is currently in progress, evaluating the use of lenzilumab in the prevention of neurotoxicity (NCT04314843).
- No randomized clinical trial has evaluated the management of neurotoxicity, making this entity an evolving field. CRS can be managed with the use of tocilizumab, an IL-6 receptor antagonist mAb that has been approved by the FDA for this indication. An increase in IL-6 is seen in the CSF of patients who develop neurotoxicity.[149] The use of IL-6 receptor antagonists for neurotoxicity without CRS is not recommended. In mice, use of tocilizumab was unable to prevent delayed lethal neurotoxicity by CAR T cells.[150] Similar results were seen in a study in humans where no benefit in neurological symptoms was seen with use of tocilizumab.[149] This perhaps is due to the inability of tocilizumab to cross the BBB.[151] In patients with neurotoxicity, dexamethasone is the preferred glucocorticoid due to its ability to penetrate the CNS.[152] For patients with severe neurological toxicities, dexamethasone 10 mg every 6 hours is recommended until symptoms improve to grade 1 or lower,[63,153] although patients with grade 4 toxicity may need pulse dose steroids followed by a taper.[63] Siltuximab, a IL-6–binding mAb can be used in steroid refractory neurotoxicity, although data for its efficacy is lacking. In mice, use of the IL-1 antagonist, anakinra, has been shown to effectively control neurotoxicity, although similar human studies are lacking.[150] The use of corticosteroids or tocilizumab has not been shown to have an effect on tumor response.[60]

BISPECIFIC T-CELL ENGAGERS

- Blinatumomab is infused continuously over a 4-week period followed by a 2-week break. A separate line should be used for infusion. The line should be labeled clearly and should not be flushed as it can cause acute toxicity.
- Patients who develop neurological toxicity should be assessed first for underlying infection, CVA, or metabolic etiologies of symptoms. Pretreatment with dexamethasone 20 mg every 6–12 hours before every step has been used successfully to prevent toxicity.[73] Pentosan polysulfate (SP54) is another agent that has been used to prevent toxicity.[73] In patients who develop seizures, antiseizure prophylaxis before re-exposure to blinatumomab has been shown to successfully prevent further seizures.[78] Treatment should be withheld for grade 3 neurotoxicity for at least 72 hours and until symptoms improve to grade 1 or lower. Treatment should be restarted at 9 μg/day. Blinatumomab should be discontinued permanently in patients who experience 2 or more seizures, in patients who experience neurological toxicity that is higher than grade 1 after withholding treatment for 1 week, in patients who develop neurological toxicity at the 9 μg/day dose, and lastly, in patients who develop grade 4 toxicity.[154]

OTHER MONOCLONAL ANTIBODIES

- **Progressive Multifocal Leukoencephalopathy**
  - Several cases of progressive multifocal leukoencephalopathy (PML) have been reported to be associated with monoclonal antibodies. In a case series of 57 patients who developed PML on rituximab, presenting complaints included confusion, incoordination, speech disturbance, and vision changes, with a median onset of 5.5 months after last rituximab dose. This condition has been associated with a 90% mortality rate.[108] Although plasmapheresis has often been used, its role is controversial and a recent study in patients who developed PML on natalizumab found no benefit of plasmapheresis.[155] Cytarabine, cidofovir, mirtazapine, mefloquine, and risperidone have all been used with sporadic benefit, and no conclusive evidence exists to support the use of these medications.[108,156] Cases of PML have also been described with BV.[97,98] Notably, JC virus DNA can be negative in the CSF in these patients.[98] This entity is associated with particularly high mortality rates.[98] In a study of 5 patients who developed PML on BV, presenting symptoms were hemiparesis, hemianopsia, aphasia, gait disturbance, and incoordination along with MRI findings of T2 hyperintensity and T1 hypointensity with enhancing lesions. Of five patients, four died and one improved with oral prednisone over 1 year.[98] The role of plasmapheresis is not well defined in this subset of patients.
- **Aseptic Meningitis**
  - Cases of aseptic meningitis with cetuximab have been reported; however, these patients have had complete recovery after symptomatic treatment and most of these patients had a negative rechallenge test.[127] This can generally be prevented by premedicating patients with antihistamines and dexamethasone 1 hour prior to infusion and utilizing slower infusion rates (5 mg/min with first infusion and 10 mg/min on subsequent infusions).[127]

Nonpharmacological Management of Toxicities

DELIRIUM

- Patients and caregivers should be made aware of the potential adverse effects, such as delirium, associated with many medications. Frequent neuro-checks should be done which can help with early detection of delirium. Standard delirium management, such as maintaining a familiar environment and enlisting the help of the caretaker/family members, can be beneficial. Maintenance of normal sleep-wake cycles and prevention of unnecessary disturbance during nighttime may also benefit these patients. In older patients, constipation, urinary retention, and pain are preventable common causes of delirium. In at-risk patients, sedative and medications with anticholinergic activity should be avoided.

NEUROPSYCHIATRIC SYMPTOMS ASSOCIATED WITH INTERFERON-α

- The presence of social support has been shown to decrease the incidence of depression in patients receiving low-dose IFN–adjuvant therapy for melanoma.[157] Fatigue is another common complaint associated with IFN-α. Regular physical activity, adequate nutrition, and maintaining a fatigue diary have been described to help patients cope with fatigue.[158]

RESPIRATORY DEPRESSION

- Patients with GBS can develop bulbar weakness, increasing their risk of aspiration pneumonia. This risk can be tempered with aggressive chest therapy (pulmonary toilet). Patients should undergo frequent spirometry as it can predict worsening respiratory status and the need for mechanical ventilation.[159]

References

1. Rosenberg SA, Yang JC, White DE, Steinberg SM. Durability of complete responses in patients with metastatic cancer treated with high-dose interleukin-2: identification of the antigens mediating response. *Ann Surg.* 1998;228(3):307–319.
2. Atkins MB, Lotze MT, Dutcher JP, et al. High-dose recombinant interleukin 2 therapy for patients with metastatic melanoma: analysis of 270 patients treated between 1985 and 1993. *J Clin Oncol.* 1999;17(7):2105–2116.
3. Fyfe G, Fisher RI, Rosenberg SA, Sznol M, Parkinson DR, Louie AC. Results of treatment of 255 patients with metastatic renal cell carcinoma who received high-dose recombinant interleukin-2 therapy. *J Clin Oncol.* 1995;13(3):688–696.
4. Sim GC, Radvanyi L. The IL-2 cytokine family in cancer immunotherapy. *Cytokine Growth Factor Rev.* 2014;25(4):377–390.
5. Hanisch UK, Quirion R. Interleukin-2 as a neuroregulatory cytokine. *Brain Res Brain Res Rev.* 1995;21(3):246–284.
6. Saris SC, Patronas NJ, Rosenberg SA, et al. The effect of intravenous interleukin-2 on brain water content. *J Neurosurg.* 1989;71(2):169–174.
7. Rosenberg SA, Lotze MT, Yang JC, et al. Experience with the use of high-dose interleukin-2 in the treatment of 652 cancer patients. *Ann Surg.* 1989;210(4):474–484; discussion 484–485.
8. Gitlitz BJ, Hoffman DM, Moldawer N, Belldegrun A, Figlin RA. Treatment of metastatic renal cell carcinoma with high-dose bolus interleukin-2 in a non-intensive care unit: an analysis of 124 consecutively treated patients. *Cancer J.* 2001;7(2):112–120.
9. Capuron L, Ravaud A, Neveu PJ, Miller AH, Maes M, Dantzer R. Association between decreased serum tryptophan concentrations and depressive symptoms in cancer patients undergoing cytokine therapy. *Mol Psychiatry.* 2002;7(5):468–473.
10. Musselman D, Royster EB, Wang M, et al. The impact of escitalopram on IL-2-induced neuroendocrine, immune, and behavioral changes in patients with malignant melanoma: preliminary findings. *Neuropsychopharmacology.* 2013;38(10):1921–1928.
11. Karp BI, Yang JC, Khorsand M, Wood R, Merigan TC. Multiple cerebral lesions complicating therapy with interleukin-2. *Neurology.* 1996;47(2):417–424.
12. Puduvalli VK, Sella A, Austin SG, Forman AD. Carpal tunnel syndrome associated with interleukin-2 therapy. *Cancer.* 1996;77(6):1189–1192.
13. Loh FL, Herskovitz S, Berger AR, Swerdlow ML. Brachial plexopathy associated with interleukin-2 therapy. *Neurology.* 1992;42(2):462–463.
14. Parker BS, Rautela J, Hertzog PJ. Antitumour actions of interferons: implications for cancer therapy. *Nat Rev Cancer.* 2016;16(3):131–144. doi:10.1038/nrc.2016.14.
15. Fritz-French C, Tyor W. Interferon-alpha (IFN alpha) neurotoxicity. *Cytokine Growth Factor Rev.* 2012;23(1–2):7–14. doi:10.1016/j.cytogfr.2012.01.001.
16. Malek-Ahmadi P, Hilsabeck RC. Neuropsychiatric complications of interferons: classification, neurochemical bases, and management. *Ann Clin Psychiatry.* 2007;19(2):113–123.
17. Hanna TP, Baetz T, Xu J, et al. Mental health services use by melanoma patients receiving adjuvant interferon: association of pre-treatment mental health care with early discontinuation. *Curr Oncol.* 2017;24(6):e503–e512.
18. Raison CL, Demetrashvili M, Capuron L, Miller AH. Neuropsychiatric adverse effects of interferon-alpha: recognition and management. *CNS Drugs.* 2005;19(2):105–123.
19. Caraceni A, Gangeri L, Martini C, et al. Neurotoxicity of interferon-alpha in melanoma therapy: results from a randomized controlled trial. *Cancer.* 1998;83(3):482–489.
20. Shakil AO, Di Bisceglie AM, Hoofnagle JH. Seizures during alpha interferon therapy. *J Hepatol.* 1996;24(1):48–51.
21. Wangensteen KJ, Krawitt EL, Hamill RW, Boyd JT. Parkinsonism in patients with chronic hepatitis C treated with interferons: case reports and review of the literature. *Clin Neuropharmacol.* 2016;39(1):1–5.
22. Lipson EJ, Drake CG. Ipilimumab: an anti-CTLA-4 antibody for metastatic melanoma. *Clin Cancer Res.* 2011;17(22):6958–6962.

23. Postow MA, Sidlow R, Hellmann MD. Immune-related adverse events associated with immune checkpoint blockade. *N Engl J Med.* 2018;378(2):158–168.
24. Ribas A, Hanson DC, Noe DA, et al. Tremelimumab (CP-675,206), a cytotoxic T lymphocyte associated antigen 4 blocking monoclonal antibody in clinical development for patients with cancer. *Oncologist.* 2007;12(7):873–883. doi:10.1634/theoncologist.12-7-873.
25. Maio M, Scherpereel A, Calabro L, et al. Tremelimumab as second-line or third-line treatment in relapsed malignant mesothelioma (DETERMINE): a multicentre, international, randomised, double-blind, placebo-controlled phase 2b trial. *Lancet Oncol.* 2017;18(9):1261–1273.
26. Longoria TC, Tewari KS. Evaluation of the pharmacokinetics and metabolism of pembrolizumab in the treatment of melanoma. *Expert Opin Drug Metab Toxicol.* 2016;12(10):1247–1253.
27. Mocellin S, Nitti D. CTLA-4 blockade and the renaissance of cancer immunotherapy. *Biochim Biophys Acta.* 2013;1836(2):187–196.
28. Blank C, Gajewski TF, Mackensen A. Interaction of PD-L1 on tumor cells with PD-1 on tumor-specific T cells as a mechanism of immune evasion: implications for tumor immunotherapy. *Cancer Immunol Immunother.* 2005;54(4):307–314.
29. Xu-Monette ZY, Zhang M, Li J, Young KH. PD-1/PD-L1 blockade: have we found the key to unleash the antitumor immune response? *Front Immunol.* 2017;8:1597.
30. Cuzzubbo S, Javeri F, Tissier M, et al. Neurological adverse events associated with immune checkpoint inhibitors: review of the literature. *Eur J Cancer.* 2017;73:1–8.
31. Makarious D, Horwood K, Coward JIG. Myasthenia gravis: an emerging toxicity of immune checkpoint inhibitors. *Eur J Cancer.* 2017;82:128–136.
32. Williams TJ, Benavides DR, Patrice KA, et al. Association of autoimmune encephalitis with combined immune checkpoint inhibitor treatment for metastatic cancer. *JAMA Neurol.* 2016;73(8):928–933.
33. Papadopoulos KP, Romero RS, Gonzalez G, Dix JE, Lowy I, Fury M. Anti-Hu-associated autoimmune limbic encephalitis in a patient with PD-1 inhibitor-responsive myxoid chondrosarcoma. *Oncologist.* 2018;23(1):118–120.
34. Raskin J, Masrori P, Cant A, et al. Recurrent dysphasia due to nivolumab-induced encephalopathy with presence of Hu autoantibody. *Lung Cancer.* 2017;109:74–77.
35. Kao JC, Liao B, Markovic SN, et al. Neurological complications associated with anti-programmed death 1 (PD-1) antibodies. *JAMA Neurol.* 2017;74(10):1216–1222.
36. Astaras C, de Micheli R, Moura B, Hundsberger T, Hottinger AF. Neurological adverse events associated with immune checkpoint inhibitors: diagnosis and management. *Curr Neurol Neurosci Rep.* 2018;18(1):3.
37. Barroso-Sousa R, Barry WT, Garrido-Castro AC, et al. Incidence of endocrine dysfunction following the use of different immune checkpoint inhibitor regimens: a systematic review and meta-analysis. *JAMA Oncol.* 2018;4(2):173–182.
38. Zhu X, McDowell MM, Newman WC, Mason GE, Greene S, Tamber MS. Severe cerebral edema following nivolumab treatment for pediatric glioblastoma: case report. *J Neurosurg Pediatr.* 2017;19(2):249–253.
39. Gerdes LA, Held K, Beltran E, et al. CTLA4 as immunological checkpoint in the development of multiple sclerosis. *Ann Neurol.* 2016;80(2):294–300.
40. Liao B, Shroff S, Kamiya-Matsuoka C, Tummala S. Atypical neurological complications of ipilimumab therapy in patients with metastatic melanoma. *Neuro Oncol.* 2014;16(4):589–593.
41. Wilson R, Menassa DA, Davies AJ, et al. Seronegative antibody-mediated neurology after immune checkpoint inhibitors. *Ann Clin Transl Neurol.* 2018;5(5):640–645.
42. Maur M, Tomasello C, Frassoldati A, Dieci MV, Barbieri E, Conte P. Posterior reversible encephalopathy syndrome during ipilimumab therapy for malignant melanoma. *J Clin Oncol.* 2012;30(6):e76–e78.
43. Sun R, Danlos FX, Ammari S, et al. Anti-PD-1 vasculitis of the central nervous system or radionecrosis? *J Immunother Cancer.* 2017;5(1):96.
44. Laubli H, Hench J, Stanczak M, et al. Cerebral vasculitis mimicking intracranial metastatic progression of lung cancer during PD-1 blockade. *J Immunother Cancer.* 2017;5:46.
45. Gu Y, Menzies AM, Long GV, Fernando SL, Herkes G. Immune mediated neuropathy following checkpoint immunotherapy. *J Clin Neurosci.* 2017;45:14–17.
46. Boisseau W, Touat M, Berzero G, et al. Safety of treatment with nivolumab after ipilimumab-related meningoradiculitis and bilateral optic neuropathy. *Eur J Cancer.* 2017;83:28–31.

47. Liewluck T, Kao JC, Mauermann ML. PD-1 inhibitor-associated myopathies: emerging immune-mediated myopathies. *J Immunother*. 2018;41(4):208–211.

48. FDA approves second CAR T-cell therapy. *Cancer Discov*. 2018;8(1):5–6.

49. Mullard A. FDA approves first CAR T therapy. *Nat Rev Drug Discov*. 2017;16(10):669.

50. Xia AL, Wang XC, Lu YJ, Lu XJ, Sun B. Chimeric-antigen receptor T (CAR-T) cell therapy for solid tumors: challenges and opportunities. *Oncotarget*. 2017;8(52):90521–90531.

51. Maus MV, Grupp SA, Porter DL, June CH. Antibody-modified T cells: CARs take the front seat for hematologic malignancies. *Blood*. 2014;123(17):2625–2635.

52. Wang Z, Han W. Biomarkers of cytokine release syndrome and neurotoxicity related to CAR-T cell therapy. *Biomark Res*. 2018;6:4.

53. Gust J, Hay KA, Hanafi LA, et al. Endothelial activation and blood-brain barrier disruption in neurotoxicity after adoptive immunotherapy with CD19 CAR-T cells. *Cancer Discov*. 2017;7(12):1404–1419.

54. Taraseviciute A, Tkachev V, Ponce R, et al. Chimeric antigen receptor T cell-mediated neurotoxicity in nonhuman primates. *Cancer Discov*. 2018;8(6):750–763.

55. Sterner RM, Sakemura R, Cox MJ, et al. GM-CSF inhibition reduces cytokine release syndrome and neuroinflammation but enhances CAR-T cell function in xenografts. *Blood*. 2019;133(7):697–709.

56. Neelapu SS, Locke FL, Bartlett NL, et al. Axicabtagene ciloleucel CAR T-cell therapy in refractory large B-cell lymphoma. *N Engl J Med*. 2017;377(26):2531–2544.

57. Schuster SJ, Svoboda J, Chong EA, et al. Chimeric antigen receptor T cells in refractory B-cell lymphomas. *N Engl J Med*. 2017;377(26):2545–2554.

58. Maude SL, Laetsch TW, Buechner J, et al. Tisagenlecleucel in children and young adults with B-cell lymphoblastic leukemia. *N Engl J Med*. 2018;378(5):439–448.

59. Hay KA, Hanafi LA, Li D, et al. Kinetics and biomarkers of severe cytokine release syndrome after CD19 chimeric antigen receptor-modified T-cell therapy. *Blood*. 2017;130(21):2295–2306.

60. Gardner RA, Finney O, Annesley C, et al. Intent-to-treat leukemia remission by CD19 CAR T cells of defined formulation and dose in children and young adults. *Blood*. 2017;129(25):3322–3331.

61. Park JH, Riviere I, Gonen M, et al. Long-term follow-up of CD19 CAR therapy in acute lymphoblastic leukemia. *N Engl J Med*. 2018;378(5):449–459.

62. Maude SL, Frey N, Shaw PA, et al. Chimeric antigen receptor T cells for sustained remissions in leukemia. *N Engl J Med*. 2014;371(16):1507–1517.

63. Neelapu SS, Tummala S, Kebriaei P, et al. Chimeric antigen receptor T-cell therapy—assessment and management of toxicities. *Nat Rev Clin Oncol*. 2018;15(1):47–62.

64. Andtbacka RH, Ross M, Puzanov I, et al. Patterns of clinical response with talimogene laherparepvec (T-VEC) in patients with melanoma treated in the OPTiM phase III clinical trial. *Ann Surg Oncol*. 2016;23(13):4169–4177.

65. Andtbacka RH, Kaufman HL, Collichio F, et al. Talimogene laherparepvec improves durable response rate in patients with advanced melanoma. *J Clin Oncol*. 2015;33(25):2780–2788.

66. Long GV, Dummer R, Ribas A, et al. Efficacy analysis of MASTERKEY-265 phase 1b study of talimogene laherparepvec (T-VEC) and pembrolizumab (pembro) for unresectable stage IIIB-IV melanoma. *J Clin Oncol*. 2016;34(15).

67. Puzanov I, Milhem MM, Andtbacka RHI, et al. Survival, safety, and response patterns in a phase 1b multicenter trial of talimogene laherparepvec (T-VEC) and ipilimumab (ipi) in previously untreated, unresected stage IIIB-IV melanoma. *J Clin Oncol*. 2015;33(15).

68. Kohlhapp FJ, Kaufman HL. Molecular pathways: mechanism of action for talimogene laherparepvec, a new oncolytic virus immunotherapy. *Clin. Cancer Res*. 2016;22(5):1048–1054.

69. Brinkmann U, Kontermann RE. The making of bispecific antibodies. *MAbs*. 2017;9(2):182–212.

70. FDA grants regular approval to blinatumomab and expands indication to include Philadelphia chromosome-positive B cell. (2018). Fda.gov. Retrieved July 1, 2018, from https://www.fda.gov/Drugs/InformationOnDrugs/ApprovedDrugs/ucm566708.htm.

71. Blinatumomab approval expanded based on MRD. *Cancer Discov*. 2018;8(6):OF3.

72. Viardot A, Goebeler ME, Hess G, et al. Phase 2 study of the bispecific T-cell engager (BiTE) antibody blinatumomab in relapsed/refractory diffuse large B-cell lymphoma. *Blood*. 2016;127(11):1410–1416.

73. Goebeler ME, Knop S, Viardot A, et al. Bispecific T-cell engager (BiTE) antibody construct blinatumomab for the treatment of patients with relapsed/refractory non-Hodgkin lymphoma: final results from a phase I study. *J Clin Oncol*. 2016;34(10):1104–1111.

74. Klinger M, Benjamin J, Kischel R, Stienen S, Zugmaier G. Harnessing T cells to fight cancer with BiTE(R) antibody constructs–past developments and future directions. *Immunol Rev.* 2016;270(1):193–208.
75. Brischwein K, Parr L, Pflanz S, et al. Strictly target cell-dependent activation of T cells by bispecific single-chain antibody constructs of the BiTE class. *J Immunother.* 2007;30(8):798–807.
76. Nagorsen D, Baeuerle PA. Immunomodulatory therapy of cancer with T cell-engaging BiTE antibody blinatumomab. *Exp Cell Res.* 2011;317(9):1255–1260.
77. Klinger M, Brandl C, Zugmaier G, et al. Immunopharmacologic response of patients with B-lineage acute lymphoblastic leukemia to continuous infusion of T cell-engaging CD19/CD3-bispecific BiTE antibody blinatumomab. *Blood.* 2012;119(26):6226–6233.
78. Topp MS, Gokbuget N, Zugmaier G, et al. Phase II trial of the anti-CD19 bispecific T cell-engager blinatumomab shows hematologic and molecular remissions in patients with relapsed or refractory B-precursor acute lymphoblastic leukemia. *J Clin Oncol.* 2014;32(36):4134–4140.
79. Klinger M, Zugmaier G, Naegele V, et al. Pathogenesis-based development of potential mitigation strategies for blinatumomab-associated neurologic events (NEs). *Blood.* 2016;128(22):1589.
80. Martinelli G, Boissel N, Chevallier P, et al. Complete hematologic and molecular response in adult patients with relapsed/refractory Philadelphia chromosome-positive B-precursor acute lymphoblastic leukemia following treatment with blinatumomab: results from a phase II, single-arm, multicenter study. *J Clin Oncol.* 2017;35(16):1795–1802.
81. Topp MS, Gokbuget N, Stein AS, et al. Safety and activity of blinatumomab for adult patients with relapsed or refractory B-precursor acute lymphoblastic leukaemia: a multicentre, single-arm, phase 2 study. *Lancet Oncol.* 2015;16(1):57–66.
82. Kantarjian H, Stein A, Gokbuget N, et al. Blinatumomab versus chemotherapy for advanced acute lymphoblastic leukemia. *N Engl J Med.* 2017;376(9):836–847.
83. Kantarjian HM, Stein AS, Bargou RC, et al. Blinatumomab treatment of older adults with relapsed/refractory B-precursor acute lymphoblastic leukemia: results from 2 phase 2 studies. *Cancer.* 2016;122(14):2178–2185.
84. Magge RS, DeAngelis LM. The double-edged sword: neurotoxicity of chemotherapy. *Blood Rev.* 2015; 29(2):93–100.
85. Peters C, Brown S. Antibody-drug conjugates as novel anti-cancer chemotherapeutics. *Biosci Rep.* 2015; 35(4):e00225.
86. Petersdorf SH, Kopecky KJ, Slovak M, et al. A phase 3 study of gemtuzumab ozogamicin during induction and postconsolidation therapy in younger patients with acute myeloid leukemia. *Blood.* 2013; 121(24):4854–4860.
87. Jen EY, Ko CW, Lee JE, et al. FDA approval: gemtuzumab ozogamicin for the treatment of adults with newly diagnosed CD33-positive acute myeloid leukemia. *Clin. Cancer Res..* 2018;24(14):3242–3246.
88. Highlights of prescribing information. https://www.accessdata.fda.gov/drugsatfda_docs/label/2018/ 125388s097lbl.pdf.
89. Accessdata.fda.gov. 2018. https://www.accessdata.fda.gov/drugsatfda_docs/label/2013/125427lbl.pdf.
90. Deng C, Pan B, O'Connor OA. Brentuximab vedotin. *Clin Cancer Res.* 2013;19(1):22–27.
91. Barok M, Joensuu H, Isola J. Trastuzumab emtansine: mechanisms of action and drug resistance. *Breast Cancer Res.* 2014;16(2):209.
92. Lee JJ, Swain SM. Peripheral neuropathy induced by microtubule-stabilizing agents. *J Clin Oncol.* 2006;24(10):1633–1642.
93. Corbin ZA, Nguyen-Lin A, Li S, et al. Characterization of the peripheral neuropathy associated with brentuximab vedotin treatment of mycosis fungoides and Sezary syndrome. *J Neurooncol.* 2017;132(3):439–446.
94. Younes A, Gopal AK, Smith SE, et al. Results of a pivotal phase II study of brentuximab vedotin for patients with relapsed or refractory Hodgkin's lymphoma. *J Clin Oncol.* 2012;30(18):2183–2189.
95. Pro B, Advani R, Brice P, et al. Brentuximab vedotin (SGN-35) in patients with relapsed or refractory systemic anaplastic large-cell lymphoma: results of a phase II study. *J Clin Oncol.* 2012;30(18):2190–2196.
96. Duvic M, Tetzlaff MT, Gangar P, Clos AL, Sui D, Talpur R. Results of a phase II trial of brentuximab vedotin for CD30+ cutaneous T-cell lymphoma and lymphomatoid papulosis. *J Clin Oncol.* 2015;33(32):3759–3765.
97. Moskowitz CH, Nademanee A, Masszi T, et al. Brentuximab vedotin as consolidation therapy after autologous stem-cell transplantation in patients with Hodgkin's lymphoma at risk of relapse or progression (AETHERA): a randomised, double-blind, placebo-controlled, phase 3 trial. *Lancet.* 2015;385(9980):1853–1862.

98. Carson KR, Newsome SD, Kim EJ, et al. Progressive multifocal leukoencephalopathy associated with brentuximab vedotin therapy: a report of 5 cases from the Southern Network on Adverse Reactions (SONAR) project. *Cancer*. 2014;120(16):2464–2471.

99. Jalan P, Mahajan A, Pandav V, Bekker S, Koirala J. Brentuximab associated progressive multifocal leukoencephalopathy. *Clin Neurol Neurosurg*. 2012;114(10):1335–1337.

100. Krop IE, LoRusso P, Miller KD, et al. A phase II study of trastuzumab emtansine in patients with human epidermal growth factor receptor 2-positive metastatic breast cancer who were previously treated with trastuzumab, lapatinib, an anthracycline, a taxane, and capecitabine. *J Clin Oncol*. 2012;30(26):3234–3241.

101. Verma S, Miles D, Gianni L, et al. Trastuzumab emtansine for HER2-positive advanced breast cancer. *N Engl J Med*. 2012;367(19):1783–1791.

102. Castaigne S, Pautas C, Terre C, et al. Effect of gemtuzumab ozogamicin on survival of adult patients with de-novo acute myeloid leukaemia (ALFA-0701): a randomised, open-label, phase 3 study. *Lancet*. 2012;379(9825):1508–1516.

103. Salles G, Barrett M, Foà R, et al. Rituximab in B-cell hematologic malignancies: a review of 20 years of clinical experience. *Adv Ther*. 2017;34(10):2232–2273.

104. Teo EC, Chew Y, Phipps C. A review of monoclonal antibody therapies in lymphoma. *Crit Rev Oncol Hematol*. 2016;97:72–84.

105. Lee HZ, Miller BW, Kwitkowski VE, et al. U.S. Food and Drug Administration approval: obinutuzumab in combination with chlorambucil for the treatment of previously untreated chronic lymphocytic leukemia. *Clin Cancer Res*. 2014;20(15):3902–3907.

106. Rizzieri D. Zevalin(®) (ibritumomab tiuxetan): after more than a decade of treatment experience, what have we learned? *Crit Rev Oncol Hematol*. 2016;105:5–17.

107. Maloney DG, Grillo-Lopez AJ, White CA, et al. IDEC-C2B8 (Rituximab) anti-CD20 monoclonal antibody therapy in patients with relapsed low-grade non-Hodgkin's lymphoma. *Blood*. 1997;90(6):2188–2195.

108. Carson KR, Evens AM, Richey EA, et al. Progressive multifocal leukoencephalopathy after rituximab therapy in HIV-negative patients: a report of 57 cases from the Research on Adverse Drug Events and Reports project. *Blood*. 2009;113(20):4834–4840.

109. Gribben JG, Hallek M. Rediscovering alemtuzumab: current and emerging therapeutic roles. *Br J Haematol*. 2009;144(6):818–831.

110. Avivi I, Chakrabarti S, Kottaridis P, et al. Neurological complications following alemtuzumab-based reduced-intensity allogeneic transplantation. *Bone Marrow Transplant*. 2004;34(2):137–142.

111. Isidoro L, Pires P, Rito L, Cordeiro G. Progressive multifocal leukoencephalopathy in a patient with chronic lymphocytic leukaemia treated with alemtuzumab. *BMJ Case Rep*. 2014:2014.

112. Bhatnagar V, Gormley NJ, Luo L, et al. FDA approval summary: daratumumab for treatment of multiple myeloma after one prior therapy. *Oncologist*. 2017;22(11):1347–1353.

113. de Weers M, Tai YT, van der Veer MS, et al. Daratumumab, a novel therapeutic human CD38 monoclonal antibody, induces killing of multiple myeloma and other hematological tumors. *J Immunol*. 2011;186(3):1840–1848.

114. Gormley NJ, Ko CW, Deisseroth A, et al. FDA drug approval: elotuzumab in combination with lenalidomide and dexamethasone for the treatment of relapsed or refractory multiple myeloma. *Clin Cancer Res*. 2017;23(22):6759–6763.

115. Richardson PG, Jagannath S, Moreau P, et al. Elotuzumab in combination with lenalidomide and dexamethasone in patients with relapsed multiple myeloma: final phase 2 results from the randomised, open-label, phase 1b-2 dose-escalation study. *Lancet Haematol*. 2015;2(12):e516–e527.

116. Taniwaki M, Yoshida M, Matsumoto Y, Shimura K, Kuroda J, Kaneko H. Elotuzumab for the treatment of relapsed or refractory multiple myeloma, with special reference to its modes of action and SLAMF7 signaling. *Mediterr J Hematol Infect Dis*. 2018;10(1):e2018014.

117. Lonial S, Weiss BM, Usmani SZ, et al. Daratumumab monotherapy in patients with treatment-refractory multiple myeloma (SIRIUS): an open-label, randomised, phase 2 trial. *Lancet*. 2016;387(10027):1551–1560.

118. Lokhorst HM, Plesner T, Laubach JP, et al. Targeting CD38 with daratumumab monotherapy in multiple myeloma. *N Engl J Med*. 2015;373(13):1207–1219.

119. Lonial S, Dimopoulos M, Palumbo A, et al. Elotuzumab therapy for relapsed or refractory multiple myeloma. *N Engl J Med*. 2015;373(7):621–631.

120. Hynes NE, Lane HA. ERBB receptors and cancer: the complexity of targeted inhibitors. *Nat Rev Cancer*. 2005;5(5):341–354.
121. Baselga J. The EGFR as a target for anticancer therapy–focus on cetuximab. *Eur J Cancer*. 2001;37 (suppl 4):S16–S22.
122. Accessdata.fda.gov.2018. https://www.accessdata.fda.gov/drugsatfda_docs/label/2012/125084s0228lbl. pdf.
123. Lo L, Patel D, Townsend AR, Price TJ. Pharmacokinetic and pharmacodynamic evaluation of panitumumab in the treatment of colorectal cancer. *Expert Opin Drug Metab Toxicol*. 2015;11(12):1907–1924.
124. Giusti RM, Shastri KA, Cohen MH, Keegan P, Pazdur R. FDA drug approval summary: panitumumab (Vectibix). *Oncologist*. 2007;12(5):577–583.
125. Hanna N, Lilenbaum R, Ansari R, et al. Phase II trial of cetuximab in patients with previously treated non-small-cell lung cancer. *J Clin Oncol*. 2006;24(33):5253–5258.
126. Saltz LB, Meropol NJ, Loehrer PJ Sr, Needle MN, Kopit J, Mayer RJ. Phase II trial of cetuximab in patients with refractory colorectal cancer that expresses the epidermal growth factor receptor. *J Clin Oncol*. 2004;22(7):1201–1208.
127. Maritaz C, Metz C, Baba-Hamed N, Jardin-Szucs M, Deplanque G. Cetuximab-induced aseptic meningitis: case report and review of a rare adverse event. *BMC Cancer*. 2016;16:384. doi:10.1186/s12885-016-2434-7. PubMed PMID: 27378078; PMCID.
128. Van Cutsem E, Peeters M, Siena S, et al. Open-label phase III trial of panitumumab plus best supportive care compared with best supportive care alone in patients with chemotherapy-refractory metastatic colorectal cancer. *J Clin Oncol*. 2007;25(13):1658–1664.
129. Hecht JR, Patnaik A, Berlin J, et al. Panitumumab monotherapy in patients with previously treated metastatic colorectal cancer. *Cancer*. 2007;110(5):980–988.
130. Hudis CA. Trastuzumab–mechanism of action and use in clinical practice. *N Engl J Med*. 2007;357(1): 39–51.
131. Swain SM, Baselga J, Kim SB, et al. Pertuzumab, trastuzumab, and docetaxel in HER2-positive metastatic breast cancer. *N Engl J Med*. 2015;372(8):724–734.
132. Piccart-Gebhart MJ, Procter M, Leyland-Jones B, et al. Trastuzumab after adjuvant chemotherapy in HER2-positive breast cancer. *N Engl J Med*. 2005;353(16):1659–1672.
133. Bookman MA, Darcy KM, Clarke-Pearson D, Boothby RA, Horowitz IR. Evaluation of monoclonal humanized anti-HER2 antibody, trastuzumab, in patients with recurrent or refractory ovarian or primary peritoneal carcinoma with overexpression of HER2: a phase II trial of the Gynecologic Oncology Group. *J Clin Oncol*. 2003;21(2):283–290.
134. Dutcher JP, Schwartzentruber DJ, Kaufman HL, et al. High dose interleukin-2 (Aldesleukin)-expert consensus on best management practices—2014. *J Immunother Cancer*. 2014;2(1):26.
135. Musselman DL, Lawson DH, Gumnick JF, et al. Paroxetine for the prevention of depression induced by high-dose interferon alfa. *N Engl J Med*. 2001;344(13):961–966.
136. Greenberg DB, Jonasch E, Gadd MA, et al. Adjuvant therapy of melanoma with interferon-alpha-2b is associated with mania and bipolar syndromes. *Cancer*. 2000;89(2):356–362.
137. Brahmer JR, Lacchetti C, Schneider BJ, et al. Management of immune-related adverse events in patients treated with immune checkpoint inhibitor therapy: American Society of Clinical Oncology Clinical Practice Guideline. *J Clin Oncol*. 2018;36(17):1714–1768. doi:10.1200/JCO2017776385.
138. Haanen J, Carbonnel F, Robert C, et al. Management of toxicities from immunotherapy: ESMO Clinical Practice Guidelines for diagnosis, treatment and follow-up. *Ann Oncol*. 2017;28(suppl_4):iv119–iv142.
139. Brown MP, Hissaria P, Hsieh AH, Kneebone C, Vallat W. Autoimmune limbic encephalitis with anti-contactin-associated protein-like 2 antibody secondary to pembrolizumab therapy. *J Neuroimmunol*. 2017;305:16–18.
140. Williams TJ, Benavides DR, Patrice K, et al. Association of Autoimmune Encephalitis With Combined Immune Checkpoint Inhibitor Treatment for Metastatic Cancer. *JAMA Neurol*. 2016;73(8):928–933. doi:10.1001/jamaneurol.2016.1399.
141. Beh SC, Greenberg BM, Frohman T, Frohman EM. Transverse myelitis. *Neurol Clin*. 2013;31(1): 79–138. doi:10.1016/j.ncl.2012.09.008. PubMed PMID: 23186897.
142. Walling AD, Dickson G. Guillain-Barre syndrome. *Am Fam Physician*. 2013;87(3):191–197.
143. Gilhus NE, Verschuuren JJ. Myasthenia gravis: subgroup classification and therapeutic strategies. *Lancet Neurol*. 2015;14(10):1023–1036.

144. Kato T, Hirose S, Kumagai S, Ozaki A, Matsumoto S, Inoko M. Electrocardiography as the first step for the further examination of cardiac involvement in myasthenia gravis. *Biomed Res Int.* 2016;2016:8058946.
145. Lau KH, Kumar A, Yang IH, Nowak RJ. Exacerbation of myasthenia gravis in a patient with melanoma treated with pembrolizumab. *Muscle Nerve.* 2016;54(1):157–161.
146. Thaipisuttikul I, Chapman P, Avila EK. Peripheral neuropathy associated with ipilimumab: a report of 2 cases. *J Immunother.* 2015;38(2):77–79.
147. Zimmer L, Goldinger SM, Hofmann L, et al. Neurological, respiratory, musculoskeletal, cardiac and ocular side-effects of anti-PD-1 therapy. *Eur J Cancer.* 2016;60:210–225.
148. Bhatia S, Huber BR, Upton MP, Thompson JA. Inflammatory enteric neuropathy with severe constipation after ipilimumab treatment for melanoma: a case report. *J Immunother.* 2009;32(2):203–205.
149. Santomasso B, Park JH, Riviere I, et al. Neurotoxicity associated with CD19-specific chimeric antigen receptor T cell therapy for adult acute lymphoblastic leukemia (B-ALL). *Neurology.* 2018;90(15 Suppl): S23.008.
150. Norelli M, Camisa B, Barbiera G, et al. Monocyte-derived IL-1 and IL-6 are differentially required for cytokine-release syndrome and neurotoxicity due to CAR T cells. *Nat Med.* 2018;24(6):739–748.
151. Nellan A, Jayaprakash N, McCully C, Widemann BC, Lee DW, Warren KE. Plasma and cerebrospinal fluid pharmacokinetics of tocilizumab in a nonhuman primate model. *AACR.* 2016:1411.
152. Balis FM, Lester CM, Chrousos GP, Heideman RL, Poplack DG. Differences in cerebrospinal fluid penetration of corticosteroids: possible relationship to the prevention of meningeal leukemia. *J Clin Oncol.* 1987;5(2):202–207.
153. Brudno JN, Kochenderfer JN. Toxicities of chimeric antigen receptor T cells: recognition and management. *Blood.* 2016;127(26):3321–3330.
154. Highlights of prescribing information. https://www.accessdata.fda.gov/drugsatfda_docs/label/2014/125557lbl.pdf.
155. Landi D, De Rossi N, Zagaglia S, et al. No evidence of beneficial effects of plasmapheresis in natalizumab-associated PML. *Neurology.* 2017;88(12):1144–1152.
156. Clifford DB. Progressive multifocal leukoencephalopathy therapy. *J Neurovirol.* 2015;21(6):632–636.
157. Kovacs P, Panczel G, Balatoni T, et al. Social support decreases depressogenic effect of low-dose interferon alpha treatment in melanoma patients. *J Psychosom Res.* 2015;78(6):579–584.
158. Nashan D, Reuter K, Mohr P, Agarwala SS. Understanding and managing interferon-alpha-related fatigue in patients with melanoma. *Melanoma Res.* 2012;22(6):415–423.
159. Lawn ND, Fletcher DD, Henderson RD, Wolter TD, Wijdicks EF. Anticipating mechanical ventilation in Guillain-Barre syndrome. *Arch Neurol.* 2001;58(6):893–898.
160. Migden MR, Rischin D, Schmults CD, Guminski A, Hauschild A, Lewis KD, Rabinowits G. PD-1 blockade with cemiplimab in advanced cutaneous squamous-cell carcinoma. *N Engl J Med.* 2018;379(4):341–351.
161. Horn L, Mansfield AS, Szczęsna A, Havel L, Krzakowski M, Hochmair MJ, Reck M. First-line atezolizumab plus chemotherapy in extensive-stage small-cell lung cancer. *N Engl J Med.* 2018;379(23): 2220–2229.
162. Paz-Ares L, Dvorkin M, Chen Y, Reinmuth N, Hotta K, Trukhin D, Voitko O. Durvalumab plus platinum–etoposide versus platinum–etoposide in first-line treatment of extensive-stage small-cell lung cancer (CASPIAN): a randomised, controlled, open-label, phase 3 trial. *The Lancet.* 2019;394(10212):1929–1939.
163. Faivre-Finn C, Vicente D, Kurata T, Planchard D, Paz-Ares L, Vansteenkiste JF, Naidoo J. LBA49 Durvalumab after chemoradiotherapy in stage III NSCLC: 4-year survival update from the phase III PACIFIC trial. *Ann Oncol.* 2020;31:S1178–S1179.
164. Powles T, Park SH, Voog E, Caserta C, Valderrama BP, Gurney H, Loriot Y. Avelumab maintenance therapy for advanced or metastatic urothelial carcinoma. *N Engl J Med.* 2020;383(13):1218–1230.

CHAPTER 21

Pulmonary Toxicities of Immunotherapy

Pradnya D. Patil, MD, FACP ▪ Tanmay S. Panchabhai, MD, FACP, FCCP

Introduction

- Cancer immunotherapy has come a long way since its inception centuries ago when, in 1777, the surgeon to the Duke of Kent injected himself with malignant cells in an effort to develop a cancer vaccine.[1] The ability to harness one's own immune system to combat malignancy has gained widespread clinical utility in the management of a broad spectrum of malignancies such as melanoma, non–small-cell lung cancer (NSCLC), renal cell carcinoma, and urothelial carcinoma, to name a few. In addition, chimeric antigen receptor CAR T-cell therapy is now approved for use in the second line setting for B-cell acute lymphoblastic leukemia and diffuse large B-cell lymphoma. Multiple ongoing clinical trials are exploring the clinical utility of immunotherapy both as monotherapy and in combination with other agents or treatment modalities such as radiation. Therefore, in the foreseeable future, it is likely that the clinical applications of these therapies will continue to expand.

- The majority of immuno-oncology agents used in clinical practice at this point target immune checkpoint pathways such as cytotoxic T-lymphocyte–associated protein 4 (CTLA-4)-B7-1/B7-2 and programmed cell death 1 transmembrane protein (PD-1)-PD-L1/PD-L2. As these are key pathways in promoting immune tolerance, monoclonal antibodies that interfere with these pathways predictably lead to toxicities which resemble autoimmune phenomenon in their clinical manifestations. Pneumonitis is among the spectrum of immune-related adverse events (irAEs) noted with these agents. Although the overall reported incidence of pneumonitis is low at 2.7% with PD-1 inhibition[2] and less than 1% in patients receiving CTLA-4 inhibitors,[3] it is one of the most feared complications because it has the potential to cause significant morbidity and, potentially, mortality. In this chapter, we describe the various clinical manifestations, pathogenesis, and management of pulmonary toxicities with immunotherapeutic agents.

Immunotherapy-related Pneumonitis

- **Epidemiology and risk factors:** Pneumonitis is the most common manifestation of pulmonary toxicity of immune checkpoint inhibitors. As mentioned above, the overall incidence of pneumonitis with the use of immune checkpoint inhibitors is less than 5% with high grade (≥grade 3) toxicities occurring in 1% to 2% of patients with CTLA-4 inhibitors, 1.1% of patients treated with PD-1 inhibitors, and in 0.4% of patients treated with PD-L1 inhibitors.[4,5] A combination of monoclonal antibodies targeting both the CTLA-4 as well as the PD-1-PD-L1/PD-L2 axes is not only associated with a higher incidence of pneumonitis (10%) versus those who received monotherapy with either agent (3%)[6] but is also more likely to be severe and resistant to therapy.[2,3]

The primary site of the tumor appears to be associated with the risk of developing pneumonitis. In a meta-analysis of 26 clinical trials of PD-1 inhibitors, the incidence of all-grade pneumonitis was significantly higher in patients with NSCLC or renal cell carcinoma than those with melanoma.[2] However, other studies have shown similar incidences of high-grade pneumonitis irrespective of the primary malignancy,[7] although the incidence of pneumonitis-related mortality appears to be higher in patients with NSCLC. In addition, in a retrospective study of patients with pneumonitis, patients with NSCLC had an earlier onset of pneumonitis in comparison to patients with melanoma. Patients with NSCLC developed pneumonitis at a median time of 2.1 months (range 0.2–27.4 months) versus 5.2 months in patients with melanoma (range 0.2–18.1 months).[8] Another meta-analysis of clinical trials using PD-1 and PD-L1 inhibitors in patients with NSCLC also revealed a significantly higher rate of pneumonitis in treatment-naïve patients in comparison to those who had received prior systemic therapy.[5] A retrospective study of 164 patients with lung cancer who were treated with a PD-1/PD-L1 inhibitor did not show any difference in the incidence of subsequent pneumonitis among patients who received thoracic radiation and those who did not.[9] However, some authors have reported radiation recall pneumonitis[10] after the use of immune checkpoint inhibitors; therefore larger studies are needed to determine the role of radiation and subsequent risk of pneumonitis with immune checkpoint inhibitors. Pneumonitis has been observed in both smokers and nonsmokers; therefore it is unclear whether there is an association between the two.[6] Current smokers and those with underlying lung conditions, however, did appear to be at an increased risk for worse clinical outcomes.[6] Many immunotherapy trials excluded patients with preexisting autoimmune conditions due to concern for exacerbation of the underlying autoimmune process. However, a retrospective study looking at outcomes in 52 patients with preexisting autoimmune disorders treated with PD-1 inhibitors showed that immunotherapy use in this patient population led to a flare of their underlying disease in 38% of the time; however, most flares were mild and did not require discontinuation of therapy. In addition, 29% of these patients developed irAEs; 10% were grade 3 and 8% were grade 4.[11] Therefore, although further clinical experience is needed in this population to evaluate the safety of immunotherapy as treatment appears to be relatively well tolerated.

- **Clinical features:** The median time to onset of pneumonitis reported in the literature is 2 to 24 months after initiation of therapy. An earlier onset may be seen in patients with NSCLC, as mentioned above, and those receiving combination therapy.[6] Due to the long half-life of immune checkpoint inhibitors, immune-related pneumonitis should be suspected in all patients presenting with new respiratory symptoms despite discontinuation of immunotherapy. Patients often present with dyspnea, cough, decreased exercise tolerance, worsening hypoxia, and occasionally, low-grade fever or chest pain. However, in one series, up to one-third of the patients were asymptomatic.[6] It is unclear if incidentally detected evidence of pneumonitis on radiography has a different clinical course or outcome than symptomatic pneumonitis. Clinically, patterns of lung involvement include organizing pneumonia, nonspecific interstitial pneumonitis, hypersensitivity pneumonitis, acute lung injury, and acute respiratory distress syndrome. Other less common clinical manifestations include sarcoidosis-like granulomatous disease[12,13] and radiation recall pneumonitis.[10] As the intrathoracic adenopathy seen with sarcoid-like reactions may be mistaken for metastatic/progressive malignancy, clinicians should be aware of the potential for this adverse effect.

- **Pathogenesis:** Immune checkpoint pathways, including the PD-1 and CTLA-4 pathways, function as naturally occurring brakes in the process of T cell activation. These are of vital importance in maintaining immune homeostasis in the body and allowing for negative regulation of autoreactive T cells. This inhibitory signal to T cells is mediated by the binding of PD-1 to its ligands PD-L1 and PD-L2 and CTLA-4 to CD80 and CD86 in the presence of T cell activation. The importance of these pathways in preventing autoimmunity is further supported by the development of severe and fatal autoimmune organ failure in CTLA-4 and PD-1 knockout mice.[14–16]

- These immune checkpoint pathways can be utilized by malignant cells to downregulate the adaptive immune response to tumors, therefore escaping immunosurveillance. Monoclonal antibodies that interfere with the binding of PD-1 or CTLA-4 with their ligands lead to the expansion of cytotoxic T cells and subsequent elimination of cancer cells. However, by interfering with the physiological mechanism for immune tolerance to self-antigens, these agents can lead to irAEs that resemble autoimmune diseases. The various pulmonary toxicities observed with immune checkpoint inhibitors are thought to be a direct consequence of this dysregulation of the immune system; however, the exact mechanism of toxicity and the role of other cells and cytokines is still unknown. As both pathways have synergistic mechanisms of action, combination immunotherapy leads to more potent activation of the adaptive immune system, therefore resulting in a higher rate of toxicity. The lower incidence of pneumonitis in patients with NSCLC treated with PD-L1 inhibitors in comparison to those treated with PD-1 inhibitors may be explained by the vital role of PD-L2 in promoting respiratory tolerance.[17] In contrast to PD-1 inhibitors which block the interaction between PD-1 and both of its ligands, selective PD-L1 inhibition could potentially still allow for the interaction of PD-1 with PD-L2 and preserve immune tolerance in the lungs.

- **Radiographic findings:** A variety of radiographic findings may be observed with pulmonary toxicities of immune checkpoint inhibitors. In one retrospective study, X-ray of the chest did not detect any abnormalities in close to 25% of patients with pneumonitis (Figs. 21.1 and 21.2); therefore computed tomography (CT) is preferred for evaluation in patients with new or worsening respiratory symptoms.[6] The most common finding on imaging is the presence of areas of ground glass attenuation, which may be diffuse or focal, along with intact bronchovascular markings. Other common findings include

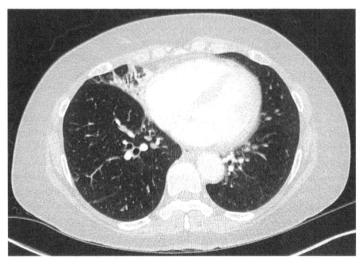

Fig. 21.1   Focal pneumonitis in a patient receiving nivolumab for advanced non–small cell-lung cancer. (Adapted with permission from Sehgal S, Velcheti V, Mukhopadhyay S, Stoller JK. Focal lung infiltrate complicating PD-1 inhibitor use: a new pattern of drug-associated lung toxicity? *Respir Med Case Rep.* 2016;19:118–120.)

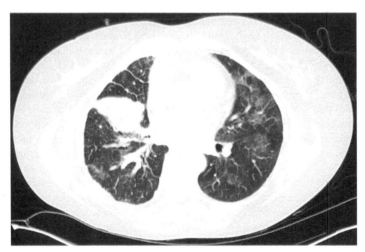

Fig. 21.2 Diffuse ground glass opacities in a patient with Stage IV non–small-cell lung cancer treated with pembrolizumab.

organizing pneumonia in which peripheral or subpleural patchy or confluent consolidations may be seen, or increased interstitial markings accompanied by septal thickening and honeycombing, which may be seen in severe cases. Other reported patterns include tree-in-bud nodularity or centrilobular nodules as may be seen with hypersensitivity pneumonitis and other nonspecific patterns.

- In a multi-institution retrospective study that evaluated various clinical features of pneumonitis associated with immune checkpoint blockade,[6] ground glass opacities were noted in 37% of the patients, hypersensitivity pattern in 22%, cryptogenic organizing pneumonia in 19%, interstitial pattern in 7%, and pneumonitis not otherwise specified was noted in 15% of patients. Focal radiographic appearances have also been reported with immune-related pneumonitis and thus clinicians should be aware of the possibility particularly because these findings masquerade as infectious pneumonia, and the correct diagnosis may be missed unless there is a high degree of suspicion.[18]
- In patients with a sarcoid-like reaction to immunotherapy, enlargement of preexisting lymphadenopathy or new lymphadenopathy may be noted on imaging. As mentioned above, unless clinicians are aware of this potential irAE, lymphadenopathy may be mistaken for disease progression and may lead to discontinuation of a potentially beneficial therapy (Fig. 21.3A and B). In a retrospective study of eight patients who developed sarcoid-like adenopathy with ipilimumab, lymphadenopathy resolved on follow-up with a median time to resolution of 3.1 months (range 1.1–5.4 months).[19]
- **Pathological findings:** Bronchoscopy with bronchoalveolar lavage with or without lung biopsy is not essential for the diagnosis of pneumonitis but may aide in the diagnosis in patients where alternate differential diagnoses such as infection or lymphangitic spread of tumor are being considered. Data regarding the histopathological findings in patients with pneumonitis is sparse. Bronchoalveolar fluid in these patients may be predominantly lymphocytic.[8] Some findings that have been noted on lung biopsy include diffuse alveolar damage, interstitial cellular infiltrate, organizing pneumonia, and eosinophilic infiltrates.[6] In patients with sarcoid-like reactions, poorly formed granulomas may be noted on biopsy.

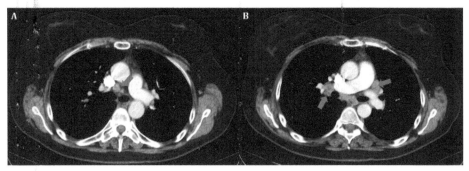

Fig. 21.3 (A and B): Mediastinal lymphadenopathy in the right paratracheal and bilateral hilar regions *(red arrows)* in a patient treated with nivolumab for metastatic melanoma. Endobronchial ultrasound-guided–transbronchial needle aspiration (EBUS-TBNA) yielded non-necrotizing granulomas.

Agents

IMMUNE CHECKPOINT INHIBITORS

- **PD-1 inhibitors:** Programmed cell death 1 (PD-1) is an inhibitory transmembrane protein that is expressed on the surface of B cells, T cells, and natural killer cells. Its action is mediated by binding to two ligands: PD-L1, which is expressed on many cells such as macrophages and dendritic cells as well as tumor cells, and PD-L2, which is usually expressed by hematopoietic cells. Monoclonal antibodies against PD-1 interfere with the binding of PD-1 to either of its ligands, therefore releasing the regulatory brakes on antitumor T cell responses. PD-1 inhibitors that are currently approved for use in clinical practice include pembrolizumab, nivolumab, and cemiplimab. PD-1 inhibitors are widely used in oncology for NSCLC, melanoma, renal cell carcinoma, advanced colon cancer with microsatellite instability, urothelial carcinoma, Merkel cell carcinoma, and head and neck cancer, and cutaneous squamous cell carcinoma to name a few. In a meta-analysis of 20 clinical trials of multiple tumor types with PD-1 inhibitors, the overall incidence of pneumonitis with monotherapy was 2.7% (95% confidence interval [CI], 1.9–3.6%). Of these, 0.8% were grade 3 or higher in severity. As mentioned above, combination with a CTLA-4 inhibitor conferred higher incidence of pulmonary toxicity. In addition, the authors also found a significantly higher incidence of all-grade and grade 3 or higher pneumonitis in patients with NSCLC than melanoma.[2]
- **PD-L1 inhibitors:** PD-L1 inhibitors are monoclonal antibodies against PD-1 which prevent the interaction between PD-1 and PD-L1. As this interaction and upregulation of PD-L1 on tumor cells is a key pathway in immune evasion by tumors, PD-L1 antibodies lead to immune reactivation and subsequent antitumor immune elimination. The PD-L1 inhibitors that have been approved for clinical use include atezolizumab, avelumab, and durvalumab. These are currently being used in NSCLC, urothelial cancer, Merkel cell carcinoma, renal cell carcinoma, triple negative breast cancer, small cell lung cancer, hepatocelluar carcinoma, and melanoma.

  Because PD-L1 antibodies still allow for the interaction between PD-1 and PD-L2, which plays a role in immune tolerance in certain organs such as the lungs, it can be hypothesized that this will lead to effective antitumor T cell activation without loss of immune tolerance and therefore lesser irAEs. It could explain the lower incidence of pneumonitis noted with PD-L1 inhibitors in comparison to that noted with PD-1 inhibitors in some studies.[5] However, others have not shown any difference in the incidence of pneumonitis between the two agents.[6] Larger studies are needed to better understand if there is a relationship between PD-1 or PD-L1 inhibition and subsequent irAEs.

- **CTLA-4 inhibitors:** CD28 is a costimulatory protein which binds to CD80 and CD86 on antigen presenting cells and results in T cell activation and expansion. CTLA-4 is an inhibitory molecule present on the surface of CD4+ and CD8+ T cells and is homologous to CD28 but binds with a much higher affinity to CD80 and CD86 than to CD28, therefore dampening the immune response. Monoclonal antibodies to CTLA-4 target this interaction and lead to enhanced antitumor T cell activity. Ipilimumab is a CTLA-4 antibody that is currently used in melanoma, NSCLC, and renal cell carcinoma and is being evaluated in other tumor types. Tremelimumab is another CTLA-4 inhibitor that is also being evaluated in clinical trials.

  The overall incidence of pneumonitis with monotherapy has been reported to be less than 1% in clinical trials.[3] However, combination with a PD-1/PD-L1 inhibitor is associated with a higher risk of pneumonitis as mentioned above.

- **Cytokines:** Cytokines play a vital role in modulating immune responses in vivo. The ability of cytokines to cause immune activation has been harnessed to promote antitumor immune responses. The cytokine that has been most widely used to date is interleukin-2 (IL-2). The role of other cytokines such as IL-15 is currently being evaluated in clinical trials.

- **IL-2:** High-dose IL-2 has been used in patients with melanoma and renal cell carcinoma and has led to durable responses in a fraction of treated patients. Although it is no longer commonly used due to the high associated toxicity and availability of alternate agents such as immune checkpoint inhibitors, clinicians may have to utilize this drug on occasion and should be aware of the potential toxicities. A major adverse effect of high-dose IL-2 is the development of capillary leak syndrome due to cytokine release. Pulmonary manifestations of this syndrome include pulmonary congestion or edema and pleural effusions in the presence of peripheral edema, generalized edema with intravascular volume depletion, and hypotension. These are usually reversible with discontinuation of therapy.[20] As IL-2 also causes profound defects in neutrophil chemotaxis,[21] infections including pulmonary infections are common and should be considered in patients with persistent fevers.

- **CAR T cells:** Chimeric antigen receptor (CAR) T cells have been successfully used in hematological malignancies and are approved for the treatment of refractory B-cell acute lymphoblastic leukemia and diffuse large B-cell lymphoma. Ongoing trials are exploring their efficacy in a variety of other malignancies. Cytokine release syndrome resulting in respiratory compromise has been noted with the use of CAR T cells.[22]

- **Oncolytic Viruses:** The most frequently used oncolytic virus in clinical practice is talimogene laherparepvec (T-VEC), which is used in the treatment of melanoma. It is an attenuated herpes simplex virus 1 which selectively replicates in and lyses tumor cells. In addition, the inactivated virus also expresses granulocyte monocyte–colony stimulating factor (GM-CSF) which increases antigen presentation and immunogenic response against the tumor.

  Although close to 30% of patients receiving this vaccine intratumorally can experience flu-like symptoms, other immune-related adverse effects including pneumonitis can be seen less frequently. Obstructive airway disease as a consequence of T-VEC therapy has been reported. In immunocompromised hosts, it can lead to disseminated herpetic infections.[23]

- **Vaccines:** The only vaccine that has been approved for use in malignancy to date is sipuleucel-T. This is a form of autologous cellular immunotherapy, wherein a patient's own dendritic cells are isolated and activated in vitro with a recombinant human fusion protein, PAP-GM-CSF, which contains an antigen specific for prostate cancer (prostatic acid phosphatase; PAP) linked to GM-CSF. These activated cells are then injected back into the host and lead to antitumor T cell responses to PAP–expressing tumor cells.

Infusion reactions accompanied by bronchospasm may be seen in up to 71% of patients, with the highest incidence seen with the second infusion. Premedication with acetaminophen and diphenhydramine reduces the likelihood of such a reaction. Up to 9.7% of patients develop flu-like symptoms and 8.7% can develop dyspnea, which is usually low grade. In addition, pulmonary emboli have been reported in postmarketing surveillance of the drug.[24]

Pharmacological Approaches for Management and Treatment

- For any patient receiving immunotherapy, the onset of new or worsening respiratory symptoms should prompt a thorough evaluation for pneumonitis. Initial workup should include a chest X-ray along with a CT scan of the chest to further define the pattern of lung involvement. Spirometry and diffusing capacity of carbon monoxide (DLCO) may be useful to determine the extent of pulmonary involvement. In addition, alternative etiologies such as infections should be ruled out by testing, for example, blood and sputum cultures, respiratory viral polymerase chain reaction, etc. In patients where the etiology is unclear, bronchoscopy with a bronchoalveolar lavage with or without a transbronchial lung biopsy can help solidify the diagnosis. In patients where the clinical and radiographic characteristics are not congruent, further tissue diagnosis with thoracoscopic approach (video assisted thoracoscopic surgery; VATS) can be considered.
- Both the American Society of Clinical Oncology and National Comprehensive Cancer Network (NCCN) guidelines recommend withholding immunotherapy for any evidence of immunotherapy-related pneumonitis, irrespective of the severity.[3,25] For patients who are asymptomatic and have limited lung parenchymal involvement (<25%, grade 1), withholding further immunotherapy and repeating a CT scan of the chest or spirometry/DLCO in 3 to 4 weeks may lead to improvement or resolution of the pneumonitis. In the interim, they should be monitored closely with weekly evaluations, including chest X-ray.[3] In such patients, immunotherapy can be resumed once there is radiographic evidence of improvement. However, if there is no clinical improvement off immunotherapy, patients should be treated with steroids in a similar fashion to those with grade 2 pneumonitis.
- For patients with grade 2 pneumonitis who are symptomatic (limiting activities of daily living) but do not require hospitalization and have involvement of 25% to 50% of the lung parenchyma, prednisone (1–2 mg/kg/day) should be initiated after ruling out infectious etiologies. These patients should be monitored very closely with physical examination and chest X-rays every 3 days. Prednisone should be tapered gradually by 5 or 10 mg/week over a period of 4 to 6 weeks.[3] If there is no improvement with oral steroids within 48 to 72 hours, patients should be admitted for closer monitoring and IV steroids. If the patient remains on steroids for over 12 weeks, appropriate prophylaxis for pneumocystis should be prescribed. Resumption of immunotherapy should only be done once symptoms have improved to grade 1 or better. Consultation with a pulmonologist is advisable.
- For grade 3 (severe symptoms with >50% lung involvement) and grade 4 (life-threatening) pneumonitis, hospital admission should be strongly considered. A thorough infectious workup and possibly empirical antibiotics should be considered in this population due to the severity of illness. In addition, methylprednisolone IV (1–2 mg/kg/day) should be initiated. After symptoms improve to grade 1 or better, corticosteroids should be tapered gradually over a 4- to 6-week period (the NCCN guidelines recommend at least 6 weeks). For steroid refractory patients who do not demonstrate any significant improvement within 48 hours, alternate immunosuppression may be considered. Some alternate drugs that have been recommended for such patients include infliximab, mycophenolate mofetil,

cyclophosphamide, or a 5-day course of intravenous immunoglobulin (IVIG).[3] Infliximab should be given as a 5 mg/kg dose IV and may be repeated in 14 days if needed. Mycophenolate can be started at 1–1.5 g twice daily followed by a taper. IVIG is given at 0.4 g/kg/day for 5 days (NCCN guidelines). Patients with grade 3 or grade 4 pneumonitis should not be rechallenged with the drug as doing so could lead to potentially fatal toxicity.

■ In theory, the use of immunosuppression during immunotherapy could interfere with the antitumor efficacy. However, current evidence suggests that immunosuppression for the treatment of an irAE does not affect antitumor efficacy.[26,27] It is therefore of utmost importance that clinicians treat symptomatic patients with immunosuppression without the fear of compromising antitumor efficacy. In fact, the development of an irAE has been shown to be associated with improved outcomes.[28,29] Therefore, it is essential that the interruption in therapy be minimized if possible, as the patients with the adverse events may be more likely to benefit from continuation of therapy.

Nonpharmacological Approaches for Management and Treatment

■ Optimal patient selection is important to reduce the risk of immune-related pneumonitis with immunotherapy. Patients with impaired lung function and underlying lung disease are at a higher risk of developing pneumonitis and the risks versus benefits of therapy should be weighed carefully prior to starting immunotherapy. For patients who require high-dose IL-2, baseline pulmonary function tests should be obtained. IL-2 use in those with significant impairment is not advisable.

■ Other nonpharmacological approaches include supplemental oxygen, management of respiratory secretions, and for those with severe respiratory impairment, invasive or noninvasive ventilation.

References

1. Ichim CV. Revisiting immunosurveillance and immunostimulation: implications for cancer immunotherapy. *J Transl Med*. 2005;3(1):8.
2. Nishino M, Giobbie-Hurder A, Hatabu H, Ramaiya NH, Hodi FS. Incidence of programmed cell death 1 inhibitor-related pneumonitis in patients with advanced cancer: a systematic review and meta-analysis. *JAMA Oncol*. 2016;2(12):1607–1616.
3. Brahmer JR, Lacchetti C, Schneider BJ, et al. Management of immune-related adverse events in patients treated with immune checkpoint inhibitor therapy: American Society of Clinical Oncology Clinical Practice Guideline. *J Clin Oncol*. 2018;36(17):1714–1768.
4. Puzanov I, Diab A, Abdallah K, et al. Managing toxicities associated with immune checkpoint inhibitors: consensus recommendations from the Society for Immunotherapy of Cancer (SITC) Toxicity Management Working Group. *J Immunother Cancer*. 2017;5(1):95.
5. Khunger M, Rakshit S, Pasupuleti V, et al. Incidence of pneumonitis with use of programmed death 1 and programmed death-ligand 1 inhibitors in non-small cell lung cancer: a systematic review and meta-analysis of trials. *Chest*. 2017;152:271.
6. Naidoo J, Wang X, Woo KM, et al. Pneumonitis in patients treated with anti-programmed death-1/ programmed death ligand 1 therapy. *J Clin Oncol*. 2017;35(7):709–717.
7. Gettinger SN, Horn L, Gandhi L, et al. Overall survival and long-term safety of nivolumab (anti-programmed death 1 antibody, BMS-936558, ONO-4538) in patients with previously treated advanced non-small-cell lung cancer. *J Clin Oncol*. 2015;33(18):2004–2012.
8. Delaunay M, Cadranel J, Lusque A, et al. Immune-checkpoint inhibitors associated with interstitial lung disease in cancer patients. *Eur Respir J*. 2017;50(2):1700050.
9. Hwang WL, Niemierko A, Hwang KL, et al. Clinical outcomes in patients with metastatic lung cancer treated with PD-1/PD-L1 inhibitors and thoracic radiotherapy. *JAMA Oncol*. 2018;4(2):253–255.

10. Shibaki R, Akamatsu H, Fujimoto M, et al. Nivolumab induced radiation recall pneumonitis after two years of radiotherapy. *Ann Oncol.* 2017;28(6):1404–1405.
11. Menzies AM, Johnson DB, Ramanujam S, et al. Anti-PD-1 therapy in patients with advanced melanoma and preexisting autoimmune disorders or major toxicity with ipilimumab. *Ann Oncol.* 2017;28(2): 368–376.
12. Montaudié H, Pradelli J, Passeron T, Lacour JP, Leroy S. Pulmonary sarcoid-like granulomatosis induced by nivolumab. *Br J Dermatol.* 2017;176(4):1060–1063.
13. Danlos FX, Pagès C, Baroudjian B, et al. Nivolumab-induced sarcoid-like granulomatous reaction in a patient with advanced melanoma. *Chest.* 2016;149(5):e133–e136.
14. Tivol EA, Borriello F, Schweitzer AN, Lynch WP, Bluestone JA, Sharpe AH. Loss of CTLA-4 leads to massive lymphoproliferation and fatal multiorgan tissue destruction, revealing a critical negative regulatory role of CTLA-4. *Immunity.* 1995;3(5):541–547.
15. Waterhouse P, Penninger JM, Timms E, et al. Lymphoproliferative disorders with early lethality in mice deficient in CTLA-4. *Science.* 1995;270(5238):985–988.
16. Nishimura H, Okazaki T, Tanaka Y, et al. Autoimmune dilated cardiomyopathy in PD-1 receptor-deficient mice. *Science.* 2001;291(5502):319–322.
17. Xiao Y, Yu S, Zhu B, et al. RGMb is a novel binding partner for PD-L2 and its engagement with PD-L2 promotes respiratory tolerance. *J Exp Med.* 2014;211(5):943–959.
18. Sehgal S, Velcheti V, Mukhopadhyay S, Stoller JK. Focal lung infiltrate complicating PD-1 inhibitor use: a new pattern of drug-associated lung toxicity? *Respir Med Case Rep.* 2016;19:118–120.
19. Tirumani SH, Ramaiya NH, Keraliya A, et al. Radiographic profiling of immune-related adverse events in advanced melanoma patients treated with ipilimumab. *Cancer Immunol Res.* 2015;3(10):1185–1192.
20. White RL, Schwartzentruber DJ, Glueria A, et al. Cardiopulmonary toxicity of treatment with high-dose interleukin-2 in 199 consecutive patients with metastatic melanoma or renal cell carcinoma. *Cancer.* 1994;74:3122–3212.
21. Klempner MS, Noring R, Mier JW, et al. An acquired chemotactic defect in neutrophils from patients receiving interleukin-2 immunotherapy. *N Engl J Med.* 1990;322:959–965.
22. Grupp SA, Kalos M, Barrett D, et al. Chimeric antigen receptor-modified T cells for acute lymphoid leukemia. *N Engl J Med.* 2013;368:1509–1518.
23. IMLYGIC (talimogene laherparepvec) prescribing information. FDA 2018. https://www.fda.gov/downloads/BiologicsBloodVaccines/CellularGeneTherapyProducts/ApprovedProducts/UCM469575.pdf.
24. PROVENGE (sipuleucel-T) prescribing information. FDA 2018. https://www.fda.gov/downloads/BiologicsBloodVaccines/CellularGeneTherapyProducts/ApprovedProducts/UCM210031.pdf.
25. NCCN website. https://www.nccn.org/professionals/physician_gls/pdf/immunotherapy.pdf.
26. Weber JS, Hodi FS, Wolchok JD, et al. Safety profile of nivolumab monotherapy: a pooled analysis of patients with advanced melanoma. *J Clin Oncol.* 2017;35(7):785–792.
27. Horvat TZ, Adel NG, Dang TO, et al. Immune-related adverse events, need for systemic immunosuppression, and effects on survival and time to treatment failure in patients with melanoma treated with ipilimumab at Memorial Sloan Kettering Cancer Center. *J Clin Oncol.* 2015;33(28):3193–3198.
28. Freeman-Keller M, Kim Y, Cronin H, Richards A, Gibney G, Weber JS. Nivolumab in resected and unresectable metastatic melanoma: characteristics of immune-related adverse events and association with outcomes. *Clin Cancer Res.* 2016;22(4):886–894.
29. Haratani K, Hayashi H, Chiba Y, et al. Association of immune-related adverse events with nivolumab efficacy in non-small-cell lung cancer. *JAMA Oncol.* 2018;4(3):374–378.

CHAPTER 22

Dermatologic Toxicities of Immunotherapy

Pradnya D. Patil, MD ■ Vamsidhar Velcheti, MD

Introduction

- Cancer immunoediting is the process by which malignant cells evade the immune system—first by incomplete elimination of tumor cells during immunosurveillance, followed by an equilibrium phase, and finally by an immune escape phase.[1] The immune escape phenomenon is mediated by a variety of interactions within the tumor microenvironment, among which immune checkpoint pathways play a prominent role. Immune checkpoint axes such as cytotoxic T-lymphocyte–associated protein 4 (CTLA-4)–B7-1/B7-2 and programmed cell death 1 transmembrane protein (PD-1)–PD-L1/PD-L2 are physiological negative regulators of activated T cells that lead to immune tolerance of normal tissues and therefore prevent autoimmunity. Because tumor cells upregulate these pathways to dampen immunosurveillance, inhibiting these axes by utilizing monoclonal antibodies has proved to be a successful therapeutic strategy for a wide range of malignancies.

- The downside to the unbridled immune activation with immune checkpoint inhibitors (ICIs) is that it can also lead to loss of immune homeostasis and result in a broad spectrum of immune-related adverse effects (irAEs). These irAEs can affect a variety of organ systems and bear a resemblance to autoimmune diseases in their clinical presentation. Dermatological irAEs are the most common irAEs reported and can be seen in 37% to 70% (all-grade) of patients treated with ipilimumab and in 17% to 37% of those receiving PD-1 inhibitors.[2] Grade 3 or higher toxicity is seen only in 1% to 3% of these patients. The incidence of cutaneous toxicities also varies according to the underlying malignancy—it appears to be more common in patients with melanoma or renal cell carcinoma in comparison to patients with non–small-cell lung cancer.[3]

  There are emerging data to suggest that the development of irAEs is associated with objective tumor responses and improved survival outcomes.[4,5] Objective response rates as high as 69% to 75% in patients who developed cutaneous irAEs with ICIs have been reported in the literature.[3] In a meta-analysis of 27 studies of patients with advanced melanoma treated with immunotherapy, the development of vitiligo as an irAE was associated with improved progression-free survival (hazard ratio [HR] 0.51; 95% confidence interval [CI] 0.32–0.82, $P < .005$) and overall survival (HR 0.25; 95% CI 0.10–0.61; $P < .003$).[6] It is therefore imperative to treat cutaneous irAEs effectively while minimizing interruption of therapy with ICIs because patients who develop irAEs appear to be more likely to derive benefit from continued treatment.

- In this chapter we describe the various clinical manifestations of cutaneous toxicities of ICIs, their pathophysiology, and approaches for their management and treatment.

Description

- **Clinical manifestations:** The time to onset of dermatological toxicities with immunotherapeutic agents is quite variable. Whereas some patients may develop cutaneous adverse events within 2 weeks of initiating therapy, others may manifest toxicities several months into their treatment. Despite the broad spectrum of dermatological reactions noted with immunotherapeutic agents, these can be classified into broad categories based on common clinicopathological features. The most commonly observed rashes are usually inflammatory in nature.[7] This category includes maculopapular rashes along with a variety of other less frequent rashes such as lichenoid, acneiform, exfoliative, dermal hypersensitivity-like, psoriasiform, or photosensitivity rashes. The common cutaneous toxicity noted with ICIs is a pruritic maculopapular rash. Maculopapular rashes tend to have an early onset into the treatment course and occur earlier with a combination of CTLA-4/PD-1 blockade than with either agent alone.[8] On examination, characteristic erythematous macules or papules are usually noted on the trunk but usually spare the hands, feet and face. Occasionally, the rash may be more prominent in sun-exposed areas. Rarely, maculopapular rashes may precede more severe cutaneous toxicities, which are described later. Lichenoid rashes are characteristically noted with PD-1/PD-L1 inhibitors rather than with CTLA-4 blockers and tend to present later. Physical examination in such cases shows flat-topped papules with visible striae which may involve the palms and soles and rarely present with mucosal lesions in the oral or genital regions.[9] Psoriasiform dermatological reactions resemble psoriasis in their manifestations and include the typical erythematous plaques covered by silvery white scales, which are preferentially located over the knees, elbows, scalp, or the intertriginous areas. Other less common forms of psoriasis, such as pustular or guttate psoriasis, or even the development of de-novo psoriatic arthritis with immunotherapy have been described.[10,11]
- **Inflammatory rashes:** Inflammatory rashes also include the potentially life threatening severe cutaneous adverse reactions (SCARs) such as drug reaction with eosinophilia and systemic symptoms (DRESS), Stevens-Johnson Syndrome/Toxic Epidermal Necrolysis (SJS/TEN), and acute generalized exanthematous pustulosis (AGEP).
  - **DRESS:** DRESS is a clinical syndrome in which patients develop a skin eruption accompanied by significant eosinophilia and organ involvement after exposure to a culprit drug. Patients often present with a morbilliform rash which progresses to a confluent erythematous rash with follicular accentuation, typically involving greater than 50% of the body surface area (BSA) and often with facial involvement. Patients have other systemic symptoms such as fever, malaise, lymphadenopathy, and other symptoms related to underlying organ dysfunction. Laboratory workup usually reveals significant eosinophilia, atypical lymphocytosis, and abnormal liver or renal function tests. Some patients may also have pulmonary involvement in the form of interstitial pneumonitis with or without pleural effusions.
  - **AGEP:** AGEP is a drug reaction characterized by the development of diffuse sterile pustules usually on top of an erythematous rash and is accompanied by systemic symptoms such as fever. The rash usually starts in the face or intertriginous areas and spreads to the trunk or limbs. Mucosal surfaces are usually spared. Patients may have facial edema and fever at presentations. Laboratory evaluations are remarkable for leukocytosis with a neutrophilic predominance.
  - **SJS and TEN:** SJS and TEN are severe cutaneous adverse effects which are a consequence of extensive keratinocyte necrosis in reaction to immunotherapy, leading to detachment of the epidermis. Based on the percentage of BSA involved, the reaction is either categorized as SJS (<10% of BSA) or TEN (>30% BSA). Patients with 10% to 30% BSA involvement have an SJS/TEN-overlap syndrome. Patients may present with a prodrome consisting of fever, flu-like symptoms, photophobia, conjunctival itching, erythematous rash, myalgias,

or arthralgias. On examination, patients usually have a painful erythematous rash in the involved areas which may evolve into vesicles or bullae with time. The palms and soles tend to be spared in this condition. A positive Nikolsky sign, in which superficial sloughing of the skin can be provoked by applying lateral pressure to the surface of apparently uninvolved skin, is classically positive. Mucosal involvement is also typical, manifesting as painful erosions in the buccal mucosa and, occasionally, with severe conjunctivitis, odynophagia, or genital erosions. Due to massive fluid and electrolyte losses and the catabolic state associated with this disorder, electrolyte imbalances as well as hypoalbuminemia are commonly noted upon laboratory evaluation. These patients are at risk of bacterial superinfection of their skin lesions and must be carefully monitored and treated for the same.

- **Rashes resembling autoimmune conditions:** Another broad category of cutaneous reactions includes rashes that resemble autoimmune dermatological conditions. Bullous pemphigoid-like reactions have been reported with PD-1/PD-L1 inhibitors but have not been reported with CTLA-4 inhibitors. The onset of blistering may be heralded by pruritis or a mild erythematous rash. On physical examination, patients often have a variable number of tense bullae which can rupture leading to moist erosions. These blisters are more commonly noted on the trunk or intertriginous areas and rarely involve mucosal surfaces. These lesions may also persist even after discontinuation of the offending immunotherapeutic agent.[12] Other reactions that resemble autoimmune conditions include dermatomyositis (serological workup may be negative for anti-Jo1 antibodies), vasculitis, and Sjogren's or sicca syndrome.[13–16]

- **Vitiligo:** Other rare cutaneous toxicities as a result of alteration of melanocytes include vitiligo, regression of melanocytic nevi, and tumoral melanosis.[7] The higher incidence of vitiligo in patients with melanoma is likely a consequence of shared antigens among melanoma cells and melanocytes.[17] Vitiligo associated with immunotherapeutic agents is usually symmetric in distribution and tends to be irreversible.

- **Other dermatological toxicities:** Other infrequently observed toxicities include alopecia, re-pigmentation of hair, and dystrophic nails.[18,19]

Diagnostic Workup

- Diagnostic workup for all patients should include thorough physical examination, including close attention to examination of mucosal surfaces. In addition, history of concomitant medications, travel, or other environmental exposures which could point towards an alternative etiology must be obtained. Routine laboratory evaluation, including a complete blood count and comprehensive metabolic panel, may be obtained for patients with higher grade toxicities. Peripheral eosinophilia has been noted in some patients with cutaneous immune related adverse effects.[20]

- Dermatological toxicity of ICIs is a clinical diagnosis; however, a biopsy may aide diagnosis in cases where the etiology is not clear or in cases that do not respond to initial therapy. A majority of patients with cutaneous adverse effects of ICIs will have a lichenoid or interface pattern on histology. This is characterized by a dense lymphocytic infiltrate that abuts or obscures the dermoepidermal junction. In patients with maculopapular rashes with ICIs, a perivascular T cell infiltrate, along with varying degrees of eosinophilic infiltrate, may be observed.[8] In patients with bullous pemphigoid, direct immunofluorescence shows immunoglobulin (Ig) G and complement 3 deposits at the basal membrane. Serum enzyme-linked immunosorbent assay (ELISA) for the pathognomonic antibodies to BP180 and BP230 can be performed to confirm the diagnosis. In patients where an autoimmune condition is suspected, workup for autoantibodies including antinuclear antibody, SS-A/Anti-Ro, SS-B/Anti-La (if predominantly photodistributed/photosensitivity), antihistone, and double-stranded DNA antibodies, is indicated.[2]

Agents and Mechanisms of Action

- **Immune checkpoint inhibitors:** Dermatological toxicities are the most commonly reported adverse effect with ICIs. These are a consequence of the dysregulation of immune tolerance mediated by physiological immune checkpoints resulting in unrestrained infiltration of activated T cells in affected organs. Although cutaneous toxicities have been observed with blockade of both the PD-1/PD-L1 pathway and the CTLA-4 pathway, there are some subtle differences in some of the clinical manifestations with agents belonging to each of those classes. For example, bullous pemphigoid-like reactions have been reported with PD-1/PD-L1 inhibitors but not with CTLA-4 inhibitors. Cutaneous toxicities are observed more frequently with CTLA-4 blockade and with combination therapy of a PD-1 and CTLA-4 inhibitor than with a PD-1 inhibitor alone.[8]
- **Cytokines:** A self-limiting pruritic erythematous macular rash is seen in most patients who receive high-dose interleukin-2 for the treatment of melanoma or renal cell carcinoma. However, in a subset of patients this reaction may be severe and may resemble one of the SCARs, such as TEN.[21]
- **Chimeric antigen receptor (CAR) T-cells:** A skin rash may be observed in 8% to 16% of patients treated with CAR T cells for refractory hematological malignancies.
- **Oncolytic viruses:** Rare side effects observed with talimogene laherparepvec (T-VEC), which is the most commonly used oncolytic virus, include rash, cellulitis, vitiligo, and exacerbation of psoriatic lesions.

Pharmacological Approaches for Management and Treatment

The severity of dermatological toxicity should be measured in accordance with the National Cancer Institute's Common Terminology Criteria for Adverse Events (NCI-CTCAE) which takes into account both the extent of the lesions and the impact on activities of daily living. Although most cutaneous adverse effects resolve with conservative management or interruption of therapy, close attention must be paid to the physical examination for all patients because innocuous clinical presentations such as pruritis or maculopapular rash may precede other potentially life-threatening SCARs.

WITHHOLDING IMMUNE CHECKPOINT INHIBITORS

For most cutaneous adverse effects that are grade 3 or higher, ICIs must be placed on hold at least until the toxicity is reduced to grade 1 or less. It is prudent to involve a dermatologist in the decision-making prior to rechallenging patients with higher grade cutaneous toxicities. For patients with grade 1 inflammatory rashes, ICIs may be continued; however, for those with grade 2 toxicity, consideration should be given to withholding ICIs until the severity is less than grade 1. On the other hand, for any patient with bullous dermatoses and greater than 10% BSA involvement, ICIs should be withheld, and may be permanently discontinued for involvement of greater than 30% BSA associated with fluid or electrolyte abnormalities. Similarly, for any patient with suspected SCAR, ICIs should be withheld immediately. A SCAR is usually considered to be a contraindication for rechallenging patients with ICIs.[2]

- **Immunosuppression:** Immunosuppression and other supportive measures form the backbone of treatment for immune-mediated cutaneous toxicities. Supportive care includes antihistamines and emollients for symptomat relief. For lower grade (1 and 2) inflammatory rashes, patients should first be treated with mild and moderate potency topical corticosteroids. If there is no improvement with this regimen, high-potency topical steroids should first be started along with oral prednisone (1 mg/kg/day), which should be tapered gradually over 4 weeks. For higher grade (3 or 4) toxicity, intravenous methylprednisolone (1–2 mg/kg/day) may be initiated and followed by a slow steroid taper upon clinical improvement. Steroid-sparing agents such as infliximab, mycophenolate mofetil, or cyclophosphamide may be used for steroid-dependent or refractory cases.[22]

- For patients with grade 2 bullous dermatoses (blisters affecting 10%–30% of BSA), high-potency topical steroids should be initiated. If there is no improvement, early initiation of 0.5–1 mg/kg/day of prednisone should be considered. For grade 3 or higher bullous dermatoses, IV methylprednisolone (1–2 mg/kg) should be initiated with a taper over at least 4 weeks. Rituximab has been used successfully for the management of bullous dermatoses and may allow for shorter courses of steroids.[23]

- For patients with severe cutaneous adverse reactions, topical treatments such as emollients, medium- to high-potency topical corticosteroids, and oral antihistamines should be initiated. Any patient with skin sloughing should be considered to have at least grade 3 toxicity and should be treated with 0.5–1 mg/kg/day of methylprednisolone. For grade 4 SCARs (sloughing/blisters involving >30% BSA), higher doses of methylprednisolone (1–2 mg/kg/day) should be considered. Intravenous immunoglobulin or cyclosporine may be used in severe or refractory cases.[2]

Nonpharmacological Approaches for Management and Treatment

- For any patient with an immune-mediated cutaneous adverse effect, skin care including topical emollients and the use of sunscreens and protective clothing to avoid sun exposure is advised. For patients with denuding cutaneous reactions (bullous dermatoses or SJS/TEN), local wound care is crucial in avoiding complications such as bacterial superinfections. For bullous dermatoses, petroleum ointment or bandages may be used over open erosions. Any patient with a grade 3 or higher SCAR should be admitted to a burn unit for intensive monitoring and treatment of associated fluid and electrolyte imbalances. In addition, aggressive wound care and prompt recognition and treatment of bacterial infections is an integral part of the management of these patients. Pain management and involvement of other specialties such as ophthalmology, urology, etc., depending on the mucosal surfaces involved, may be warranted.

- In conclusion, although most cutaneous adverse effects of immunotherapeutic agents are easily managed with a conservative approach and brief interruption of therapy, careful attention to the history and physical examination must be paid to identify patients with more severe forms of reactions that could result in significant morbidity and mortality.

References

1. Dunn GP, Bruce AT, Ikeda H, et al. Cancer immunoediting: from immunosurveillance to tumor escape. *Nat Immunol.* 2002;3(11):991–998.
2. Brahmer JR, Lacchetti C, Schneider BJ, et al. Management of immune-related adverse events in patients treated with immune checkpoint inhibitor therapy: American Society of Clinical Oncology Clinical Practice Guideline. *J Clin Oncol.* 2018;36(17):1714–1768.
3. Kaunitz GJ, Loss M, Rizvi H, et al. Cutaneous eruptions in patients receiving immune checkpoint blockade: clinicopathologic analysis of the nonlichenoid histologic pattern. *Am J Surg Pathol.* 2017;41(10):1381–1389.
4. Judd J, Zibelman M, Handorf E, et al. Immune-related adverse events as a biomarker in non-melanoma patients treated with programmed cell death 1 inhibitors. *Oncologist.* 2017;22(10):1232–1237.

5. Freeman-Keller M, Kim Y, Cronin H, et al. Nivolumab in resected and unresectable metastatic melanoma: characteristics of immune-related adverse events and association with outcomes. *Clin Cancer Res.* 2016;22(4):886–894.
6. Teulings HE, Limpens J, Jansen SN, et al. Vitiligo-like depigmentation in patients with stage III–IV melanoma receiving immunotherapy and its association with survival: a systematic review and meta-analysis. *J Clin Oncol.* 2015;33(7):773–781.
7. Curry JL, Tetzlaff MT, Nagarajan P, et al. Diverse types of dermatologic toxicities from immune checkpoint blockade therapy. *J Cutan Pathol.* 2017;44(2):158–176.
8. Sibaud V. Dermatologic reactions to immune checkpoint inhibitors: skin toxicities and immunotherapy. *Am J Clin Dermatol.* 2018;19(3):345–361.
9. Tetzlaff MT, Nelson KC, Diab A, et al. Granulomatous/sarcoid-like lesions associated with checkpoint inhibitors: a marker of therapy response in a subset of melanoma patients. *J Immunother Cancer.* 2018;6(1):14.
10. Menzies AM, Johnson DB, Ramanujam S, et al. Anti-PD-1 therapy in patients with advanced melanoma and preexisting autoimmune disorders or major toxicity with ipilimumab. *Ann Oncol.* 2017;28:368–376.
11. Bonigen J, Raynaud-Donzel C, Hureaux J, et al. Anti-PD1-induced psoriasis: a study of 21 patients. *J Eur Acad Dermatol Venereol.* 2017;31:e254–e257.
12. Naidoo J, Schindler K, Querfeld C, et al. Autoimmune bullous skin disorders with immune checkpoint inhibitors targeting PD-1 and PD-L1. *Cancer Immunol Res.* 2016;4:383–389.
13. Sheik S, Goddard AL, Luke JJ, et al. Drug-induced dermatomyositis following ipilimumab therapy. *JAMA Dermatol.* 2015;151:195–199.
14. Yamaguchi Y, Abe R, Haga N, et al. A case of drug associated dermatomyositis following ipilimumab therapy. *Eur J Dermatol.* 2016;26:320–321.
15. Le Burel S, Champiat S, Routier E, et al. Onset of connective tissue disease following anti-PD-1/PD-L1 cancer immunotherapy. *Ann Rheum Dis.* 2018;77(3):468–470.
16. Cappelli LC, Gutierrez AK, Baer AN, et al. Inflammatory arthritis and sicca syndrome induced by nivolumab and ipilimumab. *Ann Rheum Dis.* 2017;76:43–50.
17. Larsabal M, Marti A, Jacquemin C, et al. Vitiligo-like lesions occurring in patients receiving anti-programmed cell death-1 therapies are clinically and biologically distinct from vitiligo. *J Am Acad Dermatol.* 2017;76:863–870.
18. Rivera N, Boada A, Bielsa MI, et al. Hair repigmentation during immunotherapy treatment with an anti-programmed cell death 1 and anti-programmed cell death ligand 1 agent for lung cancer. *JAMA Dermatol.* 2017;153(11):1162–1165.
19. Zarbo A, Belum VR, Sibaud V, et al. Immune-related alopecia (areata and universalis) in cancer patients receiving immune checkpoint inhibitors. *Br J Dermatol.* 2017;176:1649–1652.
20. Lacouture ME, Wolchok JD, Yosipovitch G, et al. Ipilimumab in patients with cancer and the management of dermatologic adverse events. *J Am Acad Dermatol.* 2014;71:161–169.
21. Wiener JS, Tucker JA, Walther PJ. Interleukin-2-induced dermatotoxicity resembling toxic epidermal necrolysis. *South Med J.* 1992;85(6):656–659.
22. Friedman CF, Proverbs-Singh TA, Postow MA. Treatment of the immune-related adverse effects of immune checkpoint inhibitors: a review. *JAMA Oncol.* 2016;2(10):1346–1353.
23. Sowerby L, Dewan AK, Granter S, Gandhi L, LeBoeuf NR. Rituximab treatment of nivolumab-induced bullous pemphigoid. *JAMA Dermatol.* 2017;153(6):603–605.

CHAPTER 23

Cardivascular Toxicities of Immunotherapy

Shipra Gandhi, MD   Aman Gupta, MD   Pankit Vachhani, MD

Igor Puzanov, MD   Marc S. Ernstoff, MD

Introduction

Recent advances in the field of immunotherapy have revolutionized the treatment of cancer and have given hope to patients with cancers that were associated with a poor prognosis. Immune therapies have now been US Food and Drug Administration (FDA)–approved in the frontline setting for metastatic melanoma, non–small-cell lung cancer (NSCLC), renal cell carcinoma, and as second-line therapy for renal cell carcinomas, bladder cancer, Merkel cell carcinoma, gastric cancer, hepatocellular carcinoma, head and neck cancer, Hodgkin's lymphoma, and microsatellite instability-high (MSI-H) or mismatch repair deficient (dMMR) cancer. FDA–approved available immune therapies consist of immune checkpoint inhibitors (ICIs), adoptive cell transfer therapies, interferon-α (IFN-α), and interleukin-2 (IL-2). "Immune-like" therapies such as trastuzumab with cardiac side-effects have not been included in this chapter as they are discussed elsewhere. Immune therapies result in durable responses in a significant number of patients. However, varied immune-related adverse events (irAEs) may emerge as a result of nonspecific targeting of normal tissue besides the tumor tissue. The various irAEs associated with the use of ICIs include colitis, pneumonitis, hepatitis, nephritis, and uveitis, and are generally managed with high-dose glucocorticoids, at least initially. Cardiotoxic effects associated with the use of ICIs were not initially recognized but are now a well-recognized rare complication.[1] Clinically severe and even fatal cardiac events have occurred in rare instances with ICIs and, hence, it is important to detect cardiac adverse events early to initiate successful intervention. Other immune therapies are also associated with cardiac toxicities presumed to be by off-target tissue mechanisms or by cytokine release syndrome (CRS). With increasing use of ICI therapies, the incidence of immune-mediated cardiotoxicities may rise, and hence, it is necessary that emergency medicine physicians, internists, oncologists, and cardiologists be vigilant and identify early signs to improve management.

Description

IMMUNE CHECKPOINT INHIBITORS

Currently, there are several ICIs that are approved by the US FDA. Ipilimumab, an anticytotoxic T-lymphocyte-associated protein 4 (anti-CTLA-4) antibody, was the first ICI approved to be used in metastatic melanoma. Nivolumab and pembrolizumab, which target programmed cell death protein-1 (PD-1), have been approved for use in melanoma, metastatic NSCLC, head and neck squamous cell cancer, urothelial carcinoma, gastric adenocarcinoma, and dMMR solid tumors, as well as for classic Hodgkin's lymphoma. Nivolumab is also approved for use in hepatocellular carcinoma and in patients with renal cell carcinoma. The combination of nivolumab and ipilimumab has been approved by the FDA for treatment of metastatic melanoma and renal cell carcinoma. Recently, antibodies targeting the ligand of PD-1, programmed cell death protein-ligand 1 (PD-L1), have been approved, namely, atezolizumab (urothelial cancer and NSCLC), durvalumab (urothelial cancer), and avelumab (Merkel cell carcinoma and urothelial cancer), which also block the PD-1 pathway. This field is rapidly evolving as new agents and combinations continue to be made and tested.[2]

BLINATUMOMAB

Blinatumomab is a newly developed monoclonal antibody. It is a bispecific T cell engager, or BiTE, that is directed against CD19 on B lymphocytes and CD3 on T cells. This novel agent for the treatment of B-cell precursor acute lymphoblastic leukemia (ALL) has demonstrated encouraging response rates in the setting of minimal residual disease (MRD)–positive (80% complete remission) and relapsed/refractory (R/R) patients. Thus, it is approved by the FDA for the treatment of R/R, Philadelphia chromosome (Ph)-negative and positive B-cell precursor ALL in adults and children. Due to this success, the incorporation of blinatumomab in ALL patients in combination with chemotherapy, targeted therapies, and other immunotherapeutic approaches is currently being actively investigated.[3]

ADOPTIVE CELL TRANSFER

In this emerging treatment modality, T cells are isolated from a patient, genetically engineered to express either a receptor that has high affinity for specific tumor antigens (e.g., NY-ESO-1 or MAGE-A3), or a chimeric antigen receptor (CAR), and reintroduced into that patient. These affinity enhanced T cells have been used to treat multiple myeloma, melanoma, and synovial cell sarcoma, whereas CAR T cells have demonstrated efficacy primarily in the treatment of R/R ALL, chronic lymphocytic leukemia, and non-Hodgkin's lymphoma.[4] In August 2017, the FDA approved the first anti-CD19 CAR T cell product, tisagenlecleucel, for the treatment of pediatric and young adult patients with relapsed and/or refractory B-cell precursor ALL.[5] In October 2017, the FDA approved axicabtagene ciloleucel for treatment of R/R diffuse large B-cell lymphoma (DLBCL).[6]

INTERLEUKIN-2

IL-2 became the first FDA–approved immune therapy for renal cell carcinoma in 1992 and then metastatic melanoma in 1998.[7]

INTERFERON-α

The current indication for IFN-α is in the adjuvant setting for high-risk resected melanoma, and in combination with bevacizumab, for advanced renal cell carcinoma.[8]

Agents and Mechanism of Action

IMMUNE CHECKPOINT INHIBITORS

- Currently approved ICIs include anti–CTLA-4 antibodies and anti–PD-1/anti–PD-L1 antibodies.[9] CTLA-4 and PD-1, through intracellular signaling pathways, help to down-regulate T-cell function and, hence, induce apoptosis. Ipilimumab (an anti–CTLA-4 monoclonal antibody), pembrolizumab and nivolumab (anti–PD-1 monoclonal antibodies), and durvalumab and avelumab (anti–PD-L1 monoclonal antibodies), block immune checkpoints, and thereby enhance the cytotoxic immune response to cancer cells.[10]

- The irAEs secondary to ICIs, namely, colitis, hepatitis, endocrinopathies, and dermatitis, lead to significant morbidity but only cause mortality ~1% of the time. Cardiovascular complications associated with ICI treatment are potentially life threatening, with devastating clinical consequences. With increasing clinical use of ICIs and with several evolving combination treatments with ICIs, early recognition and timely intervention is required. Due to the rarity of cardiotoxicities, data are very sparse and generally include case reports or small case series.[11]

Cardiac Manifestations With Anti–CTLA-4 Treatment

Cases of fatal myocarditis, myocardial fibrosis, reversible left ventricular dysfunction, late onset pericardial effusion, cardiac tamponade, constrictive pericarditis, and Takotsubo cardiomyopathy with apical ballooning on echocardiography have all been observed with anti–CTLA-4 therapy.[11]

Cardiac Manifestations With Anti–PD-1 Treatment

Clinically significant cardiotoxic events associated with anti–PD-1 therapy include pericarditis, hypertension, atrial and ventricular arrhythmia, and myocardial infarction. A case series of melanoma patients treated with anti–PD-1 therapy showed a 1% incidence of cardiac disorders including a case of fatal ventricular arrhythmia due to myocarditis, various other arrhythmias (atrial flutter, ventricular arrhythmia), asystole due to cardiomyopathy, hypertension, myocarditis, and left ventricular dysfunction.[12] The onset of these toxicities ranged from 2 to 17 weeks after treatment. There does not appear to be any correlation between the type of anti–PD-1 therapy, tumor response, tumor type, or any particular clinical features that predispose these patients to adverse cardiac events.

Cardiac Manifestations With Combination Immune Checkpoint Inhibitors

- Toxicities associated with ICIs are enhanced with combination therapy compared with monotherapy alone. Combination ICI (ipilimumab-nivolumab) resulted in grades 3 and 4 adverse events in 55% of patients compared with 16% of patients only on nivolumab and 27% of patients only on ipilimumab.[13]
- Combination ipilimumab and nivolumab in two melanoma patients led to fulminant myositis with rhabdomyolysis, early progressive and refractory cardiac electrical instability, and myocarditis. Despite aggressive interventions with high-dose glucocorticoids and in one case, infliximab, both of the patients died.[1] Another case of myocarditis which was salvaged presented with symptoms of heart failure and left ventricular (LV) dysfunction with reduction in left ventricular ejection fraction (LVEF) from 50% to 15% after 3 combination infusions of ipilimumab and nivolumab. However, the LVEF improved to 40% after 2 months of high-dose glucocorticoids and treatment for heart failure.
- Johnson et al.[1] reported the frequency of cardiovascular complications, namely, myocarditis and myositis, in a large population extracted from the of Bristol-Myers Squibb corporate safety database. Among a total of 20,594 patients studied, 0.09% drug-related severe adverse events of myocarditis were reported. Combination therapy was associated with a higher incidence of frequent and severe myocarditis than with nivolumab alone (0.27% or 5 fatal events vs. 0.06% or 1 fatal event, $P < .001$). Mortality was high, with death occurring secondary to refractory arrhythmias or cardiogenic shock. Median time to development of myocarditis was 17 days (range, 13–64 days). Severe myositis (grade 3 to 4) also appeared more frequently when the combination of drugs was used than when nivolumab was the only agent used (0.24% vs. 0.15%). In clinical trials involving nivolumab, ipilimumab, or both, there was no routine testing for myocarditis by means of either biochemical analysis or cardiac imaging. It is important to recognize, however, that the actual incidence of cardiac

events post ICI may be more substantial than what is already known because cardiac monitoring was not a routine part of clinical trials. Also, it is important to remember that the data were collected retrospectively from a single manufacturer in the absence of prospective standardized screening of cardiac issues, and hence, it is very likely that this underrepresents the true incidence.

- A paper published in *Circulation*[14] analyzed a total of 30 patients with ICI-related cardiotoxicity which included 12 newly diagnosed patients and 24 patients with previous data that had been reported in case series. Cardiotoxicity was diagnosed at a median of 65 days (range, 2–454 days) after the initiation of ICIs, and occurred after a median of 3 infusions (range, 1–33). It was observed in the study that cardiotoxicity was higher after the first and third infusions. The most frequent clinical manifestations observed in the patients were dyspnea, palpitations, and signs of congestive heart failure. The development of LV dysfunction was observed in 79% of patients, and 14% patients developed a Takotsubo-syndrome–like appearance. Atrial fibrillation, ventricular arrhythmia, and conduction disorders were observed in 30%, 27%, and 17% of patients, respectively, who were treated with ICIs; however, after excluding the finding of LV dysfunction, they were observed to occur in 3%, 7%, and 13% of patients, respectively. Myositis was noted to develop in 23% of patients. It was also observed that cardiovascular mortality was significantly associated with conduction abnormalities (80% vs. 16%, $P = .003$) and ipilimumab-nivolumab combination therapy (57% vs. 17%, $P = .04$).

- A review of complied case reports and case series by Jain et al. revealed that the onset of cardiovascular irAEs can be seen as early as 2 weeks and as late as 32 weeks after initiation of ICI, with a median onset at 10 weeks after initiation.[15]

Mechanism of Immune Checkpoint Inhibitor–Mediated Cardiotoxicity

A plausible mechanism behind ICI-mediated myocarditis is that shared targeted antigens (epitopes)/high frequency T-cell receptors may exist among tumor cells and the cardiac myocytes that could become a target for activated T cells and thus lead to myocardial lymphocytic infiltration resulting in heart failure and several other conduction abnormalities. Among patients who died from myocarditis, autopsy showed abundant CD4+ and CD8+ T-cell infiltration of the tumor, cardiac muscle (cardiac sinus and the AV node), and skeletal muscle. These were indicative of lymphocytic myocarditis and myositis.[1] Pathology review also showed myocardial fibrosis, and cardiomyopathy predisposing to heart failure, and conduction abnormalities, including heart block and cardiac arrest.[15] Pericarditis and pericardial effusion have also been described.[16] Although rare, there has also been a case report of irAE-associated acute coronary syndrome.[17] PD-L1 expression has been noted on the membranous surface of the injured myocytes and on the infiltrating CD8+ T cells and histiocytes from the inflamed myocardium. Along with this, the over-expression of IFN-γ, granzyme B, and tumor necrosis factor-α (TNF-α), produced by the activated T cells, could also contribute to cardiac damage. On the other hand, the skeletal muscles and the tumor had negative/lower expression for PD-L1. PD-L1 upregulation in the myocardium could be a cytokine-induced cardioprotective mechanism that is abrogated by immune-checkpoint blockade. It remains undetermined as to what are the causative epitopes that are recognized by these T-cell receptors within the multitude of antigens. Mice studies have shown that genetic deletion of PD-1 in mice models results in cardiomyopathy caused by antibodies against cardiac troponin I; however, no such mechanism has been identified in humans.[18,19] Hence, Nishimura and colleagues concluded that PD-1 may be an important receptor contributing to autoimmune cardiac diseases. Several mouse models of T-cell–dependent myocarditis exist where genetic deletion of PD-L1/L2, as well as treatment with anti–PD-L1, transformed transient myocarditis into a lethal disease.[20] Preclinical studies have also shown that CTLA-4-/- mice develop severe autoimmune myocarditis mediated by CD8+ T cells, which is rapidly fatal at birth.[21]

Clinical Presentation of Immune Checkpoint Inhibitor-Mediated Cardiotoxicity

Patients may present with varied clinical manifestations and thus careful consideration must be given for this entity. Symptoms can vary from nonspecific symptoms like weakness and fatigue, to typical cardiac symptoms of chest pain, heart failure (shortness of breath, pulmonary or lower extremity edema), palpitations, irregular heartbeat, new arrhythmias (including conduction blocks), and syncope and myalgias, especially in the first few months of treatment. Patients may develop myocarditis/pericarditis along with symptoms of myositis (myalgias, rhabdomyolysis) and present with muscle pain, fevers, pleuritic chest pain, and diffuse ST elevation on electrocardiogram (ECG), and hence, these overlapping manifestations pose a challenge to the accurate diagnosis of the condition. Patients may also present with nonspecific signs of fatigue, malaise, myalgias, and/or weakness alone or along with other irAEs and symptoms may be masked by pneumonitis, hypothyroidism, or other pulmonary symptoms. Severe cases can present with cardiogenic shock or sudden death. Immune-mediated myocarditis can present as heart failure or arrhythmias. The myocarditis may be fulminant, progressive, and life threatening.[1] The dysrhythmias may present as benign supraventricular tachycardia to more fatal advanced heart blocks or ventricular tachycardia.[1] Per expert consensus, it is imperative to have high vigilance for development of cardiac symptoms in all patients, but especially in those with evidence of myocarditis, vasculitis, or myositis.[22]

Patients with known cardiac morbidities should not be denied treatment with ICI but should be carefully monitored with a low threshold of suspicion for any nonspecific presentation of cardiac irAE with the potential to cause rapid deterioration.

Referral and Consultation. Patients who present with multiple cardiovascular risk factors or established cardiovascular disease prior to starting ICIs should have a cardiology consultation prior to initiation of therapy. Any abnormal cardiac test result, in any patient, during the course of ICI treatment warrants an immediate referral to cardiology, as myocarditis can be fatal, and patients suspected with documented myocarditis should be admitted to the hospital for cardiac monitoring.[22]

BLINATUMOMAB

Tumor-specific T cells play a key role in the immune surveillance of cancer cells. This has been demonstrated by the positive correlation of CD8+ cytotoxic T cells within tumors, antitumor responses, and long-term survival.[23] BiTEs are capable of eliciting polyclonal T cell responses that are unrestricted by T cell receptor specificity, presence of major histocompatibility class (MHC), or additional T-cell co-stimuli. Blinatumomab is a BiTE which has been FDA-approved for the treatment of adult R/R Ph− B-cell precursor ALL and also for MRD-positive ALL.[3] Once CD19+ B-cells and CD3+ T cells have been linked together via blinatumomab, there is formation of a cytolytic synapse between the T cell and the cancer target cell. The cytotoxic T cell releases granzymes and perforin via exocytosis and the perforins, in the presence of calcium, bind to the target B-cell membrane, thus creating a pore for the entry of granzymes. They also release inflammatory cytokines. The granzymes activate programmed cell death. The activated T cells enter the cell cycle, expanding the T-cell compartment and, thus, increasing the number of T cells present in the target tissue.[24] T-cell activation and release of various proinflammatory cytokines results in the development of CRS. It is also important to recognize that malignant cell lysis induced by activated T cells results in development of hypocalcemia, hyperkalemia, hyperphosphatemia, and hyperuricemia and release of several proinflammatory cytokines contributing to the development of tumor lysis syndrome (TLS), a potentially life-threatening condition.

Cardiac Manifestations With Blinatumomab

A phase I/II study of blinatumomab in pediatric patients with R/R ALL in 70 patients showed that in the phase I portion, 3 patients experienced grade 4 CRS (one of which had grade 5 cardiac failure).[25,26] Severe (grade 3) CRS occurred in 2% of 189 patients who received blinatumomab for approved indication in a large phase II study; 17% of patients had any grade arrhythmias; 2% of patients developed grade 3 or higher arrhythmias; 12% of patients developed any grade hypotension; grade 3 or greater hypotension occurred in 3% of patients; any grade chest pain in 11% and 1% of patients had grade 3 or greater chest pain.[27] A study by Kantarjian et al., comparing blinatumomab with chemotherapy for advanced ALL, showed an incidence of any grade hypotension in 12% of patients, tachycardia in 6.7%, and hypertension in 6.4% of patients.[28]

Mechanism of Blinatumomab-Mediated Cardiotoxicity

Cytokine release syndrome (CRS) is mediated by the release of IL-2, TNF-α, IFN-γ, IL-6, and IL-10 from blinatumomab-engaged effector T cells. These cytokines, which reach peak on day 1 of therapy, and then decline rapidly thereafter, are responsible for the adverse effects seen in CRS. The above cytokines result in capillary leak syndrome, which results in hypotension and arrhythmias. Several cytokines have specific cardiac effects which mediate cardiac toxicity. IL-1-β and TNF-α result in a decrease in cardiac contractility, induction of fibrosis, and cardiac hypertrophy. IL-2 also results in a decrease in cardiac muscle contractility. IL-6 causes a decrease in cardiac contractility and cardiac hypertrophy induction. These proinflammatory cytokines and the subsequent elevation in nitric oxide (NO) result in both inotropic and chronotropic alterations in the myocardial excitation-contraction coupling, myocardial contractility suppression, and desensitization of the β-adrenergic receptors stimulation, thereby resulting in development of cardiac failure. Of note, the TLS induced by blinatumomab can also lead to life-threatening conditions, including cardiac failure due to hypocalcemia, hyperkalemia, and hyperuricemia, and hence, monitoring electrolytes during treatment is critical.

ADOPTIVE CELL TRANSFER

- Adoptive cell transfer (ACT) is another form of immunotherapy which has shown promise for a wide variety of solid tumors. In ACT, patients' T cells are genetically engineered to specifically target tumor cells. This is based on previous studies wherein preexisting tumor-infiltrating lymphocytes (TIL) were collected, expanded, and then reintroduced into the patient's microenvironment in the presence of IL-2 in order to stimulate their survival and expansion.[10]
- With the additional component of modification in the form of genetic engineering of the T-cell receptors (TCRs), the T cells are able to have higher affinity towards tumor antigens that are not normally well engaged by wild-type TCRs. The targeted antigens are expressed in immunologically protected germline cells but become abnormally expressed in various cancers, including NY-ESO-1 and MAGE-3.[29] ACT is currently being utilized for multiple different malignancies.[4]
- CAR T-cell therapy is a form of ACT that has been approved for B-ALL and DLBCL. In CAR T cells, the naive T cells are genetically engineered to express a CAR on the cell membrane and coupled with an external binding domain to bind to the tumor antigens (targeting CD19 on malignant cells and differentiated B-cells). In refractory B-ALL patients, CAR T-cell therapy is effective in 70% to 90% of cases.[30] IL-6 has been increasingly recognized as a key mediator of systemic toxicity associated with CAR T-cell therapy.[31]

Cardiac Manifestations of Adoptive Cell Transfer

One of the most common cardiovascular toxicities following CAR T-cell administration is tachycardia, which is frequently associated with fever. As the grade of CRS increases, hypotension, arrhythmias, and decreased ejection fraction may be seen. Grades 3 to 4 hypotension has been reported in 22% to 38% of patients. Most of these cardiovascular toxicities are reversible and can be managed with supportive care. Cardiac arrest was noted in one patient 7 days after infusion with CAR T-cell therapy with subsequent reduction in LVEF to less than 25% from baseline.[32]

Reversible reduction in ejection fraction has been reported in multiple other patients. Reversible increases in serum troponin can concomitantly occur. Asymptomatic prolongation of the QTc interval on ECG as well as atrial fibrillation have also been reported.[33] Two patients with T cells expressing receptor against MAGE-3 presented with diffuse ST elevations on an ECG and elevation of cardiac biomarkers preceding cardiopulmonary arrest. One of the patients developed a large pericardial effusion and cardiogenic shock, and ultimately died of multisystem organ failure. In both patients, robust cytokine production and T cell infiltrates were observed in the heart, with histopathological analysis demonstrating myocyte necrosis in a pattern similar to allograft rejection.

Mechanism of Adoptive Cell Transfer–Mediated Cardiotoxicity

- Most of the observed cardiac side effects appear to be secondary to the preparative regimen or IL-2, but there have been reports of significant toxicity from cross-reactivity to other normal cells with fatal consequences. A case series showed that the use of genetically modified TCR against MAGE-3, a cancer germline antigen, as mentioned above, led to the development of fatal cardiogenic shock in two patients.[34] Though cross-reactivity was thought to be the mechanism of action in these cases, there was no evidence of MAGE-3 expression on cardiac tissue. On the other hand, significant myocardial damage with T-cell infiltration targeted against titin, an unrelated myocardial protein, was observed.[35] Another case report with MART-1 TCR in melanoma resulted in neurological dysfunction and cardiac arrest 6 days after the T-cell infusion.[36] Infused T cells were noted in the cardiomyocytes, but no cross-reactivity was identified, thus suggesting that an alternate mechanism exists.
- Cardiotoxic side effects with CAR T-cell therapy are generally reversible and are part of the CRS, which is a systemic inflammatory response that correlates with the in vivo activation and proliferation of CAR T cells. It is believed that the pathophysiology for the cardiac dysfunction is similar to that of stress (stress-induced Takotsubo cardiomyopathy)[37] and sepsis.[38]
- For both CRS-mediated and off-target/cross-reactivity–mediated cardiotoxicity, the literature describing cardiovascular adverse events remains limited to case reports, and the overall incidence is yet to be defined.

INTERLEUKIN-2

Clinical data have shown a significant number of cardiac toxicities associated with the use of high-dose IL-2 (HDIL-2). IL-2 is a cytokine, or biological response modifier, produced by activated natural killer (NK) cells and promotes clonal T-cell expansion during an immune response. It also helps develop and mature T regulatory cells, promotes NK cell activity, and mediates immune tolerance by activation-induced cell death. IL-2 binds to its receptors of either high-affinity containing α(CD25)-, β(CD122)-, and γ(CD132)-chains, or low-affinity receptors that contain only α- and β-chains. This induces proliferation and differentiation of both CD4+ and CD8+ cells to effector cells or memory cells. IL-2 elicits a combination of immune responses, both activation of innate immune effectors including NK cells and macrophages, and specific immune responses mediated by T effector and memory cells for long-term control of tumor recurrence. Subsequent release of various cytokines, including other interleukins, interferons, and colony stimulating factors, is also believed to be important in induction of tumor regression.[39]

Cardiac Manifestations With Interleukin-2

The cardiac manifestations with IL-2 can range from severe hypotension (up to 65%), arrhythmias (up to 57%), and ischemia (up to 20%).[40] HDIL-2 can induce vascular leak syndrome that can result in hypotension and tachycardia.[41] Up to 10% of patients can develop arrhythmias including atrial fibrillation, which can lead to hypotension. In a series of 199 patients treated with HDIL-2 over 310 courses of therapy, 19 cases of dysrhythmias were reported that included atrial fibrillation in 16 patients (5.2%), prolonged atrial arrhythmia with hypotension in 2 patients (0.6%), and nonsustained ventricular tachycardia in 1 patient (0.3%).[41] Sinus tachycardia should be expected during therapy and is the most frequent dysrhythmia. There have been rare cases of myocardial infarction and myocarditis with IL-2 therapy.[40] Myocarditis may present with elevated cardiac enzymes in the presence of a normal ECG, patients may have fever, mild chest pain, or discomfort, and may present even days after stopping IL-2 therapy. Peripheral edema may also result from capillary leak syndrome and patients may gain 10% to 15% of their body weight due to fluid overload. Due to these toxicities, IL-2 is reserved for patients with excellent performance status and good organ function.

Mechanism of Interleukin-2–Mediated Cardiotoxicity

The previously mentioned clinical manifestations such as hypotension, tachycardia, and atrial arrhythmias are secondary to capillary leak syndrome induced by IL-2. Although these changes are secondary to cardiac stress and certain hemodynamic changes, preclinical studies have suggested that IL-2–activated lymphocytes could also directly damage endothelial cells and myocytes.[42] Myocarditis has been confirmed and myocardial infiltrating lymphocytes are seen on biopsy.

INTERFERON-α

IFN-α induces the transcription of several genes via the JAK-STAT (Janus tyrosine kinase—signal transducer and activator of transcription) and other signaling pathways.[43] The antitumor mechanism of IFN-α is the cumulative result of cytostatic, antiangiogenic, and immune-modulatory activities. The immune-modulatory effect of IFN-α includes induction of cytokines, upregulation of major histocompatibility antigen expression, enhancement of phagocytic activity of NK cells, macrophages, and augmentation of T-cell cytotoxicity against the tumor cells.[8]

Cardiac Manifestations With Interferon-α

No relationship between cardiotoxic effects and dose of IFN-α has been found. Eight phase I trials with IFN-α therapy have not reported any significant cardiotoxic adverse events. One small case series of 44 patients treated with IFN-α therapy showed that the cardiotoxic effects ranged from arrhythmia (in 25 patients), dilated cardiomyopathy (in 5 patients), ischemic heart disease (in 9 patients), and sudden death (in 22 patients).[44] Tachycardia and hypotension have been reported in 5% to 15% of IFN-α2b–treated patients during the first day of treatment.[45]

Mechanism of Interferon-α–Mediated Cardiotoxicity

In two cases of reversible cardiomyopathy in patients who received IFN-α2b, endomyocardial biopsy revealed myocardial inflammation.[46] Hypothyroidism may also be a contributing factor for cardiac dysfunction, and can have a variety of effects on the heart, such as ventricular dilation, pericardial effusion, and poor contractility.[47]

Pharmacological Approaches for Management and Treatment

IMMUNE CHECKPOINT INHIBITORS

- Due to the potential for myocarditis-related mortality, some institutions recommend monitoring troponin every week for the first 6 weeks, and then prior to each cycle for the first 12 weeks of treatment. ECG should be done at baseline and be repeated prior to every cycle for the first 12 weeks. Fig. 23.1 shows the Roswell Park Cancer Institute (RPCI) schema for monitoring patients on immune checkpoint inhibitors.

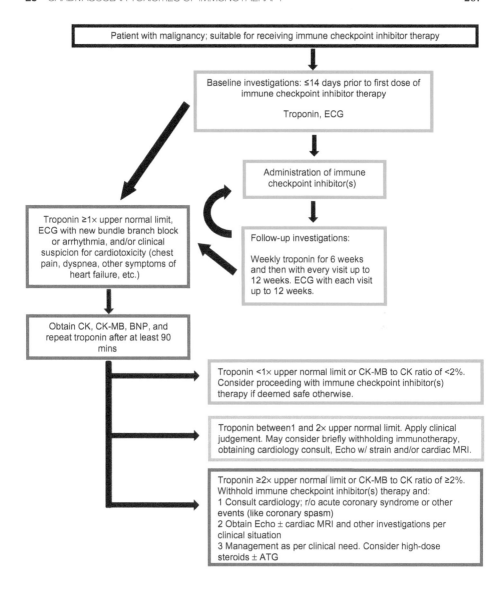

Fig. 23.1 Roswell Park Cancer Institute (RPCI) schema for monitoring patients on immune checkpoint inhibitors. *ATG,* Anti-thymocyte globulin; *BNP,* brain natriuretic peptide; *CK,* creatine kinase.

TABLE 23.1 ■ Consensus Recommendations for Pharmacological Management of Cardiotoxicity

Grade	CTCAE Description	Management	Referral
2	Abnormal screening tests with mild symptoms	• Control cardiac diseases (e.g., heart failure, atrial fibrillation) optimally • Control cardiac disease risk factors proactively (including hypertension, hyperlipidemia, discontinue smoking, and monitor diabetes)	Yes
3	Moderately abnormal testing or symptoms with mild activity	• BNP >500 pg/mL, troponin >99% institutional normal, new ECG findings (QTc prolongation, new conduction disease, or ST-T wave changes) • Consider withholding ICI • If a period of stabilization is achieved and definite cardiac toxicity was not identified, it may be reasonable to consider rechallenging the patient with ICI, with heightened monitoring. • If confirmed cardiac injury or decompensation, withhold ICI therapy until stabilized. • Optimally treat identified cardiac conditions • Consider corticosteroids if myocarditis suspected	Yes
4	Moderate to severe decompensation, intravenous medication or intervention required, life-threatening conditions	• Permanently discontinue ICI • If myocarditis is identified, consider high-dose corticosteroids (1 mg/kg methylprednisolone [IV] for at least several days) until improved to grade ≤1; after that consider at least 4–5 weeks of tapering doses. • Add additional immunosuppressive agents in severe refractory cases. • Give additional supportive treatments, including appropriate treatment of heart failure. Additional treatment of detected cardiac conditions should be provided.	Yes

BNP, Brain natriuretic peptide; *CTCAE,* Common Terminology Criteria for Adverse Events; *ICI,* immune checkpoint inhibitor.
From the consensus recommendations for pharmacological management for grades 2–4 cardiotoxicity of the SITC Toxicity Management Working Group and the ASCO Clinical Practice Guidelines.[2,22]

■ It is important to recognize that due to sparsity of data, treatment recommendations for ICI-mediated cardiotoxicity are based largely on anecdotal evidence and partly from extension of management of rejection in heart transplant patients. It is recommended that checkpoint inhibitors should be withheld for all grades of complications. The appropriateness of rechallenging remains unknown but given the gravity of cardiac complications, is currently not advised.

■ Table 23.1 lists the consensus recommendations for pharmacological management for grade 2 to 4 cardiotoxicity from the Society for Immunotherapy of Cancer (SITC) Toxicity Management Group[22] and the American Society of Clinical Oncology (ASCO) Clinical Practice Guidelines.[2]

  ■ For patients with mild to moderate symptoms (grades 2 and 3), systemic prednisone or methylprednisolone 1–2 mg/kg/day should be initiated.

  ■ For grade 3 and 4 cardiotoxicities, including cardiac decompensation, highly abnormal testing, fulminant disease, cardiogenic shock, and acute heart failure, or with life-threatening arrhythmias, in addition to steroid administration, patients should be admitted to the hospital for monitoring and management.

  ■ Cardiac symptoms (arrhythmias and heart failure) should be managed according to American College of Cardiology (ACC)/American Heart Association (AHA) guidelines.

- Patients should be considered for immediate transfer to a coronary care unit if they present with elevated troponin or with conduction abnormalities.
- Confirmed myocarditis (grade 4) should be treated emergently with high-dose corticosteroids (methylprednisolone 1 mg/kg/day for several days until toxicity ≤ grade 1, and then steroid taper over the next 4–5 weeks). As data regarding initiation of steroids in suspected myocarditis is lacking, this decision should be made on a case by case basis. Patients without an immediate response to high-dose corticosteroids may be offered early institution of cardiac transplant rejection doses of corticosteroids (methylprednisolone 1 g every day). Additional immunosuppressive therapy is generally warranted in these cases, just as for other irAEs, in the form of mycophenolate, infliximab, or anti-thymocyte globulin (ATG). Unfortunately, infliximab has been associated with heart failure and, hence, is contraindicated at higher doses than 5 mg/kg in patients with moderate or severe heart failure (NYHA class III/IV).[48] For patients with myocarditis presenting with moderate to severe heart failure, it is recommended to consider using ATG or tacrolimus (both are effective in the treatment of cardiac allograft rejection) along with high-dose steroids. It is important to consult with a cardiologist regarding the risk/benefit of continuing ICI therapy, starting steroids, or instituting other cardiac treatments.
- Other treatments such as viral-based therapy, immunoglobulins, or plasmapheresis are speculative at this point and are not included in the guidelines.[22]
- Some forms of ICI-associated cardiac toxicities are fulminant, but with appropriate intervention and cessation of checkpoint inhibitors, cardiac contractility and conduction abnormalities can improve. It is hard to predict which patients will improve or worsen. Due to the severity of the symptoms, it is important to take the patient's disease status into account before the implementation of aggressive interventions like defibrillation, resuscitation, and balloon pump placement.

BLINATUMOMAB

Prophylaxis Prior to Blinatumomab Infusion

- There is a high incidence of CRS with initial blinatumomab infusion, and hence, patients presenting with a high tumor burden, such as blast infiltration of the bone marrow greater than 50%, 15,000 blasts/μL or higher in the peripheral blood, or other signs of high leukemia load such as high lactate dehydrogenase (LDH), should be treated with steroids (generally dexamethasone 16-20 mg daily) for up to 5 days, in order to reduce this tumor load.[27]
- Premedication with dexamethasone 20 mg should be given 1 hour before treatment start to control CRS. Because of the possibility of adverse events with blinatumomab which occur during the early phase of therapy, it is recommended that patients be hospitalized for the beginning of each cycle, for each dose step, and for the start of each treatment.[27]

Treatment of Grades 2 to 4 Cytokine Release Syndrome

- **Grade 2 CRS** (hypotension – nonurgent medical intervention indicated):
  - Treat with IV fluids and one low-dose vasopressor
- **Grade 3 CRS** (hypotension – medical intervention indicated, hospitalization indicated, cardiac troponin I levels consistent with myocardial infarction):
  - Withhold blinatumomab until complete resolution. Reinitiate at 9 μg/day and dose-escalate to 28 μg/day after 7 days
  - Treat with high-dose vasopressor or multiple vasopressors
  - Corticosteroids
  - Treat with tocilizumab if refractory to steroids (experience limited)

- **Grade 4 CRS** (hypotension – life-threatening consequences and urgent intervention indicated)
  - Permanently discontinue blinatumomab
  - Treat with high-dose vasopressor or multiple vasopressors[49]
  - Corticosteroids
  - Treat with tocilizumab if refractory to steroids (limited experience)

ADOPTIVE CELL TRANSFER

Given that ACT is associated with significant CRS, the mainstay of treatment for toxicity associated with ACT is management of the underlying cytokines. Tocilizumab, an anti–IL-6 receptor antibody, has significantly reduced the severity and incidence of CRS, improving clinical outcomes.[33]

Indications for Tocilizumab[33]

- Left ventricular ejection fraction less than 40%: 4–8 mg/kg infused over 1 hour, dose not to exceed 800 mg
- If the requirement of norepinephrine (NE) for hypotension is at a dose greater than 2 μg/min for 48 hours since the first administration of NE, even if the administration of NE is not continuous
- If the systolic blood pressure (SBP) of 90 mmHg cannot be maintained with NE

Role of Steroids

Systemic corticosteroids have been used to abrogate CRS-mediated toxicities. Some evidence suggests that the use of steroids may decrease the antitumor efficacy of CAR T cells and, hence, the use of steroids is reserved for cases which are refractory to tocilizumab.[33] In these cases, methylprednisolone 1–2 mg/kg IV every 12 hours should be administered.[33]

Approach to the Management of Toxicity From ACT by Grade

Grade 2 CRS. (Responsive to fluids and low dose of NE vasopressor)[50]
- IV fluid bolus of 500–1000 mL of normal saline
- Second IV fluid bolus if SBP remains lower than 90 mmHg
- Tocilizumab 8 mg/kg IV for the treatment of hypotension refractory to fluid boluses; tocilizumab can be repeated after 6 hours if needed.
- If hypotension persists after two fluid boluses and anti–IL-6 therapy, start vasopressors, consider transfer to intensive care unit (ICU), obtain echocardiogram, and initiate other methods of hemodynamic monitoring
- If hypotension persists after 1 to 2 doses of anti–IL-6 therapy, dexamethasone can be used at a dose of 10 mg IV every 6 hours.

Grade 3 CRS. (Responsive to high doses of vasopressors or multiple vasopressors)[50]
- IV fluid boluses as needed, as recommended for the treatment of grade 2 CRS
- Tocilizumab as recommended for grade 2 CRS, if not administered previously
- Vasopressors as needed
- Transfer to ICU, obtain echocardiogram, and perform hemodynamic monitoring as in the management of grade 2 CRS
- Dexamethasone 10 mg IV every 6 hours; if refractory, increase to 20 mg IV every 6 hours

Grade 4 CRS. (Life threatening symptoms)[50]
- IV fluids, anti–IL-6 therapy, vasopressors, and hemodynamic monitoring as defined for the management of grade 3 CRS
- Methylprednisolone 1 g/day IV

INTERLEUKIN-2[51]

IL-2 is associated with several toxicities, the treatment of which is detailed below.

Hypotension

Hypotension is managed with initial intravenous fluid resuscitation with a 250ml bolus of crystalloid along with baseline fluid administration of 20-30 mL/hour with repeat fluid boluses up to 1L. Vasopressor support should be started if there is evidence of fluid overload or pulmonary edema. The two vasopressor agents commonly used are phenylephrine and dopamine. Dopamine is usually given at low doses if patients have concomitant oliguria. Phenylephrine is started at low dose (0.1 mg/kg/min) and slowly titrated until a stable blood pressure is achieved (max dose: 2 mg/kg/min). If the patient is hypotensive despite phenylephrine of 2 mg/kg/min, then phenylephrine should be discontinued, and alternative agents should be used. Once IL-2 is stopped, vasopressors are generally able be gradually weaned off within 15 to 30 minutes.[52]

Myocarditis/Myocardial Ischemia

If there is concern for potential myocarditis or ischemia, cardiac enzymes should be monitored at least daily and if elevated, IL-2 should be discontinued. Supportive care and cardiology consultation should be instituted.

Cardiac Dysrhythmias

A 12-lead ECG should be obtained. If the patient is symptomatic, cardiac enzymes should also be obtained. Sinus tachycardia generally responds to fluid challenge. If patients develop isolated PVC (premature ventricular contractions) above 10/min, bigeminy, or quadrigeminy, IL-2 doses may need to be withheld. It may also be necessary to reposition the central venous catheter in the case of minor PVCs, especially in the first 24 hours of treatment. Emergent intervention is needed if patients develop supraventricular tachycardia (SVT), atrial fibrillation with rapid ventricular response, and ventricular tachycardia. Once the patient's rhythms are converted to sinus rhythm or are rate controlled, IL-2 can be continued. Cardiac damage should be assessed if the patient has ventricular tachycardia and, in those cases, IL-2 should be discontinued.

Peripheral Edema

Careful monitoring for fluid accumulation via physical examination of daily weights is important to monitor for weight gain due to fluid administration. After stopping IL-2 treatment, patients usually return to their baseline weight. Diuretics such as furosemide can also be used if patients are very uncomfortable, but this edema is generally self-limited.

INTERFERON-α

Treatment of cardiotoxicity associated with IFN-α consists of its discontinuation and standard management of heart failure.[46] Thyroid function should also be assessed in patients with cardiotoxicity, as it may also be present. Formal cardiac evaluation of ejection fraction and other parameters is reasonable for patients whose symptoms do not resolve with conservative therapy after treatment interruption.

Nonpharmacological Approaches for Management and Treatment

IMMUNE CHECKPOINT INHIBITORS

- The SITC committee[22] and ASCO clinical practice guidelines[2] recommend monitoring of patients for the development of myocarditis during the course of treatment with checkpoint

TABLE 23.2 ■ Consensus Recommendations for Nonpharmacological Management of Cardiotoxicity

Grade	CTCAE Description	Management	Referral
1	Abnormal cardiac biomarker testing, including abnormal ECG	• Recommend baseline ECG and cardiac bio-marker assessment (BNP, troponin) to establish if there is a notable change during therapy • Mild abnormalities should be observed closely during therapy	Yes, if abnormal

BNP, Brain natriuretic peptide; *CTCAE,* Common Terminology Criteria for Adverse Events.

From the consensus recommendations for non-pharmacological management for grade 1 cardiotoxicity of the SITC Toxicity Management Working Group and the ASCO Clinical Practice Guidelines.[2,22]

inhibitors. All patients prior to beginning therapy with checkpoint inhibitors should receive testing for biomarkers which include troponin I or T (especially in patients treated with combination immune therapies), total creatine kinase (CK), and an ECG.

■ There are no specific findings for the diagnosis of myocarditis and it is generally a diagnosis of exclusion. Patients with significant cardiac history prior to initiating checkpoint inhibitors should also get an echocardiogram. If patients have abnormal tests to begin with, they should also get serial ECGs and cardiac biomarker testing, or if they develop any symptoms such as chest pain or dyspnea during the course of treatment. In these cases, cardiology consultation, brain natriuretic peptide (BNP), echocardiogram, and chest X-ray should all be obtained. Additional testing may include stress testing, cardiac catheterization, and cardiac magnetic resonance imaging (MRI).

■ Due to the possibility of arrhythmias with possible progression to life-threatening arrhythmias and heart block, continuous telemetry monitoring should be initiated. In symptomatic patients, echocardiogram should be obtained to evaluate left and right ventricular ejection fraction (with global and regional abnormalities). Cardiac MRI is very sensitive for myocarditis but endomyocardial biopsy remains the gold standard for diagnosis.[53] Endomyocardial biopsy should be considered in patients who are unstable or who have not responded to initial therapy or in cases of unclear diagnosis. In most cases, these diagnostic tests reveal the diagnosis and treatment is initiated before pathological testing is obtained.

■ Presently, there are no recommendations regarding the appropriate time interval between the tests, but patients who develop concerning symptoms during the course of ICI treatment should have chest imaging, ECG, cardiac biomarkers evaluation, and echocardiogram.[22]

■ Table 23.2 lists the consensus recommendations for nonpharmacological management for grade 1 cardiotoxicity from the SITC Toxicity Management Group[22] as well as per ASCO Clinical Practice Guidelines.[2]

ADOPTIVE CELL TRANSFER

Patients receiving CAR T-cell therapy should undergo the following supportive management[33]:

■ Stop or taper antihypertensive medications prior to cell infusion due to anticipated hypotension.

■ Vital signs should be monitored at least every 4 hours in an inpatient unit for at least 9 days following infusion.

■ Vitals signs should be monitored every 2 hours in patients with fevers and tachycardia.

- Initiate replacement IV fluids for patients with poor oral intake or high insensible losses. IV fluid boluses should be administered for patients with SBP less than their preinfusion baseline:
  - Patients with an SBP less than 80% of their preinfusion baseline and less than 100 mmHg should receive a 1L normal saline bolus.
  - Patients with an SBP less than 85 mmHg should receive a 1L normal saline bolus regardless of baseline blood pressure.
- Serum troponin level should be drawn for patients receiving more than one IV fluid bolus for hypotension, an ECG, and an echocardiogram should be performed to evaluate for cardiac toxicity.
- Patients with hypotension should be initiated on vasopressor support. Norepinephrine is the preferred first-line vasopressor. For patients on vasopressors, echocardiograms should be performed every 2 to 3 days.

INTERLEUKIN-2

Patients who are to receive IL-2 therapy should undergo a thorough cardiac evaluation with a careful history and physical examination, stress tests, ECG, and evaluation for high-risk features which may exclude patients from receiving IL-2 treatment. While receiving treatment, patients should be placed on continuous telemetry to monitor for dysrhythmias, in addition to receiving regular monitoring.[51]

References

1. Johnson DB, Balko JM, Compton ML, et al. Fulminant myocarditis with combination immune checkpoint blockade. *N Engl J Med*. 2016;375(18):1749–1755.
2. Brahmer JR, Lacchetti C, Schneider BJ, et al. Management of immune-related adverse events in patients treated with immune checkpoint inhibitor therapy: American Society of Clinical Oncology Clinical Practice Guideline. *J Clin Oncol*. 2018;36(17):1714–1768.
3. Przepiorka D, Ko CW, Deisseroth A, et al. FDA approval: blinatumomab. *Clin Cancer Res*. 2015; 21(18):4035–4039.
4. Rosenberg SA, Restifo NP, Yang JC, Morgan RA, Dudley ME. Adoptive cell transfer: a clinical path to effective cancer immunotherapy. *Nat Rev Cancer*. 2008;8(4):299–308.
5. Liu Y, Chen X, Han W, Zhang Y. Tisagenlecleucel, an approved anti-CD19 chimeric antigen receptor T-cell therapy for the treatment of leukemia. *Drugs Today (Barc)*. 2017;53(11):597–608.
6. Neelapu SS, Locke FL, Bartlett NL, et al. Axicabtagene ciloleucel CAR T-cell therapy in refractory large B-cell lymphoma. *N Engl J Med*. 2017;377(26):2531–2544.
7. Atkins MB, Lotze MT, Dutcher JP, et al. High-dose recombinant interleukin 2 therapy for patients with metastatic melanoma: analysis of 270 patients treated between 1985 and 1993. *J Clin Oncol*. 1999; 17(7):2105–2116.
8. Jonasch E, Haluska FG. Interferon in oncological practice: review of interferon biology, clinical applications, and toxicities. *Oncologist*. 2001;6(1):34–55.
9. Ledford H. Cocktails for cancer with a measure of immunotherapy. *Nature*. 2016;532(7598):162–164.
10. Papaioannou NE, Beniata OV, Vitsos P, Tsitsilonis O, Samara P. Harnessing the immune system to improve cancer therapy. *Ann Transl Med*. 2016;4(14):261.
11. Wang DY, Okoye GD, Neilan TG, Johnson DB, Moslehi JJ. Cardiovascular toxicities associated with cancer immunotherapies. *Curr Cardiol Rep*. 2017;19(3):21.
12. Zimmer L, Goldinger SM, Hofmann L, et al. Neurological, respiratory, musculoskeletal, cardiac and ocular side-effects of anti-PD-1 therapy. *Eur J Cancer*. 2016;60:210–225.
13. Larkin J, Chiarion-Sileni V, Gonzalez R, et al. Combined nivolumab and ipilimumab or monotherapy in untreated melanoma. *N Engl J Med*. 2015;373(1):23–34.

14. Escudier M, Cautela J, Malissen N, et al. Clinical features, management, and outcomes of immune check-point inhibitor-related cardiotoxicity. *Circulation.* 2017;136(21):2085–2087.
15. Jain V, Bahia J, Mohebtash M, Barac A. Cardiovascular complications associated with novel cancer immunotherapies. *Curr Treat Options Cardiovasc Med.* 2017;19(5):36.
16. Yun S, Vincelette ND, Mansour I, Hariri D, Motamed S. Late onset ipilimumab-induced pericarditis and pericardial effusion: a rare but life threatening complication. *Case Rep Oncol Med.* 2015;2015:794842.
17. Tomita Y, Sueta D, Kakiuchi Y, et al. Acute coronary syndrome as a possible immune-related adverse event in a lung cancer patient achieving a complete response to anti-PD-1 immune checkpoint antibody. *Ann Oncol.* 2017;28(11):2893–2895.
18. Nishimura H, Okazaki T, Tanaka Y, et al. Autoimmune dilated cardiomyopathy in PD-1 receptor-deficient mice. *Science.* 2001;291(5502):319–322.
19. Okazaki T, Tanaka Y, Nishio R, et al. Autoantibodies against cardiac troponin I are responsible for dilated cardiomyopathy in PD-1-deficient mice. *Nat Med.* 2003;9(12):1477–1483.
20. Lucas JA, Menke J, Rabacal WA, Schoen FJ, Sharpe AH, Kelley VR. Programmed death ligand 1 reg-ulates a critical checkpoint for autoimmune myocarditis and pneumonitis in MRL mice. *J Immunol.* 2008;181(4):2513–2521.
21. Love VA, Grabie N, Duramad P, Stavrakis G, Sharpe A, Lichtman A. CTLA-4 ablation and interleu-kin-12 driven differentiation synergistically augment cardiac pathogenicity of cytotoxic T lymphocytes. *Circ Res.* 2007;101(3):248–257.
22. Puzanov I, Diab A, Abdallah K, et al. Managing toxicities associated with immune checkpoint inhibitors: consensus recommendations from the Society for Immunotherapy of Cancer (SITC) Toxicity Manage-ment Working Group. *J Immunother Cancer.* 2017;5(1):95.
23. Nagorsen D, Baeuerle PA. Immunomodulatory therapy of cancer with T cell-engaging BiTE antibody blinatumomab. *Exp Cell Res.* 2011;317(9):1255–1260.
24. Nagorsen D, Bargou R, Ruttinger D, Kufer P, Baeuerle PA, Zugmaier G. Immunotherapy of lympho-ma and leukemia with T-cell engaging BiTE antibody blinatumomab. *Leuk Lymphoma.* 2009;50(6): 886–891.
25. von Stackelberg A, Locatelli F, Zugmaier G, et al. Phase I/phase II study of blinatumomab in pediatric patients with relapsed/refractory acute lymphoblastic leukemia. *J Clin Oncol.* 2016;34(36):4381–4389.
26. Darvishi A, Farahmand L, Jalili N, Majidzadeh AK. Blinatumomab provoked fatal heart failure. *Int Im-munopharmacol.* 2016;41:42–46.
27. Topp MS, Gökbuget N, Stein AS, et al. Safety and activity of blinatumomab for adult patients with re-lapsed or refractory B-precursor acute lymphoblastic leukaemia: a multicentre, single-arm, phase 2 study. *Lancet Oncol.* 2015;16(1):57–66.
28. Kantarjian H, Stein A, Gökbuget N, et al. Blinatumomab versus chemotherapy for advanced acute lym-phoblastic leukemia. *N Engl J Med.* 2017;376(9):836–847.
29. Jungbluth AA, Antonescu CR, Busam KJ, et al. Monophasic and biphasic synovial sarcomas abundantly express cancer/testis antigen NY-ESO-1 but not MAGE-A1 or CT7. *Int J Cancer.* 2001;94(2):252–256.
30. Jackson HJ, Rafiq S, Brentjens RJ. Driving CAR T-cells forward. *Nat Rev Clin Oncol.* 2016;13(6): 370–383.
31. Scheller J, Chalaris A, Schmidt-Arras D, Rose-John S. The pro- and anti-inflammatory properties of the cytokine interleukin-6. *Biochim Biophys Acta.* 2011;1813(5):878–888.
32. Lee DW, Kochenderfer JN, Stetler-Stevenson M, et al. T cells expressing CD19 chimeric antigen re-ceptors for acute lymphoblastic leukaemia in children and young adults: a phase 1 dose-escalation trial. *Lancet.* 2015;385(9967):517–528.
33. Brudno JN, Kochenderfer JN. Toxicities of chimeric antigen receptor T cells: recognition and manage-ment. *Blood.* 2016;127(26):3321–3330.
34. Linette GP, Stadtmauer EA, Maus MV, et al. Cardiovascular toxicity and titin cross-reactivity of affinity-enhanced T cells in myeloma and melanoma. *Blood.* 2013;122(6):863–871.
35. Cameron BJ, Gerry AB, Dukes J, et al. Identification of a titin-derived HLA-A1-presented peptide as a cross-reactive target for engineered MAGE A3-directed T cells. *Sci Transl Med.* 2013;5(197):197ra103.
36. van den Berg JH, Gomez-Eerland R, van de Wiel B, et al. Case report of a fatal serious adverse event upon administration of T cells transduced with a MART-1-specific T-cell receptor. *Mol Ther.* 2015;23(9): 1541–1550.

37. Singh K, Carson K, Shah R, et al. Meta-analysis of clinical correlates of acute mortality in Takotsubo cardiomyopathy. *Am J Cardiol*. 2014;113(8):1420–1428.
38. Romero-Bermejo FJ, Ruiz-Bailen M, Gil-Cebrian J, Huertos-Ranchal MJ. Sepsis-induced cardiomyopathy. *Curr Cardiol Rev*. 2011;7(3):163–183.
39. Krieg C, Létourneau S, Pantaleo G, Boyman O. Improved IL-2 immunotherapy by selective stimulation of IL-2 receptors on lymphocytes and endothelial cells. *Proc Natl Acad Sci U S A*. 2010;107(26):11906–11911.
40. Kragel AH, Travis WD, Steis RG, Rosenberg SA, Roberts WC. Myocarditis or acute myocardial infarction associated with interleukin-2 therapy for cancer. *Cancer*. 1990;66(7):1513–1516.
41. White Jr RL, Schwartzentruber DJ, Guleria A, et al. Cardiopulmonary toxicity of treatment with high dose interleukin-2 in 199 consecutive patients with metastatic melanoma or renal cell carcinoma. *Cancer*. 1994;74(12):3212–3222.
42. Zhang J, Yu ZX, Hilbert SL, et al. Cardiotoxicity of human recombinant interleukin-2 in rats. A morphological study. *Circulation*. 1993;87(4):1340–1353.
43. Fish EN, Platanias LC. Interferon receptor signaling in malignancy: a network of cellular pathways defining biological outcomes. *Mol Cancer Res*. 2014;12(12):1691–1703.
44. Sonnenblick M, Rosin A. Cardiotoxicity of interferon. A review of 44 cases. *Chest*. 1991;99(3):557–561.
45. Feenstra J, Grobbee DE, Remme WJ, Stricker BH. Drug-induced heart failure. *J Am Coll Cardiol*. 1999;33(5):1152–1162.
46. Khakoo AY, Halushka MK, Rame JE, Rodriguez ER, Kasper EK, Judge DP. Reversible cardiomyopathy caused by administration of interferon alpha. *Nat Clin Pract Cardiovasc Med*. 2005;2(1):53–57.
47. Klein I, Ojamaa K. Thyroid hormone and the cardiovascular system. *N Engl J Med*. 2001;344(7):501–509.
48. Kwon HJ, Coté TR, Cuffe MS, Kramer JM, Braun MM. Case reports of heart failure after therapy with a tumor necrosis factor antagonist. *Ann Intern Med*. 2003;138(10):807–811.
49. Ribera JM. Efficacy and safety of bispecific T-cell engager blinatumomab and the potential to improve leukemia-free survival in B-cell acute lymphoblastic leukemia. *Expert Rev Hematol*. 2017;10(12):1057–1067.
50. Neelapu SS, Tummala S, Kebriaei P, et al. Chimeric antigen receptor T-cell therapy—assessment and management of toxicities. *Nat Rev Clin Oncol*. 2018;15(1):47–62.
51. Marabondo S, Kaufman HL. High-dose interleukin-2 (IL-2) for the treatment of melanoma: safety considerations and future directions. *Expert Opin Drug Saf*. 2017;16(12):1347–1357.
52. Memoli B, De Nicola L, Libetta C, et al. Interleukin-2-induced renal dysfunction in cancer patients is reversed by low-dose dopamine infusion. *Am J Kidney Dis*. 1995;26(1):27–33.
53. Arangalage D, Delyon J, Lermuzeaux M, et al. Survival after fulminant myocarditis induced by immune-checkpoint inhibitors. *Ann Intern Med*. 2017;167(9):683–684.

Rheumatological Toxicities of Immunotherapy

Cassandra Calabrese, DO

Introduction

- The introduction of immune checkpoint inhibitor (ICI) therapy to treat cancer has changed the treatment paradigm for many malignancies. These agents exploit suppressor and regulatory pathways to boost integrated immunity against tumors but are associated with a unique spectrum of immune-related adverse events (irAEs) related to their untoward autoinflammatory and off-target effects. The field of irAEs from checkpoint inhibitor therapy is growing at a rapid pace and many unanswered questions remain. irAEs have been described in nearly every organ system, most commonly involving the gastrointestinal tract, skin, and endocrine system, and can range from mild and self-limiting to severe and life-threatening, often causing significant patient morbidity and even mortality.[1,2] Sometimes these irAEs require cessation of the checkpoint inhibitor.
- In addition to some of the more commonly reported irAEs, a variety of rheumatic manifestations have been described including arthralgia, inflammatory arthritis, polymyalgia rheumatica, myositis, sicca symptoms, rare reports of vasculitis, and others.[3] Rheumatic irAEs are infrequently reported in clinical trials and their descriptions are largely limited to case reports and small series. Rheumatic irAEs remain one of the most poorly understood irAEs and their true prevalence is unknown. Their natural history is also poorly defined. Whereas the more common irAEs often appear to be self-limited or resolve with effective immunosuppressive therapy, rheumatic irAEs may have a more persistent course, with some requiring treatment long after discontinuation of checkpoint inhibitor therapy.[4] Despite numerous case reports and series, the natural history of rheumatic irAEs is only starting to be elucidated. In this chapter, the current literature on rheumatic irAEs is summarized, including prevalence, clinical spectrum, diagnosis, and treatment.

Mechanism of Action

- The immune system is comprised of a system of checks and balances with many complex factors at play to maintain equilibrium. Immunological checkpoints are crucial for immune homeostasis and are involved in immune activation and deactivation. There are hundreds of known immunological checkpoints in the human immune system but the currently US Food and Drug Administration (FDA)–approved ICIs target two main immune checkpoints: cytotoxic T-lymphocyte-associated protein-4 (CTLA-4) and the programmed cell death-1 (PD-1)/PD-ligand-1 (PD-L1) pathway. CTLA-4 is primarily responsible for attenuating early activation of naïve memory T-cells in lymphoid organs. Following immune activation there is a rapid expansion of T-cells which requires two signals: (1) cognate antigen presentation by major histocompatibility complex (MHC) and (2) a co-stimulatory signal provided by engagement of CD28 on the naive T-cell with its ligand CD80/86 on

277

the antigen-presenting cell. When the immune response is no longer needed, CTLA-4 is expressed on the T-cell surface and competes for CD80/86 binding with CD28, attenuating T-cell activation.[2] The PD-1/PD-L1 pathway, on the other hand, functions in the periphery to inhibit T-cell activation at the effector stage. In certain cancers, tumor cells manipulate these pathways to evade immunosurveillance. By blocking these immunological checkpoints, ICIs harness the patient's immune system to target tumor cells. ICIs work by exploiting these suppressor and regulatory pathways to boost the integrated immune response against tumors—essentially "releasing the breaks" on immune activation and reinvigorating the immune system. This results in nonspecific immune activation that can lead to irAEs.

■ The exact pathophysiology of rheumatic irAEs, as well as irAEs involving other systems, has yet to be fully defined, as there have been few investigations into possible immunopathogenic mechanisms. It remains unclear whether rheumatic irAEs represent de novo events versus indicative of underlying immune-mediated disease. At least four candidate mechanisms have been proposed, including generalized immune activating secondary to checkpoint neutralization, direct off-target effects of checkpoint inhibitors, preexisting asymptomatic autoimmunity, and off-target effects of T-cell mediated immunity.[5] Further investigations into immunopathogenic mechanisms of rheumatic irAEs is urgently needed.

The Agents

The first ICI to be approved was ipilimumab in 2011, which blocks CTLA-4 and is indicated for metastatic melanoma.[6] Since then, six more agents have been approved for an ever-growing list of indications, including melanoma, renal cell carcinoma (RCC), non–small-cell lung cancer (NSCLC), Hodgkin's lymphoma, hepatocellular carcinoma, and many others, including a tumor agnostic indication for pembrolizumab, which is approved for treatment of microsatellite instability high or mismatch repair deficient solid tumors.[7] Agents targeting many other immunological checkpoints are currently being investigated in clinical trials for a variety of cancers and at varying stages. Ipilimumab is approved for treatment in combination with nivolumab for melanoma, NSCLC, and RCC.[8,9]

Prevalence

■ irAEs of any type are quite common, occurring in up to 90% of patients receiving CTLA-4 therapy[6] and 70% of patients receiving anti–PD-1/PD-L1 therapy,[10,11] but vary depending on tumor type. Incidence of irAEs increases when the drugs are used in combination.[2]

■ Compared with other system irAEs, the true incidence of rheumatic irAEs remains less well characterized for a variety of reasons, with the most important issue being that the Common Terminology Criteria for Adverse Events (CTCAE) used to grade adverse events is poorly applicable to rheumatic irAEs.[12] The grading system ranges from grade 1 through grade 5 (grade 1 = mild, grade 2 = moderate, grade 3 = severe, grade 4 = life-threatening, grade 5 = death). The majority of clinical trials report only events of grade 3 or higher, which generally require hospitalization. Rheumatic events such as inflammatory arthritis or polymyalgia rheumatica rarely lead to hospitalization and therefore are not captured in clinical trial data. Additionally, inflammatory arthritis does not have to require hospitalization to be severely debilitating for patients. Another reason for underreporting is that there is no standardization for coding rheumatic symptoms such that the same symptoms may be coded differently by different practitioners. For example, a swollen knee may be coded as joint pain, knee pain, knee swelling, knee effusion, or arthralgia. The creation of a more comprehensive grading system for rheumatic irAEs will facilitate earlier recognition and referral to rheumatologists, as well as more accurate reporting of their incidence and prevalence.

- The most commonly reported rheumatic irAE in clinical trials is arthralgia. A systematic review of the literature that examined reporting of irAEs secondary to ICI found that 1% to 43% of participants across 33 clinical trials developed arthralgia.[13] The true incidence of arthritis with ICI is less clear, as in that arthritis was only reported in 5 clinical trials, occurring in 1% to 7% of patients, and it is unclear how arthritis was defined in these trials. Some information on incidence of rheumatic irAEs can be gained from observational studies, including one single-center study that reported the incidence of inflammatory arthritis to be 5.1% in melanoma patients treated with anti–PD-1 therapy.[14] Other less-commonly described rheumatic irAEs such as myositis, Sjögren's syndrome, and polymyalgia rheumatica are not routinely reported in clinical trials and their incidence is largely based on case series, reports, and small retrospective studies. No large prospective studies have been conducted to help answer these questions. A systematic review and meta-analysis of irAEs was published wherein rates of certain irAEs from anti–PD-1/PD-L1 therapy in primary clinical trial data were reported.[15] Investigators found reporting of musculoskeletal events to be inconsistent. Out of 13 studies examined, 3 made no mention of musculoskeletal problems. Of the studies that did provide data, only two reported arthritis, with the remainder providing rates of arthralgia, back pain, musculoskeletal pain, and myalgia. When reported, rates of arthralgia varied across studies from 10% to 26% and 2% to 12% for myalgia.
- In general, rheumatic irAEs have been reported to occur within 12 weeks of initiation of ICI[1]; however, timing may vary from onset after the first dose to after therapy has been discontinued.[16,17]

Specific Rheumatic Immune-Related Adverse Events

INFLAMMATORY ARTHRITIS

ICI–related inflammatory arthritis has been increasingly described. One series included 30 patients with rheumatologist-confirmed inflammatory arthritis from either PD-1/PD-L1 monotherapy or anti–CTLA-4/PD-1 combination therapy.[18] They observed three major clinical phenotypes of inflammatory arthritis: a polyarticular form resembling rheumatoid arthritis with small joint involvement, a reactive arthritis-like phenotype, and a large-joint predominant seronegative spondyloarthropathy. In another case series including seven cases of ICI–related inflammatory arthritis, the median time to onset of irAE was 7.3 weeks after starting ICI, with the exception of two patients who experienced irAEs over 1 year after starting immunotherapy.[16] Rheumatic irAE led to withholding/discontinuing ICI in half of these patients. All patients required at least glucocorticoid therapy and several required further immunosuppression to treat their rheumatic irAE. Some still remained symptomatic months after their last ICI infusion. The vast majority of cases of ICI–related inflammatory arthritis are seronegative for rheumatoid factor or anti–cyclic citrullinated peptide (CCP) antibodies, although there have been rare reports of patients who developed anti–CCP-positive inflammatory arthritis who were found to be anti–CCP-positive prior to receiving ICI.[19] The most notable feature of ICI–related inflammatory arthritis is that it may persist after cessation of ICI in a large proportion of patients, oftentimes requiring long-term treatment with targeted therapies and continued follow-up with rheumatologists.[4]

SICCA SYNDROME

An entity resembling Sjögren's syndrome has been described in the setting of ICI, with atypical features including abrupt onset of severe salivary hypofunction, with xerophthalmia reported less frequently, and absence of traditional Sjögren's-related autoantibodies.[20] Cappelli et al. reported four cases of severe salivary gland hypofunction with all patients experiencing more prominent dry mouth symptoms than dry eyes.[17] One of these patients had positive anti-La/SS-B antibodies and had imaging evidence of parotitis. Another series reported five cases of sicca (two isolated cases and three in conjunction with other rheumatic irAEs) and two patients were positive for antinuclear antibodies (ANA), one in high titer (1:1280) with positive anti-Ro/SS-A antibodies.[16]

POLYMYALGIA RHEUMATICA

An entity resembling polymyalgia rheumatica (PMR) has been increasingly described in the setting of ICI therapy. In a large series of ICI-related PMR, the authors sought to identify how many cases fulfilled the 2012 European League Against Rheumatism (EULAR)/American College of Rheumatology (ACR) Criteria for PMR (Table 24.1).[21] Of 49 cases, 37 (75%) had sufficient data to reliably apply the criteria, and of these 28 (75%) fulfilled the criteria for PMR. ICI–related PMR cases share several atypical features that are often not seen in de novo PMR, including presence of inflammatory arthritis overlap features in other joints, and requirement for higher doses of glucocorticoids than typically used to treat PMR.[21]

MYOSITIS

Cases of myositis have been increasingly described in the setting of ICI, with estimated incidences of 0.76% to 1.2% of exposures to PD-L1–based therapy,[22] and also reported with combination therapy. ICI–related myositis differs from de novo inflammatory myositis in several ways, including lack of myositis-specific antibodies, higher mortality rate, and the frequent finding of concomitant myasthenia gravis and/or myocarditis—a clinical syndrome heretofore undescribed. VigiBase, a World Health Organization (WHO) database of individual safety case reports, identified 180 cases of myositis, reporting a median time to onset of 26 days after start of ICI, where 16.1% had concomitant myocarditis, 15.6% had concomitant myasthenia gravis–like symptoms, and 3.3% presented with all three, a clinical syndrome often referred to as "triple M."[23] These syndromes present as unique entities, different from spontaneous myositis and myocarditis, with a significantly higher mortality rate, with the highest mortality rates reported in cases of myositis with concomitant myocarditis.[23]

TABLE 24.1 ■ **Provisional Classification Criteria for PMR Scoring Algorithm**

	Points Without Ultrasound (0–6)	Points With Ultrasound (0–8)
Morning stiffness lasting >45 min	2	2
Hip pain or limited range of motion	1	1
Absence of RF or ACPA	2	2
Absence of other joint involvement	1	1
≥1 shoulder with subdeltoid bursitis and/or biceps tenosynovitis and/or glenohumeral synovitis and ≥1 hip with synovitis and/or trochanteric bursitis	n/a	1
Both shoulders with subdeltoid bursitis, biceps tenosynovitis or glenohumeral synovitis	n/a	1

Required to apply algorithm: age ≥50 years, bilateral shoulder aching, and abnormal CRP and/or ESR.

A score ≥4 is categorized as PMR without ultrasound, and a score of ≥5 is categorized as PMR if ultrasound findings are included.

ACPA, Anti–citrullinated protein antibody; *CRP*, c-reactive protein; *ESR*, erythrocyte sedimentation rate; *PMR*, polymyalgia rheumatica; *RF*, rheumatoid factor.

OTHERS

ICI–related vasculitis has been reported, albeit rarely. In a systematic review of ICI–related vasculitis, the majority of cases were of large-vessel vasculitis, and vasculitis involving the central and peripheral nervous system.[24] All cases resolved with either withholding ICI and/or administering glucocorticoids, and no deaths were reported. Three cases of giant cell arteritis have been described with ICI therapy: two in the setting of PMR and one isolated case.[25,26] All three cases were confirmed by temporal artery biopsy. A case of small-vessel vasculitis presenting as digital ischemia following ipilimumab therapy has been reported.[24] Retinal vasculitis has also been seen after anti–PD-1 therapy.[27,28] Other less commonly reported rheumatic irAEs include scleroderma, granulomatous/sarcoid-like lesions, and a single case of lupus nephritis after ipilimumab.[29–31]

Diagnosis and Management Strategies

- Optimal diagnosis of rheumatic irAEs remains a challenge. Referral to a rheumatologist plays a crucial role in this domain as differentiating a rheumatic irAE from other causes of rheumatic symptoms can be very challenging. As of late 2020, no criteria exist for diagnosing rheumatic irAEs of any type, and clinically validated biomarkers have yet to be identified. Whereas in some instances rheumatic irAEs may behave like traditional rheumatological disease, many case series and reports have described atypical features—for example, inflammatory arthritis or PMR cases requiring higher doses of glucocorticoids compared with patients with de novo disease.[17,21] Whereas the more common irAEs (dermatological, gastrointestinal, hepatic) are usually glucocorticoid-responsive and tend to resolve in 6 to 12 weeks,[32] many rheumatic irAEs are persistent and may require immunosuppression for symptom control long after cessation of the checkpoint inhibitor.[4]
- Although there are no evidence-based guidelines for management of rheumatic irAEs, several different management guidelines have been published, with some specifically addressing rheumatic irAEs.[32–34] These management recommendations are based on the grade of symptoms, and also include recommendations for evaluation (examination, laboratory, imaging studies) and follow-up. Recently, a EULAR task force released a consensus document on the diagnosis and management of rheumatic irAEs.[35]
- Naidoo et al. have proposed treatment recommendations for inflammatory arthritis and highlighted the frequent need for continued immunosuppression compared with irAEs involving other systems.[36] Their suggestions come in the form of an algorithm that is based on the CTCAE grading system, while acknowledging that this may underestimate severity and functional impairment of rheumatic irAEs. The first step is to assess the grade of arthritis, including the presence or absence of inflammatory symptoms (e.g., joint stiffness and swelling). Symptoms are designated grade 2 if they limit instrumental activities of daily living (ADLs). Symptoms are assigned grade 3 or higher if they limit self-care ADLs or if there is evidence of joint damage. The next step is investigation, which includes physical examination, laboratory tests, and imaging.
- In the case of unexplained rheumatic, musculoskeletal, or systemic symptoms, a complete rheumatological assessment should be performed (Box 24.1). During history taking, all patients should be asked about personal family history of autoimmune disease. Depending on the clinical scenario, other laboratory investigations may be obtained, such as testing for the presence of HLA-B27 in patients with inflammatory arthritis or other features of spondyloarthritis (uveitis, psoriasis, colitis, enthesitis). It is important to consider other differentials when evaluating for suspected rheumatic irAE, including progression of underlying malignancy, and infectious complications.

BOX 24.1 ■ Recommended Autoimmune Laboratory Tests for Patients With Suspected Rheumatic irAE

- Antinuclear antibody (ANA)
- Anti–extractable nuclear antigen panel (SSA, SSB, Jo-1, RNP, Sm, centromere, scleroderma IgG, chromatin)
- Anti–double stranded DNA antibodies
- Rheumatoid factor
- Anti–citrullinated peptide antibodies
- C-reactive protein
- Sedimentation rate

IgG, Immunoglobulin G; *Jo-1*, histidyl tRNA synthetase; *RNP*, ribonucleoprotein; *Sm*, smith; *SSA*, Sjogren's-syndrome-related antigen A; *SSB*, Sjogren's-syndrome-related antigen B.

- Depending on the physical examination, advanced imaging should be considered, especially if looking for evidence of inflammation in the joints. Imaging modalities to consider include musculoskeletal ultrasound, magnetic resonance imaging (MRI), and positron emission tomography (PET)/computed tomography (CT).
- When treating rheumatic irAEs, it is important to know when immunotherapy should be withheld, and also at what point a patient should be referred to a rheumatologist. Naidoo et al. have recommended referral to a rheumatologist if any of the following are present: patients with moderate-to-severe symptoms, symptoms lasting longer than 4 weeks, or patients requiring more than 20 mg of prednisone daily with inability to taper below prednisone 10 mg daily over a 4-week period.[36] They also recommend withholding immunotherapy for patients with grade 3 or higher disease, and to consider withholding if grade 2 inflammatory arthritis. The EULAR recommendations stress the importance of early referral to a rheumatologist.[35] The Society for Immunotherapy of Cancer (SITC) Toxicity Management Working Group published a position article and guidelines for management of irAEs in 2017 and their recommendations for inflammatory arthritis reiterate those of Naidoo et al.[33]
- The National Comprehensive Cancer Network (NCCN), in partnership with the American Society of Clinical Oncology (ASCO), published guidelines for management of immunotherapy-related toxicities which includes recommendations for diagnosis and management of inflammatory arthritis and myalgias/myositis but not for any other rheumatic irAEs.[37]
- Although glucocorticoids remain the cornerstone of treatment of rheumatic and other system irAEs, steroid-sparing, targeted therapies are often required. There has been a growing body of literature, as well as clinical experience, in the use of targeted therapies such as tumor necrosis factor alpha inhibitors and inhibitors of interleukin 6 (IL-6), amongst others.[38] Moving forward, a personalized treatment approach that takes into account the immunopathogenesis of individual irAEs has been proposed.[38]

Use of Immune Checkpoint Inhibitors in Patients With Preexisting Autoimmune Diseases

- The use of ICI in patients with preexisting autoimmune diseases (AIDs) remains an area of uncertainty both in terms of efficacy and safety. Given the nature of irAEs which are the result of dysregulation and over-activation of the immune system, there is theoretical concern that their use in such patients would result in exacerbations of the patient's underlying AID. For this reason, patients with underlying AID were largely excluded from all clinical trials that led to the approval of currently used checkpoint inhibitors, with the exception of mildly localized AID such as vitiligo.[6] This lack of data has left practitioners hesitant to treat this patient population with ICI.

- A large published series described 112 patients with preexisting AID, including rheumatoid arthritis, systemic lupus erythematous, and psoriatic arthritis, who had received ICI.[39] Flare of underlying AID was reported in 47%, a new irAE occurred in 42%, and 18% experienced both. Among these flares, 70% were considered to be mild. A prospective study from the French REISAMIC registry, where 45 patients with 53 AIDs receiving anti–PD-1/PD-L1 therapy were followed for AID flare and new irAEs.[40] Of these patients, 55% experienced an AID flare. Another notable series reported that out of 30 patients with preexisting AID receiving ipilimumab for advanced melanoma, 27% experienced AID exacerbations and 33% developed irAEs.[41]
- This raises important questions for patients with AID who develop cancer. Although our knowledge is largely based on small cases series, it seems that most AID flares in the setting of ICI therapy are manageable with appropriate treatment and thus a preexisting diagnosis of AID is not a contraindication to receipt of ICI therapy. However, this may depend on the severity of the underlying AID. Ultimately, treating the patient's malignancy should be the main goal, thus highlighting the importance of multidisciplinary care by oncologists, rheumatologists, and other subspecialists.

Conclusion

The use of ICIs to treat cancer is a rapidly growing field. Moving forward, these drugs will continue to be approved for a wider range of malignancies, meaning an ever-growing number of patients will be receiving ICIs. As a result, the incidence of rheumatic irAEs is going to rise, and these patients will increasingly come in to contact with health care professionals, not only in the oncology setting but in family practice, emergency rooms, and many subspecialties. It is important for health care providers in all fields to have an awareness of rheumatic irAEs so that they may aide in the optimal management of these patients, including referral to rheumatologists and other appropriate subspecialists.

References

1. Michot JM, Bigenwald C, Champiat S, et al. Immune-related adverse events with immune checkpoint blockade: a comprehensive review. *Eur J Cancer.* 2016;54:139–148.
2. Boutros C, Tarhini A, Routier E, et al. Safety profiles of anti-CTLA-4 and anti-PD-1 antibodies alone and in combination. *Nat Rev Clin Oncol.* 2016;13(8):473–486.
3. Kostine M, Rouxel L, Barnetche T, et al. Rheumatic disorders associated with immune checkpoint inhibitors in patients with cancer-clinical aspects and relationship with tumour response: a single-centre prospective cohort study. *Ann Rheum Dis.* 2018;77(3):393–398.
4. Braaten TJ, Brahmer JR, Forde PM, et al. Immune checkpoint inhibitor-induced inflammatory arthritis persists after immunotherapy cessation. *Ann Rheum Dis.* 2020;79:332–338.
5. Calabrese LH, Calabrese C, Cappelli LC. Rheumatic immune-related adverse events from cancer immunotherapy. *Nat Rev Rheumatol.* 2018;14(10):569–579.
6. Hodi FS, O'Day SJ, McDermott DF, et al. Improved survival with ipilimumab in patients with metastatic melanoma. *N Engl J Med.* 2010;363(8):711–723.
7. Marcus L, Lemery SJ, Keegan P, Pazdur R. FDA approval summary: pembrolizumab for the treatment of microsatellite instability-high solid tumors. *Clin Cancer Res.* 2019;25(13):3753–3758.
8. Larkin J, Chiarion-Sileni V, Gonzalez R, et al. Combined nivolumab and ipilimumab or monotherapy in untreated melanoma. *N Engl J Med.* 2015;373(1):23–34.
9. Motzer RJ, Tannir NM, McDermott DF, et al. Nivolumab plus ipilimumab versus sunitinib in advanced renal-cell carcinoma. *N Engl J Med.* 2018;378(14):1277–1290.
10. Topalian SL, Hodi FS, Brahmer JR, et al. Safety, activity, and immune correlates of anti-PD-1 antibody in cancer. *N Engl J Med.* 2012;366(26):2443–2454. doi:10.1056/NEJMoa1200690.
11. Brahmer JR, Tykodi SS, Chow LQM, et al. Safety and activity of anti-PD-L1 antibody in patients with advanced cancer. *N Engl J Med.* 2012;366(26):2455–2465.

12. Common Terminology Criteria for Adverse Events (CTCAE) v4.0. https://www.acrin.org/Portals/0/Administration/Regulatory/CTCAE_4.02_2009-09-15_QuickReference_5x7.pdf.

13. Cappelli LC, Gutierrez AK, Bingham CO 3rd, Shah AA. Rheumatic and musculoskeletal immune-related adverse events due to immune checkpoint inhibitors: a systematic review of the literature. *Arthritis Care Res (Hoboken)*. 2017;69(11):1751–1763.

14. Buder-Bakhaya K, Benesova K, Schulz C, et al. Characterization of arthralgia induced by PD-1 antibody treatment in patients with metastasized cutaneous malignancies. *Cancer Immunol Immunother*. 2018;67(2):175–182.

15. Baxi S, Yang A, Gennarelli RL, et al. Immune-related adverse events for anti-PD-1 and anti-PD-L1 drugs: systematic review and meta-analysis. *BMJ*. 2018;360(k793):1–13.

16. Calabrese C, Kirchner E, Kontzias K, Velcheti V, Calabrese LH. Rheumatic immune-related adverse events of checkpoint therapy for cancer: case series of a new nosological entity. *RMD Open*. 2017;3(1):e000412.

17. Cappelli LC, Gutierrez AK, Baer AN, et al. Inflammatory arthritis and sicca syndrome induced by nivolumab and ipilimumab. *Ann Rheum Dis*. 2017;76(1):43–50.

18. Cappelli LC, Brahmer JR, Forde PM, et al. Clinical presentation of immune checkpoint inhibitor-induced inflammatory arthritis differs by immunotherapy regimen. *Semin Arthritis Rheum*. 2018;48(3):553–557.

19. Belkhir R, Le Burel S, Dunogeant L, et al. Rheumatoid arthritis and polymyalgia rheumatica occurring after immune checkpoint inhibitor treatment. *Ann Rheum Dis*. 2017;76(10):1747–1750.

20. Warner BM, Baer AN, Lipson EJ, et al. Sicca syndrome associated with immune checkpoint inhibitor therapy. *Oncologist*. 2019;24(9):1259–1269.

21. Calabrese C, Cappelli LC, Kostine M, Kirchner E, Braaten T, Calabrese L. Polymyalgia rheumatica-like syndrome from checkpoint inhibitor therapy: case series and systematic review of the literature. *RMD Open*. 2019;5(1).

22. Liewluck T, Kao JC, Mauermann ML. PD-1 inhibitor-associated myopathies: emerging immune-mediated myopathies. *J Immunother*. 2018;41(4):208–211.

23. Anquetil C, Salem JE, Lebrun-Vignes B, et al. Immune checkpoint inhibitor–associated myositis: expanding the spectrum of cardiac complications of the immunotherapy revolution. *Circulation*. 2018;138(7):743–745.

24. Daxini A, Cronin K, Sreih AG. Vasculitis associated with immune checkpoint inhibitors—a systematic review. *Clin Rheumatol*. 2018;37(9):2579–2584.

25. Goldstein BL, Gedmintas L, Todd DJ. Drug-associated polymyalgia rheumatica/giant cell arteritis occurring in two patients after treatment with ipilimumab, an antagonist of CTLA-4. *Arthritis Rheumatol*. 2014;66(3):768–769.

26. Micaily I, Chernoff M. An unknown reaction to pembrolizumab: giant cell arteritis. *Ann Oncol Off J Eur Soc Med Oncol*. 2017;28(10):2621–2622.

27. Manusow JS, Khoja L, Pesin N, Joshua AM, Mandelcorn ED. Retinal vasculitis and ocular vitreous metastasis following complete response to PD-1 inhibition in a patient with metastatic cutaneous melanoma. *J Immunother Cancer*. 2015;2(1):41.

28. Theillac C, Straub M, Breton AL, Thomas L, Dalle S. Bilateral uveitis and macular edema induced by nivolumab: a case report. *BMC Ophthalmol*. 2017;17(1):227.

29. Barbosa NS, Wetter DA, Wieland CN, Shenoy NK, Markovic SN, Thanarajasingam U. Scleroderma induced by pembrolizumab: a case series. *Mayo Clin Proc*. 2017;92(7):1158–1163.

30. Tetzlaff MT, Nelson KC, Diab A, et al. Granulomatous/sarcoid-like lesions associated with checkpoint inhibitors: a marker of therapy response in a subset of melanoma patients. *J Immunother Cancer*. 2018;6(1):14.

31. Fadel F, El Karoui K, Knebelmann B. Anti-CTLA4 antibody-induced lupus nephritis. *N Engl J Med*. 2009;361(2):211–212.

32. Brahmer JR, Lacchetti C, Schneider BJ, et al. Management of immune-related adverse events in patients treated with immune checkpoint inhibitor therapy: American Society of Clinical Oncology Clinical Practice Guideline. *J Clin Oncol*. 2018;36(17):1714–1768.

33. Puzanov I, Diab A, Abdallah K, et al. Managing toxicities associated with immune checkpoint inhibitors: consensus recommendations from the Society for Immunotherapy of Cancer (SITC) Toxicity Management Working Group. *J Immunother Cancer*. 2017;5(1):1–28.

34. Martins F, Sykiotis GP, Maillard M, et al. New therapeutic perspectives to manage refractory immune checkpoint-related toxicities. *Lancet Oncol*. 2019;20(1):e54–e64.

35. Kostine M, Finckh A, Bingham CO, et al. EULAR points to consider for the diagnosis and management of rheumatic immune-related adverse events due to cancer immunotherapy with checkpoint inhibitors. *Ann Rheum Dis.* April 2020:annrheumdis-2020-217139.
36. Naidoo J, Cappelli LC, Forde PM, et al. Inflammatory arthritis: a newly recognized adverse event of immune checkpoint blockade. *Oncologist* 2017;22(6):627–630.
37. Thompson JA. New NCCN guidelines: recognition and management of immunotherapy-related toxicity. *J Natl Compr Canc Netw.* 2018;16(55):594–596.
38. Esfahani K, Elkrief A, Calabrese C, et al. Moving towards personalized treatments of immune-related adverse events. *Nat Rev Clin Oncol.* 2020;17:504–515.
39. Tison A, Quéré G, Misery L, et al. Safety and efficacy of immune checkpoint inhibitors in patients with cancer and preexisting autoimmune disease: a nationwide, multicenter cohort study. *Arthritis Rheumatol.* 2019;71(12):2100–2111.
40. Danlos F-X, Voisin A-L, Dyevre V, et al. Safety and efficacy of anti-programmed death 1 antibodies in patients with cancer and pre-existing autoimmune or inflammatory disease. *Eur J Cancer.* 2018;91:21–29.
41. Johnson DB, Sullivan RJ, Ott PA, et al. Ipilimumab therapy in patients with advanced melanoma and preexisting autoimmune disorders. *JAMA Oncol.* 2016;2(2):234–240.

CHAPTER 25

Mechanisms of Radiation-Related Toxicities

Christopher W. Fleming, MD ■ Mohamed Abazeed, MD, PhD

Introduction

Radiotherapy comprises the delivery of ionizing radiation, most commonly in the form of X-rays, for the treatment of malignant or benign neoplasms. Radiotherapy induces DNA damage either through direct ionization or through the generation of intermediary reactive oxygen species.[1] Left unrepaired, this damage can lead to normal and tumor cell death via apoptosis, mitotic catastrophe, autophagy, or terminal growth arrest/senescence.[2] Deficiencies in DNA repair, a hallmark of some cancers, can sensitize these tumors to death after irradiation, in part accounting for the favorable therapeutic ratio of radiotherapy. However, DNA repair within normal cells can be incomplete or can be overwhelmed by the dose of radiotherapy delivered, leading to the development of radiation-induced toxicities.

Types of Radiation-Related Toxicities

- Radiotherapy is a local treatment and therefore adverse effects are generally expected within tissues in closest proximity to the irradiated volume. For example, radiotherapy to the pelvis may result in cystitis, enteritis, proctitis, or bone marrow suppression, but it will not typically cause toxicity in distant organs (e.g., lung). Similarly, in the treatment of pituitary adenomas, cumulative dose to the optic nerves and chiasm will be the major consideration during the treatment planning process to prevent optic neuritis or subsequent blindness. In addition to direct organ damage, there is a risk of secondary malignancy postirradiation. The relationship between the distance from the irradiated volume and risk of secondary malignancy is represented by an inverted U-shape. That is, the risk is lower in the high-dose irradiated volume, increases at intermediate distances from the target volume within a relatively lower dose region, and decreases at greater distances from the treated organ (e.g., increased risk of breast cancer after radiation for mediastinal Hodgkin's lymphoma).[3]
- Radiation toxicities are generally categorized as acute, occurring during or within a few weeks of radiotherapy, or late, occurring months to years after treatment. Acute toxicities are mainly mediated by the adverse effects of radiotherapy upon the endothelium, leading to vascular permeability, edema, and lymphocyte adhesion and infiltration.[4] Soon after irradiation, endothelial cells have changes in their physiological appearance and exhibit alteration in synthesis and secretion of growth factors, chemoattractants, and injury markers such as interleukin (IL)-1, IL-6, and tumor necrosis factor-alpha.[5] This process produces an inflammatory response resulting in the recruitment and activation of neutrophils and eosinophils,[6] which culminates in endothelial apoptosis mediated by the activation of sphingomyelinases, the generation of ceramide, and the activation of various caspases.[7]
- Late toxicities are primarily attributed to the depletion of tissue-specific stem cells and the generation of fibrosis through the excessive production of fibrocytes. Although the inciting

molecular reactions take place shortly after radiation exposure, the cellular events and tissue remodeling processes take place over a period of years. Ionizing radiation also induces premature terminal differentiation of progenitor fibroblasts to fibrocytes through an imbalance of inflammatory regulators, particularly transforming growth factor (TGF)-β.[5] TGF-β overexpression has been linked to late effects throughout many organ sites, attributed to the induction of excess collagen synthesis and the inhibition of matrix metalloproteinases.[8] This excessive fibrosis also leads to late vascular effects including capillary collapse, thickening of basement membrane, telangiectasias, and loss of stem cell clonogenic capacity. Tissue-specific stem cells have been shown to reverse this process by normalizing proinflammatory cytokine levels, promoting revascularization, and upregulating antioxidant enzymes, assuming they remain intact after exposure to radiotherapy.[6]

Genetic Determinants of Radiation Toxicity

Though the likelihood of adverse radiation effects is generally dependent on the cumulative radiation dose, a small number of patients develop toxicity after only mild exposure. Genetic syndromes such as ataxia telangiectasia, Fanconi's anemia, and Bloom syndrome are known to confer significant radiosensitivity, though the exact mechanisms remain poorly understood.[9] Systemic diseases such as scleroderma, systemic lupus erythematosus, and inflammatory bowel disease are also known to confer sensitivity to radiation, presumably due to a baseline proinflammatory state that exacerbates acute and, relatedly, late toxicities of radiotherapy.[10] However, a majority of patients who exhibit hypersensitivity to irradiation have no identifiable causative mutation or comorbid condition, suggesting that individual sensitivity is contingent on numerous genes with variable penetrance.[9] In addition to normal tissue sensitivity, recent studies indicate a genetic basis for the sensitivity of tumors to irradiation.[11] Biomarkers from these and similar studies could offer an opportunity to personalize radiation doses, which can in turn lead to appropriate deescalation strategies for individual patients.

Technical Advances in Precision Radiotherapy Can Reduce Toxicity

- Advancements in radiation technology have increased safety by reducing radiation doses to normal tissue. Three examples (not exhaustive) of these advances include intensity-modulated radiotherapy (IMRT), image-guided radiotherapy (IGRT), and motion management. IMRT, a highly conformal radiation technique, is characterized by two main features: intensity modulation and reverse planning. The intensity of the radiation beam is modulated with the use of multi-leaf collimators (MLCs) within the head (gantry) of the linear accelerator. Reverse planning utilizes planning software to optimize MLC positioning at each gantry angle. IGRT utilizes imaging, most commonly cone beam computed tomography (CT), at the time of radiation treatment to ensure the patient is aligned correctly and the treatment will be delivered to the desired area. Motion management (i.e., breath hold or 4-dimensional CT scanning) can further reduce the size of radiation volumes by reducing uncertainty in tumor position during treatment.
- Whereas technical advancements aim to control toxicity by increasing the conformality of radiation plans, dose and fractionation are commonly altered as well in an effort to reduce side effects. Fractionation is a critical variable for managing toxicity within the irradiated field. Early radiobiological studies showed that a single fraction of radiotherapy separated into multiple smaller fractions would result in considerably less toxicity due to DNA repair and repopulation between fractions.[12] Hence, radiotherapy has traditionally been delivered as daily treatments lasting multiple weeks. The advancements in radiotherapy detailed above

permit the implementation of highly conformal plans. Treatments may now be safely delivered in as few as one to five fractions, for example, stereotactic body radiotherapy (SBRT).[13] However, there remain many clinical scenarios where organs at risk lie in close proximity to the target volume, such that treatments may still require reduced total dose or an increase in the number of fractions in order to safely treat patients.

- Particle therapy is another means used to reduce dose to normal tissue. External beam radiotherapy is most commonly delivered with megavoltage X-rays, which are attenuated as they pass completely through the patient. Charged particles such as electrons and protons possess a dosimetric benefit of delivering the majority of radiation by a certain depth, practically eliminating exit dose. Electrons are commonly used in practice but are limited by their superficial penetration. Proton therapy is becoming increasingly utilized in large centers, and randomized trials through multiple organ sites are ongoing to assess the clinical benefit of protons versus photon therapy.[14–17]

Medical Therapies Alter Radiation Response

- Various medical therapies have been investigated for their potential to improve the therapeutic index of radiotherapy. Radiosensitizing agents, most commonly cytotoxic chemotherapy, are given concurrently with radiotherapy in the curative treatment of many cancers throughout the body.[18] These agents interact with radiation in additive and synergistic ways, and hence can increase tumor kill but may exacerbate toxicities. Antagonistic interactions between drugs and radiation are characteristics of radiation protectors. Amifostine is a radioprotectant that has been shown to reduce xerostomia and mucositis in head and neck cancers, though some concerns have been raised about a potential to protect tumor cells as well.[19]
- Other systemic agents have been used to treat late toxicities of radiotherapy, though data supporting their efficacy is limited. Pentoxyphylline is an antiinflammatory drug that improves blood flow to irradiated tissues and has been used in combination with the antioxidant vitamin E to treat late radiation fibrosis.[20] Hyperbaric oxygen is thought to counteract the late effects of radiation by promoting reoxygenation and revascularization.[21]

Conclusions

Radiotherapy is the targeted delivery of ionizing radiation for the treatment of benign and malignant neoplasms. Radiotherapy primarily exerts its effect via DNA damage. Acute vascular injury can lead to local inflammation. Excessive fibrosis and loss of tissue-specific stem cells is sine qua non of late radiation effect. Individual sensitivity to radiotherapy is generally unknown prior to radiation, and most likely a polygenic trait. Finally, toxicity can be mitigated with highly conformal treatment delivery, alterations in dose and fractionation, particle therapy, and adjunctive systemic therapies.

References

1. Baskar R, Dai J, Wenlong N, Yeo R, Yeoh KW. Biological response of cancer cells to radiation treatment. *Front Mol Biosci.* 2014;1:24.
2. Thoms J, Bristow RG. DNA repair targeting and radiotherapy: a focus on the therapeutic ratio. *Semin Radiat Oncol.* 2010;20(4):217–222.
3. Ng J, Shuryak I. Minimizing second cancer risk following radiotherapy: current perspectives. *Cancer Manag Res.* 2015;7:1–11.
4. Jaenke RS, Robbins ME, Bywaters T, Whitehouse E, Rezvani M, Hopewell JW. Capillary endothelium. Target site of renal radiation injury. *Lab Invest.* 1993;68(4):396–405.
5. Rodemann HP, Blaese MA. Responses of normal cells to ionizing radiation. *Semin Radiat Oncol.* 2007;17(2):81–88.

6. Wei J, Meng L, Hou X, et al. Radiation-induced skin reactions: mechanism and treatment. *Cancer Manag Res.* 2019;11:167–177.

7. Li YQ, Chen P, Haimovitz-Friedman A, Reilly RM, Wong CS. Endothelial apoptosis initiates acute blood-brain barrier disruption after ionizing radiation. *Cancer Res.* 2003;63(18):5950–5956.

8. Martin M, Lefaix J, Delanian S. TGF-beta1 and radiation fibrosis: a master switch and a specific therapeutic target? *Int J Radiat Oncol Biol Phys.* 2000;47(2):277–290.

9. Travis EL. Genetic susceptibility to late normal tissue injury. *Semin Radiat Oncol.* 2007;17(2):149–155.

10. Chon BH, Loeffler JS. The effect of nonmalignant systemic disease on tolerance to radiation therapy. *Oncologist.* 2002;7(2):136–143.

11. Yard BD, Adams DJ, Chie EK, et al. A genetic basis for the variation in the vulnerability of cancer to DNA damage. *Nat Commun.* 2016;7:11428.

12. Ng WL, Huang Q, Liu X, Zimmerman M, Li F, Li CY. Molecular mechanisms involved in tumor repopulation after radiotherapy. *Transl Cancer Res.* 2013;2(5):442–448.

13. Tsang MW. Stereotactic body radiotherapy: current strategies and future development. *J Thorac Dis.* 2016;8(Suppl 6):S517–S527.

14. Dose-escalated photon IMRT or proton beam radiation therapy versus standard-dose radiation therapy and temozolomide in treating patients with newly diagnosed glioblastoma. https://clinicaltrials.gov/ct2/show/NCT02179086.

15. Radiation therapy with protons or photons in treating patients with liver cancer. https://clinicaltrials.gov/ct2/show/NCT03186898.

16. Comparing proton therapy to photon radiation therapy for esophageal cancer. https://clinicaltrials.gov/ct2/show/NCT03801876.

17. Comparing photon therapy to proton therapy to treat patients with lung cancer. https://clinicaltrials.gov/ct2/show/NCT01993810.

18. Lawrence TS, Blackstock AW, McGinn C. The mechanism of action of radiosensitization of conventional chemotherapeutic agents. *Semin Radiat Oncol.* 2003;13(1):13–21.

19. Gu J, Zhu S, Li X, Wu H, Li Y, Hua F. Effect of amifostine in head and neck cancer patients treated with radiotherapy: a systematic review and meta-analysis based on randomized controlled trials. *PLoS One.* 2014;9(5):e95968.

20. Ozturk B, Egehan I, Atavci S, Kitapci M. Pentoxifylline in prevention of radiation-induced lung toxicity in patients with breast and lung cancer: a double-blind randomized trial. *Int J Radiat Oncol Biol Phys.* 2004;58(1):213–219.

21. Bennett MH, Feldmeier J, Hampson NB, Smee R, Milross C. Hyperbaric oxygen therapy for late radiation tissue injury. *Cochrane Database Syst Rev.* 2016;4:CD005005.

CHAPTER 26

Mucosal and Esophageal Toxicites of Radiation Therapy

Nitika Thawani, MD ▦ Shilpa Vyas, MD

Introduction

▪ Oral and esophageal mucosal injuries are inevitable postradiation changes, encountered with daily radiation therapy. Mucositis has remained a morbid side effect of radiation therapy since its first clinical use as an agent effective against cancer. Mucosal injury is generally the first change that is observed as the radiation beam enters human tissues. Alimentary mucositis (AM) is the recommended term to describe cancer therapy–associated mucosal injury of the alimentary tract (mouth to anus). This unifying term acknowledges the similarities along the entire gastrointestinal (GI) tract while allowing for regional differences that require discussion of oral and GI mucositis separately at times, based on pathophysiological responses, clinical characteristics, and management options. In almost all patients, AM is associated with considerable pain and thus can significantly impair quality of life and, in neutropenic patients, mucositis represents a clinically significant risk factor for sepsis.[1] Furthermore, in some patients, AM becomes a dose-limiting toxicity, slowing or preventing continuation of selected cancer therapies, including accelerated fractionation and hyperfractionation in radiotherapy and interventions that combine chemotherapy and radiotherapy.

▪ The major determinants of mucosal injury are total dose of radiation, daily radiation dose, and concurrent chemotherapy, in addition to an individual's inherent sensitivity to radiation. The incidence of AM is governed by these previously mentioned factors. Lower grade reactions are extremely common in nearly all patients receiving radiation with an incidence of almost 80% to 100%, with almost a third of these patients experiencing severe mucosal injury.[2,3]

Description

▪ Clinically, mucositis usually begins with mucosal congestion and erythema, which progresses through white, elevated, desquamative patches that are painful to contact pressure. Following this, the patches may coalesce and, eventually, there is development of painful, contiguous, pseudomembranous lesions (Fig. 26.1) with associated dysphagia and decreased oral intake. The nonkeratinized mucosa in the oral cavity and GI tract is at the highest risk of being affected by the radiation-related reaction. Mucosal lesions usually heal within 2 to 3 weeks. The clinical course of AM may sometimes be complicated by local infection, particularly in immunosuppressed patients. Fungal infections such as candidiasis, and viral infections, such as herpes simplex virus (HSV) can sometimes be superimposed on oral mucositis, complicating its course by delaying healing.

▪ The sequence of events that occurs during radiation therapy for head and neck cancer reflects the different kinetics of the cell populations involved[4]:
  ▪ **Week 1:** The first week is characterized by slight focal hyperemia and edema caused by dilatation of capillaries in sensitive patients. Sensitivity may be associated with alcohol or tobacco use, chemotherapy, infection (oral candidiasis, HSV), or immunosuppression (such as HIV).

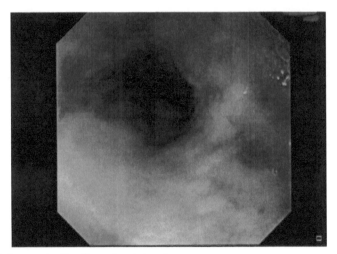

Fig. 26.1 Radiation esophagitis with confluent ulceration.

- **Week 2:** The second week is characterized by increasing pain and loss of desire to eat. Sense of taste is altered; bitter and acid flavors are most changed, with less change with salty and sweet tastes. Erythema and edema increase, and early desquamative mucositis occurs. Basal cell division has been affected; this layer is being denuded, and vasculoconnective tissue damage becomes apparent. Mucositis is patchy during this time.
- **Week 3:** The third week is characterized by mucositis and swelling with depletion of gland secretions leading to difficulty in swallowing. Mucositis plaques are confluent. Impairment of taste acuity occurs during the third week of a multifraction radiotherapy regime.
- **Week 4:** The fourth week is characterized by further progression of signs previously seen signs. Confluent mucositis sloughs, resulting in denuded lamina propria. Mucosa becomes covered by fibrin and polymorphonuclear leukocytes.
- **Week 5:** Maximal radiation damage becomes apparent by the fifth week. There is extreme sensitivity to touch, temperature, and grainy food. Recovery of epithelial layer may begin during therapy.
- **Posttherapy:** After therapy concludes basal cells migrate into the area and proliferate. In 2 to 4 weeks, complete resolution is observed.
- Defining the epidemiology of mucositis has been confounded historically by a number of variables, including underreporting, differences in terminology used to describe it, differences in assessment techniques and scales, and the correlation between mucositis and other clinically important sequelae. Multiple scoring systems for AM have been devised over the years with the goal of providing a uniform system which is objective, validated, and reproducible across all clinical situations and applications. The two most commonly used scoring systems in the field of radiation oncology include the ones formulated by the National Cancer Institute (Common Terminology Criteria for Adverse Events - CTCAE), and the Radiation Therapy Oncology Group (RTOG) scales for the purpose of uniform reporting throughout the globe.[5,6] Regardless of the scale used, increasing evidence confirms the importance of training and standardization for improving the accuracy and consistency of mucositis assessment.
- The RTOG and NCI–CTCAE scoring systems for mucositis and esophagitis, are given in Tables 26.1 and 26.2.

TABLE 26.1 ■ RTOG and NCI–CTCAE Scoring System for Mucositis

Source	Grade 1	Grade 2	Grade 3	Grade 4	Grade 5
RTOG	May experience mild pain not requiring analgesic	Patchy mucositis may have a serosanguinous discharge. May experience pain requiring analgesics, <1.5 cm, noncontiguous	Confluent fibrinous mucositis/may include severe pain requiring narcotics, >1.5 cm, contiguous	Necrosis or deep ulceration, ± bleeding	Death
NCI–CTCAE	Painless ulcers, erythema or mild soreness	Painful erythema, edema or ulcers, but can eat	Painful erythema, edema or ulcers cannot eat	Requires parenteral or enteral support	Death

NCI–CTCAE, National Cancer Institute–Common Terminology Criteria for Adverse Events; *RTOG*, Radiation Therapy Oncology Group.

TABLE 26.2 ■ RTOG and NCI–CTCAE Scoring System for Esophagitis

Source	Grade 1	Grade 2	Grade 3	Grade 4	Grade 5
RTOG	Mild dysphagia or odynophagia, topical anesthetics or NSAIDs, soft diet	Moderate dysphagia or odynophagia, narcotic analgesics, puree or liquid diet	Severe dysphagia or odynophagia, dehydration or weight loss >15%, IV fluids, NGT, TPN	Complete obstruction, ulceration, perforation, fistula	Death
NCI–CTCAE	Asymptomatic	Symptomatic, altered eating/swallowing; IV fluids <24 h	Symptomatic, inadequate oral caloric/fluid intake, need IV fluids > 24 h, TPN	Life-threatening (obstruction, perforation)	Death

NCI–CTCAE, National Cancer Institute–Common Terminology Criteria for Adverse Events; *NGT*, nasogastric tube; *NSAID*, nonsteroidal antiinflammatory drug; *RTOG*, Radiation Therapy Oncology Group; *TPN*, total parenteral nutrition.

Risk Factors

■ As mentioned previously, there are certain risk factors directly associated with the incidence and severity of mucositis, which can be categorized as treatment- or patient-related. Treatment-related risk factors include the type of ionizing radiation, the volume of irradiated tissue, the dose per day, and cumulative dose. Lower energy radiation used for head and neck cancer results in higher surface dose compared with the higher energy radiation used for deeply situated tumors at other sites. The higher radiation doses needed for head and neck cancer, in the order of over 5000 cGy has been directly responsible for causing mucosal injury.[2,3] Any altered fractionation with dose fractions above 200 cGy or more than one fraction of radiation a day can also increase the risk of mucosal toxicity.[7-10] It has been noted in a considerable number of clinical trials that the severity of acute normal tissue responses, particularly oral mucositis, is significantly increased when the overall treatment time is shortened.[11] It is important to note that the incidence and severity of acute mucosal toxicity has not been significantly decreased by the introduction of newer techniques in radiation therapy. Using a different modality, such as proton therapy for head and neck radiation, has also not resulted in any significant mucosal sparing or decreased mucosal toxicity so far. Additional treatment in the form of concurrent chemotherapy is also a significant contributor to acute mucositis.

■ Patient-related factors play an equally important role when it comes to increased risk of mucosal injury. Any genetic changes that cause DNA repair deficiencies can inherently predispose the carrier to radiation sensitivity. There are reports of serious grade 5 toxicity with primarily homozygotes with DNA repair disorders, such as ataxia-telangiectasia (A-T), Nijmegen breakage syndrome (NBS), and Fanconi's anemia (FA) being the most common ones.[12] There is a high suspicion of a larger number of likely heterozygotes of these same disorders which have a higher risk of developing radiation-related toxicity due to their radiosensitivity. There appear to be additional risk factors (e.g., genetic polymorphisms) in some cohorts that account for the degree of clinical expression of mucosal injury. Further study of these more recently defined factors will likely strategically advance the pathobiological model in relation to clinical expression of the toxicity. Among other more common patient-related risk factors, comorbidities (e.g., malnutrition) can contribute important risk. Smoking is another important factor that can lead to both increasing the risk of mucosal toxicity and delaying its healing. In addition, patients who develop clinically significant salivary hypofunction/xerostomia due to head and neck radiation and/or antiemetic drugs may experience increased discomfort from oral mucositis.

Mechanism of Action

■ Mucositis has been known from the very beginning of the use of radiation in the treatment of cancer. However, the biological complexities underlying mucosal barrier injury have only recently been appreciated. Historically, mucositis was viewed solely as an epithelium-mediated event due to radiation toxicity on dividing epithelial stem cells.[13] The epithelial surface of the alimentary tract has a rapid turnover rate, predisposing it to be at a high risk of injury from ionizing radiation. It was previously believed that radiation resulted in direct damage to the basal epithelial cell layer leading to the loss of the reproductive capacity of the epithelium, further resulting in clonogenic cell death, atrophy, and consequent ulceration. However, there have been more recent findings confirming the involvement of submucosal cells and the extracellular matrix, which is not explained by the simpler previous theory of epithelial damage alone. Continued experimental evidence supports the involvement of virtually all of the cells and tissues of the oral mucosa, including the extracellular matrix, in barrier injury. There is evidence of microvascular endothelial and connective tissue damage which seems to precede epithelial changes.[14,15] There is also evidence of decreased incidence of mucosal toxicity with inhibition of platelet aggregation which supports the involvement of endothelial cells and platelets in radiation-induced mucositis.[16] The sequence of cell and tissue changes further implies that nothing occurs within the mucosa as a biologically isolated event. Rather, it appears that interactions among the various mucosal components, including those influenced by the oral environment, collectively lead to mucositis. There is also evidence of increased proinflammatory cytokines with anticancer treatment leading to increased mucosal toxicity in animal and human studies.[15,17] There is evidence of similar pathogenesis for both oral mucositis and esophagitis,[18] with direct damage to dividing cells, apart from decrease in the proliferative capacity of connective tissue cells within the lamina propria, leading to increased vascular permeability and an inflammatory infiltrate and causing tissue ischemia along with fibrosis.

■ From a radiobiology standpoint, the initiating event for radiation-induced mucosal injury is direct DNA damage to basal epithelial cells and cells in the underlying tissue. Radiation causes DNA-strand breaks as well as non–DNA injury initiated through a variety of mechanisms, most commonly with reactive oxygen species (ROS). Several injury-producing pathways involving multiple transcription factors are activated which leads to the upregulation of genes that modulate the damage response. Of the transcription factors that may be significant, nuclear factor-κB (NF-κB) has many of the characteristics that suggest that it may be a key element in the genesis of mucositis. NF-κB is activated by either radiotherapy or chemotherapy, is detectable in stressed mucosa, and can respond differently to varying challenges. Once activated, NF-κB leads to the upregulation of many genes, including those that result in the production of the proinflammatory cytokines tumor necrosis factor-α (TNF-α), interleukin (IL)-1β, and IL-6, with the potential to elicit a broad range of tissue responses, including apoptosis.[10] Agents known to attenuate the expression of both these cytokines have demonstrated efficacy in the prevention of both experimental[15] and clinical[19] mucositis. These signaling molecules also participate in a positive-feedback loop that amplifies the original effects of radiation. There is synchronous direct and indirect damage to epithelial stem cells which result in a loss of renewal capacity. Acute mucositis results from the loss of squamous epithelial cells owing to the sterilization of mucosal stem cells and the inhibition of transit cell proliferation.[20] This leads to a gradual linear decrease in epithelial cell numbers. Normally, oral mucosal cells have a rapid turnover rate of 1 to 2 weeks, which is reduced with radiation therapy, interfering with recovery of mucosal damage.[20] Poor nutritional status further interferes with mucosal regeneration by decreasing cellular migration and renewal. As one advances in the course of radiation, the initial erythema/mucosal congestion transforms into patchy or confluent mucositis when the delicate balance between cell death and cell regeneration is altered, resulting in partial or complete denudation. As the mucositis becomes more severe, pseudomembranes and ulcerations develop.

- There is a higher chance of developing secondary infections with damaged mucosal surfaces, which would otherwise form the primary barrier to protect any penetration by microorganisms. There is loss of "colonization resistance" which is a potent defense mechanism used by homeostatic microbial communities which prevents colonization by exogenous pathogens.[21] When oral tissues are irradiated, the colonization resistance is practically abolished. Irradiation mucositis is caused by a combination of alteration of the normal oral microflora with concomitant changes in the tissues. However, healing eventually occurs when cells regenerate from the surviving mucosal stem cells.

- To summarize, the following are the stages of pathogenesis of mucositis, based on evidence available date[20]:

  - **Initiation of tissue injury:** Radiation and chemotherapy induces cellular damage resulting in the death of the basal epithelial cells. The generation of ROS by radiation or chemotherapy is also believed to exert a role in the initiation of mucosal injury. These small highly reactive molecules are by-products of oxygen metabolism and can cause significant cellular damage. The consistent reports of ROS generation after exposure to stomatotoxic agents[22] and the results of studies that demonstrate successful attenuation of mucosal injury by agents that effectively block or scavenge oxygen-free radicals[23] suggest a significant role for ROS in injury induction.

  - **Upregulation of inflammation via generation of messenger signals:** In addition to causing direct cell death, free radicals activate second messengers that transmit signals from receptors on the cellular surface to the inside of cell. ROS stimulates secondary mediators of injury, including transcription factors such as NF-κB. This leads to upregulation of genes producing proinflammatory cytokines, including the genes for TNF-α, IL-1β, and IL-6, leading to tissue injury and apoptosis of cells within the submucosa and primary injury of cells within the basal epithelium. Other genes also are upregulated, leading to the expression of adhesion molecules, cyclooxygenase-2 (COX-2), and subsequent angiogenesis. ROS and anticancer drugs can also activate enzymes (sphingo-myelinase and ceramide synthase) that catalyze ceramide synthesis, complementing the ceramide pathway which appears to work in parallel, or sequentially, to induce primary apoptosis.[24]

- **Signaling and amplification:** During this phase, one of the consequences of upregulation of proinflammatory cytokines, such as TNF-α, is a series of positive feedback loops that serve to amplify and prolong tissue injury through their effects on transcription factors and on the ceramide and caspase pathways. Consequently, gene upregulation occurs with resultant increases in injurious cytokine production. Because the damaging events are focused in the submucosa and basal epithelium, the clinical appearance of the mucosal surface remains deceptively normal.
- **Ulceration and inflammation:** The ulcerative phase is a result of cell injury and death of the basal epithelial stem cells after the prior phases. This phase is generally markedly symptomatic. The ulcers serve as a nidus for bacterial colonization, and secondary infection is common. The cell wall products from bacteria penetrate the submucosa and further exacerbate the condition by stimulating infiltrating macrophages to produce and release additional proinflammatory cytokines, further amplifying and accelerating local tissue damage.[15,20]
- **Healing:** This phase starts with a signal from the extracellular matrix and is characterized by epithelial proliferation, as well as cellular and tissue differentiation,[15] restoring the integrity of the epithelium, and reestablishment of the local microbial flora. The mucosa regains its normal appearance with, however, significant alterations in the environment. There is residual angiogenesis, which puts patients at increased risk of future episodes of oral mucositis.
- The pathobiology of mucositis shows that it is the culmination of a series of biologically complex and interactive events that occur in all tissues of the mucosa. Although the complete definition of mucositis as a biological process remains a work in progress, the current understanding of cellular and molecular events that lead to mucosal injury has provided a number of potential interventional targets. Consequently, for the first time, directed, biologically rational therapies are now in various stages of development. Furthermore, mechanistically based risk prediction and disease monitoring appear to be realistic goals for the future.

Pharmacological Approaches for Management and Treatment

The clinical management for oral mucositis and esophagitis can be categorized into agents for the therapeutic management of mucositis, pain control, control of infections, and dry mouth.

- **Therapeutic agents for oral mucositis and esophagitis:** This class of medications include medications which may be used to decrease the chance of developing oral mucositis or to shorten the duration of oral mucositis in patients receiving chemotherapy and radiation therapy.
  - **Anti-inflammatory/immunomodulatory agents:**
    - **Benzydamine hydrochloride 0.15%:** Benzydamine hydrochloride is a nonsteroidal anti-inflammatory mouth rinse that is recommended for use to prevent and/or relieve the pain and inflammation associated with oral mucositis in patients who are receiving moderate doses of radiation therapy for head and neck cancer.[25] It inhibits proinflammatory cytokines including TNF-α. In a phase III trial, benzydamine hydrochloride mouth rinse reduced the severity of mucositis in patients with head and neck cancer undergoing radiation therapy of cumulative doses of up to 50 Gy radiation therapy.[19]

Indomethacin: Indomethacin is a nonsteroidal anti-inflammatory drug which inhibits prostaglandin synthesis and is noted to delay the onset of mucositis.

Prednisone: A short course of systemic prednisone (40 to 80 mg daily for up to 1 week) has been helpful in reducing inflammation and discomfort.

- **Cytoprotective agents**
  - **Amifostine:** Amifostine is a cytoprotectant agent that may help to reduce the incidence and severity of chronic or acute xerostomia in patients who are receiving radiation therapy for head and neck cancer. It is a phosphorothioate (a radiation protection agent) and is thought to act as a scavenger for harmful ROS that are known to potentiate mucositis.[26] However, because of insufficient evidence of benefit, various guidelines do not recommend the use of this agent in oral mucositis in chemotherapy or radiation therapy patients. The use of amifostine, however, has been recommended for the prevention of esophagitis in patients receiving chemoradiation for non–small-cell lung cancer.[27]
  - **Sucralfate:** Sucralfate is a cytoprotective agent used for GI ulcerations. It is a basic aluminum salt of sucrose octasulfate and may be useful in reducing symptoms and discomfort and help healing by coating the esophagus. Studies have been negative in the radiation arena for oral mucositis, and a new randomized controlled trial of sucralfate in radiation treatment has confirmed this lack of benefit, showing no difference between micronized sucralfate and salt and soda mouth washes.[28] However, some patients with severe esophagitis may derive symptomatic benefit.

- **Growth factors**
  - **Palifermin**: Palifermin is a recombinant human keratinocyte growth factor-1, which can increase epithelial cell proliferation, and has been used for the management of oral mucositis. Recent evidence shows that intravenous recombinant palifermin significantly reduced incidence of World Health Organization (WHO) grade 3 and 4 oral mucositis in patients with hematological malignancies (e.g., lymphoma and multiple myeloma) receiving high-dose chemotherapy and total body irradiation before autologous hematopoietic stem cell transplantation.[29,30] Palifermin is also known to prevent oral mucositis in patients with head and neck cancer undergoing radiation and chemotherapy, according to two randomized trials.[31–33] There is a theoretical concern that these growth factors may promote growth of tumor cells, which may have receptors for the respective growth factor. However, one recent study found no significant difference in survival between subjects with colorectal cancer receiving palifermin compared with placebo at a median follow-up duration of 14.5 months.[31,34] Further studies are ongoing to confirm the safety of epithelial growth factors in the solid tumor setting, including patients receiving radiation therapy for head and neck cancer.

- **Agents used for pain control:** In general, topical analgesics provide rapid but temporary relief to a localized area. Oral opioids and opioid-containing combinations may be necessary for more moderate or persistent pain. Analgesics should be given at regular intervals for moderate and severe pain.
  - **Topical analgesics/anesthetics:**
    - **Magic mouthwash:** Magic mouthwash is the most commonly prescribed medication for oral mucositis and esophagitis. It is made up of lidocaine, diphenhydramine, and magnesium aluminum hydroxide, in equal amounts. Patients are asked to swish and gargle for 1 minute, and then swallow immediately before each meal. Similar preparations have been made with readily available ingredients for patients who have oral thrush. This is commonly known as the GI Cocktail (1 tbsp. [15 mL] Cherry Maalox [analgesia] + 1 tsp. [5 mL] Nystatin [antifungal] + 1/2 tsp. [2 mL] Hurricane Liquid [analgesia] original flavor).

- **Oxethazaine aluminum/magnesium hydroxide (Mucaine) analgesic/antacid Combination:** This combination is useful for esophagitis and should be taken 10 to 15 minutes before meals and at bedtime.
- **Lidocaine HCl 2%:** Oral lidocaine is usually swished in the mouth and spat out, up to 6 times daily. It may be swallowed slowly if there is also pharyngeal involvement; however, this can impair the swallowing reflex and may increase the risk of aspiration. Given this risk, it should be used carefully.
- **Benzocaine:** Benzocaine is used as an adhesive paste as a topical anesthetic for local application to affected ulcerations.
- **Systemic analgesics:**
  - **Acetaminophen/codeine:** Acetaminophen with codeine is an opioid-containing analgesic in tablet form, prescribed during early mucositis when patients can still swallow medication.
  - **Liquid acetaminophen/codeine:** The aforementioned combination is also available in a liquid formulation that is used for severe mucositis-induced odynophagia.
  - **Morphine:** Morphine is an opioid available in tablet, liquid, or IV formulations.
  - **Hydromorphone HCl:** Hydromorphone is a particularly potent opioid that is available in both enteral and parenteral formulations.
  - **Transdermal fentanyl:** Fentanyl patches are opioid analgesics used for stable and chronic pain as it is available as a skin patch to be replaced every 72 hours. Note that parenteral forms of fentanyl are also available; however, these are very short acting.
  - **Patient-controlled analgesia:** Some patients with very severe mucositis may require systemic opioids administered continuously via patient-controlled analgesia (PCA) pumps.
- **Oral infection management:** Depending on the causative organism, an antifungal, antiviral, or antibacterial can be used and can be administered either topically or systemically. The systemic route is most useful for patients at risk of serious infections (e.g., patients with myelosuppression).
  - **Antifungals:** If symptoms of mucositis start earlier in the course of radiation therapy, get worse suddenly, or persist a long time after treatment completion, a candidal (monilial fungal) infection may be present, which can be effectively treated with multiple antifungal agents.
    - Nystatin oral suspension is one of the most commonly used agents to prevent and treat candidiasis in the mouth and esophagus. The usual instructions entail to swish in mouth for 5 minutes, then spit out or swallow. Patients should avoid eating for at least 30 minutes after use.
    - Fluconazole is a commonly used systemic treatment for fungal infections.
    - Other agents to treat oral candidiasis include ketoconazole, amphotericin, and itraconazole.
  - **Antivirals:**
    - Acyclovir ointment is used as a topical therapy for herpes labialis.
    - Acyclovir, famciclovir, and valacyclovir are used for systemic herpes treatment. Note that short courses of these agents can also be used for herpes labialis.
  - **Antibacterials:** Oral decontamination has historically been shown to reduce infection of the oral cavity by opportunistic pathogens.[35] Furthermore, it can also reduce the risk of systemic sepsis from resident oral and/or opportunistic pathogens. In the past, some commonly used selective oral decontamination agents included chlorhexidine gluconate mouth rinse to suppress oral microflora and prevent dental plaque formation. Later, given some evidence suggesting lack of benefit of chlorhexidine, this agent fell out of favor.[36] Antimicrobial lozenges in patients receiving radiation for cancers of head and neck were then assumed to provide effective mucositis prevention. Addition

of ciprofloxacin or ampicillin with clotrimazole to sucralfate had shown reduction in mucositis.[37] However, a few recent studies of oral lozenges that contained polymyxin, tobramycin, and amphotericin B or bacitracin, clotrimazole, and gentamicin showed no improvement in the incidence or severity of radiation-induced mucositis.[38,39] Despite the often-postulated role of infection in the pathogenesis of mucositis, there is no conclusive evidence for the use of antibiotics in the prevention of radiation-induced mucositis. They might be still useful in cases of severe mucositis and would be recommended if suspicion for bacterial infection is high.

■ **Agents for dry mouth:** In cancer therapy, patients often develop transient or permanent xerostomia and hyposalivation. Hyposalivation can further aggravate inflamed tissues, increase risk for local infection, and make mastication difficult. Many patients also complain of a thickening of salivary secretions, because of a decrease in the serous component of saliva.

　■ Products to moisturize dry mouth include prescription or over-the-counter mouth rinses, artificial saliva, or moisturizers to lubricate the mouth. Mouthwashes designed for dry mouth, especially ones with xylitol, can be effective, such as Biotene Dry Mouth Oral Rinse or Act Dry Mouth Mouthwash, which also offer protection against tooth decay. Saliva substitutes (e.g., Moi-Stir) are available as sprays or swabs to be used as needed. SalivaMAX is an artificial saliva that is used to relieve acute and chronic symptoms of xerostomia and mucositis. It is a supersaturated calcium phosphate powder that, when dissolved in water, creates a solution with a high concentration of electrolytes similar to that of natural saliva.

　■ Cholinergic agents are prescribed as necessary. Commonly prescribed agents include pilocarpine (Salagen) or cevimeline (Evoxac) to stimulate saliva production.

Nonpharmacological Approaches for Management and Treatment

■ Nonpharmacological interventions for oral mucositis and esophagitis include general healing measures, nutritional support, oral hygiene, oral decontamination, and interventions for palliation of dry mouth.

■ Frequent use of a gentle mouthwash may help reduce discomfort or pain. A solution of baking soda and salt dissolved in warm water may be used instead of commercial mouthwashes, which may be irritating to the oral mucosa.

■ **Nutritional support:** All patients should be screened for nutritional risk and early enteral nutrition should be initiated in the event that swallowing difficulties develop. A soft diet or liquid diet is more easily tolerated than a normal diet when oral mucositis is present; gastrostomy tube placement may be beneficial, particularly when there is severe mucositis.

■ **Oral hygiene:** Proper oral care reduces some of the oral toxicity of radiation therapy. Multiple studies have demonstrated that maintenance of good oral hygiene can reduce the risk and severity of oral mucositis. Alcohol-containing mouthwashes should be avoided as these can cause further irritation. The importance of effective oral hygiene should be stressed with recommendations for use of a standardized oral care protocol, including brushing with a soft toothbrush, flossing, and the use of nonmedicated rinses (for example, saline or sodium bicarbonate rinses).[40,41]

■ **Oral decontamination:** Oral decontamination is achieved by maintaining a good oral hygiene. Apart from pharmacological measures, some over-the-counter products like Cepacol Lozenges, Chloraseptic spray and lozenges, or the use of tea for swishing and gargling may help. Oral Balance is a dental gel that moistens the mouth while sores are healing and also has enzymes that help control oral bacteria. Saline mouthwashes are also preferred for their antiseptic properties.

- **Palliation of dry mouth:** Sipping of water or ice chips throughout the day to moisten the mouth, in addition to drinking water during meals to aid chewing and swallowing, are beneficial techniques that should be relayed to patients.
  - Breathing through the nose rather than through the mouth is encouraged. Patients may even need to seek treatment for snoring if it causes them to breathe through their mouth during the night.
  - Chewing sugar-free gum or sucking on sugar-free hard candies may help stimulate salivary flow and improve symptoms of dry mouth.
  - Some over-the-counter saliva substitutes that contain xylitol (such as Mouth Kote or Oasis Moisturizing Mouth Spray), carboxymethylcellulose, or hydroxyethyl cellulose (such as Biotene OralBalance Moisturizing Gel) are recommended. Products that contain xylitol may also help prevent cavities.
  - Simple measures like adding moisture to the air at night with a room humidifier, or moisturizing lips to soothe dry or cracked areas, can be helpful.
  - Avoidance of products that can make xerostomia symptoms worse is also important. These include caffeine, tobacco, and alcohol, which can cause dryness and irritation. Over-the-counter antihistamines and decongestants can worsen dry mouth as well.
- **Newer developments in radiation therapy:** With the use of newer modalities in radiation treatment, there are multiple ways to reduce the incidence of oral mucositis and esophagitis. Various steps can be taken to decrease toxicity in normal tissues, including precise treatment planning and irradiation techniques, selective decreased volume receiving higher doses dictated by estimated cell burden, and maneuvers to exclude sensitive organs (oral mucosa and esophagus) from the irradiated volume. With the emphasis on organ preservation, treatment planning is critical to achieve maximum tumor control probability (TCP) with the least side effects and satisfactory cosmetic results. Some recent changes in the field of radiation oncology, which have led to some reduction in the incidence and severity of oral mucositis and esophagitis, include:
  - The use of **custom-made, intraoral prosthesis** to exclude uninvolved tissues from the treatment portals or to provide shielding of tissues within the treatment area to aide with mucosal sparing.[42]
  - **Computed tomography (CT)-based simulation** and target delineation (Fig. 26.2) for accurate definition of the tumor and subclinical disease has led to better sparing of non-tumor tissue with smaller target margins.
  - **Treatment planning with intensity-modulated radiation therapy (IMRT)** utilizes inverse planning algorithms which allow for the generation of a plan after taking into account the tolerance doses of organs at risk. The usual dose constraint used for oral cavity is a mean dose of 40 Gy or less to 30 Gy or less, depending on the proximity of the target volume to the same.[43] The esophagus dose constraints include a mean dose of 34 Gy or less. With IMRT, the volume receiving 35 Gy is 50% or less, the volume receiving 50 Gy is 40% or less, and the volume receiving 70 Gy is 20% or less.[43] The ultimate goal for planning is to reduce the exposure of the mucosa to the minimum possible, taking special care to avoid having hotspots in the uninvolved mucosa.
  - The use of daily **cone-beam imaging** for treatment verification has led to use of even smaller margins, minimizing exposure to uninvolved mucosa, which potentially leads to less mucositis.
  - **Photobiomodulation by low-level laser therapy (LLLT):** In the last decade, LLLT has been used both to prevent and treat oral mucositis induced by various antineoplastic

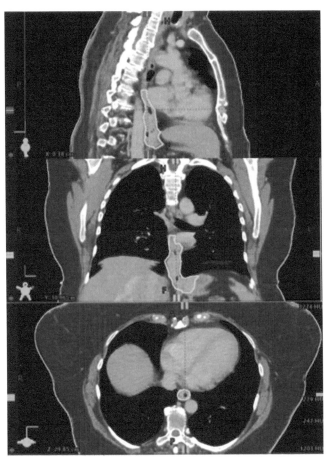

Fig. 26.2 Delineation of the esophagus to allow sparing during dose calculation.

therapies.[44-46] It consists of the specific application of a monochromatic light source of a narrow high-density spectrum with wavelength ranging from visible red to infrared. LLLT changes mitochondrial respiration and leads to increased adenosine triphosphate production, which produces intracellular ROS. These changes result in fibroblast proliferation, collagen synthesis, and adjustment of inflammatory response, as well as enhancement of angiogenesis and tissue repair.[47] It is believed that LLLT acts in a beneficial and noninvasive way, being also able to induce biological effects like analgesia and aid in tissue repair through increased vascularization, cellular motility, and reepithelialization.[48-50] It is currently under further investigation and seems to hold promise for the future.

- **Identification of genetic disorders leading to radiosensitivity:** Common characteristic phenocopies among genetic disorders like A-T, NBS, and FA can help physicians diagnose or suspect potentially radiosensitive individuals before radiotherapy is recommended or initiated. Delineation of predictive models that could enhance the ability of clinicians to identify prospectively which patients are at highest risk for development of clinically significant AM are under investigation.

References

1. Elting L, Cooksley C, Chambers M, Cantor SB, Manzullo E, Rubenstein EB. The burdens of cancer therapy: clinical and economic outcomes of chemotherapy-induced mucositis. *Cancer.* 2003;98(7): 1531–1539.
2. Trotti A, Bellm LA, Epstein JB, et al. Mucositis incidence, severity and associated outcomes in patients with head and neck cancer receiving radiotherapy with or without chemotherapy: a systematic literature review. *Radiother Oncol.* 2003;66(3):253–262.
3. Vera-Llonch M, Oster G, Hagiwara M, Sonis S. Oral mucositis in patients undergoing radiation treatment for head and neck carcinoma. *Cancer.* 2006;106(2):329–336.
4. Hall EJ, Giaccia AJ. *Radiobiology for the Radiologist.* 7th ed. Philadelphia: Lippincott, Williams & Wilkins; 2012.
5. Cox JD, Stetz J, Pajak TF. Toxicity criteria of the Radiation Therapy Oncology Group (RTOG) and the European Organization for Research and Treatment of Cancer (EORTC). *Int J Radiat Oncol Biol Phys.* 1995 Mar 30;31(5):1341-1346. doi: 10.1016/0360-3016(95)00060-C. PMID: 7713792.
6. U.S. Department of Health and Human Services. Common Terminology Criteria for Adverse Events (CTCAE) Version 4.0. 2009. https://evs.nci.nih.gov/ftp1/CTCAE/CTCAE_4.03/Archive/CTCAE_4.0_2009-05-29_QuickReference_8.5x11.pdf.
7. Fu KK, Pajak TF, Trotti A, et al. A Radiation Therapy Oncology Group phase III randomized study to compare hyperfractionation with two variants of accelerated fractionation to standard fractionation radiotherapy for head and neck squamous cell carcinoma: first report of RTOG 9003. *Int J Radiat Oncol Biol Phys.* 2000;48(1):7–16.
8. Johnson CR, Schmidt-Ullrich R, Wazer DE. Concomitant boost technique using accelerated superfractionated radiation therapy for advanced squamous cell carcinoma of the head and neck. *Cancer.* 1992;69(11):2749–2754.
9. Horiot J, Fur RL, N'Guyen T, et al. Hyperfractionated compared with conventional radiotherapy in oropharyngeal carcinoma: an EORTC randomized trial. *Eur J Cancer Clin. Oncol.* 1990;26(7):779–780.
10. Logan RM, Gibson RJ, Sonis ST, Keefe DM. Nuclear factor-kappa B (NF-kappa B) and cyclooxygenase-2 (COX-2) expression in oral mucosa following cancer chemotherapy. *Oral Oncol.* 2007;43(4):395–401.
11. Dobrowsky W, Naudé J, Widder J, et al. Continuous hyperfractionated accelerated radiotherapy with/without mitomycin C in head and neck cancer. *Int J Radiat Oncol Biol Phys.* 1998;42(4):803–806.
12. Pollard JM, Gatti RA. Clinical radiation sensitivity with DNA repair disorders: an overview. *Int J Radiat Oncol Biol Phys.* 2009;74(5):1323–1331.
13. Lockhart PB, Sonis ST. Alterations in the oral mucosa caused by chemotherapeutic agents: a histologic study. *J Dermatol Surg Oncol.* 1981;7(12):1019–1025.
14. Paris F, Fuks Z, Kang A, et al. Endothelial apoptosis as the primary lesion initiating intestinal radiation damage in mice. *Science* 2001;293(5528):293–297.
15. Sonis ST, Peterson R, Edwards L, et al. Defining mechanisms of action of interleukin-11 on the progression of radiation-induced oral mucositis in hamsters. *Oral Oncol.* 2000;36(4):373–381.
16. Wang J, Albertson CM, Zheng H, Fink LM, Herbert JM, Hauer-Jensen M. Short-term inhibition of ADP-induced platelet aggregation by clopidogrel ameliorates radiation-induced toxicity in rat small intestine. *Thromb Haemost.* 2002;87:122–128.
17. Hall PD, Benko H, Hogan KR, Stuart RK. The influence of serum tumor necrosis factor-alpha and interleukin-6 concentrations on nonhematologic toxicity and hematologic recovery in patients with acute myelogenous leukemia. *Exp Hematol.* 1995;23(12):1256–1260.
18. Squier CA, Kremer MJ. Biology of oral mucosa and esophagus. *J Natl Cancer Inst Monogr.* 2001;2001(29):7–15.
19. Epstein JB, Silverman S, Paggiarino DA, et al. Benzydamine HCl for prophylaxis of radiation-induced oral mucositis. *Cancer.* 2001;92(4):875–885.
20. Sonis ST, Elting LS, Keefe D, et al. Perspectives on cancer therapy-induced mucosal injury: pathogenesis, measurement, epidemiology, and consequences for patients. *Cancer.* 2004;100(9):1995–2025.
21. Dörr W, Emmendörfer H, Haide E, Kummermehr J. Proliferation equivalent of accelerated repopulation in mouse oral mucosa. *Int J Radiat Biol.* 1994;66(2):157–167.
22. Gaté L, Paul J, Ba GN, Tew KD, Tapiero H. Oxidative stress induced in pathologies: the role of antioxidants. *Biomed Pharmacother.* 1999;53(4):169–180.

23. Culy CR, Spencer CM. Amifostine: an update on its clinical status as a cytoprotectant in patients with cancer receiving chemotherapy or radiotherapy and its potential therapeutic application in myelodysplastic syndrome. *Drugs.* 2001;61(5):641–648.

24. Maddens S, Charruyer A, Plo I, et al. Kit signaling inhibits the sphingomyelin-ceramide pathway through PLCγ1: implication in stem cell factor radioprotective effect. *Blood.* 2002;100(4):1294–1301.

25. Lalla RV, Sonis ST, Peterson DE. Management of oral mucositis in patients who have cancer. *Dent Clin North Am.* 2008;52(1):61–77.

26. Mantovani G, Macciò A, Madeddu C, et al. Reactive oxygen species, antioxidant mechanisms and serum cytokine levels in cancer patients: impact of an antioxidant treatment. *J Environ Pathol Toxicol Oncol.* 2003;22(1):17–28.

27. Bensadoun RJ, Schubert MM, Lalla RV, Keefe D. Amifostine in the management of radiation-induced and chemo-induced mucositis. *Suppor Care Cancer.* 2006;14(6):566–572.

28. Dodd MJ, Miaskowski C, Greenspan D, et al. Radiation-induced mucositis: a randomized clinical trial of micronized sucralfate versus salt and soda mouthwashes. *Cancer Invest.* 2003;21(1):21–33.

29. Niscola P, Scaramucci L, Giovannini M, et al. Palifermin in the management of mucositis in hematological malignancies: current evidences and future perspectives. *Cardiovasc Hematol Agents Med Chem.* 2009;7(4):305–312.

30. Spielberger R, Stiff P, Bensinger W, et al. Palifermin for oral mucositis after intensive therapy for hematologic cancers. *N Engl J Med.* 2004;351(25):2590–2598.

31. Brizel DM, Murphy BA, Rosenthal DI, et al. Phase II study of palifermin and concurrent chemoradiation in head and neck squamous cell carcinoma. *J Clin Oncol.* 2008;26(15):2489–2496.

32. Le Q-T, Kim H, Schneider CJ, et al. Palifermin reduces severe mucositis in definitive chemoradiotherapy of locally advanced head and neck cancer: a randomized, placebo-controlled study. *J Clin Oncol.* 2011;29(20):2808–2814.

33. Henke M, Alfonsi M, Foa P, et al. Palifermin decreases severe oral mucositis of patients undergoing postoperative radiochemotherapy for head and neck cancer: a randomized, placebo-controlled trial. *J Clin Oncol.* 2011;29(20):2815–2820.

34. Rosen LS, Abdi E, Davis ID, et al. Palifermin reduces the incidence of oral mucositis in patients with metastatic colorectal cancer treated with fluorouracil-based chemotherapy. *J Clin Oncol.* 2006;24(33):5194–5200.

35. Spijkervet FK, Van Saene HK, Van Saene JJ, et al. Effect of selective elimination of the oral flora on mucositis in irradiated head and neck cancer patients. *J Surg Oncol.* 1991;46(3):167–173.

36. Foote RL, Loprinzi CL, Frank AR, et al. Randomized trial of a chlorhexidine mouthwash for alleviation of radiation-induced mucositis. *J Clin Oncol.* 1994;12(12):2630–2633.

37. Matthews RH, Ercal N. Prevention of mucositis in irradiated head and neck cancer patients. *J Exp Ther Oncol.* 1996;1(2):135–138.

38. Stokman MA, Spijkervet FK, Burlage FR, et al. Oral mucositis and selective elimination of oral flora in head and neck cancer patients receiving radiotherapy: a double-blind randomised clinical trial. *Br J Cancer.* 2003;88(7):1012–1016.

39. El-Sayed S, Nabid A, Shelley W, et al. Prophylaxis of radiation-associated mucositis in conventionally treated patients with head and neck cancer: a double-blind, phase III, randomized, controlled trial evaluating the clinical efficacy of an antimicrobial lozenge using a validated mucositis scoring system. *J Clin Oncol.* 2002;20(19):3956–3963.

40. Yoneda S, Imai S, Hanada N, et al. Effects of oral care on the development of oral mucositis and microorganisms in patients with esophageal cancer. *Jpn J Infect Dis.* 2007;60(1):23–28.

41. McGuire DB, Correa ME, Johnson J, Wienandts P. The role of basic oral care and good clinical practice principles in the management of oral mucositis. *Support Care Cancer.* 2006;14(6):541–547.

42. Kaanders JH, Fleming TJ, Ang KK, Maor MH, Peters LJ. Devices valuable in head and neck radiotherapy. *Int J Radiat Oncol Biol Phys.* 1992;23(3):639–645.

43. Marks LB, Ten Haken RK, Martel MK. Guest editors introduction to QUANTEC: a user's guide. *Int J Radiat Oncol Biol Phys.* 2010;76(3 suppl):S1–S2.

44. Lino MD, Carvalho FB, Oliveira LR, et al. Laser phototherapy as a treatment for radiotherapy-induced oral mucositis. *Braz Dent J.* 2011;22(2):162–165.

45. Antunes HS, Herchenhorn D, Small IA, et al. Phase III trial of low-level laser therapy to prevent oral mucositis in head and neck cancer patients treated with concurrent chemoradiation. *Radiother Oncol.* 2013;109(2):297–302.

46. Sonis ST, Hashemi S, Epstein JB, Nair RG, Raber-Durlacher JE. Could the biological robustness of low level laser therapy (Photobiomodulation) impact its use in the management of mucositis in head and neck cancer patients. *Oral Oncol.* 2016;54:7–14.
47. Moshkovska T, Mayberry J. It is time to test low level laser therapy in Great Britain. *Postgrad Med J.* 2005;81(957):436–441.
48. Lisboa de Castro JF, Gomes Henriques ÁC, Cazal Lira C, de Andrade Santos RN, Anderson de Barros Matos J, Carneiro do Nascimento S. Effect of laser therapy on laryngeal carcinoma cell proliferation (H.Ep-2). *Braz Res Pediatr Dent Integr Clin.* 2014;14(4):275–282.
49. Amadori F, Bardellini E, Conti G, Pedrini N, Schumacher RF, Majorana A. Low-level laser therapy for treatment of chemotherapy-induced oral mucositis in childhood: a randomized double-blind controlled study. *Lasers Med Sci.* 2016;31(6):1231–1236.
50. Melo Jr WA, da Silva Jr EF, Calista AA, et al. Laser therapy in prevention and treatment of oral mucositis in pediatric oncology. *J Nurs UFPE.* 2016;10(10):2404–2411.50 7.

CHAPTER 27

Dermatologic Toxicities of Radiation Therapy

Nitika Thawani, MD ▨ Subhakar Mutyala, MD

Introduction

- Radiation dermatitis is one of the earliest known side effects of radiation. Almost all patients receiving radiation therapy have some changes in the skin. Acute and/or chronic skin changes may occur, which may have implications for quality of life during and after completion of radiation. These dermatological reactions may lead to delay in treatment or diminished cosmesis and functional deficits.
- Radiation is used as adjuvant therapy after surgery in many situations such as after breast conserving therapy or mastectomy to reduce the risk of local recurrence for breast cancer, or as definitive treatment for early stage medically inoperable lung cancer concurrent with chemotherapy for locally advanced lung cancer, as well as with or without chemotherapy in the treatment of sarcomas, thymomas, and lymphomas. Radiation is also used as external beam radiation therapy or brachytherapy for the treatment of skin cancers. These broad indications increase the sheer numbers of potential patients, many of whom will develop some form of radiation dermatitis.
- Radiation effects to the skin are usually unavoidable, as the radiation must enter, exit, or be deposited near the skin to reach the target volume. Skin cells, because they originate from a rapidly reproducing differentiated stem cell, are relatively radiosensitive. The side effects can sometimes lead to interruption of therapy and be dose-limiting for tumor control and thus prevention and treatment strategies become extremely important.
- In this chapter, we will discuss the clinical manifestations, mechanism of action, treatment, and prevention of radiation dermatitis.

Description

The earliest reports of radiation-induced skin changes date back to 1896, nine months after Roentgen's discovery, when Clarence E. Dally, a colleague of Thomas Edison participating in fluorescent lamp construction, developed epilation, skin ulceration of the hands and arms, carcinoma, and ultimately died in 1904 due to metastasis.[1] This phenomenon of radiation dermatitis may be produced by both diagnostic and therapeutic radiation equipment.

TIMING

Radiation dermatitis typically occurs within 90 days of starting treatment. The specific skin changes depend upon the radiation dose and include erythema, edema, pigment changes, hair loss, and dry or moist desquamation. Late stage or chronic radiation dermatitis typically presents months to years after radiation exposure. It is characterized by dermal fibrosis and poikilodermatous changes, including hyper- and hypopigmentation, atrophy, and telangiectasias.[2]

CLINICAL PRESENTATION

In order to be defined as radiation dermatitis, the skin reaction must occur within or at the margin of the radiotherapy field. Features of dermatitis are dose dependent. Early changes noted in the skin are: erythema at doses of 2 Gy or higher, dry desquamation at doses of 12–20 Gy, moist desquamation at greater than 20 Gy, and necrosis at 35 Gy or higher.[3] All patients do not experience all acute skin reactions; however, there may be a combination of reactions occurring simultaneously in the radiation field.

Late radiation changes are progressive and may begin to appear 10 weeks after the radiation. Reactions may progress slowly and subclinically, beginning months to years following treatment. Changes may include photosensitivity, hyper- or hypopigmentation, atrophy, fibrosis, telangiectasia, ulceration, and necrosis.

GRADING AND SEVERITY

The grading and severity of radiation dermatitis is reflected in Table 27.1.

DIAGNOSTIC EVALUATION

The diagnosis of acute radiation dermatitis is clinical, based upon the findings of the skin changes.[4–6]
1. **Mild dermatitis** (Common Terminology Criteria for Adverse Events [CTCAE] grade 1) is characterized by mild blanchable erythema or dry desquamation. The onset is typically within days to weeks of initiating therapy and symptoms generally dissipate within a month. Pruritus and hair loss are commonly associated symptoms.
2. **Moderate dermatitis** (CTCAE grade 2) is characterized by painful erythema and edema that may progress to focal loss of epidermis and moist desquamation, usually limited to skin folds. Moist desquamation is characterized by epidermal necrosis, fibrinous exudates, and often considerable pain. Bullae, if present, may rupture or become infected. This reaction usually peaks 1–2 weeks after the end of treatment.
3. **Severe dermatitis** (CTCAE grades 3 and 4) is characterized by confluent moist lesions which can become secondarily infected. Pain is usually severe.

Chronic radiation dermatitis is characterized by sustained loss of certain skin structures such as sebaceous glands, hair follicles, and nails; as well as textural changes to the skin.[4,7] Atrophy of the epidermis and dermis may be observed, although some patients may develop induration and thickening of the dermis. Telangiectasia may occur as a result of blood vessel dilatation, while damage to blood vessels may also result in tissue hypoxia, predisposing the patient to development of skin ulceration and/or chronic wounds. Radiation induced fibrosis is a potentially serious consequence of radiation that may cause poor cosmesis, lymphedema, skin retraction, persistent hyperpigmentation, and joint immobility.[7–9]

Pathogenesis

The pathogenesis of radiation dermatitis is complex but is often characterized by the following findings[10–12]:
- Erythema: increased blood supply via the dermal vascular plexus
- Dry desquamation: inability of basal cells to replicate quickly enough to replenish the damaged squamous epithelium
- Moist desquamation: focal loss of epidermis with a serous drainage and exudate
- Alopecia: loss of hair follicles
- Telangiectasias: dilated superficial blood vessels
- Fibrosis and contraction: tightening of skin secondary to injury to fibroblasts
- Radiation necrosis: dermal ischemia and impairment of the reparative process

TABLE 27.1 ■ CTCAE V4.0 Skin Toxicity Grading Criteria

	Grade 1	Grade 2	Grade 3	Grade 4	Grade 5
Skin and subcutaneous tissue disorders – Other, specify	Asymptomatic or mild symptoms; clinical or diagnostic observations only; intervention not indicated	Moderate; minimal, local, or noninvasive intervention indicated; limiting age-appropriate instrumental ADL	Severe or medically significant but not immediately life-threatening; hospitalization or prolongation of existing hospitalization indicated; disabling; limiting self-care ADL	Life-threatening consequences; urgent intervention indicated	Death
Skin atrophy		Covering <10% BSA; associated with telangiectasias or changes in skin color	Covering 10%–30% BSA; associated with striae or adnexal structure loss	Covering >30% BSA; associated with ulceration	
Skin hyperpig-mentation		Hyperpigmentation covering <10% BSA; no psychosocial impact	Hyperpigmentation covering >10% BSA; associated psychosocial impact	-	
Skin hypopig-mentation		Hypopigmentation or depigmentation covering <10% BSA; no psychosocial impact	Hypopigmentation or depigmentation covering >10% BSA; associated psychosocial impact		
Skin infection		Localized, local intervention indicated	Oral intervention indicated (e.g., antibiotic, antifungal, antiviral)	IV antibiotic, antifungal, or antiviral intervention indicated; radiological or operative intervention indicated	Death
Skin ulceration		Combined area of ulcers <1 cm; nonblanchable erythema of intact skin with associated warmth or edema	Combined area of ulcers 1–2 cm; partial thickness skin loss involving skin or subcutaneous fat	Combined area of ulcers >2 cm; full-thickness skin loss involving damage to or necrosis of subcutaneous tissue that may extend down to fascia	Death
Dry skin		Covering <10% BSA and no associated erythema or pruritus	Covering 10%–30% BSA and associated with erythema or pruritus; limiting instrumental ADL	Covering >30% BSA and associated with pruritus; limiting self-care ADL	-

ADL, Activities of daily living; *BSA,* body surface area; *CTCAE,* Common Terminology Criteria for Adverse Events; *IV,* intravenous.

Radiation dermatitis is the overall result of injury to multiple skin structures including epidermal keratinocytes, dermal fibroblasts, cutaneous vasculature, and hair follicles. It interferes with maturation, reproduction, and the repopulation of these cells and is the result of direct tissue injury, as well as inflammation recruited to the injured skin. DNA damage is mediated by the production of free radicals. Leukocytes and other immune cells migrate from the circulation to the skin. Increased release of cytokines and chemokines has been associated with acute radiation dermatitis. Production of reactive oxygen species cause further damage to the skin. This process triggers vasodilatation, increased vascular permeability, and recruitment of inflammatory cells. The immune cells secrete proinflammatory cytokines such as transforming growth factor beta which cause fibroblast differentiation into myofibroblasts, and subsequently produce collagenous and smooth muscle actin, resulting in much of the observed findings in fibrosis.[13]

Factors Influencing the Onset, Duration, and Intensity of the Radiation Dermatitis

- **Patient-related factors**
  - Skin folds provide a warm, moist environment compounded by friction with movement, all of which contribute to an increased risk for skin breakdown. Fig. 27.1 depicts radiation toxicity within a skin fold. These lesions can frequently become desquamative as shown in Fig. 27.2.

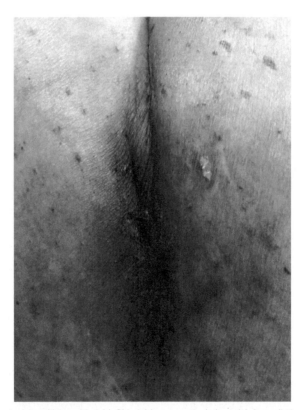

Fig. 27.1   Radiation toxicity within a skin fold. Skin folds are particularly at risk for radiation toxicity.

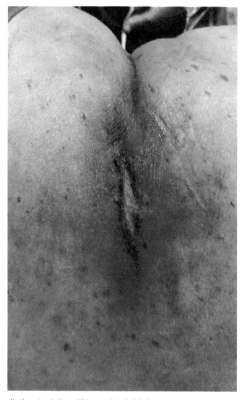

Fig. 27.2   Desquamative radiation toxicity within a skin fold due to increased friction and excessive moisture.

- Some types of skin tolerate radiation better than others. The skin of the scalp has the greatest tolerance, followed in decreasing order by the face, neck, trunk, ears, groin, and extremities.
- Age, skin integrity at the initiation of treatment, nutritional status, and comorbidities such as vascular disease may influence the risk of dermatitis.
- Some autoimmune diseases, such as scleroderma, are associated with a heightened response to radiation.
- Individuals with ataxia telangiectasia (AT) and hereditary nevoid basal cell carcinoma syndrome (Gorlin syndrome) are at increased risk for radiation dermatitis.
- **Treatment-related factors:**
  - Beam type influences the risk of dermatitis. Electrons are associated with increased risk of skin reactions, whereas photons are generally deposited below the skin, resulting in fewer acute skin reactions.
  - Use of tissue equivalent materials may cause bolus dosing in close proximity to the skin, which will increase the severity of skin reactions.
  - Previous radiation therapy to the same field or concurrent chemotherapy increases the risk of skin reactions.
  - External beam radiation is associated with less skin toxicity as opposed to surface brachytherapy.
  - The cumulative dose to the skin impacts the risk of dermatitis dramatically.
- **Consequential late effects:** In intensive fractionation protocols, stem cell populations are depleted below the levels needed for tissue restoration. Therefore an early reaction in a

rapidly proliferating tissue may result in a chronic injury. This is called a consequential late effect.[14] Examples include fibrosis or necrosis of skin after desquamation and acute ulceration. A relation between acute moist dermatitis and late telangiectasias as a result of consequential reaction is reported for the skin.

■ **Radiation recall reaction:** This is a poorly understood, uncommon, and unpredictable phenomenon that is characterized by an acute inflammatory reaction confined to previously radiated areas and triggered by the administration of a precipitating systemic agent (example alkylating agents include docetaxel, dacarbazine, etoposide, 5-fluorouracil, trastuzumab, nivolumab, and others)[15–19] after radiation treatment. The precise mechanism is unknown, although various hypotheses have been proposed. The mechanism appears to be related to a priming effect created by cytotoxic therapy, which then suffers a second insult from radiation and results in a secondary process of cellular damage causing radiation recall dermatitis.

Pharmacological Approaches for Management and Treatment

The key in managing skin reactions is to prevent the development of severe grade 3 to 4 dermatitis. Different modalities have been recommended, depending upon the severity of the dermatitis. It is of utmost importance to maintain skin hydration, as this improves epithelialization and hence moisturizers, barrier creams, aloe vera, lanolin, and steroid creams are used extensively.[20,21]

■ **Aloe vera:** A systematic review of the literature emphasized that there is no evidence from clinical trials to suggest that topical aloe vera is effective in preventing or minimizing radiation-induced skin reactions.[22] However, prophylactic use appears to be effective in delaying radiation dermatitis, especially in the head and neck cancer population.[23]

■ **Steroids:** Steroid ointments have been tried owing to their antiinflammatory properties. Studies have shown topical steroid application may reduce symptoms of burning, itchiness, and clinical erythema and may delay the progression of skin reactions. A randomized controlled trial reported no benefit in terms of severity of dermatitis with the use of 1% methylprednisolone cream.[11] However, it has been useful in ameliorating dermatitis-related symptoms in patients.

■ **Other topical agents:** Many other topical agents have been investigated, but data are limited or conflicting with respect to efficacy compared to best supportive care, and thus use is recommended based on anecdotal evidence.

■ **Treatment of desquamation**
   ▪ When radiation dermatitis becomes more significant, particularly if dry and moist desquamation develops, additional strategies of wound care may be beneficial.[24] Key measures include keeping the site clean and moist, protecting the area from contamination and infection, and addressing pain management. A moist environment encourages migration of keratinocytes in the wound bed to help promote healing. Saline soaks to the area of skin sensitivity can be cleansing and comforting. Application of dressings may also serve to reduce further contact or mechanical injury to the wound site, while promoting healing. Some of the most frequently used dressings include hydrocolloid or hydrogel dressings, soft silicone dressings, and silver-based dressings or ointments. The data are mixed regarding the absolute benefit and time to complete wound healing with use of various products. But in general, these agents help to provide barrier protection and have a soothing and cooling effect that mediates discomfort.

■ **Treatment of late skin reactions**
   ▪ Polyurethane dressings appear to be effective in all stages of skin toxicity, from prevention to management of late toxicities.[25]

BOX 27.1 ■ **Recommendations for Supportive Care During and After Treatment With Radiation**

During treatment

■ Using lukewarm water, gently wash the area using fingertips. Rinse well and pat dry with a soft cloth.
■ Avoid harsh soap. Use neutral soaps.
■ Do not apply any ointment cream or lotion, deodorant, perfume, cologne, powder, cosmetics, or home remedy to the skin unless specifically instructed to do so. Kitchen cornstarch may be used in place of deodorant to decrease itching.
■ Apply water-soluble lubricant to reduce itching and discomfort 2–3 times per day. Avoid applying right before radiation treatment.
■ Avoid shaving if possible. Use an electric shaver if shaving is necessary.
■ Avoid extreme temperatures to the skin in the treatment area.
■ Avoid tight-fitting clothing made of irritating fabric. Clothes made of cotton or cotton blends are preferred.
■ Avoid exposing skin to sun. Always apply sunscreen with SPF 15 or higher.
■ Drink 8–10 glasses of water every day.
■ Do not apply taper adhesive bandage to the skin in the radiation field.

After treatment

■ Continue to follow the above guidelines for 1 month after the completion of treatment.
■ Continue using an unscented hydrophilic emollient 2–3 times daily.
■ Massage with vitamin E oil >3 years.
■ Always avoid exposing previously radiated skin to sun. If unavoidable, use sunscreen with SPF 15 or greater.

■ Several small randomized trials have suggested that prolonged treatment with pentoxifylline in combination with vitamin E for up to 3 years may be helpful for the treatment of subcutaneous radiation-induced fibrosis. However, the optimal dose and duration of therapy has not been determined.[26,27] It is also unclear whether this therapy should be continued indefinitely to maintain benefit.

■ Grade 4 radiation dermatitis is fortunately rare. Patients presenting with full-thickness skin necrosis and ulceration should be treated on a case-by-case basis. They may require discontinuation of radiation therapy and a multidisciplinary approach, involving wound care, radiation oncology, and dermatology. Treatment may include surgical debridement, full-thickness skin grafts, or myocutaneous or pedicle flaps. Other treatments that have been investigated include laser or light therapy, hyperbaric oxygen, and use of other selected pharmacological agents, but strong evidence of efficacy to advocate for any of these specifically is lacking.

■ **Supportive care approaches:** Various supportive care strategies for use during and after radiation treatment are outlined in Box 27.1.

Nonpharmacological Approaches for Management and Treatment

Several techniques that have been utilized in radiation treatment planning have shown to reduce permanent skin toxicity. Contouring the skin as a 3- to 5-mm rind on the external body surface and limiting the dose to this region of the skin, especially in patients who undergo repeat treatment with radiation, reduces the incidence of skin toxicity. Utilization of multiple beams as well as beam modulation, as in intensity-modulated radiation therapy (IMRT), spreads the integral skin dose and thus reduces the incidence of skin toxicity. Accounting for the attenuation of doses

---

BOX 27.2 ■ Dose Constraints for Skin During Planning

Stereotactic Body Radiation Therapy (SBRT)

1 Fraction – 0.035 cc <26 Gy, 23 Gy <10 cc
3 Fractions – 0.035 cc <33 Gy, 30 Gy <10 cc
4 Fractions – 0.035 cc <36 Gy, 33.2 Gy <10 cc
5 Fractions – 0.035 cc <36.2 Gy, 33.2 Gy <10 cc
8 Fractions – 0.035 cc <45.6 Gy, 43.2 Gy <10 cc
External Beam Radiation Therapy
Max dose <100 Gy BED 2

BED, Biologically effective dose.

---

through the immobilization devices and including them in dose calculation allows for assessment of actual skin dose and reduces the incidence of dose buildup on the skin. Scanning patients with tissue equivalent bolus allows more real-life dose calculation and avoidance of hotspots on the skin which can also be helpful. Dose constraints for skin should be taken into account when planning radiation treatments, as these can also help mitigate radiation dermatitis. (Box 27.2).

References

1. Sansare K, Khanna V, Karjodkar F. Early victims of X-rays: a tribute and current perception. *Dentomaxillofac Radiol*. 2011;40(2):123–125.
2. Brown KR, Rzucidlo E. Acute and chronic radiation injury. *J Vasc Surg*. 2011;53(1 suppl):15S–21S.
3. Jaschke W, Schmuth M, Trianni A, Bartal G. Radiation-induced skin injuries to patients: what the interventional radiologist needs to know. *Cardiovasc Intervent Radiol*. 2017;40(8):1131–1140.
4. Hymes SR, Strom EA, Fife C. Radiation dermatitis: clinical presentation, pathophysiology, and treatment 2006. *J Am Acad Dermatol*. 2006;54(1):28–46.
5. McQuestion M. Evidence-based skin care management in radiation therapy: clinical update. *Semin Oncol Nurs*. 2011;27(2):e1–17.
6. Salvo N, Barnes E, van Draanen J, et al. Prophylaxis and management of acute radiation-induced skin reactions: a systematic review of the literature. *Curr Oncol*. 2010;17(4):94–112.
7. Spalek M. Chronic radiation-induced dermatitis: challenges and solutions. *Clin Cosmet Investig Dermatol*. 2016;9:473–482.
8. Dyer BA, Hodges MG, Mayadev JS. Radiation-induced morphea: an under-recognized complication of breast irradiation. *Clin Breast Cancer*. 2016;16(4):e141–e143.
9. Laetsch B, Hofer T, Lombriser N, Lautenschlager S. Irradiation-induced morphea: x-rays as triggers of autoimmunity. *Dermatology*. 2011;223(1):9–12.
10. Simonen P, Hamilton C, Ferguson S, et al. Do inflammatory processes contribute to radiation induced erythema observed in the skin of humans?. *Radiother Oncol*. 1998;46(1):73–82.
11. Schmuth M, Sztankay A, Weinlich G, et al. Permeability barrier function of skin exposed to ionizing radiation. *Arch Dermatol*. 2001;137(8):1019–1023.
12. Rupprecht R, Lippold A, Auras C, et al. Late side-effects with cosmetic relevance following soft X-ray therapy of cutaneous neoplasias. *J Eur Acad Dermatol Venereol*. 2007;21(2):178–185.
13. Muller K, Meineke V. Radiation-induced alterations in cytokine production by skin cells. *Exp Hematol*. 2007;35(4 suppl 1):96–104.
14. Bentzen SM, Overgaard M. Relationship between early and late normal-tissue injury after postmastectomy radiotherapy. *Radiother Oncol*. 1991;20(3):159–165.
15. Sakaguchi M, Maebayashi T, Aizawa T, Ishibashi N. Docetaxel-induced radiation recall dermatitis with atypical features: a case report. *Medicine (Baltimore)*. 2018;97(36):e12209.
16. Rouyer L, Bursztejn AC, Charbit L, Schmutz JL, Moawad S. Stevens-Johnson syndrome associated with radiation recall dermatitis in a patient treated with nivolumab. *Eur J Dermatol*. 2018;28(3):380–381.

17. Mehta K, Kaubisch A, Tang J, Pirlamarla A, Kalnicki S. Radiation recall dermatitis in patients treated with sorafenib. *Case Rep Oncol Med*. 2018;2018:2171062.
18. Barco I, Fraile M, Vidal M, et al. Tamoxifen induced radiation recall dermatitis in a breast cancer patient. *Breast J*. 2018;24(4):662–663.
19. Kumar V, Meghal T, Wu E, Huang Y. Radiation recall dermatitis consecutive to cabozantinib use. *Am J Ther*. 2019;26(4):e559–e561.
20. Bernier J, Russi EG, Homey B, et al. Management of radiation dermatitis in patients receiving cetuximab and radiotherapy for locally advanced squamous cell carcinoma of the head and neck: proposals for a revised grading system and consensus management guidelines. *Ann Oncol*. 2011;22(10):2191–2200.
21. Bernier J, Bonner J, Vermorken JB, et al. Consensus guidelines for the management of radiation dermatitis and coexisting acne-like rash in patients receiving radiotherapy plus EGFR inhibitors for the treatment of squamous cell carcinoma of the head and neck. *Ann Oncol*. 2008;19(1):142–149.
22. Richardson J, Smith JE, McIntyre M, Thomas R, Pilkington K. Aloe vera for preventing radiation-induced skin reactions: a systematic literature review. *Clin Oncol (R Coll Radiol)*. 2005;17(6):478–484.
23. Rao S, Hegde SK, Baliga-Rao MP, Palatty PL, George T, Baliga MS. An aloe vera-based cosmeceutical cream delays and mitigates ionizing radiation-induced dermatitis in head and neck cancer patients undergoing curative radiotherapy: a clinical study. *Medicines (Basel)*. 2017;4(3).
24. Patel AN, Varma S, Batchelor JM, Lawton PA. Why aqueous cream should not be used in radiotherapy-induced skin reactions. *Clin Oncol (R Coll Radiol)*. 2013;25(4):272.
25. Fernandez-Castro M, Martin-Gil B. [Effectiveness of topical therapies in patients with breast cancer that experience radiodermatitis. a systematic review]. *Enferm Clin*. 2015;25(6):327–343.
26. Kaidar-Person O, Marks LB, Jones EL. Pentoxifylline and vitamin E for treatment or prevention of radiation-induced fibrosis in patients with breast cancer. *Breast J*. 2018;24(5):816–819.
27. Magnusson M, Höglund P, Johansson K, et al. Pentoxifylline and vitamin E treatment for prevention of radiation-induced side-effects in women with breast cancer: a phase two, double-blind, placebo-controlled randomised clinical trial (Ptx-5). *Eur J Cancer*. 2009;45(14):2488–2495.

CHAPTER 28

Pulmonary Toxicities of Radiation Therapy

Nitika Thawani, MD ▪ Tanmay S. Panchabhai, MD

Introduction

- Radiation is an integral component of many patients' treatment regimens. The goal of radiation therapy is to deliver a dose to the target while sparing the normal tissue so that the treatment can be well tolerated. Treatment toxicity is caused by dose to the normal organs that receive radiation as bystanders. All lung and mediastinal tumors have an adjacent boundary with the normal lung and thus pulmonary toxicity is fairly common. The lung is one of the most sensitive organs to ionizing radiation and thus pulmonary toxicity from radiation is seen in 5% to 50% of patients receiving radiation for lung cancer.

- Radiation is used as a single modality treatment for early-stage medically inoperable lung cancer in the form of stereotactic body ablative radiotherapy (SBRT) mainly because these patients are unable to tolerate surgery secondary to poor pulmonary lung function and low pulmonary reserve. SBRT has recently become increasingly utilized due to excellent local control rates, improved survival, and its noninvasive nature. It is used in conjunction with chemotherapy for locally advanced lung cancer, especially when nodal metastasis is present. Concurrent chemotherapy and radiation have shown improved survival for both non–small-cell lung cancer (NSCLC) as well as small-cell lung cancer (SCLC), thus supporting its use; however, it comes at the price of increased rates of toxicities with concurrent treatment compared to sequential chemotherapy and radiation. Radiation has also been utilized for palliation of symptoms from lung tumors in the advanced disease setting for airway obstruction, dysphagia, hemoptysis, and superior vena cava syndrome. Both brachytherapy and external beam radiation have been utilized for palliation of symptoms.

- Even with conformal techniques, such as three-dimensional (3-D) conformal radiation and the more modern intensity modulated radiation therapy (IMRT), planned with accurate assessment of target and organ at risk (OAR) motion with four-dimensional (4-D) computed tomography (CT) scans and delivered with image-guided radiation therapy (IGRT) and gating techniques, pulmonary toxicity still continues to be the main dose-limiting toxicity for thoracic radiation therapy both for primary cancers like NSCLC and SCLC as well as sarcomas, lymphomas, and other mediastinal tumors such as thymomas.

- With the popularization of SBRT for primary as well as secondary malignancies of the lung and varying fractionation and dose schedules being utilized, the understanding of radiation-induced lung diseases is a focus of research. Side effects that are usually not noted with conventional fractionation are now being noted with SBRT. Some notable examples are bronchial necrosis and fistula formation.

- This chapter focuses on radiation-induced pneumonitis and the changing patterns of toxicity with advanced radiation modalities like SBRT, IMRT, and brachytherapy. The mechanisms of action, various factors affecting the development of pneumonitis, and strategies for reducing the incidence of pneumonitis, and the pharmacological and nonpharmacological interventions to treat pneumonitis are discussed in this chapter.

Characteristics of Radiation-induced Lung Injury

Radiation-induced lung injury was first described in 1898. It was then subdivided in 1925 into radiation pneumonitis and radiation fibrosis. Both types of lung injury are observed in patients who have undergone thoracic radiation treatment for lung, breast, or hematological malignancies. Radiation-induced damage to lung parenchyma remains a dose-limiting factor in chest radiotherapy.

- **Timing:** Symptoms caused by acute radiation pneumonitis usually develop approximately 4 to 12 weeks following radiation; various symptoms of fibrotic radiation pneumonitis usually develop after 6 to 12 months.
- **Clinical presentation:** The signs and symptoms of the two phases of radiation pneumonitis (acute and fibrotic) are similar, although fever is less likely to occur in the fibrotic phase. The following signs and symptoms have been described:

Symptoms

- A nonproductive cough which may occur during therapy as a manifestation of bronchial mucosal injury or later as a manifestation of fibrosis.
- Dyspnea may occur only with exertion or may be described as an inability to take a deep breath.
- Fever is usually low grade but can be more pronounced in severe cases.
- Chest pain may be pleuritic or substernal and can mimic cardiac chest pain.
- Malaise and weight loss may be observed.
- Physical signs include the following:
  - A pleural rub may be heard.
  - Dullness to percussion may be detected as a result of a pleural effusion that is seen in about 10% of patients.
- **Grading and severity:** Tables 28.1 and 28.2 describe the grading and severity of radiation pneumonitis.
- **Diagnostic evaluation:** Radiation pneumonitis is usually a diagnosis of exclusion. It should be suspected when a patient who has undergone thoracic radiation develops symptoms or signs such as shortness of breath, cough, fever, or malaise in weeks to months after radiation therapy. Appropriate evaluation is designed to assess the severity of respiratory impairment,

TABLE 28.1 ■ **Commonly Utilized Acute Pneumonitis Grading Criteria**

Scale	Grade 1	Grade 2	Grade 3	Grade 4	Grade 5
RTOG	Mild symptoms of dry cough or dyspnea on exertion	Persistent cough requiring narcotic, antitussive agents/ dyspnea with minimal effort but not at rest	Severe cough unresponsive to narcotic antitussive agent or dyspnea at rest/clinical or radiological evidence of acute pneumonitis/ intermittent oxygen or steroids may be required	Severe respiratory insufficiency/ continuous oxygen or assisted ventilation	Death
CTCAE	Asymptomatic; clinical or diagnostic observations only; intervention not indicated	Symptomatic; medical intervention indicated; limiting instrumental ADL	Severe symptoms; limiting self-care ADL; oxygen indicated	Life-threatening respiratory compromise; urgent intervention indicated (e.g., tracheotomy or intubation)	Death

ADL, Activities of daily living; *CTCAE,* Common Terminology Criteria for Adverse Events; *ROTG,* Radiation Therapy Oncology Group.

TABLE 28.2 ■ Commonly Utilized Chronic Pulmonary Fibrosis Grading Criteria

Scale	Grade 1	Grade 2	Grade 3	Grade 4	Grade 5
RTOG	Asymptomatic or mild symptoms (dry cough); slight radiographic appearances	Moderate symptomatic fibrosis or pneumonitis (severe cough); low-grade fever; patchy radiographic appearances	Severe symptomatic fibrosis or pneumonitis; dense radiographic changes	Severe respiratory insufficiency/continuous oxygen/assisted ventilation	Death
CTCAE	Mild hypoxemia; radiological pulmonary fibrosis	Moderate hypoxemia; evidence of pulmonary hypertension; radiographic pulmonary fibrosis 25%–50%	Severe hypoxemia; evidence of right-sided heart failure; radiographic pulmonary fibrosis >50%–75%	Life-threatening consequences (e.g., hemodynamic/ pulmonary complications); intubation with ventilatory support indicated; radiographic pulmonary fibrosis >75% with severe honeycombing	Death

CTCAE, Common Terminology Criteria for Adverse Events; *ROTG,* Radiation Therapy Oncology Group.

to determine the correspondence of the radiographic changes with the radiation therapy portal, and to exclude other possible etiologies, such as infection, thromboembolic disease, drug-induced pneumonitis, spread of the underlying malignancy, tracheoesophageal fistula, exacerbation of underlying chronic obstructive pulmonary disease (COPD), interstitial lung disease, or heart failure.

■ **Chest radiography:** Perivascular haziness is an early radiation-induced abnormality, often progressing to patchy alveolar filling densities. Radiographs taken during the chronic phase may show volume loss with coarse reticular or dense opacities. A straight-line effect which does not conform to anatomical units but rather to the confines of the radiation field is virtually diagnostic of radiation-induced lung injury. However, conformal and stereotactic treatment strategies, such as 3-D conformal radiation therapy, SBRT, and tomography, do not cause this straight-line radiographic finding due to the complex distribution of the radiation dose. With these techniques, a focal area of opacity with ill-defined margins is seen in the radiated region.

■ **Chest CT:** Chest CT (Fig. 28.1) is more sensitive than chest radiography for detecting lung injury following radiation treatment and is often obtained in the evaluation of the patient with increased dyspnea or cough following radiation therapy, especially when other causes such as infective pneumonia or pulmonary thromboembolism have been ruled out. The key step in the evaluation of radiation pneumonitis is the comparison of the pretreatment CT images, containing rate deviation dosimetric information, with diagnostic CT images obtained at the time of symptom presentation by the radiation oncologist. Lung involvement in CT images of radiation pneumonitis typically aligns closely with the radiated area.

■ **Pulmonary function testing (PFT):** PFT can be helpful in differentiating whether symptoms are due to a flare of COPD or an interstitial process, and to determine the severity of respiratory impairment. In patients with radiation-induced lung injury, PFTs generally demonstrate a reduction in lung volumes—that is, total lung capacity (TLC), forced vital capacity (FVC), residual volume (RV), diffusion capacity, and lung compliance.

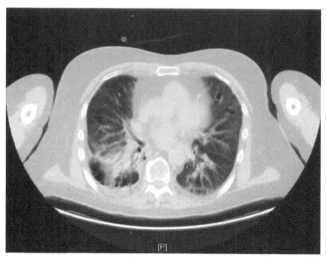

Fig. 28.1 CT chest depicting post-radiation pneumonitis 6 months after radiation therapy.

- **Mechanism of action:** The risk of radiation-induced lung toxicity for each individual patient remains unclear. At the cellular level, radiation activates free radical production, leading to DNA damage, apoptosis, cell cycle changes, and reduced cell survival all of which may contribute to the development of radiation-induced lung toxicity.
  - **Phases of evolution of radiation pneumonitis[1]:**
    1. **Immediate phase** is characterized by Hyperemic, congested mucosa with leukocytic infiltration and increased capillary permeability resulting in pulmonary edema. Exudative alveolitis is accompanied by tracheobronchial hypersecretion and degenerative changes in the alveolar epithelium and endothelium. Type I alveolar epithelial cells are sloughed and alveolar surfactant levels increased.
    2. **Latent phase** with thick secretions accumulated due to the increase in number of goblet cells combined with ciliary dysfunction.
    3. **Acute exudative phase** clinically observed as radiation pneumonitis. It consists of sloughing of endothelial and epithelial cells with narrowing of the pulmonary capillaries and microvascular thrombosis.
    4. **Intermediate phase** where there may be resolution of alveolar exudate and dissolution of the hyaline membranes or there may be collagenous deposit shown by fibroblasts which results in thickening of the interstitium.
    5. **Final phase** consists of fibrosis that may be evident as early as 6 months but can progress over years. There is an increase in the number of myofibroblasts within the interstitial and alveolar spaces along with an increase in the collagen deposition. This results in anatomic narrowing of the alveolar spaces which further results in diminishing lung volume and distortion of normal lung architecture.
- **Immunology of radiation-mediated lung injury:** In general, fractionated radiation therapy is considered to be immunosuppressive and thus may contribute to the radiation-mediated lung toxicity. Pulmonary fibrosis in lung cancer patients also appears to be at least partly driven by immunological effects. It is observed that about 15% of patients receiving high-dose radiation therapy for lung cancer develop pneumonitis.[2] Transforming growth factor-β (TGFβ) and interleukin (IL)-8 have been reported to predict radiation pneumonitis in some studies,[3] highlighting the role of cytokines in the pathogenesis of this disease.

Risk of Pneumonitis With Various Treatment Modalities

- **Risk of pneumonitis with conventional radiation therapy:** In general, the risk of pneumonitis is related to clinical patient factors, inherited biological factors, tumor factors, dosimetric parameters, and other variables.[4] Older patients are believed to have poor tolerance of radiation therapy and are often given less aggressive treatment. Age should be considered a risk factor for radiation-induced lung toxicity but a clear cut-off value may not exist owing to heterogeneity amongst older patients. The effect of sex is also not clear. There are two types of preexisting lung disease that might influence the risk of radiation-induced lung injury: interstitial lung disease and COPD. Clinically, acute exacerbation of preexisting lung disease following radiation can confound the definitive diagnosis of radiation pneumonitis. Other factors that influence the development of radiation-induced lung disease include pulmonary function, tumor factors, and tumor location, especially when the lower part of the lung is included in the radiation field. Tumor volume and tumor stage increase the risk of pneumonitis, with more advanced tumors being associated with increased risk. History of previous radiation, previous chemotherapy, concurrent chemotherapy, and individual biological factors or genetic phenotypes all increase risk of pneumonitis.
- **Risk of pneumonitis with SBRT:** The overall grade of radiation-induced lung toxicity is relatively low after thoracic SBRT. Older age and larger tumor size are significant adverse risk factors for radiation pneumonitis. Lung dosimetry (specifically the volume of lung receiving 20 Gy) and mean lung dose also significantly affect radiation pneumonitis risk. An analysis of 88 published studies with 7752 patients receiving SBRT reported 9% grade 2 and 1.8% grade 3 toxicity.[5]
- **Risk of pneumonitis with concurrent chemoradiotherapy:** For patients with unresectable locally advanced NSCLC, concurrent chemoradiotherapy improves overall survival as compared with sequential chemotherapy and radiation therapy, but is associated with higher rates of toxicities. In the Radiation Therapy Oncology Group (RTOG) trial 9410, higher than grade 3 acute pulmonary toxicity occurred in 9%, 4%, and 2% of patients in sequential chemoradiation, concurrent chemoradiation with daily radiation, and concurrent chemoradiation and twice daily radiation therapy groups, respectively.[6]
- **Risk of pneumonitis with concurrent targeted therapy and immunotherapy with radiation therapy:** There are increasing reports in the literature of increased radiation-induced pulmonary toxicity with the combination of BRAF inhibitors and radiation. Consensus guidelines recommend withholding BRAF inhibitors and/or MEK inhibitors for at least 3 days before and after fractionated radiation and at least 1 day before and after stereotactic radiation.

  Radiation pneumonitis is also noted to recall with immunotherapy drugs like nivolumab, EGFR–inhibitors such as erlotinib, and other chemotherapeutic agents like gemcitabine and adriamycin.[7,8]

Pharmacological Approaches for Management and Treatment

Radiation-induced pneumonitis is a relatively early event evident in most radiation-exposed patients, and is observed within 2 to 4 months of treatment, but can lead to fibrosis at later timepoints. Several cytokines and inflammatory molecules in radiated tissues play a role in the development of pneumonitis and fibrosis. Although certain cytokines may be exploited as biomarkers, they also appear to be a potential target of intervention at transcriptional level. Initiation and progression of pneumonitis and fibrosis are thus dynamic processes occurring a few months to a year after radiation of lung tissue. Currently available treatment strategies attempt to limit the effect of radiation pneumonitis on patient symptoms, but also attempt to decrease cancer-directed treatment interruptions.

Tissue toxicity in the lungs and its progression in local/regional areas require specific treatment that is also decided by the physiological status of the patient. The most common form of radiation pneumonitis is referred to as bronchiolitis obliterans organizing pneumonia (BOOP), which is an inflammatory response of the tissues. Pneumonitis is subcategorized into organizing pneumonia and secondary organizing pneumonia. The term BOOP is used for the nonidiopathic forms, such as radiation-therapy BOOP,[9] which is characterized by a specific pulmonary lesion with a typical pathological pattern. The treatment for radiation pneumonitis, BOOP, and other radiation-induced lung tissue damage is generally centered around immunosuppressants and antihypertensives.

- **Steroids:** Steroids are the mainstay of treatment for radiation-induced lung injury. The most commonly utilized drug is prednisone, at a dose of 1 mg/kg (up to 60 mg) administered orally for 2 weeks. This is followed by a slow tapering over several weeks.
- **Other immunosuppressants:** In patients who cannot tolerate steroids or have refractory disease, other immunosuppressive agents such as azathioprine and cyclosporine can be considered; however, evidence for their use is limited to case reports.[10] Other experimental agents which have been studied include amifostine and pentoxifylline. Amifostine was found to reduce rates of radiation pneumonitis when given daily before radiotherapy in a randomized control trial of patients with advanced lung cancer.[11] Subsequent studies did not confirm this finding, and thus guidelines have not recommended its use.[12] In a small, randomized, placebo-controlled trial of 40 patients, pentoxifylline given 3 times daily during radiotherapy was shown to decrease the rates of late pulmonary injury.[13]
- **Angiotensin-converting enzyme (ACE) inhibitors:** ACE inhibitors are effective in mitigating radiation-induced pneumonitis and have been shown in trials to have variable success. ACE inhibitors are believed to act by decreasing the vascular remodeling and the levels of TGFβ.

Nonpharmacological Approaches for Management and Treatment

The dose and volume of the lung irradiated are important parameters in the pathogenesis of radiation pneumonitis. Many studies have evaluated the correlation of dose to toxicity as well as techniques to reduce excess radiation exposure by normal tissues.

- **Dosimetric correlates:**
  - The most frequently correlated parameters in most studies are of validated V20 (the volume of lung receiving 20 Gy) and mean lung dose, though several other variables have also shown to be predictive including the volume of the lungs receiving greater than 5 Gy (V5), 13 Gy (V13), 25 Gy (V25), and 30 Gy (V30).[14] In a study of patients receiving conventionally fractionated radiotherapy published by Graham and colleagues,[15] the V20 was found to predict the development of grade 2 or higher pneumonitis as follows:
    - V20 less than 22%: 0% risk by 24 months
    - V20 22% to 31%: 7% risk by 24 months
    - V20 32% to 40%: 13% risk by 24 months
    - V20 greater than 40%: 36% risk by 24 months
  - Thus, the best-known strategies for reducing radiation-induced lung injury are those that limit the radiation dose and volume of the normal lung tissue. Advances in radiation treatment planning techniques of delivery allow control of the dose delivered to the normal lung. Various strategies have been proposed to reduce the volume of the lung receiving radiation dose.

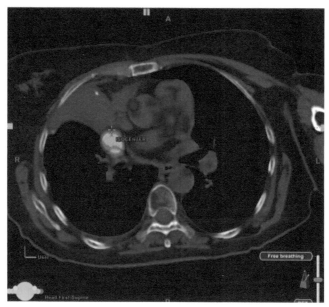

Fig. 28.2   Positron emission tomography/computed tomography (PET/CT) fusion for target delineation.

- **Simulation:** More sophisticated radiation therapy technologies, such as 4-D imaging, permit an improvement in its therapeutic goals, allowing for the design of personalized treatment planning that delivers adequate doses directed at the target while sparing the surrounding critical normal tissues.[16]
- **Radiation treatment planning:** In addition to using positron emission tomography (PET)-CT imaging (Fig. 28.2) for developing treatment plans, the technique of "dose painting" is being investigated. This involves the application of varying radiation dosage to the tumor based on tumor homogeneity identified by fluorodeoxyglucose (FDG) imaging. Others are investigating the utility of PET-CT imaging during treatment to detect areas of resistance so that boost doses may be applied to more resistant tumor regions.[17]

References

1. Rubin P, Casarett GW. Respiratory system. In: Rubin P, Casarett GW, eds. *Clinical Radiation Pathology*. Philadelphia: WB Saunders; 1968.
2. Abid SH, Malhotra V, Perry MC. Radiation-induced and chemotherapy-induced pulmonary injury. *Curr Opin Oncol*. 2001;13(4):242–248.
3. Stenmark MH, Cai XW, Shedden K, et al. Combining physical and biologic parameters to predict radiation-induced lung toxicity in patients with non-small-cell lung cancer treated with definitive radiation therapy. *Int J Radiat Oncol Biol Phys*. 2012;84(2):e217–e222.
4. Kong FM, Wang S. Nondosimetric risk factors for radiation-induced lung toxicity. *Semin Radiat Oncol*. 2015;25(2):100–109.
5. Zhao J, Yorke ED, Li L, et al. Simple factors associated with radiation-induced lung toxicity after stereotactic body radiation therapy of the thorax: a pooled analysis of 88 studies. *Int J Radiat Oncol Biol Phys*. 2016;95(5):1357–1366.
6. Curran WJ Jr, Paulus R, Langer CJ, et al. Sequential vs. concurrent chemoradiation for stage III non-small cell lung cancer: randomized phase III trial RTOG 9410. *J Natl Cancer Inst*. 2011;103(19):1452–1460.

7. Shibaki R, Akamatsu H, Fujimoto M, Koh Y, Yamamoto N. Nivolumab induced radiation recall pneumonitis after two years of radiotherapy. *Ann Oncol.* 2017;28(6):1404–1405.

8. Korman AM, Tyler KH, Kaffenberger BH. Radiation recall dermatitis associated with nivolumab for metastatic malignant melanoma. *Int J Dermatol.* 2017;56(4):e75–e77.

9. American Thoracic Society European Respiratory Society. American Thoracic Society/European Respiratory Society international multidisciplinary consensus classification of the idiopathic interstitial pneumonias. This joint statement of the American Thoracic Society (ATS), and the European Respiratory Society (ERS) was adopted by the ATS board of directors, June 2001 and by the ERS Executive Committee, June 2001. *Am J Respir Crit Care Med.* 2002;165(2):277–304.

10. McCarty MJ, Lillis P, Vukelja SJ. Azathioprine as a steroid-sparing agent in radiation pneumonitis. *Chest.* 1996;109(5):1397–1400.

11. Antonadou D, Coliarakis N, Synodinou M, et al. Randomized phase III trial of radiation treatment +/- amifostine in patients with advanced-stage lung cancer. *Int J Radiat Oncol Biol Phys.* 2001;51(4):915–922.

12. Hensley ML, Hagerty KL, Kewalramani T, et al. American Society of Clinical Oncology 2008 clinical practice guideline update: use of chemotherapy and radiation therapy protectants. *J Clin Oncol.* 2009;27(1):127–145.

13. Lauterbach R, Pawlik D, Zembala M, et al. Pentoxyfylline in and prevention and treatment of chronic lung disease. *Acta Paediatr Suppl.* 2004;93(444):20–22.

14. Palma DA, Senan S, Tsujino K, et al. Predicting radiation pneumonitis after chemoradiation therapy for lung cancer: an international individual patient data meta-analysis. *Int J Radiat Oncol Biol Phys.* 2013;85(2):444–450.

15. Graham MV, Purdy JA, Emami B, et al. Clinical dose-volume histogram analysis for pneumonitis after 3D treatment for non-small cell lung cancer (NSCLC). *Int J Radiat Oncol Biol Phys.* 1999;45(2):323–329.

16. Chang JY, Cox JD. Improving radiation conformality in the treatment of non-small cell lung cancer. *Semin Radiat Oncol.* 2010;20(3):171–177.

17. Feng M, Kong FM, Gross M, Fernando S, Hayman JA, Ten Haken RK. Using fluorodeoxyglucose positron emission tomography to assess tumor volume during radiotherapy for non-small-cell lung cancer and its potential impact on adaptive dose escalation and normal tissue sparing. *Int J Radiat Oncol Biol Phys.* 2009;73(4):1228–1234.

CHAPTER 29

Cardiovascular Toxicities of Radiation Therapy

Shyamal Patel, MD ▪ Nitika Thawani, MD

Introduction

- Cardiovascular disease and cancer are the top two causes of global mortality, accounting for 46% of deaths worldwide.[1] To complicate matters further, cancer treatment has led to a significant increase in the global incidence of cardiovascular disease. A mainstay of cancer treatment is radiation therapy (RT). Its success with and without systemic therapy as an effective modality in Hodgkin's and non-Hodgkin's lymphomas, breast cancer, and lung cancer, for example, has led to improved survival rates. There were an estimated 16.9 million American cancer survivors in 2019[2] and this number is expected to grow to 26 million by 2040.[3] This increase in survivorship will continue to lead to an increase in manifestations of various cardiovascular toxicities.

- Compared with nonirradiated patients, patients who have received mediastinal radiation have a 2% higher absolute risk of cardiac toxicity and death at 5 years and 23% increased absolute risk after 20 years.[4] Cardiovascular disease associated with RT presents via a spectrum of disorders. This is thought to reflect the differing radiosensitivities of involved cells and tissues. Coronary artery atherosclerosis, valvular disease, pericardial disease, cardiomyopathy, and autonomic dysfunction represent the main clinical manifestations of radiation-induced cardiovascular disease (RICD).

- Late cardiac toxicity has been notably described in pediatric patients receiving mediastinal radiation for lymphomas. Given that these patients have curable cancers and live for decades after initial treatment with radiation with or without chemotherapy, they have a greater potential for the development of RICD. Although not as prevalent, cardiovascular toxicity has also been described in women with breast cancer receiving adjuvant RT. As cure rates are high, women live long enough for cardiac toxicity to be exhibited.

- Advances in modern chest radiotherapy techniques have led to the development of newer considerations in radiation oncology. Beyond the initial radiation course with or without systemic therapy, the implementation of reirradiation as well as stereotactic body RT have led to unique clinical situations requiring careful thought. Although the clinical manifestations of cardiotoxicity may remain similar, the nuances provided by possible cardiac cell regeneration and hypofractionation serve to make an already complex situation even more challenging in terms of safely delivering therapies.

- In this chapter, we will review the clinical manifestations of cardiovascular toxicity and the mechanistic changes associated with such toxicities. We will then review preventative methods including published dose constraints for the major cardiovascular organs and discuss management options and considerations.

Description

- Radiation-induced cardiovascular toxicity has become an important issue as outcomes have improved with advances in thoracic RT. Risk factors for the development of toxicity include younger age at time of RT (<50), higher cumulative dose of RT (>30 Gy), volume of heart irradiated, higher dose per fraction (>2 Gy/day), anterior or left chest irradiation, presence of tumor in the mediastinum, concurrent cardiotoxic systemic therapy, and preexisting cardiovascular disease as well as cardiovascular risk factors.[5]

■ Cardiotoxicity manifests itself in a number of ways. The tissues affected include the pericardium, coronary arteries, the myocardium, the valves, the cardiac electrical conduction system, and the great vessels of the chest.[6] Whereas acute effects can manifest themselves during RT or weeks to months after RT, long-term effects are demonstrated years to decades later. Table 29.1 shows the various toxicities and associated early and late effects. Although pericarditis is the most common manifestation of RICD, ischemic heart disease is the most common cause of cardiac death in patients who have undergone RT. The risk of RICD relates to both the dose and duration of RT.

Symptoms

The clinical presentation of RICD is similar to that of cardiac disease unrelated to RT, which makes it difficult to differentiate the two. It is important to assess the risk factors and the timeframe for development in diagnosing radiation-induced cardiotoxicity.

Syndrome	Clinical Presentation
Acute pericarditis	Chest pain, fever, pericardial rub
Chronic pericarditis	Dyspnea, hypotension, thready pulse
Cardiomyopathy	Dyspnea, fatigue, weakness, edema, pulmonary edema
Valvular disease	Dyspnea, symptoms of valvular regurgitation/stenosis
Coronary artery disease	Chest pain/tightness/heaviness, dyspnea, fatigue
Conduction abnormalities	Palpitations, dizziness, dyspnea, chest discomfort

Screening and Diagnostic Workup

■ The initial evaluation of the patient involves a complete history and physical examination, together with a history of prior RT and prior systemic therapy, with close attention to cumulative cardiovascular radiation dose and volume of cardiac tissue irradiated in addition to cumulative dose of systemic therapy received. Subsequent workup depends on the symptoms and history but all include an electrocardiogram (ECG) with echocardiography with or without the following (depending on scenario): chest X-ray, cardiac enzymes, chest computed tomography (CT), cardiac magnetic resonance imaging (MRI), angiography, and Holter monitoring.

■ The most common screening tool for detection and monitoring of RICD is echocardiography. The European Association of Cardiovascular Imaging and the American Society of Echocardiography recommends comprehensive screening and risk-factor modification for patients, in addition to baseline transthoracic echocardiography (TTE) to detect cardiac abnormalities prior to RT.[7] They recommend careful annual symptom screening and an annual TTE if a murmur is detected. At 5 years, a TTE is recommended for high-risk asymptomatic patients, stress echocardiography or stress cardiac MRI, and repeat TTE at 5-year intervals. At 10 years, TTE is recommended for non–high-risk patients with repeat TTE at 5-year intervals.

TABLE 29.1 ■ Cardiotoxicity With Early and Late Effects[5,7]

Early	Late
Pericarditis	Pericarditis
Acute exudative pericarditis, rare—occurs during RT—reaction to necrosis/inflammation of tumor adjacent to the heart	Delayed chronic pericarditis—weeks to years after RT—extensive fibrous thickening, adhesions, chronic constriction, and chronic pericardial effusion—observed in up to 20% of patients within 2 years
Delayed acute pericarditis—within weeks—manifests as asymptomatic pericardial effusion or symptomatic pericarditis. Cardiac tamponade, rare. Spontaneous clearance of effusion can take up to 2 years	Constrictive pericarditis seen in 4%–20% of patients and is dose-dependent and related to presence of pericardial effusion in delayed acute phase
Cardiomyopathy	Cardiomyopathy
Acute myocarditis—radiation-induced inflammation with transient repolarization abnormalities and mild myocardial dysfunction	Diffuse myocardial fibrosis (after >30 Gy) with systolic/diastolic dysfunction, conduction abnormalities, and autonomic dysfunction
	Restrictive cardiomyopathy—advanced myocardial damage due to fibrosis with severe diastolic dysfunction and heart failure signs and symptoms
Valvular Disease	Valvular Disease
No immediate effects	Valve apparatus and leaflet thickening, fibrosis, shortening, and calcification on mostly left-sided valves
	Valve regurgitation > valve stenosis
	Stenosis more commonly affects aortic valve
	Valve disease increases significantly after 20 years
Conduction System Disease	Conduction System Disease
No immediate effects	Right bundle branch block most common
	Prolongation of the corrected QT interval
	Atrioventricular nodal bradycardia, heart block, sick sinus syndrome
Coronary Artery Disease	Coronary Artery Disease
No immediate effects—perfusion defects can be seen in ~50% of patients 6 months after RT, sometimes a/w wall-motion abnormalities and chest pain	Accelerated CAD appearing at younger age
	Patients <50 tend to develop CAD in first 10 years, patients >50 have longer latency
	Coronary ostia and proximal segments typically involved
	CAD doubles risk of death via myocardial infarction
Carotid Artery Disease	Carotid Artery Disease
No immediate effects	RT–induced lesions more extensive, involve longer segments, and atypical areas of carotid segments
Vascular Disease	Vascular Disease
No immediate effects	Atherosclerotic calcifications of ascending aorta and aortic arch

a/w, Associated with; *CAD,* coronary artery disease; *RT,* radiation therapy.

Imaging

■ **Echocardiography:** Features of RICD on echo include biventricular systolic and diastolic dysfunction, multivalvular involvement with mixed valvular dysfunction, prominent calcification (pericardial, valvular, annular, aortomitral curtain, and aortic), wall motion abnormalities associated with coronary artery disease, and pericardial constriction.[8] Valvular regurgitation is more common than stenosis.

- **Coronary computed tomographic angiography (CTA):** This can be useful for its negative predictive value in that no coronary calcification is indicative of a very low chance of coronary artery disease (CAD). CTA can be used for the evaluation of aortic, valvular, myocardial, and pericardial calcification and for preoperative assessment in patients undergoing cardiac surgery. CT can provide information regarding mediastinal and pulmonary fibrosis, and single photon emission CT, as well as positron emission tomography, have been utilized to assess myocardial ischemia.[8]
- **Cardiac magnetic resonance (CMR):** CMR allows for the simultaneous analysis of functional and structural data, enabling detection of RICD involving the coronary arteries, the valves, and the myocardium, as well as the pericardium. Cine imaging allows assessment of ventricular volumes and regional wall motion abnormalities, whereas late gadolinium enhancement allows for visualization of scar and viable tissue as well as regional nonischemic fibrosis.[8]
- **Cardiac catherization:** Invasive catheterization allows for confirmation of findings seen in noninvasive imaging. Left-heart catheterization evaluates coronary artery stenosis severity and disease extent, whereas right-heart catheterization allows for calculation of intracardiac and pulmonary pressures.
  Evaluation for pulmonary disease: Patients with RICD should also be evaluated for concurrent pulmonary disease via clinical evaluation, chest X-ray, pulmonary function tests, and dedicated high-resolution chest CT. This is because concurrent pulmonary disease is independently associated with reduced survival in RICD.[9]

Grading

The grading of RICD can be performed with the use of Common Terminology Criteria for Adverse Events (CTCAE) version 5.0.[10] This grading system is described in detail elsewhere in this book. Each component of RICD is analyzed individually and graded accordingly.

Mechanisms of Action

- RICD occurs via differing mechanisms based on the sequelae in question. The major mediator of RICD is the formation of fibrosis in both acute and chronic settings, which can affect all cardiac tissues including the pericardium, the myocardium, the coronary arteries, and conductive tissue, as well as the great vessels.
- **Acute phase:** In the acute phase, radiation to cardiac tissues results in acute inflammation via tumor necrosis factor (TNF), interleukin-1 (IL-1), IL-6, and IL-8 leading to vasodilation and vascular permeability. This results in neutrophil infiltration and the release of profibrotic cytokines such as platelet-derived growth factor (PDGF), transforming growth factor (TGF)-β, fibroblast growth factor (FGF), insulin-like growth factor (IGF), and connective tissue growth factor (CTGF).[11] Subsequently, the coagulation cascade is initiated and degradation of the endothelial basement membrane begins, allowing for the clearance of injured tissue. The acute phase spans minutes to several days.
- **Late phase:** In the late phase, radiation-induced upregulation of c-Myc, c-Jun, TGF-β, IL-4, and IL-13 lead to further development of fibrosis.[12,13] Radiation additionally can induce premature differentiation of fibroblasts, leading to the development of fibrocytes that in turn produce higher levels of collagen. This results in chronic collagen deposition within cardiac tissue leading to fibrotic scar tissue and reducing the heart's elasticity and, eventually, function.[14] In radiation-induced vascular disease, NF-κβ plays a large role by upregulating proinflammatory cytokines and adhesion molecules in the endothelium, leading to the recruitment of inflammatory cells to the site of vascular injury.[15]

- DNA damage response, chronic oxidative stress/hypoxia, epigenetic regulation, and telomere extension have also been found to be involved in the formation of radiation-induced fibrosis and RICD.[12,14,16] Other chronic changes include microvascular injury and neovascularization, which affect conductive tissue and the pericardium, as well as atherosclerosis, which affects the coronary arteries as well as the great vessels. Table 29.2 describes the mechanisms related to various components of RICD.

TABLE 29.2 ■ **Mechanistic Changes Leading to RICD**

Type of Cardiovascular Toxicity	Developmental Mechanisms
Pericardial disease	microvascular damage episodic ischemia inflammation fibrotic build-up effusions long-term fibrosis thickened pericardium constrictive pericarditis and cardiac tamponade
Myocardial disease	cardiomyocyte hypoxia and hypertrophy fibrotic build-up reduced elasticity decreased distensibility reduced ejection fraction perfusion defects
Valvular disease	leaflet fibrosis valve calcification valve thickening valve regurgitation valve stenosis reduced ejection fraction
Vascular disease	Tunica intima—endothelial cells leukocyte adhesion coagulative changes inflammatory changes fatty streak formation atherosclerotic lesions plaque build-up, growth, and rupture myocardial infarction Tunica media—smooth muscle cells acute vasculitis (occasional) smooth muscle replaced with fibrous tissue Tunica externa acute vasculitis (occasional)
Conduction disease	fibrotic build-up adjacent to conductive system fibrotic build-up in the myocardium

RICD, Radiation-induced cardiovascular disease.

Adapted from Spetz J, Moslehi J, Sarosiek K. Radiation-induced cardiovascular toxicity: mechanisms, prevention, and treatment. *Curr Treat Options Cardiovasc Med.* 2018;20(4):31.

Pharmacological Approaches for Management and Treatment

- The various pharmacological and invasive options for its management and treatment depend on the specific manifestation of RICD. These treatments typically are the same regardless of whether the cardiac disease is attributable to RT. Patients with RICD benefit from evaluation and management by a cardio-oncologist, if available. Although surgical options often are the most effective in addressing some of these issues, survival rates in patients with RICD are often worse than in those who have not been irradiated.[17]
- **Acute pericarditis** is often self-limiting but can also be treated with nonsteroidal anti-inflammatory drugs and diuretics.
- **Chronic pericarditis** and cardiac tamponade are more serious and are treated with loop diuretics and pericardiocentesis or pericardiectomy.
- **Cardiomyopathy** can lead to congestive heart failure and is treated with loop diuretics, angiotensin converting enzyme inhibitors (ACEIs), nitroglycerin, inotropic agents, and vasodilators. Cardiac transplantation remains as a possible option.
- **Valvular disease** depends on whether the condition is stenosis or regurgitation and can be managed with ACEIs and/or β-blockers if asymptomatic or minimally symptomatic. If more significant symptoms, patients may require mechanical intervention, which could entail percutaneous therapy versus surgical valve repair or replacement.
- **Coronary artery disease** is treated with ACEIs, β-blockers, antiplatelet therapy, angioplasty, stenting, or coronary artery bypass grafting.
- **Conduction abnormalities** can be managed via antiplatelet therapy, antiarrhythmic drugs, catheter ablation, and pacemaker placement.
- **Vascular disease** is often treated with antiplatelet therapy (aspirin), omega-3 fatty acids, and statins, which may help modulate NF-κβ activity.

Nonpharmacological Approaches for Management and Treatment

- Preventative measures for reducing the risk of RICD revolve around limiting both the radiation dose to the heart and the volume of heart irradiated. In an extensive case-control study of over 2000 women with breast cancer who underwent RT, the risk of developing significant RICD increased linearly with the mean dose to the heart by 7.4% per gray (Gy) with no upper threshold.[18] A similar linear radiation dose–response relationship was demonstrated in survivors of Hodgkin's lymphoma who had developed coronary heart disease.[19] In the randomized trial of standard versus high-dose chemoradiation for locally advanced non–small-cell lung cancer (RTOG 0617), the heart V50 Gy (volume of the heart which receives 50 Gy) was found to significantly correspond with survival where a V50 less than 25% versus a V50 greater than 25% led to 2-year survival rates of 45% versus 26%.[20] In a retrospective study of advanced stage lung cancer patients, associations were noted between all-cause death rate and conduction or ischemic/pericarditis-like changes on ECG at 6 months, and between higher death rate and heart or left atrial volumes receiving 63 to 69 Gy.[21]
- The volume of heart irradiated also plays a role in the development of RICD. For example, subcarinal blocking was found to decrease the relative risk of death from cardiac causes in Hodgkin's patients; valvular dysfunction was increased in patients receiving internal mammary node RT in breast cancer patients; and the rate of pericarditis was reduced by shielding the left ventricular and subcarinal areas.[22–24]
- **Radiation techniques:** Various techniques have been developed over the years to help reduce radiation dose to the heart. In breast cancer, the use of deep inspiration breath hold can serve

TABLE 29.3 ■ Radiation Dose Constraints for Cardiac Organs

	QUANTEC 2010[27] (conventional fractionation)	RTOG 0617 (conventional fractionation for lung)	Darby et al.[18] (Conventional Fractionation for Breast)	RTOG 0813 (SBRT for Central Lung ca, 5 fx)	RTOG 0631 (SBRT for Spine, 1 fx)	NRG BR001 (SBRT, 3 fx)
Heart	V25 < 10% (< 1% risk cardiac mortality at 15 years)	V60 < 33% V45 < 67% V40 < 100%	Mean < 2 (10% increased risk coronary event)	V32 < 15 cc Dmax 105%	V16 <15 cc Dmax 22 Gy	V24 < 15 cc Dmax 30 Gy
Pericardium	Mean < 26 V30 < 46% (< 15% risk pericarditis)			V32 < 15 cc Dmax 105%	V16 <15 cc Dmax 22 Gy	V24 < 15 cc Dmax 30 Gy
Great Vessels				V47 < 10 cc Dmax 37 Gy	V31 < 10 cc	V39 < 10 cc Dmax 45 Gy

Dmax, Maximum dose; fx, fractions; NRG, XXX; NSABP, National Surgical Adjuvant Breast and Bowel Project; GOG, Gynecologic Oncology Group; QUANTEC, Quantitative Analyses of Normal Tissue Effects in the Clinic; RTOG, Radiation Therapy Oncology Group; SBRT, stereotactic body radiation therapy.

to push the heart inferiorly and posteriorly away from the chest wall and the tangent fields. Additionally, the utilization of a prone setup for left-sided cancers or women with pendulous breasts can serve to significantly reduce dose to the heart. In lung cancer, appropriately defining margins can reduce cardiac dose. This can be accomplished by using a four-dimensional simulation scan to develop planning target volumes (PTVs) with appropriate internal target volumes (ITVs) defining the true extent of tumor motion. Advancements in the field have led to widespread use of intensity-modulated radiation therapy (IMRT) and the more recent implementation of volumetric arc therapy (VMAT), which can reduce dose to critical organs such as the heart by modulating dose during treatments. In the management of lymphoma, there has been a paradigm shift with a concurrent reduction in radiation dose needed for cure and a limitation in radiation volume through the involved-site RT technique.[25]

■ **Radiation dose constraints:** Table 29.3 shows published dose constraints for cardiac organs and their corresponding clinical situations. Of note, great vessel constraints for conventional fractionation are not shown as the great vessels have historically tolerated conventionally fractionated treatments with or without chemoradiation therapy without specifically being constrained. However, constraining them becomes important in the case of reirradiation. In a retrospective analysis of 35 patients treated with two rounds of external beam radiation that included aorta in both treatments, there was a 25% rate of grade 5 toxicity for patients receiving 120 Gy or greater raw composite dose versus 0% in patients receiving less than 120 Gy.[26]

References

1. Han X, Zhou Y, Liu W. Precision cardio-oncology: understanding the cardiotoxicity of cancer therapy. *NPJ Precis Oncol.* 2017;1(1):31.
2. American Cancer Society. *Cancer Treatment & Survivorship Facts & Figures 2019–2021*: Atlanta; 2019. https://www.cancer.org/research/cancer-facts-statistics/survivor-facts-figures.html.
3. Bluethmann SM, Mariotto AB, Rowland JH. Anticipating the "silver tsunami": prevalence trajectories and comorbidity burden among older cancer survivors in the United States. *Cancer Epidemiol Biomarkers Prev.* 2016;25(7):1029–1036.

4. Galper SL, Yu JB, Mauch PM, et al. Clinically significant cardiac disease in patients with Hodgkin lymphoma treated with mediastinal irradiation. *Blood*. 2011;117(2):412–418.
5. Donnellan E, Phelan D, Collier P, Desai M, Griffin B, McCarthy CP. Radiation-induced heart disease: a practical guide to diagnosis and management REVIEW. *Cleve Clin J Med*. 2016:83.
6. Moreira LAR, Silva EN, Ribeiro ML, Martins Wde A. Cardiovascular effects of radiotherapy on the patient with cancer. *Rev Assoc Med Bras*. 2016;62(2):192–196.
7. Lancellotti P, Nkomo VT, Badano LP, et al. Expert consensus for multi-modality imaging evaluation of cardiovascular complications of radiotherapy in adults: a report from the European Association of Cardiovascular Imaging and the American Society of Echocardiography. *Eur Hear J—Cardiovasc Imaging*. 2013;14(8):721–740.
8. Desai M. Expert analysis: radiation associated cardiac disease. American College of Cardiology. https://www.acc.org/latest-in-cardiology/articles/2017/06/13/07/13/radiation-associated-cardiac-disease.
9. Desai MY, Karunakaravel K, Wu W, et al. Pulmonary fibrosis on multidetector computed tomography and mortality in patients with radiation-associated cardiac disease undergoing cardiac surgery. *J Thorac Cardiovasc Surg*. 2014;148(2):475–481.e3.
10. National Institute of Health. *Common Terminology Criteria for Adverse Events (CTCAE) Version 5.0*. 2017.
11. Yarnold J, Vozenin Brotons MC. Pathogenetic mechanisms in radiation fibrosis. *Radiother Oncol*. 2010;97(1):149–161.
12. Spetz J, Moslehi J, Sarosiek K. Radiation-induced cardiovascular toxicity: mechanisms, prevention, and treatment. *Curr Treat Options Cardiovasc Med*. 2018;20(4):31.
13. Madan R, Benson R, Sharma DN, Julka PK, Rath GK. Radiation induced heart disease: pathogenesis, management and review literature. *J Egypt Natl Canc Inst*. 2015;27(4):187–193.
14. Taunk NK, Haffty BG, Kostis JB, Goyal S. Radiation-induced heart disease: pathologic abnormalities and putative mechanisms. *Front Oncol*. 2015;5:39.
15. Weintraub NL, Jones WK, Manka D. Understanding radiation-induced vascular disease. *J Am Coll Cardiol*. 2010;55(12):1237–1239.
16. Bhattacharya S, Asaithamby A. Ionizing radiation and heart risks. *Semin Cell Dev Biol*. 2016;58:14–25.
17. Wu W, Masri A, Popovic ZB, et al. Long-term survival of patients with radiation heart disease undergoing cardiac surgery. *Circulation*. 2013;127(14):1476–1484.
18. Darby SC, Ewertz M, McGale P, et al. Risk of ischemic heart disease in women after radiotherapy for breast cancer. *N Engl J Med*. 2013;368(11):987–998.
19. van Nimwegen FA, Schaapveld M, Cutter DJ, et al. Radiation dose-response relationship for risk of coronary heart disease in survivors of Hodgkin lymphoma. *J Clin Oncol*. 2016;34(3):235–243.
20. Speirs CK, DeWees TA, Rehman S, et al. Heart dose is an independent dosimetric predictor of overall survival in locally advanced non-small cell lung cancer. 2017;12(2):293-301.
21. Vivekanandan S, Landau DB, Counsell N, et al. The impact of cardiac radiation dosimetry on survival after radiation therapy for non-small cell lung cancer. *Int J Radiat Oncol Biol Phys*. 2017;99(1):51–60.
22. Hancock SL, Tucker MA, Hoppe RT. Factors affecting late mortality from heart disease after treatment of Hodgkin's disease. *JAMA*. 1993;270(16):1949–1955.
23. Hooning MJ, Botma A, Aleman BMP, et al. Long-term risk of cardiovascular disease in 10-year survivors of breast cancer. *JNCI J Natl Cancer Inst*. 2007;99(5):365–375.
24. Carmel RJ, Kaplan HS. Mantle irradiation in Hodgkin's disease. An analysis of technique, tumor eradication, and complications. *Cancer*. 1976;37(6):2813–2825.
25. Hoskin PJ, Díez P, Williams M, Lucraft H, Bayne M. Recommendations for the use of radiotherapy in nodal lymphoma. *Clin Oncol*. 2013;25:49–58.
26. Evans JD, Gomez DR, Amini A, et al. Aortic dose constraints when reirradiating thoracic tumors. *Radiother Oncol*. 2013;106(3):327–332.
27. Marks LB, Yorke ED, Jackson A, et al. Use of normal tissue complication probability models in the clinic. *Radiat Oncol Biol*. 2010;76(3 suppl):S10–S19.

Page numbers followed by "*b*", "*f*" and "*t*" indicate boxes, figures and tables respectively.